A Textbook of
Medical Practice

A Textbook of Medical Practice

Edited by

J. Fry, P. S. Byrne
and S. Johnson

MTP

Published by
MTP Press Limited
St. Leonard's House,
Lancaster
England

ISBN-13:978-94-011-5904-3   e-ISBN-13:978-94-011-5902-9
DOI: 10.1007/978-94-011-5902-9

Typeset by Santype International (Coldtype Division)
Salisbury, Wilts.

Contents

Contributors

H. W. K. Acheson, O.B.E., M.B., Ch.B., F.R.C.G.P.
  Department of General Practice, University of Manchester, Darbishire House Health Centre, Upper Brook Street, Manchester, M13 0FW
D. Brooks, M.D., F.R.C.G.P., D.Obst.R.C.O.G.
  133 Manchester Old Road, Middleton, Manchester
Professor P. S. Byrne, C.B.E., M.B., Ch.B., F.R.C.G.P.
  Department of General Practice, University of Manchester, Darbishire House Health Centre, Upper Brook Street, Manchester, M13 0FW
S. Carne, M.B., B.S., F.R.C.G.P.
  The Grove Health Centre, Goldhawk Road, London, W12 8EJ
J. Fry, M.D., F.R.C.S., F.R.C.G.P.
  138 Croydon Road, Beckenham, Kent
I. Gregg, M.A., B.M., B.Ch., F.R.C.G.P.
  Department of Clinical Epidemiology in General Practice, Cardio-Thoracic Institute, Fulham Road, Brompton, London, SW3 6HP
G. W. Hickish, V.R.D., M.B., Ch.B., D.Ch., M.R.C.G.P.
  1 Oakwood Road, Highcliffe, Christchurch, BH23 5NY
S. Johnson, B.Sc., Ph.D.
  Chapel Gate, Kirklands Road, Over Kellet, Carnforth, Lancashire
Professor J. D. E. Knox, M.D., F.R.C.P.(Edinburgh), F.R.C.G.P.
  Department of General Practice, The University, Dundee
G. Lloyd, B.Sc., M.B., Ch.B., M.R.C.O.G., F.R.C.G.P.
  Department of General Practice, University of Manchester, Darbishire House, Upper Brook Street, Manchester, M13 0FW
J. S. Norell, M.B., B.S., M.R.C.G.P.
  58 Roman Way, London, N7 8XF
H. T. N. Sears, M.D., F.R.C.P.Lond., M.R.C.G.P.
  Danecroft, Holmes Chapel, Cheshire CW4 7ED
M. K. Thompson, M.B., B.Chir., M.R.C.G.P.
  24 Frystone Avenue, Croydon, CR0 7HL
G. B. Walker, M.B., Ch.B., D.R.C.O.G.
  27 Pinewood Avenue, Bolton le Sands, Lancashire
C. A. H. Watts, O.B.E., M.D., F.R.C.G.P.
  2 Tower Gardens, Ashby de la Zouche, Leicestershire

Professor E. Wilkes, O.B.E., M.A., M.B., B.Chir., F.R.C.P., F.R.C.G.P., M.R.C.Psych,, D.Obst.R.C.O.G.
Department of Community Medicine, University of Sheffield, Beech Hill Road, Sheffield, S10 2RX

Preface

It is accepted now that a primary level of medical care is essential in all health systems. Whatever the form and structure of a national health care system, the clinical medical problems in primary care will be similar, namely, to assess, diagnose and manage the various common ills of humanity and to provide long term and continuing personal care and support for individuals living in a known community.

In most societies the family is still the most important fundamental base for sound social and communal life and it is on the basis of care for the common illnesses and problems of the family that the specialty of family medicine or family practice has evolved and developed. It is the oldest specialty in medicine but has only lately begun to be researched, taught and organised in modern ways.

Family medicine is now a part of the curriculum of many medical schools. It has its own special postgraduate training programme and it is developing its own body of research and investigations. As a discipline of medicine it has its own special characteristics and requirements for good practice. Nowhere do the art and science of medicine require more care in their close integration and harmony for the sake of the patient.

There is a special knowledge and understanding required of the common diseases encountered in this field. It is not sufficient to accept and translate the experience and dictates of hospital specialists to family practice. The standard and traditional medical textbooks written by specialists from other fields are only partially useful and it is for this reason that we have brought together a group of family physicians to write on their special field.

Our book is a textbook on the common clinical problems in family medicine. Our emphasis has been on a sound clinical and common sense approach to problems and diseases encountered by family physicians all over the world. Reading the book our colleagues in family medicine anywhere should at once feel that the problems which we describe are just those that they meet in their own practices and we hope that our shared experiences may help them to understand better and to strive together for our common goal — better care for our patients.

The authors are all active family practitioners. They are generalists caring for families but they have all made special studies and have some special experience in the subjects on which they write. The team that we have collected is a group of individuals with their own bents and beliefs developed through years of practical experience, study, research and teaching, and this shows in their contributions.

As editors we have not sought to produce dull uniformity of presentation. Apart from general instruction and guidance we have allowed each contributor to write in his personal way and to present his views as he chooses. This may make for differences in style and approach but we believe that our readers will appreciate the personal flavours of each chapter and that it will add to their interest.

We have not intended to produce a book that is dogmatic and blindly authoritative. There will be many who will not agree with all the views and suggestions put forward. This has been our intention — to present together the collected practical experiences of colleagues whom we know and respect and whom we know are good doctors and who base their knowledge on supportive personal research and study. We hope that their views will create some differences of opinion that will lead to further thought, discussion and research.

What is needed more than anything in our common field of family practice is new thinking and questioning on long held beliefs and attitudes. We hope that our book will help to stimulate our readers, to foster more critical and questioning attitudes on the work that we do and to help to create and promote better care for our patients.

John Fry
Patrick S. Byrne
Susan Johnson

Preface

It is accepted now that a primary level of medical care is essential in all health systems. Whatever the form and structure of a national health care system, the clinical medical problems in primary care will be similar, namely, to assess, diagnose and manage the various common ills of humanity and to provide long term and continuing personal care and support for individuals living in a known community.

In most societies the family is still the most important fundamental base for sound social and communal life and it is on the basis of care for the common illnesses and problems of the family that the specialty of family medicine or family practice has evolved and developed. It is the oldest specialty in medicine but has only lately begun to be researched, taught and organised in modern ways.

Family medicine is now a part of the curriculum of many medical schools. It has its own special postgraduate training programme and it is developing its own body of research and investigations. As a discipline of medicine it has its own special characteristics and requirements for good practice. Nowhere do the art and science of medicine require more care in their close integration and harmony for the sake of the patient.

There is a special knowledge and understanding required of the common diseases encountered in this field. It is not sufficient to accept and translate the experience and dictates of hospital specialists to family practice. The standard and traditional medical textbooks written by specialists from other fields are only partially useful and it is for this reason that we have brought together a group of family physicians to write on their special field.

Our book is a textbook on the common clinical problems in family medicine. Our emphasis has been on a sound clinical and common sense approach to problems and diseases encountered by family physicians all over the world. Reading the book our colleagues in family medicine anywhere should at once feel that the problems which we describe are just those that they meet in their own practices and we hope that our shared experiences may help them to understand better and to strive together for our common goal — better care for our patients.

The authors are all active family practitioners. They are generalists caring for families but they have all made special studies and have some special experience in the subjects on which they write. The team that we have collected is a group of individuals with their own bents and beliefs developed through years of practical experience, study, research and teaching, and this shows in their contributions.

As editors we have not sought to produce dull uniformity of presentation. Apart from general instruction and guidance we have allowed each contributor to write in his personal way and to present his views as he chooses. This may make for differences in style and approach but we believe that our readers will appreciate the personal flavours of each chapter and that it will add to their interest.

We have not intended to produce a book that is dogmatic and blindly authoritative. There will be many who will not agree with all the views and suggestions put forward. This has been our intention — to present together the collected practical experiences of colleagues whom we know and respect and whom we know are good doctors and who base their knowledge on supportive personal research and study. We hope that their views will create some differences of opinion that will lead to further thought, discussion and research.

What is needed more than anything in our common field of family practice is new thinking and questioning on long held beliefs and attitudes. We hope that our book will help to stimulate our readers, to foster more critical and questioning attitudes on the work that we do and to help to create and promote better care for our patients.

John Fry
Patrick S. Byrne
Susan Johnson

1

Introduction: Levels of Medical Care

J. Fry

We are living in a changing world. The 20th Century has been involved almost continuously in social, political and economic conflicts on national and international scales. In the midst.of such conflicts there have been major changes in medical care that have influenced the development and evolution of the form and structure of medical care services throughout the world.

There have been dramatic advances in medicine and in social and public health and as a result we now live longer than ever before and in greater health and comfort. Medical advances have come step in step with those in other sciences and as a result we now have a situation when more and more is demanded and expected of the medical profession to achieve almost the impossible in curing many, if not most, diseases.

Medical advances have led to increasing specialisation within medicine and it has become fashionable to assume that good care for almost any but the simplest of disorders requires care by a 'specialist'. This is a false assumption that has led to many difficulties and errors. Good medical care requires good generalists who can provide care for the non-specialist problems of the diseases that so commonly occur and who can assess the individual's needs for specialist care, only when and where this becomes necessary.

Paradoxically, there has never been a greater need for good generalists in primary care in the community and in the hospitals, for unless they are able to protect the specialists from non-specialist problems the specialists will be ill—used and wasted.

With better schooling, with the explosion of mass communication through all the media and with more and more world travel by ordinary people we now have a better educated and informed public than ever before. This public is an expectant and demanding one. It expects good health and long life and is demanding good medical care for all as a human and civic right and not as a selective acquisition of those who can afford to pay for it.

With advances and progress, the costs of good modern medical health care have risen to levels well beyond the pockets of ordinary people. The provision and distribution of medical health care today demands national government involvement in organisation and financing.

Such involvement by government creates many problems. It raises new difficulties between an historically independent medical profession and governments that have to exercise controls and directives. It creates problems of endeavouring to achieve good care at minimum cost and this leads to difficulties in deciding on priorities, quality and standards of care. It raises dilemmas such as those of trying to create a national medical system that is effective, efficient, economic and satisfactory for the consumer and satisfying, rewarding and stimulating for the medical profession. It raises issues such as the encouragement and development of good doctor-patient relations, good personal care and the maintenance of 'clinical freedom'.

SYSTEMS OF MEDICAL CARE

Such basic issues and problems are common to all systems and have to be tackled in every national situation. The type of system of medical care that each nation will create will depend on factors outside medicine.

A national health service will be influenced by political, social, philosophical and economic factors. It will be influenced by local and national geography. It will be influenced by the educational development of the people. It will, in the end, be influenced by the views and attitudes of the local medical profession, but such views and attitudes are bound to carry less and less weight as medicine becomes more and more technically advanced, more specialised and more costly putting it right outside the private pocket.

In spite of the possible different systems of medical and health care in the world there are within all systems certain common and inevitable levels of care, levels of administration and levels of disease.

There are, within all systems, levels of self-care, of primary (first-contact) professional medical and social care, of general specialist care at hospitals (and other institutions) and of super-specialist care. These levels of care require increasingly large units of population to make them administratively efficient, and these units progress in size from the family for self-care, the neighbourhood-locality for primary care, the district for general specialist care and the region for super-specialist care.

PRIMARY CARE – AN ESSENTIAL LEVEL

In each and every system of medical care there has to be a level of primary care. There has to be a primary physician (or other professional worker) of first-contact to whom the sick patient can turn in the first instance. This primary physician has similar roles, functions and features in all systems, yet he may be labelled differently in various systems. In Britain he is called a general practitioner, in the USA he may be a family physician or he may be a specialoid internist or paediatrician and in the USSR he may be a therapist[1].

Whatever his label he is an essential and inevitable member of the medical establishment. He is the foundation on which the rest of the system is firmly based. The quality of a health and medical care system depends on the quality and morale of primary medical care. It is a false economy to neglect primary medical care and self-care and to devote more resources on specialist hospital services, on the assumption that good specialist services can neutralise, overcome and compensate for poor primary care. This is a hypothesis full of waste and inefficiency. All levels of care are part of a whole system and all must achieve and maintain high standards in a sound system.

From the medical manpower point of view, primary care is the largest level of care. In a developed society more than half of all physicians are likely to be working as primary physicians, general practitioners, family physicians or whatever name or title is given to them. As a corollary it is an inevitable fact of medical life that more than half of all medical students in any year, or any decade, will become primary physicians.

For all these reasons family medicine, general practice or primary medical care is an important branch of medicine.

FEATURES, ROLES AND FUNCTIONS

The primary physician in all systems has certain similar features, roles and functions. That must be recognised if he is to be provided with the right facilities and support to enable him to provide good care for his patients.

His roles are to act as the physician-of-first-contact and as such he has the special responsibilities and difficulties of making the initial assessment and diagnosis of the presenting problem, be it emotional, physical, or social, and of organising the initial management.

To carry out this role he has to provide direct access to his patients. There is much more to this than is at first apparent. If he is to provide such direct access he has to organise his services so that he, or his personal deputy, is available and accessible during 24 hours a day. If his services are to be fully available they must also be freely available without artificial economic and other barriers such as distance, transport and time.

The most characteristic features of the primary physician are that he lives and works in a relatively small and static community and that he is able, therefore, to provide long-term and continuing care for his patients for as long as he or they remain together in a professional relationship.

As a result of this, the primary physician is well able to practise as a personal physician and as a family physician in the truest sense. In a stable community he comes to know his patients, and they to know him over many years and generations, and he scarcely needs to read through the notes that he accumulates over the years. He knows his patients and their families as soon as they walk into his consulting room.

Such important roles and functions will develop only if the primary physician is able to work as a generalist caring for the whole family and for all their medical problems rather than as a specialoid when the primary physician restricts and confines his work to certain disease groups such as emotional disorders, gynaecology or obstetrics, skin diseases or even surgery.

Working as he does with a relatively small community (often 2000—3000 persons in a developed society), the primary physician's spectrum of morbidity will be inevitably that which occurs in a population of this size (see Chapter 3). He will be involved with the diseases that commonly occur, with the mass of more minor disorders, with the early diagnosis of major diseases, with the long-term care of chronic disorders, with the social pathology that intrudes on medical care and with the personal and family factors and characteristics that so intertwine disease, its manifestations and management.

The primary physician functions as an all-round and all-purpose pro-fessional, using many skills and techniques. He has to be an excellent clinician, good in diagnosis and in applying sound and common sense care. He has to be intensely interested in and concerned for human beings as individuals and as members of the local community, He has to act not only as a personal and family physician but also as a public and community physician concerned with the general health and social welfare of his population. He has to be concerned with prevention as well as with treatment of established disease.

He has to deploy his skills as a local diplomat, as a coordinator and manipulator of available services for his patients' benefit, as a protector of his patients from unnecessary and hazardous procedures and situations, and as an economist in the widest sense ensuring that resources are being used efficiently and effectively.

PRIMARY MEDICAL CARE AS A SPECIALITY

To carry out his roles and functions well the primary physician has become a 'specialist' and his field of work a 'specialty'. This means that there is an accepted core of knowledge and expertise that can be defined and distinguished, which can be studied and researched, and taught.

Family medicine, general practice, primary care or whatever title we give it, certainly fulfils these criteria. It has its own core of well-defined diseases and problems (see Chapter 3). It has its own roles, functions and features and it requires its own special expertise and methodology. It offers special opportunities for research and study and its researches have added to our understanding of disease and its processes. Particular opportunities exist for the study of those diseases that are rarely seen other than in primary care, such as the common respiratory and gastro-intestinal infections, the common skin disorders and the common emotional disorders. The long-term study of the natural history, course and outcome of disease cannot be researched elsewhere[2].

The past decade has seen a dramatic growth and development in the number of University departments of family medicine and in the postgraduate vocational training (or residency) programmes for training young doctors in the specialty, and in the spread of continuing education for more senior practitioners. It has been demonstrated amply that it is a subject that can be taught.

FUTURE TRENDS IN ORGANISATION AND DEVELOPMENT

The present is the forerunner of great potential evolution and development in this field. There are many experiments and exercises taking place as a result of which future changes may take place. Some of these can be highlighted in a series of questions and answers.

Who? Who should provide the first-contact care? The days of the single-handed do-it-all-himself physician are past. Good primary care has to be provided by a team of physician, nurse, social worker and secretary. The roles and functions of each and all of these have to be worked out. There are probably many functions and roles that can be shared out in such a team.

Where? Primary care has to involve care in the home, in the community, at work, in the hospital as well as in the physician's consulting room. The good physician has to extend his interests and involvement in his patients' welfare well beyond his own office.

Why? If there is no sound level of primary medical care the whole system becomes inefficient. More and more conditions are taken to the next level, the hospital, adding to expense, with less than good care. It is essential for a primary physician to provide first contact and continuing care on a personal and family basis.

When? The challenge is how to organise primary care to provide continuing direct access on a 24 hour a day basis. This can be done most easily by close cooperation with colleagues.

What? The type of care provided by the primary physician includes the traditional approach of diagnosis, assessment and treatment. In addition there is the element of long-term personal care and support over many years, often for conditions that are not strictly curable but which certainly benefit from relief and comfort.

One of the current debates is whether the primary physician should be a 'generalist' or 'specialoid'. This has to be resolved by each system in relation to other levels of care, but it seems at present most economic and effectual for him to act as a 'generalist'.

How? There is concern about the type and quality of care being provided by the primary physician and some measures of quality have to be evolved by which standards can be assessed and improved. Such assessments will have to be related to the three phases of care, the structure of the system, the process of the care given and the outcome.

References

1. Fry, J. (1969). In *Medicine in Three Societies*, (Lancaster: MTP Press).
2. Fry, J. (1974). *Common Diseases*, (Lancaster: MTP Press).

2

Clinical Methods

P. S. Byrne

It is important to appreciate that family practitioners are concerned with whole person medicine. Factors causing or influencing illness may be discovered in the patient's psyche as well as in his soma, in his family, his home, his work-situation and in his local and wider environment. Thus organic disease must be regarded as only a part of the patient's total illness.

The succeeding chapters of this book deal with the more common diseases as revealed by morbidity studies. In almost every instance there are some general considerations which apply and these are briefly described here. They will be considered under the headings: the special circumstances of family practice; the available facilities; the needs of family practice.

SPECIAL CIRCUMSTANCES

The Time Scale

The first consideration is that of the time scale of disease and the operational time scale of the family practitioner. Even in crisis medicine, a knowledge of the natural history of disease is essential. Few diseases in fact produce crises until they have been diagnosable for some time. Chronic bronchitis for example has a natural history in the individual patient of 20–30 years. There must be a time interval of a year or two from a quiet onset before the clinical diagnostic features are clearly present. Yet some will make a 'probability' diagnosis earlier than others. The advantage of this to the patient lies not in the fact that he may be 'cured' but that as early as possible he may be advised and helped to avoid some of the respiratory insults, such as smoking, which environment and infection can produce. The necessary health education of the patient, with encouragment for 'self-help', must not be neglected. With each such insult the process of deterioration of the patient is accelerated.

Index of Suspicion

An important part of our effective clinical armamentarium is that high index of suspicion which stems from experience and a knowledge of epidemiology, and thus an increased capacity to make a diagnosis based on probability. To be clinically effective does not always require an accurate clinico-pathological diagnosis. There can be just as valid a base for decision-making without the application of a specific diagnostic label. We might call this base our 'operational' diagnosis. Thus if one sees a child of 2 with an acute abdomen it is necessary to decide that the child requires admission to hospital, for observation and perhaps laparotomy. The definitive diagnosis of strangulation of a Meckel's diverticulum is unlikely to be made, even in hospital, until laparotomy. Our proper attempts to relieve cardiac arrest by external cardiac massage owe little to an accurate aetiological diagnosis.

Place of Treatment
There is a changing picture of the locus for treatment of many diseases. Diabetes mellitus and pernicious anaemia were once 'hospital' diseases. Now most patients suffering from either condition may be both diagnosed and treated by the family practitioner. Increased diagnostic and therapeutic facilities (to be discussed later) mean that more diseases begin to fall into the potential care of the family practitioner in his surgery, in the patient's home or in the 'community' or 'cottage' hospital. The more effective we family practitioners are, the more will the hospital consultants be enabled to fulfil their chosen task of being specialists.

Consulting Times
Our consulting time scale varies from one practioner to another. Many consult at five-minute intervals, some at ten minutes or more. It is interesting to reflect how short a time is allotted to patients in Britain compared with Holland, North America, Australia, New Zealand and other European countries. If we adopt the basic principle of Weed[1] that one cannot rationally treat a patient until his problems have been identified, we would take longer over our consultations, but after a year of crucifixion we should discover, hopefully, that many of our patients were understood, stabilised or cured, and that our work-load was substantially less than before. Nobody has yet carried out the essential basic tests to discover whether the outcome of the common diseases differ in any of the systems and whether the duration of individual consultations is an influencing factor.

It may be that each of us has discovered an optimum personal tempo for work and for its sessional duration. It is also true that we may aggregate a series of short consultations over a period into an effective whole, which we may call the 'extended' consultation. It is important that we combine these factors to help define the problems of the patient in sufficient detail to permit rational therapy.

The Consultation

Sir James Spence said 'The essential unit of medical practice is the occasion when, in the intimacy of the consulting room or sick room, a person who is ill or believes himself to be ill seeks the advice of a doctor whom he trusts. This is a consultation. . . . The purpose of the consultation is that the doctor, having gathered his evidence shall give explanation and advice'.

This is still substantially true, yet is too broad a definition. The consultation contains intellectual process and format and a wide range of clinical and behavioural skills and is subject to modifications dependent on the goals of the participants, the factor of time, the national system of health care, as well as local environmental circumstance. The temporal factor is important. Many of us use the 'short' and the 'long' consultation.

The 'short' consultation is the norm. It is used for the routine follow-up and for the 'repeat' consultation which we know represents about two-thirds of all our consultations. It may also be used as a first consultation with a new patient, or for a new episode of illness reported by a familiar patient. In these instances it may provide all the time required for that patient and his problems. It may also serve to identify the need for more time and hence lead to a 'long' consultation of twenty minutes or more. With some few patients the need for a 'long' consultation may be immediately apparent. On these rare occasions perhaps the immediate need should be met immediately.

The time involved in the 'short' consultation is from five to ten minutes. This time, precious both to doctor and patient, must be used to the best advantage for each. We have been undertaking in Manchester a study of the consultation based on a verbal behavioural analysis of audio-tapes of actual surgery consultations conducted by family practitioners.

The five-minute consultation may be regarded as an average only, yet the results of this study suggest that this time is too short. We have all experienced the 'by the way, doctor' situations; those times when the patient at the apparent end of a consultation starts all over again with this challenging remark. Some 95 per cent of them occur in the five-minute consultation, in particular on those occasions when the doctor has failed to enquire or to determine why the patient has come. Moreover nearly all the patently dysfunctional consultations, those in which neither doctor nor patient either demonstrate or achieve defined goals, occur also within the five-minute format. What seems to be certain is the need for flexibility, for the capacity to adapt to the patient's needs, to personal matters, to the overall constraints of work-load.

The Family

Our patients have to be seen and treated in the context of their family and its environment. Kay[2] studied staphylococcal infections within the family, demonstrating the sites and patterns of cross infection. Many instances of disease and its pattern in the family have been demonstrated[3]. We know of the need to examine all members of the family when one is revealed to suffer from oxyuris infection, scabies or impetigo, yet we do not frequently enough explore the possible background of family stress. Selye[4] demonstrated how, for some months after acute stress, various members of a family could show a clustering of episodes of organic disease apparently disconnected. Hagerty[5] found that, in children suffering from acute tonsillitis, compared with a group of normal controls, a history of acute family stress in the previous week occurred five times as often in the sufferers as it did in the controls. The stress might for example have been an examination, an accident or a bereavement and not necessarily have directly affected the sufferer.

These examples of 'family illness' are environmental in origin; the effects of living together. The same may be said to some extent of the 'husband and wife' diseases, when each is found to suffer from, say, hypertension, chronic bronchitis, or malnutrition. Our knowledge of the domestic and environmental circumstances of our patients should help us to recognise early, and to be prepared for the possibilities of, such conditions as malnutrition or hypothermia.

Many battered children and wives have continued to be maltreated because we, among others, have accepted at face value the causes of bruising and injury advanced to us, often by the batterer. Those who undertake home visits may see evidence of potential trauma in a variety of environmental dangers.

Hereditary disease is another area of disease in the family, and here we need to be aware how and from whom we may seek genetic counselling if it appears to be required.

The Environment
Most of us family practitioners spend a substantial part of our working life in the same practice. We are thus ideally placed to learn a great deal of the local industrial, climatic, and environmental factors of illness in our patients. It is always worth while to have visited the premises of the major local industries so that we may learn of the nature of our patients' occupations and their inherent hazards.

Now that the aeroplane is one of its fastest vectors, we have to be on the watch for exotic disease. In practice Maegraith's[6] three questions are still important. Where have you been? When were you there? How long did you stay there? A few people die each year in the UK from falciparum malaria because these questions were not asked.

Consultation Techniques
It is too early to comment on the attempts being made in many places to define and teach new consultation techniques. What must be said is that the well-tried techniques and format of sound traditional clinical medicine must always be

practised. To take a proper history, to conduct an appropriate examination and to undertake necessary investigations, to make a diagnosis, to propose therapy or referral, even to exhibit the 'masterly inactivity' of careful observation, to manage the patient and the family — all these are the components of sound clinical medicine.

FACILITIES

It was A. J. Cronin in his novel *The Citadel* (1937) who made his central character, the practioner Manson, demand passionately that the doctor be provided with the necessary tools for him to practise scientific medicine. Today in many countries the family practioner has ample diagnostic resources. He has full open-access to the various laboratory and radiological departments, and often to electrocardiography and electroencephalography. He has available a wide range of 'do-it-yourself' equipment, such as 'peak flow' meters, spirographs, equipment for hearing testing, spectrometers and machines for estimating haemoglobin and other blood constituents. There are a number of dipsticks, disposable vaginal and procto-scopes, and his own microscope. He has a stethoscope, auroscope, ophthalmoscope and other instruments of his choice. All these instruments however require to be accurate and 'zeroed' — even the humble sphygmomanometer, especially the aneroid type. We may seek assistance from the technicians of the firms who supply our equipment, but the hospital technicians are themselves usually most helpful.

Investigation
There is evidence, too, that the pick—up rate of abnormal radiological and pathological findings is highest in those investigations requested by family practioners, although the reasons for this are not clear. There are some points which should be made about our use of investigations. Thus we may not wish to undertake any investigation unless:

1. it is calculated to assist us in confirming or excluding a presumptive diagnosis;
2. we will understand the meaning of whatever result is obtained;
3. understanding the results, we have the capacity to use them in treatment or management.

There is, however, great professional satisfaction to be derived from the painstaking 'work up' of a patient even if the patient has then to be referred to hospital. Hence we may wish on occasion to act in defiance of 3 above, and may well be better clinicians by so doing.

We must distinguish between the common use of the departments of pathology and radiology in our hospitals as service departments alone, and the more interesting cooperation with the pathologist and the radiologist as consultant specialists. These colleagues are as interested as we are in good clinical medicine. It is often profitable to discuss with them clinical problems and their potential for help in solutions.

Relations with Consultants

Referrals to hospital for 'in' or 'out' patient facilities are made easier if we seek a working relationship with the consultants of our local hospitals. Most of them are prepared to indicate those times when they least mind being available to discuss clinical problems. These times may even coincide with our own, while a reputation for meaningful clinical communication is a useful one for the family practitioner to acquire.

Such relationships do not simply happen. They are to be sought and earned on both sides. Postgraduate medical centres provide an excellent forum for discussion and the development of relationships. Young practioners, new in an area, are well advised to seek such opportunities where they exist. Apart from the usual social relationships deriving from professional contacts, a group of practitioners may invite consultants for a meal and in the post-prandial atmosphere determine a *modus vivendi et operandi.*

There are several valid reasons for referral:

1. when we have not yet achieved a diagnosis and require help;
2. when a diagnosis having been made, the hospital services are required for treatment, e.g. acute appendicitis.

These two may be regarded as technical reasons, but there are two further equally important reasons for referral:

3. when the diagnosis made is one of lethal potential, so that, especially for a young patient, it is felt necessary to have a second opinion in order that no stone may be conceived to be unturned;
4. when the patient, or sometimes a relation like the aunt who was a nurse in World War II, insists on a second opinion.

Referral should never be a matter of 'opting out'. Although it may be argued that this ensures the patient's safety we should practise to the best of our ability.

Whatever the reasons for our referral of a patient we should be clearly aware of them and indicate them to the consultant. We might indicate whether we are

1. seeking an opinion on a specific stated point(s);
2. that we are asking the consultant to take over the care of the patient; or
3. that we are suggesting shared care on a continuing basis.

The latter may be required for a patient who is diabetic and difficult to stabilise, or for some patients with depressive illness for example.

When a choice of consultants is available we often adopt a policy of 'horses for courses'. We select a particular consultant for a particular patient. Some surgeons are known to be at their best in elective planned surgery, others at improvisation in acute complicated conditions. Our general physicians tend to have sub-specialist skills in cardiology or neurology for example. Consultants are also themselves persons with personalities. Some adopt the same whole person approach to patients as do we ourselves. Others are less sensitive to any factor of illness other than the organic, and indeed, the more technology is used in a speciality, the more likely this is to be so. Nevertheless we take into account all these factors when deciding to whom we will refer our patient.

NEEDS

Prescribing
There are many questions to be asked about the rationale of much of our therapy, of our use of drugs in particular. Assuming that we all prescribe, in, say, acute lower urinary tract infections, according to the sensitivity to drugs of the infecting organism as demonstrated by the laboratory, how valid is our reliance? Where is the evidence? It is well known that clinical success may often occur following the *in vivo* administration of a drug which the laboratory *in vitro* findings suggest would be ineffective.

Why do upwards of two-thirds of all patients leave our consulting room clutching a prescription?[7] It seems unlikely that all are necessary and there is much hard evidence to show how large a proportion of the drugs prescribed are either not collected[8] from the pharmacist, or if collected left to languish in bathroom cupboards.

An important study of long-term prescribing is described by Balint[9]. This study revealed that many patients were taking a variety of nostrums regularly and unchanged over long periods — in one instance sixteen years. The rationale for their original prescription was obscured by time if indeed there had ever been one. The problem in each case was to attempt to stop prescribing what now seemed to be unnecessary.

Perhaps we should listen more to clinical pharmacologists and to our own and our colleagues' experience, than to the eulogies of the 'reps' of the pharmaceutical industry. Excluding conditions such as epilepsy and diabetes which require long-term therapy *ab initio* it is perhaps no bad thing to prescribe defined courses of drugs once we have decided that a prescription is required at all.

That it is often more time-consuming to explain to the patient why he does not need a prescription than it is to issue one is a poor excuse which may be held to derive from the constraints of the five-minute appointment. Perhaps we need a strict pruning of the national available pharmacopeia to remove the plethora of choices from the indistinguishable. It is an area which needs to be covered more in continuing education.

Quality Management

We as professionals must be concerned with the quality of our care of patients. We must learn how to monitor, evaluate and audit the quality of our care. The major difficulty is that there are no agreed existing yardsticks against which we may measure our own performance. An urgent major need is the setting up of a considered series of studies out of which the clinical yardsticks may be produced. Such studies, once begun, would need to be continuous, for it seems certain that the optimum measures now may be different, in many areas, from those of ten years hence. This is a huge task, but one which would, if successful, improve the capacity of our profession both in the actual quality of care and in the dilution of our professional isolation. We would be able then to compare our own performance with the contemporary professional standards of our colleagues.

Despite this need it is still possible for us to use our own good clinical records to consider clinical outcomes. When we have referred a patient to a consultant we may reflect, on receipt of the latter's letter, what did he do which we could not? What did he discover in the history, or in the ensuing examination, which we failed to discover? It is possible by using simple disease indexes like the Walford[10] to review the clinical outcomes of groups of patients suffering from the same condition, hypertension, or depression for example. How effective was our therapy? Were there any consistent patterns of features of the disease, of therapy, of clinical outcome, and did some therapies appear to be more advantageous than others?

Comparisons may be made with partners and other family practitioners. This type of study is of great value, for in some common diseases such as ischaemic heart disease and stroke, it has been noted that there is a significant difference in the age groups of sufferers between hospital and family practice studies[11]. There are still many useful contributions to the natural history of disease yet to come from family practice.

While many of our trainees in family practice are quick to appreciate how little their previous medical education has prepared them, we have too little hard evidence as yet on which we may base rational educational programmes. However important the psycho-social factors of illness may be, it is organic disease which is still the greatest killer and incapacitator. Even in its minor common presentations such as lower urinary tract infection and upper respiratory tract infections, we are still given to unjustifiable and expensive therapy. We must make more, wider and continuing contributions to its study.

There is no such person as an average family practitioner[12]. This book would seek to present what in North America would be called the 'core knowledge' required for all family practitioners. Yet each of we family practitioners is in a unique environmental and personal context. Each has to learn to practise, within the needs and constraints of his personal situation. Thus the common 'core' is for all, but our personal, physical and preferential circumstances demand a wider range of knowledge and skills. What that range shall be is the decision of the individual, and in consequence it will vary a great deal from practice to practice. Some may wish, or find it necessary, to be more skilled and practised in gynaecology, in occupational health, in exotic or zootic diseases, in psychological medicine, or in the diseases of poverty or affluence. Thus each must fulfil the requirements laid down by his environment and his personal choice, but all must be based on a minimum common 'core'.

Health Centres and Health Teams

There is at the present time a growing bandwagon of support for health centres and health teams. We assume that the quality of the care provided from the health centre, and by the team, is higher than that provided by a single-handed family practitioner practising from less sophisticated surroundings. There is not, however, one piece of objective evidence which supports this assumption. It is high time that attempts were made to achieve it, if indeed the assumption is true. The work of Cartwright[13] and others suggests that the patient's view may well be just the opposite. While the health teams have an important and not yet fully determined role to play, we, the family practitioners, are the only trained clinicians in the team. This is our basic role and we must fulfil it to the best advantage.

References

1. Weed, L. (1969). *Medical Records, Medical Education and Patient Care*, (Press of Cape Western Reserve University).
2. Kay, C. R. (1962). *Brit. med. J.* 2, 1048.
3. Spence, J., Walton, W. S., Miller, F. J. W., Court, S. D. M. (1954). *A Thousand Families in Newcastle upon Tyne*, (Oxford: Oxford University Press).
4. Selye, H. (1957). *The Stress of Life*, (Longmans, Green and Co.).
5. Hagerty, R. J., Alpert, J. P. (1963). *Postgrad. Med.* 34, 228.
6. Maegraith, B. (1963). *Exotic Diseases in Practice*, (London: Heinemann).
7. Elective study by a medical student in Darbishire House (1973). (unpublished).
8. Lloyd. G. (1973). M.D. Thesis. Self-Titration: A Study of Long Term Prescribing in a British National Health Service Practice.
9. Balint, M. (1970). *Treatment or Diagnosis*, (London: Tavistock Publications).
10. Walford, P. A. (1963). The Practice Index. *J. roy. Coll. gen. Practit.* 6, 225.
11. Acheson, J., Acheson, H. W. K., Tellwright, J. M. (1968). *J. roy. Coll. gen. Practit.* 16, 428.
12. The Future General Practitioner (1973). Published by British Medical Journal for the Royal College of General Practitioners.
13. Cartwright, A. (1967). *Patients and Their Doctors*, (London: Routledge and Kegan, Paul).

3

Common Diseases

J. Fry

If good care is to be provided in family practice, then it is necessary to understand the nature of disease and the general social setting. Unless we learn and appreciate this, care will be based unrealistically on traditions derived from specialist hospital practice taught in medical schools on conditions and situations very different from those that exist in family practice.

As noted in Chapter 1, the special features of primary care practice are first-contact and long-term care of individuals and families in small and relatively static communities. This does not mean that these communities are small and isolated units but rather that within any community a primary physician attracts to himself a population group of 2000—3000 persons for whom he provides the roles and functions of personal and family physician.

These features of primary care lead inevitably to a special spectrum of disease morbidity and mortality. The types of diseases and allied problems will be those that are likely to occur in a relatively small (2000—3000 persons) population.

This being so there will be a predominance of more minor and less dramatic diseases, of long-term chronic and degenerative conditions of ageing and of social and socio—medical problems, and only a few and occasional cases of the more major and more dramatic conditions encountered in hospital practice.

HEALTH AND DISEASE

Before the nature, content and problems of common diseases are discussed it is necessary first to consider 'health' and its criteria.

If the World Health Organization's (WHO) definition of 'health' as 'a state of complete physical, mental and social well-being and not merely an absence of disease'[1] is accepted then there are probably few of us who are 'healthy' at any time. It has been estimated that only 10 per cent of us are 'healthy' in WHO terms at any time and another 25 per cent in 'good health'[2,3].

Health is a highly subjective state that is coloured and influenced by many personal and environmental factors and any attempts at more definite objective measurements are fraught with difficulties.

A pyramid of health and disease can be devised and flow between each level is highly influenced by local and subjective factors.

A level of sub-health, or pre-symptomatic phase of disease, can be postulated. This is the state of quiet and incipient disease with no symptoms but with possible signs if they are searched for. This is the level of possible pre-symptomatic diagnosis and screening for early signs of undetected disease. It is uncertain how effective and useful are the applications of this philosophy into medical practice. It is uncertain whether intensive and expensive screening exercises are worthwhile[4].

Once symptoms are present, the individual is presented with the choice of self-treatment or of seeking professional advice. In fact, approximately three out of every four symptoms are self-treated and self-medicated by the individual and family. It is just as well that this is so for otherwise the medical services would be overwhelmed by the demands for care.

The decision to seek medical attention and to cross the threshold of care into the medical care system means that it is the primary physician who is usually consulted. It is on the basis of these decisions that the pattern of disease in primary care is based. It is the individual patient and his family who take the first step to seek care and there are many factors that will influence the decision.

It is well known that different families and individuals have different patterns and rates of attendance in primary care. There are some who are frequent attenders and others who are rarely seen from year to year. In my own practice a survey of infrequent attenders showed that they differed considerably from the average and frequent attenders. They were not more healthy but they were much more self-reliant and self-confident and less appreciative of, and overwhelmed by, the potentials of the medical profession.

The attendance patterns of individuals are influenced by their beliefs and attitudes to the possible 'cure' for their complaints, by their beliefs that the physician can relieve these symptoms better than they can themselves, and by their hope for comfort from the physician, even if cure and relief are not possible. They are influenced by the knowledge and understanding of the individual of what is 'normal' and of the nature and course of common diseases and their potential for cure. They are influenced also by their personal tolerance of the symptoms and discomfort that they are suffering. These factors are all amenable to influence by the physician and his team and with good relations and health education the attendance rates and use of medical services can be developed and controlled by the physician.

The flow between primary care and hospital specialist care depends usually on the primary physician's actions. Referrals of patients to hospitals vary considerably between practitioners[5] and appear to be influenced by the age, experience, and attitudes of the primary physician and on the facilities that he has for investigating and hospitalising his own patients. The rates depend also on the system of remuneration and on the financial incentives that exist for admitting patients to hospital or for treating them in the community.

COMMON DISEASES

The nature and extent of the common diseases depend on the level of care that is being observed. Thus, what is common in a super-specialist unit may be rare in a general hospital unit. What is common in hospital is rare in family practice and what is seen commonly by a primary physician may be a rare experience for a family. The 'commonness' of disease depends on the size of the population at risk and on the pre-selection of the clinical material. The super-specialist unit may deal only with cases of a single rare disease from a population of 5 million persons, the general specialist surgical unit in a district hospital will deal with all the herniae, breast lumps and acute abdomens from a population of 250 000 persons and a family practitioner will see all those 70 per cent of his 2500 patients who decide to consult him in any year.

To give some idea of the number of conditions that may be expected to be encountered at the various levels of care, the following tables are presented.

SELF CARE

In a survey, it was found[2] that the most common disorders complained of by a random sample of the population were, in order: respiratory disorders; nervous and emotional symptoms; aches and pains in joints, back and feet, and disorders of the gastro-intestinal symptoms (Table 3.1).

Most of the common symptoms recorded in Table 3.1 are either suffered without special treatment or self-medication may be carried out. Few of these would be taken to the primary physician.

Self-care is an important level of care that has been neglected by the medical profession. It offers considerable opportunities for research and experiment to determine whether better self-care and health maintenance. may lead to better health, earlier medical advice for appropriate conditions and more discriminating use of the medical services by the public.

PRIMARY CARE

The family practitioner is responsible on average for a population of 2500 people. In Table 3.2 are shown, the numbers of persons in such a population

Table 3.1   Common symptoms in a sample of adults (after Dunnell, K. and Cartwright, A. 1972[2]).

	Symptoms	Percentage reporting symptoms in a two-week period prior to survey
Respiratory	Cough, catarrh or sputum	32
	Colds or influenza	18
	Breathlessness	15
	Sore throats	12
Nervous and emotional	Headaches	38
	Sleeplessness	16
	Tiredness	16
	Eye strain	14
Rheumatic	Aching limbs and joints	29
	Backache	21
	Painful feet or corns	19
Digestive	Indigestion	18
	Constipation	10
	Diarrhoea	3
	Vomiting	3
	Weight problems	10
Accidents		9
Average number of symptoms reported per person		3.9

who will consult their family practitioner in a typical year in Britain and in the USA.

These illustrative numbers show the range of disease in family practice. In a year about 1850 of the 2500 persons at risk will consult the family practitioner. In a year he probably will carry out some 7000–10 000 consultations either at his consulting room or in his patients' homes. Probably only one-tenth of the volume of his work is now home visits. In the USA few home visits are done. Each day he will see some 20–40 patients and in addition he will probably also undertake other medical work on some days in hospitals or elsewhere.

GENERAL DISTRICT HOSPITAL

The types of cases that are seen at a local district hospital represent those requiring the facilities of a hospital in a population of around 250 000, which is the planned population for a district hospital.

This being so, the likely number of cases admitted to such a hospital would be as shown in Table 3.3

Table 3.2   Common diseases seen in a year in typical family practices of 2500 persons in the UK[6] and USA.[7],[8]

Diseases		Persons consulting per year in a population of 2500	
		UK	USA
Minor	Upper respiratory infections	500	400
	Emotional disorders	300	300
	Acute gastrointestinal disorders	250	200
	Skin diseases	225	200
Major	Pneumonia and acute bronchitis	50	35
(new cases)	Myocardial infraction	7	10
	New cancers	5	7
	Acute appendicitis	5	8
	Strokes	5	7
	Severe depression	12	10
	Suicide attempts	3	3
	Suicide	(1 every 4 years)	
Chronic	Arthritis	100	100
	Mental illness	75	
	Chronic bronchitis	50	20
	Heart failure	45	60
	High blood pressure	25	75
	Asthma	25	25
	Peptic ulcer	15	20
	Epilepsy	10	10
	Diabetes	10	20
	Parkinsonism	3	3
	Multiple sclerosis	2	2
	Chronic pyelonephritis	(less than 1)	
Social	Severe physical handicap	70	65
Problems	Broken bones	50	60
	Severe mental handicap	10	10
	Divorce	3	6
	Illegitimate births	3	3
	Committed to prison	2	3

SOME PROBLEMS IN THE CARE OF COMMON DISEASES

Having noted the types and frequency of the common diseases that are seen in family practice, it is necessary now to consider and examine some of the problems that face the physician in caring for them.

There has been a lack of research and study of the common diseases and we know relatively little of their nature, course, outcome and effective management. Most are benign; they are either short and self-limiting or chronic

Table 3.3   Numbers of persons likely to be admitted annually to a District Hospital
caring for 250 000 persons.

Diseases	Number of persons hospitalised per year (per 250 000 at risk).
Myocardial infarctions	250
Cancers	600
Acute appendicitis	500
Strokes	300
Haemorrhoids	300
Herniae	300
Pneumonia and bronchitis	750
Suicide attempts	250

causing discomfort and disability, but not necessarily death. In view of our uncertainty of the true causes or of the real natural history of these common diseases, it is scarcely surprising that their management tends to be somewhat irrational and inadequately based on controlled trials and scientific evidence. There is great need to study these common diseases further in the context of family practice.

Respiratory Conditions

The common respiratory conditions account for between one-quarter and one-third of all the work in family practice. Their prevalence is influenced by the season: they are more frequent in winter than in summer, but even so they are by no means infrequent in summer months. Taken as a group, respiratory disorders affect most young children (under 10) and the elderly (over 60), but persons at all ages are liable to suffer from common acute respiratory infections.

In addition to the problem of sheer numbers of cases, the common respiratory infections present other issues. Their aetiology and pathogenesis are uncertain. Similar clinical symptoms of acute respiratory tract irritation and inflammation may be caused by microorganisms, bacteria or viruses, by allergic reactions in hypersensitive individuals, by inhaled atmospheric pollutants such as dust, fog or chemical irritants, or through nervous reactions in persons who are emotionally sensitive.

Even when and where the probable causal microorganism is isolated it is impossible to relate the clinical features in the patient to specific characteristics of the infecting organism. The practising physician is at a loss to try and make an accurate aetiological diagnosis from the clinical appearances and symptoms. Pathological and radiological investigations are of little help.

The real problem in management is to decide on the use of various drugs and other physical measures in treating these common respiratory diseases. If we are unsure of the causes, how can we be efficient in applying treatment? The answer is that we are not efficient, but, nevertheless, we seem to be effective. The facts are that most persons suffering from acute respiratory infections get better quickly. Whether this is the natural history of the condition or whether it is influenced by the use of specific antibiotics or other therapeutic measures is uncertain. Those clinical trials that have been carried out suggest that there is no difference between antibiotics and symptomatic measures in the recovery rates from common respiratory infections.

Whilst we need to pursue research to determine the causes of common respiratory infection, it is more urgent to carry out controlled clinical trials to determine whether specific antibiotics are really required to treat these conditions.

Emotional and Mental Disorders

The various forms of emotional and mental disorders constitute the second largest group of conditions in family practice. Approximately 15—20 per cent of all the work is concerned with these disorders.

The practical problems relating to this group are difficulties of initial diagnosis, the difficulties of understanding the nature and causes of the conditions and of their course, and the difficultes of management and deciding whether psychotropic drugs are likely to be beneficial and how the patient, his family and environment might be managed and supported.

In the care and management of persons with emotional and mental disorders it is necessary to understand and to help and support the individual and his family, possibly over many years because it is likely that those liable to these disorders are vulnerable individuals who will require regular and long-term help and care.

In the management of these disorders it is frustrating for the physician to seek a 'cure' for his patient. It is far better in those emotionally vulnerable individuals to accept that no cure will ever be possible but that with personal and family support and understanding the physician will be able to do much to help keep these persons at terms with themselves, their family and their environment.

Skin Disorders

Disorders of the skin are another group of common diseases encountered in primary care practice. The difficulties here are those of lack of adequate training in dermatology and uncertainty on the part of the primary physician in the diagnosis of the various rashes and skin blemishes that his patients bring to him. The few weeks as an undergraduate and the few more weeks as a trainee are certainly not sufficient to make him adept and confident in diagnosing and managing skin disorders. Thus, since there is so much uncertainty still of the nature and causation of skin diseases, treatment tends to be rather unscientific and uncertain. Fortunately there are the corticosteroids which when applied to many rashes cause dramatic and rapid relief and they are the most widely used preparations in dermatology.

Paediatrics, Geriatrics, Gynaecology and Obstetrics

The practice of child care, of geriatrics, of gynaecology, and of obstetrics now require considerable knowledge and expertise of social issues, problems and resources. They demonstrate the importance of the need to establish close links and understanding between social and medical services, in all districts.

Many of the problems, not only in these groups but in all of family practice, are created through social troubles, and their management will require attempts at resolving or ameliorating the social troubles that result.

Within an ageing society, the disorders of ageing and degeneration pose their own particular difficulties. We know little of the ageing processes and certainly not enough to halt or delay their progression. We are faced therefore with the end results of worn joints that cause arthritic pain and disabilities; with furred up and weak arteries leading to myocardial ischaemia and cardiac failure, to strokes from cerebral thrombosis or haemorrhage and damage to the brain, to eye and kidney disturbances from atherosclerotic ischaemia and of intermittent claudication or sometimes gangrene of the legs, and with chronically irritated bronchial and lung linings from years of smoking cigarettes and breathing polluted air that may lead to chronic bronchitis and bronchial cancer.

The primary physician has to become expert in caring for the disorders of old age, for some 15 per cent of his practice will be over 65 years of age.

AN APPROACH

These problems of the common diseases demand a systematic and realistic approach if the primary physician is to be able to cope with the numbers and with the issues raised.

First, it is essential that the *disease* is understood as best as one can with the present state of knowledge.

The physician needs to know its epidemiology, whom it affects, when and where and if possible, why? He must know its clinical presenting symptoms and signs from which he can proceed to a reasonably certain and accurate diagnosis, supported if necessary, by investigations.

Before considering the treatment and management, the physician should attempt to make an assessment of the *patient* as an individual and of his family and environment, where appropriate. It is as a result of such an assessment that the patient and his problems will be able to be managed in the most satisfactory manner. Special personal or family situations may require quite different forms of management in different individuals with the same disease.

Before engaging in any therapeutic exercise it is important for the physician to appreciate and understand the *natural history of the disease.* Many common diseases will clear up and resolve spontaneously without attempts at specific therapies. It is as well therefore always to pause before writing out a prescription for antibiotics, for psychotropic drugs, for hypotensives, for anti-inflammatory drugs and other specific or pseudo-specific drugs — because they may not be necessary or helpful and they may, in fact, be harmful in the side effects that they may cause.

The good therapist should come to know well by experience the few drugs that he customarily uses. It is far better to know a few drugs well than to dabble with many.

The good physician also must know the potentials of the *local facilities* that are available and may have to be called into use, coordinated or manipulated for his patient's good. He should know the qualities of his specialist colleagues to whom he may refer his patients. He should know the hospitals and their qualities and deficiencies. He should know the skills and experience of local paramedical workers such as nurses, health visitors, social workers and the various social and voluntary agencies.

The good physician must know, above all else, *his own strengths and weaknesses* and what it is reasonable for him to undertake and what he should not attempt.

References

1. Introducing WHO (1976). (Geneva: World Health Organization).
2. Dunnell, R. and Cartwright, A. (1972). *Medicine Takers, Prescribers and Hoarders,* (London: Routledge and Kegan Paul).
3. Wadsworth, M. E. J., Butterfield, W. J. H. and Blaney, R. (1971). *Health and Sickness, The Choice of Treatment,* (London: Tavistock Publications).
4. Nuffield Provincial Hospitals Trust (1968). *Screening in Medical Care*, (Oxford: Oxford University Press).
5. McLachlan, G. (ed.) (1966). In *Problems and Progress in Medical Care*, (Oxford: Oxford University Press).
6. Fry, J. (1974). *Common Diseases*, (Lancaster: MTP Press).
7. Marshland, D. W. *et al.* (1976). *J. fam. Pract.* **3**, 25.
8. Marsh, G. N. *et al.* (1976). *Brit. med. J.* **1**, 1321.

4

Acute Respiratory Infections

J. Fry

There are a number of reasons why the common acute respiratory infections are important to the family practitioner.

First, they are the largest single clinical group in everyday practice throughout the year all over the world.

Second, they are an amorphous and confusing collection of symptoms that make clear clinical diagnosis and definition difficult, and because of this they abound with many multiple labels and name-tags. These may be descriptive or unsuccessful attempts at a pathological or aetiological terminology.

Third, is our lack of understanding of the nature of many of the clinical syndromes. There is little correlation between the bacteriological, virological and pathological findings and the clinical features. In fact, even when intensive efforts have been made in family practice[1,2] or in hospital[2,3] to establish the aetiology of the conditions it has been found possible in only about 20 per cent of cases.

Fourth, because of our lack of proper understanding of these conditions it is impossible to develop sound rational treatments for them. Two examples illustrate this point:

1. Although it has been shown that only a few of these common infections are caused by organisms that are sensitive to antibiotics, nevertheless it has become customary that the majority of these common infections are treated with antibiotics.

2. The other example is the traditional custom of treating recurrent attacks of respiratory illness in children by removing their tonsils and adenoids. (This is discussed in chapter 10).

CLASSIFICATION

Even with these problems and difficulties some attempt at classification is necessary if these common acute respiratory infections are to be described and considered. A reasonable division is as follows. It is a modification of that proposed by the Medical Research Council[2].

1. Colds, coughs and catarrh (CCC)
2. Influenza
3. Acute throat infections
4. Laryngitis and croup
5. Acute chest infections
6. Acute otitis media

Having listed these conditions as apparent separate entities it must be said that their clear distinction is often more apparent than real and that these acute conditions often are linked and associated with chronic conditions such as the catarrhal child syndrome and chronic bronchitis. Each of them will now be considered in detail with the exception of otitis media which is fully discussed in chapter 10.

COLDS, COUGHS AND CATARRH (CCC)

Nature

The main symptoms are *rhinitis* causing nasal discharge and blockage; a *cough* that is dry at first and later becomes productive but without any physical signs in the chest; variable degrees of *malaise* and *fever*.

Aetiology

It is generally assumed that the CCC syndrome is caused by viruses but intensive studies using modern virological techniques can at best detect unknown viruses in about 20—25 per cent. Higher isolation rates are obtained in young children than in adults[4].

The most likely viruses to be isolated in this syndrome are rhinoviruses, para-influenzae viruses and adenoviruses. In hospital practice, but not in family practice, the respiratory syncytial viruses are often isolated in infants with common upper respiratory infections.

No bacteria have any special primary aetiological role but the beta haemolytic streptococci, the pneumococci and *Haemophilus influenzae* may at times cause secondary infections.

The *pathology* is that of a diffuse non-specific inflammatory reaction to virus infection. The discharges from the nasal and bronchial mucosae will be mucoid initially becoming muco-purulent later. This purulent appearance of the nasal discharge or sputum does not necessarily indicate a secondary bacterial infection, since in most of those investigated with muco-purulent sputum no specific bacteria or viruses will be isolated.

Assessment

It is important to appreciate the unitary nature of the respiratory tract and to anticipate spread of infection from the nose to the sinuses, ears and lower respiratory tract in certain vulnerable individuals. More than usual concern should be paid to those with underlying chronic respiratory conditions, such as chronic bronchitics or those with congested lungs associated with cardiac failure, and children who seem never to be free from coughs or colds.

Differentiation from vasomotor rhinitis and other allergic nasal syndromes should be considered (see p. 141–147) in those with recurrent and persistent symptoms.

Management

These are self-limiting benign conditions and as such should be managed with simple, safe and pleasant measures. There are no specific antibiotics known to shorten and improve the course of these conditions. Since prophylactic antibiotics are of doubtful and unproved value even in vulnerables, it may be best to wait and see rather than use them blindly or haphazardly.

Future Needs

Little is known of the nature and epidemiology of this syndrome and it is in family practice that more studies are required. In particular studies are needed on families and individuals who appear to be particularly vulnerable to CCC.

INFLUENZA

Aetiology

There is a world of difference between sporadic cases of 'flu' – used as a convenient label for any acute febrile illness that cannot be placed in any other clinical category – and 'epidemic influenza' caused by the specific myxoviruses of influenza. When used at all 'influenza' should be restricted to the latter type of epidemic cases.

Attacks of epidemic influenza tend to occur every 2–3 years in a practice and every 30 years or so a major pandemic with a new virulent mutant strain of influenza A explodes and causes much world wide chaos and havoc. The last major pandemic was in 1957—8, with the Asian Flu epidemic caused by influenza A 2 (Hong Kong) variety of virus. In Britain alone it is estimated to have caused 10 million known cases (out of a population of 50 million) with 5000 deaths and a national cost of £100 million.

The cause of influenza is infection with one of the influenza viruses which are a sub-group of the myxoviruses. There are three main serotypes, A, B and C. Serotype A is the one responsible for most major epidemics, serotype B causes moderate local epidemics or sporadic cases and serotype C rarely produces more than occasional sporadic cases.

Over the years with repeated epidemics a considerable herd immunity is developed and relatively few persons succumb in any epidemic. However, influenza A virus has the ability to develop new mutant strains and when such a virulent strain arrives it spreads on a world wide basis with a huge prevalence and a more than usual proportion of complications and deaths.

Pathology

The chief pathological effects of infection with influenza virus are an acute inflammation of the upper respiratory tract with possible spread to the lungs and bronchi.

The earliest changes are acute inflammation of the mucosa caused by the virus but secondary infection with bacteria may occur leading to sinusitis, otitis media or pneumonia. It is possible that influenza may cause an encephalitis, but infection of other organs and structures by influenza viruses is extremely unlikely.

Prevalence and Extent of Infuenza Epidemics

Over 25 years in my practice there have been 11 epidemics of influenza[5]. The age-prevalence rates of those infected in any epidemic differed somewhat depending on the immune state of the population. The highest prevalence rates were found in children and young adults. Prevalence rates in the elderly were low. This low frequency in the elderly was probably because they mixed less socially and were less exposed to cross-infection. It is possible that old persons as a group have higher levels of immunity because of their longer experience with more epidemics.

Clinical Features

The clinical spectrum of influenza is wide. At one end of the spectrum are the mild and sub-clinical cases with few symptoms. These are known to occur because of rising antibody titres in such persons during surveys that have been carried out. At the other extreme is the rare but occasional fulminating case of such severity that death may occur within a couple of days.

The most usual clinical presentation is of an abruptly sudden onset with malaise, fever, cough, raw throat and coryza. Aching of the eyes, head, back and limbs is characteristic. There may be vomiting and diarrhoea but 'gastric flu' is a description of a type of epidemic influenza. Profuse sweating is common, a picture of intense misery and malaise is present for 2—3 days, followed by a slow improvement.

Complications

Influenza is a condition with a low case fatality rate. In my practice it has been 2 per 1000. Over a period of 25 years this represents 8 persons, of whom 6 were over the age of 70.

Chest complications (bronchitis and pneumonia) occurred in 13 per cent of all those seen with influenza during 1950—1975 and the age distribution of these complications indicated an increasing liability with increasing age.

Complicating pneumonia or bronchitis in influenza are generally non-dramatic happenings. The usual story is that, instead of the victim beginning to feel better and improving after a few days, the cough becomes worse and more productive and the feeling of malaise continues. On examination there are localised areas of rales, or more diffuse rhonchi, in the chest. Chest radiography will confirm patchy consolidation in the lung fields.

The more rare and more severe type of complicating chest infection is of a rapidly deteriorating condition with breathlessness, collapse and shock, with generalised moist sounds in the chest and with early evidence of cardiac failure. These serious complications tend to occur in elderly persons with some established chronic cardiac or respiratory conditions.

Acute otitis media, sinusitis and *laryngitis* are occasional complications, the former occurring mainly in children and the latter two mainly in adults.

Encephalitis and other neurological complications can occur but have not been seen in my practice during the 25 year period. However, as with other virus diseases, such as hepatitis, influenza can precipitate a depressive condition which may persist long after the precipitating fever has gone. Occasionally the depression may be severe enough to require physical treatment, especially when it occurs in persons prone to depression; for example, following bereavement. (This is discussed in greater detail in chapter 22).

Diagnosis and Investigations

The diagnosis of influenza is probably only accurate during a known epidemic that has been confirmed by a regional or national influenza centre.

Virological tests for influenza are not practical in everyday normal practice. The results take too long to arrive in order to influence the management of the patient. Culture of influenza viruses is not easy or reliable and tests for rising levels of influenzal antibodies in the patient's serum will take at least two weeks because of the time interval required between the two blood tests.

The only investigation that may be required is a chest radiograph in those patients with influenza in whom cough and malaise persist and in whom a low grade pneumonia is a possibility.

Management

The Uncomplicated Case

Since most cases of influenza are uncomplicated and benign and do not require any specific remedies, relief can be obtained by hot drinks, linctuses and analgesics.

If the case is not improving after 3—4 days then a physician's opinion and assessment are necessary.

The Complicated Case

Chest complications such as pneumonia or bronchitis should be treated with antibiotics such as the tetracyclines, ampicillin, or intramuscular penicillin. Some of the elderly with known cardiac disease may also develop cardiac failure and require oxygen, diuretics and digoxin.

There is a case for giving patients with known chronic heart or chest disorders prophylactic antibiotics as soon as they start influenza or if there is a case in their place of residence.

Influenza Vaccines

There are a number of commercial vaccines against influenza. They are advertised as being of considerable value in the prevention of influenza. Their practical value is much more limited. They may not contain sufficient antigenic material in the correct form to create sufficient artificial immunity against a forthcoming epidemic. The protection is relatively short-lived being for a few months only. Since the vaccines are prepared from chicken eggs they may cause reactions in persons sensitive to egg protein.

Nevertheless there may be a place for giving influenza vaccines to members of the practice team and to some other key members of the community.

The case of giving severe chronic bronchitics and others with serious cardiac disorders preventive vaccines is less strong. Most of these persons will be restricted and house bound and will not mix enough to run risks of acquiring influenza. There may be a case for vaccinating anyone with a history of severe depression being precipitated by an attack in influenza.

Effects of an Influenza Epidemic on a Practice

The effects of an influenza epidemic on an area or on a practice are dramatic and disrupting. Not only are large numbers of persons disabled and unable to work but some of these will be physicians, nurses and other medical staff, causing extra strains on those who remain at their posts.

There is usually some warning that an influenza epidemic is coming from reports in the news media. There is a slow beginning with a few typical but sporadic cases. By the end of the second or third week from the onset of the epidemic the work load of the practice in terms of telephone and office consultations and home and hospital visits will have trebled or quadrupled. Whole families and other closed communities go down with the infection within a short period.

Once begun the epidemic tends to affect school children at an early stage and then spread to their families. The peak of the epidemic is reached within a month and then a slow decline begins. A typical epidemic in a practice lasts for 2−3 months.

Practice Preparations for an Influenza Epidemic

Steps can be taken to ease the coming work load before an influenza epidemic arrives. There is usually a warning period during which preparations can be made.

A practice policy of managing normal cases of influenza should be agreed on and all members of the practice team informed so that they can advise those who phone in for help. Arrangements should be made to prescribe or provide simple medications to relieve symptoms. Arrangements should be made with the local social security departments to provide certification for unfitness for work without necessarily seeing the patients at once. Plans should be made for visiting those at home, these visits can be made by nurses rather than by doctors. Plans should be made with local social and welfare services to provide extra help for those families who are stricken down.

Since there will be extra patients with cardio-respiratory complications admitted to local hospitals, plans for managing these and for some agreed collaborative policies between hospital specialists and family practitioners should be laid before the epidemic arrives.

Whatever policies are agreed there should be some attempt at establishing good communications with the public and providing information on how cases can be self-managed.

ACUTE THROAT INFECTIONS

Nature of the Condition

The clinical syndrome of sore throat, malaise, fever and redness and swelling of the tonsils and oro-pharynx is a common one. This clinical condition has a number and a mixture of causes. It should be stated at once that it is generally not possible clinically to arrive at an accurate aetiological diagnosis merely by looking at the throat and listening to the history. Even with full supporting investigations, pathogenic organisms will be detected in only about one-half of the cases.

Sore throat may be part of a more general upper respiratory infection as in influenza (pp. 27–30) or the CCC syndrome (page 26) and it may be a prominent feature of uncommon disorders such as glandular fever (infectious mononucleosis) or very rare conditions such as agranulocytosis or leukaemia.

The acute sore throats under discussion here are those where the local symptoms of throat soreness are unassociated with other respiratory symptoms and where there is no evidence of any associated serious general disease.

They may be labelled as *acute tonsillitis* (when the condition appears confined to swelling, redness and exudate or ulceration of the tonsils with tender swelling of the upper cervical lymph glands) or *pharyngitis* (when the inflammatory reaction is more generalised and affects the posterior oropharynx and the soft palate as well as the tonsils). It is not clear whether these different clinical appearances signify different conditions with different causes.

Aetiology

The causes of acute throat infections are many. When a consecutive series of such cases is swabbed and the swabs examined for bacteria and viruses, the usual experience is that pathogenic bacterial organisms are found in up to 40 per cent of specimens, viruses may be grown in up to 20 per cent and in 40 per cent no pathogenic organisms and no underlying disease, such as glandular fever, is found.

These findings may mean that our methods of investigations are faulty, that is of taking and transporting the specimens and of isolating and culturing the possible organisms. This certainly may apply to the detection of viruses because our techniques and methods are relatively new, but this cannot be the explanation for the low isolation rate of bacteria.

It may be that merely swabbing the surface of an inflamed throat with a sterile swab cannot be an adequate method of collecting evidence of the cause of the infection and we may need to develop better methods of collecting material to provide proof of the causes. It may be that the causal agents are still undetectable by our presently available methods or it may be that there are other pathological mechanisms at work that we have not elucidated.

Whatever the explanations, the facts are that we are able to establish the causes of acute throat infection in only about one-half of those who are intensively investigated and we must be honest enough to accept this when we consider the treatment.

Of the organisms detected and the other underlying causes (Table 4.1) it is evident the beta haemolytic streptococci are the largest single detectable cause.

It is not proven whether bacteria such as *Haemophilus influenzae* or pneumococci are pathogenic as causes of sore throats and they are not therefore usually put forward as pathogens. Other organisms that cause sore throats on occasions are organisms of Vincent's angina and *Candida albicans*.

The viruses most often detected in acute sore throats are adenoviruses, rhinoviruses and enteroviruses, but these do not add up to more than 20 per cent of all cases (Table 4.1).

Epidemiology

The age-prevalence of acute throat infections shows two peaks, one in early childhood (3—8 years) and the other in the late teens and early twenties. It is likely that these peaks represent distinct clinical disorders. In early childhood the rise in prevalence is part of the catarrhal child syndrome, when all respiratory infections are frequent. The second peak, in the teens and early twenties, is smaller. This is the time when glandular fever (see page 156) occurs but there is also an increase in the other more common types of acute sore throat. The explanations are most likely to be some characteristic immunological responses specifically related to the age of those affected. Acute sore throats are rare in infants and in the elderly.

The frequency of occurence of acute sore throats depends on how widely the definition is interpreted. In a developed society, a family practitioner, with

Table 4.1   Acute sore throat — known causes.

Cause	Per cent
Beta haemolytic streptococci	35
Other organisms such as Vincent's angina and Candida albicans	3
Adenoviruses, rhinoviruses and enteroviruses	20
General disorders such as glandular fever	2
No detectable cause	40

a practice of about 2500 persons, may expect to see and treat 100—150 new cases each year. Recurrent attacks may occur in some individuals, particularly at the two peak periods of prevalence.

Seasonal variations in prevalence are less notable with acute sore throats than with other common respiratory infections. There is a fairly constant prevalence rate throughout the year but small epidemic peaks may occur at any time, particularly in hot dry weather.

Clinical Features

The clinical features in acute throat infections may be:

1. pain and soreness of the throat;
2. general malaise and fever;
3. redness and swelling of the fauces;
4. enlargement of cervical glands;
5. rash;
6. complications of the disease or the treatment.

Pain and Soreness of the Throat

These are first symptoms. They may range from a tightness and soreness of the throat on swallowing, particularly towards the end of the day, to pain and discomfort of such severity that not even spittle can be swallowed and the patient presents a pathetic and disturbing picture of lying in bed severely ill with discharge drooling from the mouth. Symptoms of such severe degree usually occur only in adults and denote either a complication such as quinsy (peritonsillar abscess) or some systemic disorder such as severe glandular fever, agranulocytosis, leukaemia or even a malignant neoplasm of the throat. In the past, a really ill child with a sore throat suggested the likelihood of diphtheria.

It must be appreciated that whilst acute throat infections are unusual in infancy, young children cannot localise the discomfort and complain of 'a sore throat'. In them the presentation is one of a sudden febrile illness often with abdominal pains, vomiting and dehydration.

General Malaise and Fever

The extent of general systemic disturbance will vary with the severity of infection, its nature and the individual affected. Many will be little affected and the condition will be no more than a nuisance. Generally there is less systemic disturbance with viral infections and where no specific causes are found than in infections with beta haemolytic streptococci. Although diphtheria is now a great rarity it must still be remembered as a possibility when there is more toxaemia than expected.

Some cases of glandular fever may be associated with considerable illness but many of the young adults who are found to be suffering from glandular fever appear little affected.

Redness and Swelling of the Fauces
The local appearances in acute throat infections comprise redness, swelling and possibly exudate and ulceration.

There may be a diffuse redness and swelling of the posterior pharyngeal wall, the faucial pillars and the soft palate with some punctate erythema or larger patches of submucosal purpura on the soft palate. This is the picture of *pharyngitis*.

In *acute tonsillitis* there is more localised swelling and redness of the tonsils. There may be an exudate covering the tonsils and this may be greyish and diffuse or whitish-yellow within the tonsillar crypts giving the appearance of ulceration. There may be actual areas of ulceration with a dirty grey-brown slough in cases of Vincent's angina which is usually associated with an ulcerative gingivitis. In *Candida albicans* infections there are white creamy patches of exudate that can be removed readily from the surface of the tonsils. In diphtheria (see page 562) the appearance may range from swollen oedematous fauces to a diffuse area of inflammation and swelling with confluent adherent and tough exudate. In quinsy (peritonsillar abscess) there is considerable localised red swelling of the soft palate above and laterally to the affected tonsil with marked tenderness and associated trismus.

In the ordinary and common types of acute tonsillitis both tonsils are affected although the extent of the inflammatory changes may vary. When only one tonsil is affected with swelling, redness and pain suspicion should be roused of early quinsy, or infection by Vincent's angina organisms, or even the rare possibility of a tonsillar neoplasm.

These clinical descriptions are appropriate and necessary but accurate diagnosis of the causal type of infection from the appearances of the throat is not possible with any accuracy. Ross[6], in a study of sore throats in family practice in Edinburgh, found that practitioners were accurate on only one-half occasions when they attempted to decide from appearances of the throat on the probable organisms causing the infection.

Enlargement of Cervical Lymph Glands
The upper cervical lymph glands are often enlarged and tender during acute throat infections. However, cervical glands are normally palpable in young children between 3 and 8 years. Swelling and tenderness the neck glands are likely to be more marked in beta haemolytic streptococcal infections than viral infections. In glandular fever there is more widespread swelling of other lymph glands in the posterior triangle of the neck, the axillae and groins. Persistence of

swelling of the cervical glands after the clearing of the throat infection is of little significance, but these cases should be followed up to exclude the possibility of their being early reticuloses such as lymphadenoma or even the now rare cervical gland tuberculosis.

Rash

A rash may be associated with an acute throat infection. A diffuse erythematous rash over most of the body may be a part of a streptococcal infection. This is 'Scarlet fever' but there is not need now to treat these cases any differently from other cases of streptococcal infections. They carry no greater risks or hazards. Macular or papular pink rashes may occur as part of a viral syndrome, usually one of the entero viruses, and here there often is associated redness of the eyes with conjunctival infection.

Rashes may occur from sensitivities to drugs. If ampicillin is used in cases of glandular fever a diffuse deep red macular rash will appear on the trunk and limbs in 4 cases out of 5. There may be similar skin sensitivities to other antibiotics and to analgesics such as aspirin.

Complications

The likely course of an acute throat infection is for improvement to begin after 2—3 days and for complete resolution within a week. Complications are unusual and infrequent.

Quinsy occurs as a complication in less than 1 per cent of cases. It is more likely in adults. The history is of a sore throat that, instead of improving after the expected few days, continues with increasing pain on one side and difficulty in swallowing. Inspection of the throat may be difficult because of trismus, but when visible there is oedema and redness above and outside the tonsil with considerable cervical gland enlargement.

In a few cases *cervical adenitis* may proceed to cellulitis and abscess formation. This is rare and when it occurs the pus must always be examined for tubercle bacilli.

Remote complications, probably from abnormal antigen—antibody reactions, include erythema nodosum, acute nephritis and rheumatic fever. These conditions occur 1 or 2 weeks after the original throat infection and these occurrences are unrelated to the severity of infection. They occur probably only in association with streptococcal infections. There is no proof that they can be prevented by treatment of all sore throats with antibiotics.

Erythema nodosum is annoying and uncomfortable but benign. Red, bumpy swellings appear on the front of the lower legs. They persist for a few weeks and then disappear. Erythema nodosum may occur also from other causes such as sensitivity to drugs, in sarcoidosis and in primary tuberculosis.

Acute nephritis is rare. In my practice I have seen 5 cases over 25 years and only 2 of these were associated with a preceding acute throat infection. This is a rate of less than 1 per 1000 cases of acute throat infections. It used to be customary to test the urine for albumen for all persons who had suffered from acute throat infections to pick up early or missed cases of renal damage but since the condition is so rare this seems an unnecessary routine.

Rheumatic fever is potentially one of the most dangerous results of a streptococcal infection, leading to endocarditis and valvitis and scarring and damage of the heart valves. It is a possibility when flitting limb pains are reported. It was and still is very much a socially orientated disease being more frequent in lower social areas. I have seen no cases in 25 years of practice in spite of very selective use of antibiotics.

There is certainly no reason to assume that the rarity of rheumatic fever has been because of the general use of antibiotics. It is more likely to be due to changes in the pathogenicity of the haemolytic streptococcus. There are still many cases of streptococcal sore throats untreated by antibiotics and many of those who are treated take the drugs for just a few days until symptoms clear and certainly not for the full recommended prophylactic duration of 10 days. A reversal of this trend of reduced pathogenicity may occur at sometime in the future with the associated hazards to joints, kidneys and heart valves.

Investigations

Although the policy of perfection may be to swab all sore throats *before* specific treatment is given and to wait for the results to decide on the appropriate antibiotic, in practice this is quite an unreal and impossible procedure.

Examination of *throat swabs* for pathogenic bacteria or viruses may be useful and necessary when the appearance of the throat is unusual and the possibility of some condition such as diphtheria is being considered. Throat swabs may be useful also during epidemics of sore throats in closed communities such as boarding schools, to plot the course of the infections and to assess the success of the preventive measures being taken.

Examination of the *blood* is necessary if the condition is slow in clearing and when glandular fever or some other possible blood disorder such as agranulocytosis or leukaemia are being considered. The essential tests are examination of the white blood cells and the monospot or Paul-Bunnell test (for glandular fever). When rheumatic fever and nephritis are suspected, measurements of the anti-streptolysin titre beginning two weeks after the onset of the infection may reveal high and rising titres.

Examination of the *urine* for albumen should be carried out whenever nephritic complications are a possibility (see page 327).

Assessment

When presented with a patient with an acute sore throat assessment should consider the following:

1. What is the likely nature and type of the condition? Is it of the usual pattern or are there some special unusual features that require special investigation and management?
2. How severely ill is the patient? Can the condition be left to run its own natural course? Should special treatment be given? Should the patient be hospitalised?
3. Are specific antibiotics required and, if so, which?
4. What, if any, investigations are indicated?
5. Are any measures required to prevent spread of infection within the family, or household or community?
6. What special arrangements for follow-up are needed and what steps need to be taken to prevent or control further attacks?

Management

Acute throat infections are common conditions of children and young adults. For various reasons, such as improved social conditions and lower virulence of the pathogens, they are now much more benign than in the past. Their natural course is for a self-limiting condition lasting up to a week with few complications. Even with intensive investigations the probable causal organisms can be detected in only about one-half of the cases.

These facts need reiteration as we come to consider the management.

General Measures

Relief of symptoms can be achieved by simple analgesics, such as soluble aspirin or paracetamol, given every 2 or 3 hours. Gargles, lozenges and hot drinks have their supporters and can all be recommended since they are safe and give the patient something to do.

Antibiotics

It is difficult to arrive easily at any policy on the use of antibiotics for acute throat infections that is rational, logical and acceptable. The facts are that these are benign and self-limiting conditions and that only a minority have been shown to be caused by antibiotic-sensitive organisms. Nevertheless we do have available potent and safe specific antibiotics that have achieved an omnipotent status on the assumption that they can control these infections, shorten the period of disability and prevent complications. It must be acknowledged that there are no objective facts based on reliable trials to support these beliefs.

The policy for the use of antibiotics in acute throat infections has to be developed by each practitioner. My own approach is to assess each situation individually using the following guide lines as indications for use of antibiotics:

1. If the patient with an acute throat infection is not seriously distressed or disturbed then I would treat with simple analgesics for a few days. If there is no improvement or if there is deterioration after 2 days then I would prescribe antibiotics.
2. If the patient with an acute throat infection appears severely ill when first seen, with high fever and general illness and toxaemia and considerable discomfort, then I would use antibiotics at once.
3. If there is a history of previous recurrent sore throats, or of some other serious illness or chronic ill health, then these are other factors that would suggest early use of antibiotics.
4. Social factors and the ability of the mother or other persons to cope with the illness, may also influence early use of antibiotics. Thus if the child or young adult is from a socially deprived family and/or if the mother is known from expereince to be a 'non-coper' then antibiotics may be indicated early.

In my own practice I find that with such a selective and discriminating approach I use antibiotics in no more than one third of acute throat infections.

The antibiotic of choice for acute throat infections is still penicillin. It should be administered by intramuscular injection in those who are severely ill either as a single magna-dose of a combined short and long acting penicillin, or as crystalline penicillin G (1 mega unit) twice daily for 2—3 days followed by oral penicillin V. In those less severely ill, oral penicillin V should be used for at least 5—7 days (In adults 250 mg 6 hourly and in children between 3 and 10 125 mg 6 hourly). Where the infection is caused by a penicillin sensitive organism there should be a good and evident response within 2—3 days. In those who have a history of sensitivity to penicillin then erythromycin is a reliable alternative.

In Vincent's angina, the infection will respond to penicillin or to metronidazole. Infections with Candida albicans will clear with local applications of nystatin.

Throat infections in glandular fever are not responsive to antibiotics and if ampicillin is used there is a great likelihood of skin rashes developing. (The management of glandular fever is discussed in Chapter 10, page 156).

Quinsy should be treated with penicillin by intramuscular injection. In most cases the peritonsillitis should resolve quickly without any need to drain any peritonsillar abscess.

Tonsillectomy
The merits and de-merits of tonsillectomy, with or without adenoidectomy, are still being hotly debated. Removal of chronically infected tonsils liable to

recurrent infection is a sound approach. However, the problem is how to decide when tonsils are chronically diseased. Appearances are no guide, nor is the presence of enlarged and palpable cervical glands. The decision is best made individually relying on the frequency and severity of recurrent attacks.

The results of tonsillectomy for recurrent attacks of tonsillitis are usually good but there are some persons who continue to suffer from sore throats even after removal of the tonsils and adenoids.

Tonsillectomy and adenoidectomy are further discussed in Chapter 10, page 154.

Follow-up

No special follow-up care is indicated for most of those who suffer a throat infection. There is a small group of children and young adults who pass through a period when they appear liable to suffer frequent recurrent attacks. The choice in these is between tonsillectomy or early administration of penicillin during an attack.

LARYNGITIS AND CROUP

Nature of the Conditions

Acute infection of the larynx presents as two common syndromes, that of *croup* in children and *acute laryngitis* in adults.

Pathologically the two conditions are similar in that they produce an acute inflammation of the larynx with redness and swelling and this results in the clinical features of cough, hoarseness and breathing difficulties. All these features are more striking and dramatic in children because of the small size of their larynges and a small amount of swelling can cause appreciable laryngeal obstruction.

The *causes* of acute laryngitis are usually viral. In the Medical Research Council Survey[2], positive virus isolations in acute laryngitis were obtained in 10—15 per cent of adults and in 30—40 per cent of children. The most frequent viruses isolated were the parainfluenzae group in children and the rhinoviruses in adults.

The *age-prevalence* rates show that at no age does the annual rate exceed 5 per cent of those at risk and that the highest rates are in children in their first 3 years of life.

The *course* of these acute infections is for a short, sharp acute illness of a few days followed by a slower period of recovery over another week or two.

The chief complication is acute laryngeal obstruction in young children. Although it rarely is dangerous, the risk of suffocation makes management of children at home with croup a worrying affair.

Clinical Features

Acute Laryngitis in Adults

This condition is characterised by sudden onset with a raw throat, hoarseness and a dry cough. Dyspnoea is not a feature and fever and general malaise are not prominent. There may be a generalised redness of the fauces. The larynx, if visualised, shows swelling and redness of the vocal cords and adjacent structures. After a few days the condition begins to resolve and the hoarseness should have disappeared completely within 2 weeks. If it has not then it is essential that an expert view of the larynx should be obtained to exclude other possible causes of persistent hoarseness, such as neoplasms.

Croup or Acute Laryngo-Tracheo-Bronchitis in Children

This is common and in certain children it is a recurring condition from infancy until they appear to outgrow the tendency to suffer attacks at 3–4 years of age. It is also a condition that tends to run in families and boys are more often affected than girls. The onset may follow a common upper respiratory infection but often there is no obvious precipitating factor, and the precise cause is not known. Some specific allergy or local laryngeal anomaly or both may be responsible for the condition.

The classical presentation is for the child to awake in the early hours of the night, often between midnight and 2 am, frightened and distressed by a croaky barking and seal-like cough that is made worse as the child cries. There is a variable degree of difficulty with breathing. Most children affected are not breathless when they are quiet and not crying. However, in some there is considerable distress with stridor and recession of the chest on inspiration. With serious laryngeal obstruction there is general restlessness and there may be frank cyanosis or a grey pallor. No abnormalities are generally notable on examination of the throat and the chest is usually clear of adventitious sounds.

A rare and dangerous condition, *acute epiglottitis* caused by *Haemophilus influenzae* presents similarly but on examination of the throat the swollen and red epiglottis may be seen as a red cherry like swelling behind the tongue.

The *course* of croup in most children is for the distress to subside once the child has settled and is asleep and for the symptoms to improve as daybreak approaches. The croaky cough will continue for a week or so.

The possibility of a diphtheric membrane being responsible for stridor must always be borne in mind even though it's incidence is rare. Malformation of the vocal cords and an aortic ring (an arterial ring pressing on the trachea) are other rare causes of croup. Foreign bodies in the larynx or trachea must always be considered in a child with persistent stridor and this problem is considered in more detail in chapter 10, page 161.

Diagnosis and Investigation

The diagnosis of *acute laryngitis* in adults presents few difficulties. It is important to re-examine the diagnosis when hoarseness persists or when the attacks are recurrent. This is further discussed in chapter 10, page 156. Chronic laryngeal irritation through excessive smoking or talking may be a cause, but laryngeal neoplasms may cause similar symptoms. Angioneurotic oedema as part of generalised hypersensitivity may cause sudden laryngeal obstruction but with no cough or hoarseness.

Croup also presents few diagnostic difficulties. The chief problem in these children is the decision as to whether they should be admitted to hospital in case the laryngeal obstruction becomes more serious. The possibility of an inhaled foreign body should be remembered in the atypical case.

Apart from referral of adults with persistent hoarseness for a laryngeal examination by a specialist there are no special investigations that are helpful in these cases.

Management

Acute Laryngitis in Adults

This is a benign condition requiring relief but little else. Hot drinks, steam inhalations, lozenges and linctuses will help to relieve the discomfort. Antibiotics are not indicated since there is no evidence that the condition is caused by organisms sensitive to antibiotics.

Croup in children

This is a mild condition in 9 cases out of 10, but the occasional case can cause great anxiety. The danger is of laryngeal obstruction, suffocation and death. The management of laryngeal obstruction is discussed in Chapter 10, page 161. It would be quite wrong to advocate admission to hospital of all children with croup. This would be a waste of resources and also create unnecessary anxiety for the parents and the child.

How then are we to decide which cases of croup can be managed at home? It is necessary that the parents are prepared to care for the child at home and that the home conditions are good. The danger signs which suggest that the child should be admitted to hospital are:

1. development of cyanosis or grey-pallor with drowsiness or increasing restlessness;
2. signs of exhaustion;
3. toxaemia which suggests the possibility of acute epiglottitis;
4. increasing anxiety in the parents or unwillingness of the physician to provide the necessary care at home

At home the most useful forms of therapy are reassurance and support for the parents by the physician. Hot drinks relieve the child's discomfort and maintain hydration. Sedatives are useful where the child is anxious and distressed, but they must not be too strong to cause drowsiness and confusion, chloral and promethazine are suitable. There is no proof that steam inhalations help or that antibiotics are helpful unless there is the possibility of secondary bacterial infection. Most cases will begin to improve quite quickly spontaneously.

Management in hospital will consist of administration of oxygen and close observation to decide if and when intubation or tracheostomy are necessary.

ACUTE CHEST INFECTIONS

The newcomer to family practice soon discovers that the gulf between the neatly organised and well defined and labelled conditions of hospital practice and the vague and indeterminate disorders of family practice is greatest when he comes to try and diagnose, define and label the acute chest infections. In many ways he has to unlearn what he learnt in his hospital training and develop a new and more practical approach in family practice.

There are more than 100 synonyms attempting to describe the various acute infections of the lungs and bronchi, and this shows the lack of correlation between our understanding of their pathology and our attempts at diagnosis and management.

Acute chest infections are important in family practice, since they are by far the largest group of major life-threatening diseases that the family physician encounters and because, even in these days of availability of antibiotics, they have a case mortality rate of around 5 per cent.

Nature of the Condition

The acute chest infections are a definable syndrome with a sudden onset and symptoms of an infection of the chest, that is, cough, purulent sputum, fever and general malaise. There may be chest pain and breathlessness depending on the site, nature and extent of the infection. There usually are abnormal physical signs in the chest, which can be separated into a number of clinical groups (see below). The chest radiograph may confirm the physical findings. It may reveal fresh and unexpected evidence of lung involvement or it may appear normal and not correlating with abnormal physical signs.

The patho-physiological effects of a chest infection result in some degree of respiratory failure that depends on the basic functional state of the lungs in the patient affected and on the degree and extent of the infection. An extensive infection superimposed on an already damaged and vulnerable respiratory tract will lead to the triad of carbon dioxide retention, anoxaemia and acidaemia. Obstruction of the pulmonary circulation by the inflammatory process may lead to back pressure strain on the heart resulting in right sided heart failure (*cor pulmonale*).

Aetiology

It is presumed that acute chest infections are caused by bacterial or viral organisms but even with intensive investigations a definite aetiological cause can be identified in only about one-third of the cases seen in family practice[1] and in hospitals[3]. A classification based on a precisely defined aetiology is not possible in practice, although there are some clinical features that are characteristic of some special types of chest infections.

The bacteria most likely to be found are pneumococci and *Haemophilus influenzae*. Less common are staphylococci, streptococci, *Klebsiella pneumoniae* (Friedlander's Bacillus) and tubercle bacilli. The viruses found in acute chest infections are the influenza viruses, the para-influenza viruses and the respiratory syncytial viruses. Less common are the ornithosis-psittacosis group and the organisms causing Q-fever (*Rickettsia burnetti*) and *Mycloplasma pneumoniae*.

There is another important causal factor to remember in acute chest infections and that is that infection may be secondary to some local or general cause. Chest infections may be secondary to some bronchial obstruction caused by a neoplasm or foreign body or a stenosis following trauma or old tuberculosis.

Acute chest infections often complicate chronic bronchitis (see page 66), are frequent in the catarrhal child syndrome, and are a feature of the rare condition of fibro-cystic disease in children. They are also more frequent in persons prone to asthma or sinusitis.

Excessive tobacco smoking will predispose to chest infections as will poor social conditions such as inferior housing, inadequate nutrition or bad working conditions.

Clinical Features

A practical clinical classification of acute chest infection is essential and the following, which is a mixture of presenting physical signs and a pathological terminology, has been found useful in practice:

1. acute bronchitis
2. acute bronchiolitis
3. pneumonia

4. pleurisy
5. other types of acute chest infection
6. Specific types caused by specific organisms

Acute Bronchitis

Acute bronchitis or 'acute wheezy chest' is the condition where, in addition to the common symptoms of cough, infected sputum, fever, malaise and breathlessness, there are present, diffuse and bilateral wheezes (rhonchi) which may be interspersed with occasional moist sounds (rales). There are no radiographic abnormalities in these cases.

The degree of breathlessness will depend on the amount of bronchial obstruction and on the previous state of the patient's pulmonary function.

This is the most frequent type of acute chest infection and accounts for about 50 per cent of all such cases. It can occur at all ages but is most frequent in the first decade and in the over sixties.

Bronchiolitis

Bronchiolitis is the label given to an acute illness, usually in infants or young children. The acute illness generally follows a minor upper respiratory infection with onset of fever, breathlessness, harsh dry cough and diffuse and generalised rales on both sides of the chest. In infants pulmonary distension and costal recession may occur from the obstruction of the bronchioles. It is a potentially dangerous condition in infants.

Some chronic bronchitics may also develop a similar condition with an acute onset, breathlessness and cough with cyanosis. Diffuse rales are heard at both bases. This is probably a mixture of acute chest infection and cardiac failure.

Pneumonia

'Pneumonia' is a convenient term for a more localised infection with possible signs of consolidation, either clinically or radiographically.

Two clinical types can be recognised:

1. The most frequent is the patient who during an acute respiratory infection is more unwell than expected or continues to remain unwell with a persistent productive cough; on examination there is an area of some diminished air entry and resonance at one or other lung base, but the most characteristic sign is an area of inspiratory moist sounds in the affected area. The patient is generally not very ill or distressed and the condition resolves in 1–2 weeks. These cases account for over one-third of all acute chest infections.

Chest radiography shows patchy areas of consolidation and collapse in the affected part but there may be no abnormal findings in spite of clinical signs being present. This type of condition occurs most often in children, but it is found also in adults at all ages.

Some would term this 'pneumonitis' but it is difficult to separate it from the better general label of pneumonia.

2. The other type of pneumonia is the more severely ill patient with signs of clinical consolidation in the chest, with dullness, diminished air entry and bronchial breathing. These cases are now rare and account for only 1–2 per cent of all acute chest infections. Chest radiograph will show extensive lobar or lobular consolidation.

Pleurisy
The chief feature of acute pleurisy is sharp pain in the chest on inspiration with a pleural rub heard at the same site. There is variable general upset.

Other Types of Acute Chest Infection
There are cases where the chief signs and features are of *lung collapse* or *pleural effusion*, or even *lung abscess* but these are most unusual in family practice and will be picked up as the result of chest radiography. Empyemas and lung abscesses may occur once or twice in a practitioner's professional life-time.

Specific Types Caused by Specific Organisms
Note should be taken of some acute chest infections caused by specific organisms.

Pneumococci often mixed with *Haemophilus influenzae* will cause the types described but characteristically pneumococci are associated with lobar pneumonia. The clinical features here are sudden onset, severe illness with high fever and rigors. A sharp and painful cough with rusty sputum. Pleuritic chest pain and signs of local consolidation. Labial herpes is common. Confusion and delirium may occur especially in the elderly.

Staphylococci may cause pneumonia in infants and young children as part of a septicaemia and may be complicated by a pyopneumothorax. Staphylococci may also complicate influenza and cause secondary pneumonias.

Friedlander's pneumonia (*Klebsiella pneumoniae*) is a rare infection with extensive consolidation, abscesses and empyema and tends to affect alcoholic 'drop outs' and the destitute.

Pulmonary tuberculosis should still be remembered as a possible cause of a refractory pneumonia particularly in elderly male chronic bronchitics.

Mycoplasma pneumoniae may be responsible for epidemics of pneumonia particularly in closed communities.

Investigations

Most patients with acute chest infections do not need to be intensively investigated. The course of most cases is satisfactory with a recovery expected within 2–3 weeks. It is when the presentation is unusual or the course slow or atypical that further investigations are necessary. The adult whose productive cough continues after the acute episode should be investigated to exclude possible underlying causes such as a bronchial neoplasm or pulmonary tuberculosis. The child with recurring chest infections should be investigated more to reassure the parents than in the expectation of discovering anything abnormal.

Chest Radiography
This is the most useful investigation but in a series from my practice[1] we found abnormalities on chest radiography in only one-half of all acute chest infections investigated.

The value of chest radiography is to confirm and localise the lesions, to assess progress and to exclude any other unexpected pulmonary pathology.

As a rule those patients who are being managed at home can have their radiography postponed until they can attend the local unit. However it is possible in the British National Health Service for a portable chest radiograph to be carried out in the patient's home by a radiologist. This should be done if progress is slow or complicated.

Examination of the Sputum for Causal Organisms
This has limitations. The appearance of a purulent sputum does not necessarily mean that pathogenic organisms will be discovered. In only about one quarter of those tested does sputum examination provide useful information.

Blood Examination
Examinations for white blood cell count, erythrocyte sedimentation rate (ESR), viral antibodies or for other reasons is rarely helpful in diagnosis and management. Routine blood tests in these cases are not necessary.

Respiratory Function Tests
These tests can be done by the family practitioner and are useful in monitoring the functional progress. They are particularly helpful in assessing the progress in patients with chronic respiratory disorders such as asthma and chronic bronchitis. They are discussed in detail in Chapter 5.

Assessment and Diagnosis

Four aspects should be considered in assessing a case of acute chest infection:

1. The diagnosis has to be confirmed. In most instances this is not difficult given of the characteristic signs and symptoms and help from radiography. Conditions that cause difficulties are the patient with

acute left ventricular heart failure where cough, breathlessness and moist sounds in the chest are present. Here the sudden breathlessness is the main feature, there is no history or symptom of a chest infection, but there is usually a history of previous hypertension or coronary artery disease.

2. Underlying conditions such as bronchial neoplasms, tuberculosis or chronic bronchitis should be considered in the appropriate age groups, that is middle aged and elderly men.

3. A decision has to be made on what investigation should be carried out and when, bearing in mind their low rates of positive findings.

4. The presenting condition should be related to the patient's personal, family and social background and to the natural history of the condition. Catarrhal children will pass through a period of recurrent respiratory infections until they 'grow out of them' naturally around 7—8 years of age. Asthmatics and chronic bronchitics are liable to suffer bouts of acute chest infection. Heavy smokers are another vulnerable group and there is no doubt that some families are more liable to suffer from respiratory infections than others.

Management

Hospitalization

Having made a diagnosis of an acute chest infection the first question to be considered is whether the patient should be hospitalised or managed at home. Most acute chest infections are not severe and it should be possible to treat them at home. In my own practice my hospitalization rate for patients with acute chest infections is only 10 per cent.

The decision on whether to treat the patient at home will depend on the severity of the illness, and obviously those who are seriously ill should be admitted to a hospital with facilities for intensive care. It will depend on whether there is someone to nurse the patient at home and on the home conditions.

If the patient lives alone and/or the home conditions are inadequate, then admission to hospital is necessary. It will depend on the wishes of the patient and the family and on whether the physician, himself, is prepared to and capable of managing the patient at home.

Antibiotics

Most acute chest infections will be treated with an antibiotic but it must be pointed out that specific causal organisms that are sensitive to antibiotics will only rarely be found on investigation.

Antibiotics are prescribed on the assumption that most infections are caused by pneumococci and *Haemophilus influenzae.* The choice of antibiotic will be a personal matter for the physician. At present the most popular choices are penicillin, either crystalline penicillin by intramuscular injection, oral penicillin V (for children) or ampicillin, as the current choice for a broad spectrum penicillin (see page 70).

The tetracyclines are less popular than they were in the past but are still being prescribed for the case of acute infection in chronic bronchitics. Co-trimoxazole is usually reserved as a second choice when there has been poor response to a penicillin or a tetracycline. Of course there are many other antibiotics available and used effectively by practitioners.

In some acute chest infections antibiotics may not be necessary. In catarrhal children the acute chest infection will often settle within a few days on simple non-specific measures. Asthmatics and chronic bronchitics will suffer some acute infective episodes that will settle spontaneously. The decision on the use of antibiotics must be made individually in each case.

Other Treatments

Symptomatic measures such as cough medicines are traditional but their worth has never been proved.

Antispasmodics may be helpful when wheezing is prominent and ephedrine, salbutamol, aminophylline or corticosteroids may be used (see page 70).

Oxygen will be of great value in chronic bronchitics or those with associated heart failure.

Diuretics and digoxin may be required in cases of heart failure.

Physiotherapy is useful in assisting expectoration by postural drainage in children and chronic bronchitics.

Follow-up

All patients with acute chest infections should be followed-up until their chests have returned to normal. In an uncomplicated case this takes up to 2 or 3 weeks. If clearance has occurred by this time no further measures are required. Those whose progress is slower require further investigation.

Those with chronic respiratory conditions in whom the acute infection is but an episode will require long-term supervision and support. The parents of catarrhal children must be reassured and encouraged and arrangements made to see the child regularly during the vulnerable period. Adults with chronic bronchitis or asthma and others liable to suffer from chest infections should also be seen regularly in order to provide some health education. Smoking should cease. Occupational hazards such as dusts, poor ventilation and cold should be avoided if possible. Antibiotics may be supplied to be taken early in an attack. Objective assessments should be made by regular tests of respiratory function.

References

1. Batty-Shaw, A. and Fry, J. (1955). *Brit. med. J.* 2, 1577.
2. Medical Research Council (1973). *Postgrad. med. J.* 49, 749.
3. Holland, W. W., Tanner, E. I., Pereira, M. S. and Taylor, C. E. D. (1960). *Brit. med. J.* 1, 1917.
4. Poole, P. M. and Tobin, J. O. H. (1973). *Postgrad. med. J.* 49, 778.
5. Fry, J. (1974). *Common Diseases*, (Lancaster: MTP Press).
6. Ross, P. W. (1971). *Practitioner* 207, 659.

5

Disorders of Pulmonary Function: Assessment and Measurement

I. Gregg

INTRODUCTION

Many diseases of the chest can be regarded as having two components — disorder of structure and disorder of function. Only during the last twenty five years or so has the importance of the latter been fully appreciated. Previously, medical thought had been preoccupied with disorder of structure, because it was this that largely determined the outcome of tuberculosis and pneumonia — then the two most common potentially lethal diseases of the chest.

The introduction of auscultation enabled the clinician not only to distinguish between different types of structural disorder (for instance, bronchiectasis, cavitation and consolidation) but also to make some estimate of their severity in terms of the amount of lung tissue involved. Later, the greater precision afforded by radiography served only to enhance this preoccupation with the pathological varieties and anatomical extent of diseases of the chest.

With the advent of chemotherapy and the decline in mortality from tuberculosis and pneumonia which followed it, chronic chest diseases, notably asthma, chronic obstructive bronchitis and emphysema, began to assume greater prominence. With this came the realisation that in these, and in some other diseases of the chest, disordered function was often of greater importance than structural damage.

Hutchinson as long ago as 1844, made a classical study of vital capacity and its relationship to lung disease, but it was not until the middle of the present century that tests of pulmonary function began to come into general use. The last twenty years have seen the introduction of a large number of tests by which different aspects of pulmonary function can be measured. Although some of these are extremely complex and require the facilities of specially equipped laboratories for their performance, others have now come into routine use in hospitals and chest clinics, while an increasing number of family practitioners have discovered the value of simple tests of pulmonary function in the diagnosis, assessment and management of asthma and chronic obstructive bronchitis.

FUNDAMENTAL ASPECTS OF PULMONARY PHYSIOLOGY

Pulmonary function is less complex than that of, say, the liver or kidneys[1]. The fundamental purpose of respiration is to exchange oxygen and carbon dioxide between the body and the external air. To achieve this, three requirements must be fulfilled: there must be a large surface area of a very thin membrane across which both gases can easily diffuse into and out of the blood; there must be an adequate blood supply to this membrane; the air which is brought into contact with the membrane must be continually replaced.

It follows that there are three basic ways in which respiratory function can be disturbed. These are termed disorders of:

1. *ventilation*, in which there is interference with the conduction of air between the atmosphere and the alveolar-capillary membrane,
2. *diffusion*, in which there is impedance to diffusion across the membrane or inadequacy of its surface area, and
3. *perfusion*, in which there is impairment of the blood supply to and from the membrane.

It must be emphasised, however, that in many diseases of the respiratory system more than one type of disorder may be present.

The respiratory system is so designed that it can meet the body's requirements of oxygen uptake and carbon dioxide elimination over a wide range of activity, from a state of complete rest to extreme physical exertion. Various mechanisms ensure that the partial pressures of oxygen (pO_2) and carbon dioxide (pCO_2) in the arterial blood are kept within a very narrow range.

Considerable disturbance of function must have occurred before the lungs become unable to fulfil their primary function of maintaining the levels of pO_2 and pCO_2 within their normal range. *Respiratory insufficiency* is said to be present if ordinary exercise (such as climbing stairs or walking at a brisk pace) causes a fall of pO_2. If the blood gases cannot be maintained at normal levels even when the patient is at rest he is said to be in *respiratory failure*.

In all cases of respiratory insufficiency and failure there is an abnormally low pO_2 (hypoxaemia): in some cases there is in addition an abnormally high pCO_2 (hypercapnia). The distinction between these two types of respiratory failure carries important implications in their management. If hypoxaemia alone is present oxygen can be given with complete safety, whereas if hypercapnia is also present oxygen must only be given under strict control.

Disorders of Ventilation

Delivery of air to the alveolar-capillary membrane requires, first, the provision of a conducting system whereby atmospheric air is distributed uniformly to the alveoli and, secondly, a 'bellows' mechanism which causes air to flow into and out of the lungs. Therefore, there are two ways in which ventilation can be disturbed: those disorders which interfere with the conduction of air are termed *obstructive* while those which impair the bellows function of the lungs are termed *restrictive*.

Obstructive Disorders of Ventilation
Obstructive disorders of ventilation are the most common of all diseases of the respiratory system. Airways obstruction is the cardinal disorder in chronic obstructive bronchitis, emphysema and asthma. By definition, airways obstruction in asthma is *reversible*, whereas in chronic obstructive bronchitis and in emphysema it is mainly *irreversible*, being caused by structural damage of the airways.

Airways obstruction is easily measured by simple instruments and by their use it is possible to distinguish between reversible and irreversible airways obstruction. Two instruments are suitable for use under the conditions of family practice and they will be described in detail in a later section of this chapter.

Restrictive Disorders of Ventilation
Restrictive disorders of ventilation are found in a wide variety of diseases which involve the chest wall or the lungs themselves. Scoliosis, fibrosis of the pleura and gross obesity all restrict the expansion of the thorax. In sarcoidosis, alveolitis and pneumoconiosis the lungs are abnormally rigid due to inflammatory changes or fibrosis of the alveoli. Interference of the nerve supply to the respiratory muscles, as in poliomyelitis and phrenic nerve palsy, also causes a restrictive disorder.

Disorders of Diffusion

In this type of disorder the alveolar-capillary membrane is less permeable as a result of inflammation or fibrosis (as in sarcoidosis and alveolitis), or the alveoli become filled with exudate or transudate (as in pneumonia and pulmonary oedema), or there is a reduction of the total surface area of the alveolar-capillary membrane (as in emphysema). It has already been noted that those diseases in which there is inflammation or fibrosis of the alveolar–capillary membrane also give rise to a restrictive ventilatory disorder.

Disorders of diffusion are readily detectable and measured by tests which can be performed in any hospital department of pulmonary physiology, but there is no test which is suitable for family practice. However, in many cases the pathological processes which give rise to impairment of diffusion give rise to physical signs which can be detected on clinical examination.

Disorders of Perfusion

In this type of disorder there is interference of the blood supply to the alveolar-capillary membrane. The most common cause is obstruction of the pulmonary arteries by one or more large emboli or multiple small emboli. The most commonly used investigations when a disorder of perfusion is suspected are angiography and lung scanning.

Ventilation–Perfusion Imbalance

The maintenance of normal respiration depends upon there being a proper balance between ventilation and perfusion. In chronic obstructive bronchitis some alveoli receive no air but remain adequately perfused, this situation giving rise to what is essentially a right to left shunt: other alveoli are ventilated but are not perfused, as a result of which some of the work of ventilation is wasted and in effect there is an increase in dead space. Imbalance between ventilation and perfusion is the most common cause of cyanosis in chronic lung disease.

CLINICAL MANIFESTATIONS OF DISORDERED PULMONARY FUNCTION

Only abnormalities of ventilation can be detected and measured by tests which are suitable for use in family practice. To identify other types of disordered function, the family practitioner must rely upon the findings of clinical examination.

Dyspnoea

Dyspnoea is the most important symptom complained of by patients whose pulmonary function is abnormal. Its subjective nature makes if one of the most difficult of all symptoms to evaluate. The act of respiration is not normally consciously perceived and therefore dyspnoea is essentially a state of abnormal proprioception.

The manner in which the patient describes the sensation of dyspnoea may give some indication of the underlying abnormality of function. A history of episodic breathlessness associated with wheeze and occurring equally at rest or on exercise is suggestive of reversible airways obstruction. Breathlessness whose occurrence is clearly dependent upon the degree of exertion suggests that the patient has chronic respiratory insufficiency, either due to irreversible airways obstruction or to an abnormality of diffusion or a combination of these, the most common causes being chronic obstructive bronchitis, emphysema, left ventricular heart failure, sarcoidosis and alveolitis.

Central Cyanosis

Central cyanosis is most easily detected by examining the tongue. The ability to recognize cyanosis varies between clinicians, and it is more difficult in artificial light. Its presence indicates that the blood is less than 80 per cent saturated with oxygen, and because of the shape of the oxygen dissociation curve, this means that there must have been a severe fall in pO_2. It should be noted that a moderate degree of hypoxaemia can occur without cyanosis. The most common cause of cyanosis is severe chronic obstructive bronchitis (the 'blue bloater').

The Manner of Breathing

The manner of breathing often reflects the type of disordered function which is present. Prolonged exiration occurs as a result of airways obstruction. Breathing with pursed lips is characteristic of patients with severe long-standing airways obstruction with air trapping and is seen commonly in patients with severe emphysema. Tachypnoea is especially liable to occur with disorders of diffusion or perfusion, for instance in pneumonia, alveolitis and pulmonary infarction. It is also a characteristic feature of patients with emphysema occurring in the absence of chronic obstructive bronchitis (the 'pink puffer').

The shape and movements of the chest may help to distinguish between obstructive and restrictive types of ventilatory disorder. If the abnormality is due to airways obstruction, the chest will be maintained in a position of hyperinflation. On the other hand, deformity of the chest is usually associated with a restrictive disorder of ventilation. In both types of ventilatory disorder there is reduced expansion of the thorax, despite the use of the accessory muscles of respiration and there is often recession of the intercostal spaces on inspiration.

Neurological Features

Restlessness, mental confusion and a coarse tremor commonly occur with carbon dioxide retention and are an indication of severe respiratory failure.

Auscultation

Auscultation is of very limited value for assessing the degree of severity of disordered function. However, it may be an invaluable guide to the type of disorder present. Wheeze or rhonchi are an indication that the calibre of small airways has been reduced almost to the point of closure. Grossly diminished breath sounds are suggestive of emphysema, in which condition the amount of air flow may be so reduced that it is insufficient to generate any sound. Crepitations are miniature explosions which occur when there is a sudden equalisation of gas pressure in deflated regions of the lungs. They are characteristic of many diseases in which parts of the lungs are deflated — notably pneumonia, alveolitis, sarcoidosis and pulmonary oedema — in all of which the predominant abnormality of function is a reduction of diffusion.

TESTS OF VENTILATORY FUNCTION

Disordered ventilation is the only form of abnormal pulmonary function which can be detected and measured by instruments that are suitable for use in family practice. There are two instruments available — the Vitalograph and the Wright peak flow meter. Whereas the former will identify and measure both obstructive and restrictive disorders, the peak flow meter only provides a measure of airways obstruction. However, because airways obstruction is far commoner than any other type of disordered function, being the fundamental abnormality in chronic obstructive bronchitis, emphysema and asthma, this limitation of the peak flow meter is not of great importance.

The use of instruments to measure airways obstruction is as relevant to the identification and treatment of chronic obstructive bronchitis and asthma as is the sphygmomanometer to the diagnosis and management of hypertension. Both the Vitalograph and the peak flow meter measure a single, forced expiration: whichever is used, it is of the utmost importance that the subject who is being tested understands what he has to do and is persuaded to make a maximum effort.

The Vitalograph

The Vitalograph is essentially a dry spirometer which provides a recording of the whole of a subject's forced expiration. The expired air inflates an internal rubber bellows which causes a stylus to write on a recording chart. The latter is carried on a frame which begins to move laterally at a constant speed as soon as the subject's expired air enters the bellows. From the tracing (spirogram) it is simple to measure the volume of air expelled in the first second of expiration (the forced expiratory volume in one second or FEV_1) and the total amount of air expelled up to the point when the subject can expire no further (the forced vital capacity or FVC).

In normal subjects the FEV_1 should be at least 70 per cent of the FVC, which should be attained within four seconds. In obstructive disorders both FEV_1 and FVC are reduced but the latter is relatively less so and hence the FEV_1/FVC ratio is abnormally low (i.e., less than 70 per cent). On the other hand, in restrictive disorders, although FEV_1 and FVC are both reduced, the ratio between them usually remains normal.

The Wright Peak Flow Meter

The Wright peak flow meter was originally introduced as a test of ventilatory function for use in epidemiological surveys. It has come to be used increasingly widely by clinicians in hospitals, chest clinics and family practice. It is an outstanding example of an instrument which meets all the special requirements of the family practitioner, being portable and not requiring electrical power for its operation. The test itself is rapidly performed and the result can be read immediately. Its use should be regarded as an essential part of the clinical examination of all patients suspected of having asthma, chronic bronchitis or emphysema.

The subject makes a short, forced expiration into the meter. This causes an internal vane to rotate and with it a needle on the dial of the instrument. The needle comes to rest on the scale which indicates the subject's peak expiratory flow (PEF) in litres per minute (l/min).

The Relative Merits of the Vitalograph and Peak Flow Meter

Both instruments are highly accurate and as an index of airways obstruction there is little to choose between FEV_1 and PEF: in fact there is a close correlation between the two measurements.

Whereas the peak flow meter provides only a measure of airways obstruction, the Vitalograph enables the clinician to identify restrictive ventilatory disorders as well, because it gives the additional measurement of FVC. Furthermore, the Vitalograph provides a written tracing which can be kept as a permanent record. Analysis of the shape of a spirogram gives valuable information, although considerable experience is required for its interpretation.

Apart from the much smaller cost of the peak flow meter, perhaps its greatest advantage is that the test takes so little time to perform and the result is obtained immediately. This is of particular value in the management and follow-up of patients with asthma, in whom repeated measurements are essential as a guide to progress (see Chapter 7).

The Evaluation of FEV_1 and PEF

It is essential to realise that there is no absolute range of normal values of FEV_1 or PEF, unlike the situation which obtains in the case of, say, blood urea and blood sugar — these being very largely independent of the age or other characteristics of the subject in whom they are estimated.

Both FEV_1 and PEF are influenced by the dimensions of the thorax and the power of the muscles used in making a forced expiration. Because there is a broad correlation between standing height and the dimensions of the thorax and because height is so conveniently measured, it is used as one of the indices for the evaluation of both FEV_1 and PEF. Men have higher values of FEV_1 and PEF than women of corresponding height, whose chest volume is smaller and whose respiratory muscles are less powerful. For the same reason, a broad muscular subject is likely to have a higher FEV_1 or PEF than a tall thin subject whose chest volume is smaller.

As well as height and sex, age has to be taken into account in the prediction of FEV_1 and PEF. During adolescence there is a steep rise in both, reaching a maximum at about the age of 25 years. Thereafter, in normal subjects, there is only a gradual fall with advancing age.

Some guide to the values of FEV_1 or PEF which a subject should be capable of achieving can be obtained either from tables of predicted values or from nomograms. From these a predicted normal value can be found for any subject of given sex, age and height, against which the subject's observed value can be compared. Only if the latter is more than two standard deviations less than predicted can it be regarded as being abnormal.

The standard deviation is a measure of the scatter around the mean regression and in the case of FEV_1 and PEF a large part of this scatter can be accounted for by differences of body build and musculature between individuals of the same age and height. Clearly, the larger the scatter is, the less discriminatory will the normal values be, and observed values in some subjects who are in fact abnormal may nevertheless fall within the normal range.

Normal values of FEV_1 and PEF have been derived from studies of large numbers of supposedly normal subjects. In almost every case, however, smokers were not excluded from the normal series provided that they denied having chronic or persistent expectoration. There is now considerable evidence that some smokers and ex-smokers, even though they have no symptoms of mucus hypersecretion, nevertheless have lower values of FEV_1 or PEF than persons who have never smoked. Therefore, the inclusion of smokers in a normal series has two important consequences. First, the mean value of FEV_1 or PEF of the whole series is lowered and, secondly, the scatter of values around the mean is increased.

Normal Values of FEV_1

The makers of the Vitalograph provide a manual for users of the instrument which includes nomograms for predicting FEV_1 in subjects of both sexes. These were derived from the findings of a small series of healthy factory workers and pensioners in West Germany, from which, however, smokers were not excluded. A high standard deviation of FEV_1 was found in both sexes, and as a result the 'normal range' of FEV_1 is very wide and it becomes progressively less discriminatory with increasing age. Thus, in a man aged 60 years an observed value of FEV_1 would have to be less than 48 per cent of the predicted value before it fell outside the normal range, while in a woman of the same age it would be abnormal only if it were less than 41 per cent of the predicted value.

Normal Values of PEF

Most of the published normal values of PEF were derived from studies which included smokers. In calculating the regression of PEF on age it was assumed that PEF begins to fall in a linear fashion from the age of 20 years. The distributors of the Wright peak flow meter provide a nomogram of normal values, based on the findings of PEF in normal subjects over the age of 15 years who satisfied stringent criteria of normality as well as being lifelong non-smokers. In both sexes the regression of PEF on age is curvilinear. A large difference between the sexes emerges at puberty and this is due to the more powerful muscular forces and the larger chest volume of males.

Because of the comparatively small standard deviation in both sexes, an observed value of PEF of less than 80 per cent of predicted falls outside the normal range, irrespective of the subject's age or height. A simple guide to apply in the evaluation of an observed PEF is that in men it should be within 100 1/min and in women within 90 1/min of the predicted value.

Normal values of FEV_1 and PEF in children aged 5—18 years can be found from a nomogram, also provided by the distributors of the Wright meter, based on the findings in a large series of normal children.

The Limitations of Normal Values

Because of the wide range of normal values, even in series which have a comparatively small standard deviation, some subjects who are in fact abnormal may nevertheless have an FEV_1 or PEF which lies within the normal range. For instance, a man at the age of 20 years might have had a PEF about two standard deviations *above* the predicted value. Over the course of the next twenty years his PEF could fall by almost 200 1/min, yet at the age of 40 years he could still have a PEF which was within the normal range, being just less than 2 standard deviations *below* that predicted.

If an observed value of PEF can be compared with the highest value which the patient has previously achieved this provides a more realistic guide to what he should be capable of achieving.

REVERSIBILITY OF AIRWAYS OBSTRUCTION

Some patients with asthma do not have typical, paroxysmal episodes of wheezing but are persistently short of breath. If they are smokers and they are found to have an abnormally low FEV_1 or PEF, it is only too easy to conclude that they have chronic obstructive bronchitis. While some part of their airways obstruction may be irreversible, there may also be a large reversible component which, having once been identified, can then be treated. Therefore, FEV_1 or PEF should be measured at one minute intervals after the inhalation of isoprenaline from a metered aerosol. If airways obstruction is readily reversible there is an immediate improvement which continues until it reaches a maximum within about five minutes.

Refractory Airways Obstruction

It is important to realise that, even if little or no increase in FEV_1 or PEF is brought about by isoprenaline it is still possible that the patient's airways obstruction is refractory rather than irreversible. The distinction between refractory and irreversible airways obstruction can only be made with certainty by giving corticotrophin or steroids in high dosage for several days, provided that such a trial is clinically justified. If this treatment does not bring about improvement of FEV_1 or PEF it can be concluded that the patient's airways obstruction is irreversible.

USES OF TESTS OF VENTILATORY FUNCTION BY THE FAMILY PRACTITIONER

There are three principal uses which the family practitioner can make of tests of ventilatory function:

1. in the differential diagnosis of patients with dyspnoea,
2. in the detection of chronic obstructive bronchitis in its early stages
3. the management of asthma.

The Differential Diagnosis of Patients with Dyspnoea

Although chronic obstructive bronchitis, emphysema and the combination of these two diseases are the most common causes of dyspnoea, this symptom may be due to an abnormality of pulmonary function other than airways obstruction, or it may be cardiac in origin. Therefore, the finding of a normal or only slightly reduced FEV_1 or PEF in a patient who complains of dyspnoea indicates that his principal abnormality is not ventilatory in nature. The possibility that he has an abnormality of either diffusion or perfusion should be considered and confirmatory evidence of this may be found in the history, on physical examination, in a chest radiograph or after referral for more detailed pulmonary function tests.

Not uncommonly patients complain of dyspnoea which is thought to have no organic basis. Sometimes, patients with severe emphysema are mistakenly believed to be neurotic and are referred to specialists with the object of reassuring the patient that he has no organic disease. Such a mistake would be unlikely to occur if the patient's PEF had been measured and found to be severely reduced. On the other hand, patients who do have spurious dyspnoea, due to chronic anxiety tension, usually complain of a sensation of being unable to take an adequately full breath and enquiry usually elicits the fact that they sigh frequently. The finding of a normal PEF in such a patient is valuable confirmatory evidence that his dyspnoea is not organic in origin, while the knowledge that his PEF is normal may help the patient to accept reassurance that his lungs are not diseased.

Detection of Early Chronic Obstructive Bronchitis

The identification of those who have a slight to moderate degree of airways obstruction can be made by means of the techniques outlined above. Selective screening of people who are at special risk may reduce the impact of chronic obstructive bronchitis which is usually not diagnosed until it has reached an advanced stage (see Chapter 6).

Management of Asthma

If the family practitioner possesses a peak flow meter and is prepared to make frequent measurements of PEF in his patients with asthma, he can manage this disease as effectively as a hospital outpatient clinic. By means of serial measurements of PEF a patient's progress can be followed and his response to treatment can be assessed objectively (see Chapter 7).

Reference

1. Cotes, J. E. (1975). *Lung Function, Assessment and Application in Medicine*, 3rd Ed., (Oxford: Blackwell Scientific Publications).

6

Chronic Bronchitis

I. Gregg

INTRODUCTION

The natural history of chronic bronchitis usually extends over many years of a patient's lifetime. In some it begins in childhood as recurrent wheezy bronchitis. The first recognizable symptom in adulthood is a chronic productive cough which all too often is dismissed as 'just the normal smoker's cough'. A long latent period ensues in which there is a gradual progressive increase in airways obstruction, due to structural damage of the bronchi. During this period the patient usually has recurrent episodes of acute bronchitis. For many years he is not aware of any shortness of breath, but eventually the amount of damage to the bronchi is such that he begins to be short of breath on ordinary exertion.

In the advanced stages of the disease disability from shortness of breath becomes increasingly severe, limiting everyday activities until the patient becomes dyspnœic even at rest. After a shorter or longer period of respiratory crippledom, death occurs as a result of respiratory or cardiac failure.

In the UK chronic bronchitis is one of the foremost public health problems[1]. Its importance for the family practitioner lies in the following:

1. a large number of his older patients will have chronic bronchitis and in some it will cause disablement long before they reach retiring age;
2. acute episodes of infection occurring in the course of the disease are among the most common conditions which the family practitioner has to treat and require an understanding of the principles underlying the choice of antibiotics;
3. in the management of the advanced stages of the disease there is much that the family practitioner and his team can do to make the patient's life more tolerable;
4. no one has a better opportunity than the family practitioner to recognize chronic bronchitis in its early stages, long before it has given rise to any disability, and to institute preventive measures which may arrest further progress of the disease.

DEFINITION AND CLASSIFICATION

It is important to be clear about what is meant by the term 'chronic bronchitis'. Clinicians tend to restrict their use of the term to patients who have some degree of disability, either from shortness of breath or because they are subject to recurrent episodes of acute bronchitis. Epidemiologists, on the other hand, define the disease without any reference to disability.

For epidemiological purposes, any person who regularly expectorates sputum, at least during the winter months, and has done so for the last two years can be deemed to have 'chronic bronchitis'. Therefore, anyone with a smoker's cough which is accompanied by only a minimal amount of sputum on most days during the winter fulfils the criteria of the definition, even though his pulmonary function may be entirely normal. The British Medical Research Council suggested that this form of the disease should be classified as 'simple chronic bronchitis', whereas patients who have impairment of ventilatory function in addition to persistent expectoration should be regarded as having 'chronic obstructive bronchitis'.

AETIOLOGICAL FACTORS

Although chronic bronchitis is such a common disease, surprisingly there are still a number of aspects of its pathogenesis which are still not understood. For instance, it is not known why the prevalence and mortality from chronic obstructive bronchitis in the United Kingdom is so much higher than elsewhere. Nor is it known why only a small proportion of those with simple chronic bronchitis develop progressive impairment of ventilatory function, leading eventually to disability.

Because epidemiological methodology is so well suited to the study of environmental agents, a great deal is now known about the effects of atmospheric pollution and smoking in the pathogenesis of chronic bronchitis. However, the operation of environmental agents does not fully explain several problems relating to its inception and progress. For instance, some persons who live in the country and have never smoked become disabled by the disease, whereas some heavy smokers who live in polluted cities have normal ventilatory function and may not even have symptoms of mucus hypersecretion. This strongly suggests that host factors modify the noxious effects of environmental agents, presumably by making some persons more susceptible and others more resistant to them.

Irritation of the Bronchi

The inhalation of any irritant into the bronchi leads to hypersecretion of mucus. The greater part of the mucus which is expectorated originates from glands within the walls of the larger bronchi. Deeper inhalation of irritants into the smaller, distal airways causes metaplasia of the epithelium with replacement of ciliated columnar cells by goblet cells. In normal subjects few goblet cells are found in the bronchioles, whereas in patients with chronic bronchitis they may be more numerous than ciliated cells. Although goblet cells secrete relatively much less mucus than the glands in the large airways the presence of mucus in small calibre airways must have a more pronounced effect upon air flow.

Many epidemiological surveys have investigated the role of agents which irritate the bronchi — notably atmospheric pollution, smoking and certain occupational dusts and fumes.

Atmospheric Pollution

The examination of mortality statistics in various countries reveals large differences in the death rates from chronic bronchitis: these are undoubtedly real, for they remain after every allowance has been made for differences in terminology and diagnostic habit. It is believed that there are two principal reasons why chronic bronchitis is so common in the UK; first, the habit (until recently) of burning coal in open grates for domestic heating, and second, the climatic conditions which are particularly liable to temperature inversions, as a result of which atmospheric pollutants are trapped at a low level. Over the last twenty years, as a result of the Clean Air legislation, there has been a considerable reduction in the levels of atmospheric pollution caused by smoke in most cities.

Epidemiological surveys have compared the prevalence of symptoms of mucus hypersecretion and dyspnoea in various parts of the world. One study examined the prevalence of symptoms in men, aged 45 to 64 years, living in three different areas of the UK (rural areas, county towns and cities) and that of men of a similar age living in Berlin, a city with low levels of atmospheric pollution in New Hampshire, USA. Little difference was found between any of the areas in the UK and Berlin in the prevalence of cough and phlegm. On the other hand, a marked rural to urban gradient was found in the prevalence of breathlessness, that in Berlin being approximately the same as that in the rural areas of the UK. These findings have been interpreted as evidence for atmospheric pollution being a contributory factor in chronic obstructive bronchitis.

Smoking

Studies of symptom prevalence have a more limited value than studies which compare ventilatory function in different populations. A study which compared British postal workers with men in the American postal service showed that at all levels of smoking, from non-smokers to heavy smokers, the mean forced expiratory volume in one second (FEV_1) of men in the United States was higher than that of men in the British county towns, and this in turn was higher than that of men in London. Furthermore, the differences in FEV_1 between the three areas were greater than those between non-smokers and heavy smokers. This suggests that smoking is less important than area of residence.

As yet, no epidemiological survey has shown there to be a relationship between smoking consumption and impairment of ventilatory function. Although the part which smoking may play in causing progressive airways obstruction is still far from clear, smoking is certainly of great importance as a factor which causes irritation of the bronchi and therewith mucus hypersecretion. In both sexes there is a close correlation between smoking consumption and the prevalence of expectoration. Thus, at least 25 per cent of men and women below 30 years of age who regularly smoke more than ten but less than twenty cigarettes a day have expectoration on most days during the winter months, and therefore would fulfil the criteria of the definition of chronic bronchitis. In smokers of the same age who smoke more than thirty cigarettes a day, the proportion who have expectoration rises to more than 50 per cent. Even so, a small number of persons who have never smoked will be found to have expectoration, while some heavy smokers deny any symptoms of mucus hypersecretion. This suggests that there are host differences in susceptibility to bronchial irritation .

One important aspect of smoking often overlooked is the depth of inhalation. A study carried out by the Tobacco Research Council showed that the depth of inhalation correlated closely with the amount smoked, this being particularly well seen in men who smoked cigarettes. Thus, heavy smokers not only tend to expose their bronchi to more irritation but they also tend to inhale smoke to a deeper level. This may be of considerable importance because it seems probable that mucus secreted in small calibre airways causes airways obstruction. That this may be reversible is suggested by the improvement in ventilatory function which usually occurs when smoking is given up, and also by evidence from bronchographic studies.

It is possible, that tobacco smoke inhaled deeply into the distal airways has other noxious effects apart from stimulating mucus hypersecretion: there is evidence that nitrogen dioxide, which is one of the many constituents of tobacco smoke, has a directly damaging effect upon the region of the lung where the bronchioles join the alveoli; experiments have shown that cigarette smoke and nitrogen dioxide cause emphysema.

Constitutional Predisposition

It has already been emphasised that only a small proportion of persons with simple chronic bronchitis develop airways obstruction. Therefore, it would appear that some factor other than mucus hypersecretion must be responsible for the development of chronic obstructive bronchitis.

The well-recognized preponderance of males with chronic obstructive bronchitis may be as much a reflection of a genetic predisposition as it is of the male's generally greater exposure to irritation from smoking and occupational dusts and fumes and the fact that boys are more prone than girls to recurrent wheezy bronchitis may be a display of this same constitutional factor operating in earlier life. The well-attested familial incidence of chronic obstructive bronchitis is also suggestive of a genetic predisposition.

Infection

Clinicians cannot but be impressed by how frequently patients with chronic bronchitis are subject to acute exacerbations, often occurring shortly after an upper respiratory infection. The patient himself often describes this course of events as 'a cold going onto the chest'.

Undoubtedly, the majority of episodes of acute lower respiratory infection are initiated by viruses, of which a large number of different types are now known to be capable of infecting the respiratory tract. Whereas in normal subjects viral infection may be restricted to the upper respiratory tract, in the chronic bronchitic it usually affects the lower respiratory tract also within a few days, the sputum becomes purulent, indicating the occurrence of secondary bacterial infection.

Haemophilus influenzae and pneumococci are the commonest organisms which are isolated from sputum in acute exacerbations. Both these organisms are found as commensals in the upper respiratory tract of normal persons. It would seem that viral infection activates a persistent, latent bacterial infection of the bronchi. The lower respiratory tract is normally protected by the cough reflex and by mucociliary clearance, so that in a normal subject the bronchi are sterile below the main carina. If these defence mechanisms have been impaired – for instance by smoking, or if there is pre-existing structural damage of the bronchi, *Haemophilus influenzae* can establish itself in the lower respiratory tract and may persist there indefinitely.

THE DEVELOPMENT OF AIRWAYS OBSTRUCTION

By the time a patient first notices that he is short of breath during everyday exertion (usually between the ages of 45–60 years), his peak expiratory flow (PEF) will be considerably impaired and almost certainly below 250 l/min. Clearly, there must have been a long latent period during which airways obstruction was present but was not sufficiently severe to cause breathlessness on ordinary exertion. All the evidence suggests that in patients who eventually become disabled by chronic obstructive bronchitis there is an insidious fall of ventilatory function throughout adult life.

The Role of Infection

For many years it was believed that the structural damage of the bronchi which gave rise to progressive airways obstruction was caused by the acute episodes of infection which punctuate the course of chronic obstructive bronchitis. There is, however, a great deal of evidence against this inference. In the first place, no prospective study has shown that a permanent, stepwise deterioration of FEV_1 or PEF occurs in association with episodes of acute lower respiratory infection. Secondly, the widespread use of antibiotics for some twenty years has had no discernible impact upon mortality from chronic obstructive bronchitis.

This has led some authorities to assert that bronchial infection plays no part in the pathogenesis of chronic obstructive bronchitis. Although clearly the role of infection is far less straightforward than was formally believed, it cannot be lightly dismissed. A survey carried out within the author's own practice has shown that, in both sexes, by far the most significant of all the factors examined for their association with impairment of PEF was a previous history of lower respiratory infection (defined as episodes during which there had been an increase of cough or sputum and abnormal signs had been heard in the chest on auscultation).

It would seem, therefore, that those who are susceptible to acute episodes of lower respiratory infection are the ones most liable to develop progressive airways obstruction. It is not clear whether pre-existing airways obstruction predisposes to recurrent episodes of infection, or whether the liability to these episodes is merely an index of the operation of some other, as yet unknown host factor, which is also responsible for the development of airways obstruction.

During the last few years several studies have shown that ventilatory function is often impaired in adolescents and in young adults who have had recurrent bronchitis in childhood. These findings suggest that in childhood, as in adulthood, the liability to lower respiratory infection is associated with the development of airways obstruction: it is possible that this association is a reflection of the same host factor operating at different ages. In any case, a history of recurrent bronchitis during childhood would seem to be indicative of a constitutional liability to develop chronic obstructive bronchitis later in life. Such a liability might be expected to be enhanced by environmental agents, particularly smoking, thus leading to an accelerated rate of decline of ventilatory function.

DIAGNOSIS

No difficulties arise over the recognition of patients with advanced chronic obstructive bronchitis. By the time this state is reached, however, the disease is incurable and the most that can be done for such patients is to provide symptomatic relief and to try and prevent still further deterioration. Clearly, it is all important to identify the disease at a much earlier stage when preventive measures might have a greater prospect of success.

Differential Diagnosis

Habitual expectoration and shortness of breath occur in many other chronic chest diseases, notably bronchiectasis, tuberculosis, sarcoidosis and fibrosing alveolitis. Chest radiography will usually enable these diseases to be distinguished from chronic obstructive bronchitis.

The most difficult problem of differential diagnosis is that of recurrent wheezy bronchitis in patients with late onset asthma who have not previously been subject to the intermittent, paroxysmal attacks of wheeze which are characteristic of 'typical' asthma. The possibility that a patient has asthma rather than chronic obstructive bronchitis should be considered if his symptoms have begun recently and he has not previously been a heavy smoker. The methods of distinguishing reversible, refractory and irreversible airways obstruction by measurements of PEF are described in Chapter 5, page 60.

The possibility of other diseases co-existing with chronic bronchitis should be borne in mind. Heavy smokers should have a chest radiograph periodically to exclude carcinoma. Although tuberculosis has become much less common among young adults in some areas of the world, its incidence is higher in immigrant populations – especially those from Asia, and it is still encountered in elderly men whose cough is attributed to 'just bronchitis'. Chronic left-sided heart failure gives rise to expectoration, shortness of breath and wheeze which may be superimposed upon the symptoms of chronic obstructive bronchitis. Its presence can be confirmed by the improvement which occurs with diuretic therapy.

Recognition of 'Early' Chronic Obstructive Bronchitis

The people who are at special risk of developing airways obstruction and in whom selective screening is likely to prove rewarding are:

1. those with a familial history of chronic bronchitis,
2. heavy smokers who inhale deeply,
3. those with a history of recurrent bronchitis during childhood and/or adulthood.

By the use of the peak flow meter or the Vitalograph (see Chapter 5) the family practitioner can readily identify those who already have a slight to moderate degree of irreversible airways obstruction which has not given rise to breathlessness.

A considerable degree of airways obstruction may be found in patients who have never been aware of any shortness of breath. Disability is seldom found in patients whose PEF is greater than 250 l/min., while in those who are severely disabled (respiratory cripples) PEF is usually less than 150 l/min.

Having identified persons with a slight to moderate degree of irreversible airways obstruction, every effort should be made to prevent further deterioration of function by the preventive measures outlined below.

PREVENTIVE MEASURES

The importance of preventive measures applies equally at all stages of the disease from the time at which it is first identified, before it gives rise to breathlessness, and to the terminal stage of severe disability.

By far the most important aspect of prevention is to reduce as far as possible any further irritation of the bronchi. The patient must understand the importance of giving up smoking completely, not merely reducing the amount smoked. It is unwise to make any promise that once smoking has been given up there will be any immediate improvement. Indeed, patients should be warned that at first they may find it more difficult to expectorate without the habitual irritation caused by smoking.

If a patient has an occupation which is either dusty or exposes him to fumes or damp, the question of alternative employment must be considered. The difficulties involved in this are discussed more fully later in this chapter.

TREATMENT

Measures to Promote Bronchial Clearance

One of the chief problems in the management of advanced chronic bronchitis is to prevent retention of mucus within the airways. Patients find this most troublesome on awaking and the sensation of being congested is one of the reasons why patients seek relief by smoking their first cigarette of the day, the acute irritation of the bronchi being virtually a process of purgation.

Bromhexine has been shown to reduce the viscosity of sputum and it has been claimed that its use enables patients to expectorate more easily. However, most trials have shown that the clinical benefits which bromhexine confers are small, at any rate in the dose in which it is generally prescribed.

Expectorants have long held a hallowed place in the prescribing of family practitioners. It is doubtful whether they have any value and it is certain that most do not promote expectoration. The inhalation of steam, while not being very convenient, is of value. Probably the best expectorant is Mistura Sodium Chloride taken in hot water.

Antibiotics

The antibiotic of first choice for the treatment of acute exacerbations is either ampicillin, amoxycillin, or oxytetracycline. It is doubtful whether any other antibiotic has real advantages over these three for the treatment of the majority of episodes of acute bronchitis.

If the patient has a high fever and there are signs suggestive of consolidation, the possibility of acute lobar pneumonia should be considered. Penicillin, ampicillin or amoxycillin should be given in preference to oxytetracycline in case the organism is a resistant pneumococcus[2]. During epidemics of influenza A virus the possibility of secondary staphylococcal pneumonia should be remembered. This is one situation in which laboratory examination of sputum and sensitivity tests are indicated. The role of antibiotics in the management of acute episodes of chest infections is also discussed in Chapter 4.

It has been claimed that by giving bromhexine concurrently with oxytetracycline, the latter's efficacy is enhanced by greater penetration into sputum but as yet there is no convincing evidence to substantiate this claim.

It is common practice to give patients a reserve supply of an antibiotic, sufficient for at least 48 hours, so that they can start taking it on their own initiative at the first onset of symptoms suggestive of an impending exacerbation.

Some patients have persistently purulent sputum or they have such frequent exacerbations that it is difficult to know when one ends and the next begins. In such patients, it is convenient to prescribe antibiotics on a continuous long-term basis — for instance, throughout the winter. There is no evidence that long-term antibiotic treatment reduces the number of acute exacerbations although it may shorten their duration. Surprisingly, side-effects from repetitive or long-term treatment with antibiotics rarely occurs. The fear of monilial infection has been exaggerated. It is unnecessary to prescribe routinely either nystatin or vitamin B supplements, and it is doubtful whether they are even indicated when antibiotics are given on a long-term basis.

Bronchodilators

Although the major component of airways obstruction in chronic obstructive bronchitis is irreversible, there is usually a small reversible component caused by bronchial muscle constriction and relief of this is beneficial.

Bronchodilator therapy can be given orally or in the form of suppositories or aerosols. The most frequently prescribed tablets and capsules contain ephedrine, theophylline and a barbiturate. Ephedrine is a relatively weak bronchodilator and in elderly bronchitics it may cause urinary retention. The long-term administration of a barbiturate is undesirable. Various forms of theophylline are prepared in tablet form, but all are relatively weak broncho-- dilators in doses which do not cause gastric irritations. Aminophylline supposi- tories are limited in their usefulness to patients who are confined in bed or who are breathless at night, and their prolonged use may give rise to proctitis.

Bronchodilator drugs are more effective when given as an aerosol than in tablet form. Self-administered metered aerosols are of particular value to patients who are subject to wheeze. Aerosols containing bronchodilators, such as salbutamol, isoetharine and terbutaline, which have a selective action on bronchial beta-receptors, are not only the most effective but also carry the least dangers of cardiotoxicity — an important consideration in elderly patients who may have ischemic heart disease in addition to chronic bronchitis. Broncho- dilators are also discussed in management of asthma (Chapter 7, pages 92 and 100).

Steroids

Steroids have no place in the treatment of chronic obstructive bronchitis. However, in patients who have a marked liability to wheeze and who therefore may have late onset asthma a trial of steroids is justified. If there is no clear improvement of PEF within a week of starting steroids in high dose, this form of treatment should be withdrawn.

Drug Treatment for Respiratory Cripples

Respiratory failure occurs when so much structural damage has been caused that the lungs cannot maintain adequate respiration for the patient's metabolic requirements, even when at rest. Two consequences ensue. First, there is a fall in the level of oxygen in the blood and a rise in that of carbon dioxide. Second, the respiratory centre becomes insensitive to changes in the levels of oxygen and carbon dioxide which in a normal person would stimulate it and lead to an increase in the rate and depth of ventilation and the restoration of the blood gases to normal levels.

Respiratory failure is a dangerous situation, which requires urgent treatment in hospital so that measurements of blood gases are made and oxygen can be given under strict control. Signs of respiratory failure which indicate the need for urgent admission are cyanosis, shallow respiration, drowsiness, headache, irritability and a coarse tremor.

Chronic hypoxaemia causes pulmonary hypertension and sooner or later most patients with advanced chronic obstructive bronchitis show signs of right sided heart failure (*cor pulmonale*). This should be treated with diuretics.

Drugs which stimulate the respiratory centre when given intravenously have been prepared in tablet form. Dichlorphenamide and cropropamide have been advocated as long-term respiratory stimulants but there is no convincing evidence that either is of value when given orally.

Domiciliary oxygen therapy is a controversial subject. Paradoxically, the patient has a chronic need for more oxygen than he can obtain from atmospheric air, yet the uncontrolled adminstration of oxygen carries dangers of carbon dioxide narcosis because of the insensitivity of the respiratory centre. A small number of intelligent patients can obtain benefit from lightweight, portable oxygen cylinders which they recharge themselves from a 48 cu. ft cylinder kept at home.

THE MANAGEMENT OF ADVANCED CHRONIC BRONCHITIS

General Measures

All the preventive measures which have been outlined already apply with equal force to the patient who has an advanced stage of the disease. He should be told of the importance of heating his bedroom, staying indoors during foggy weather, and whenever possible avoiding situations in which he is likely to come into contact with respiratory infections. Because it has been shown that respiratory viruses are often introduced by young children into the home, visits by grandchildren who have recently begun a cold or cough are inadvisable.

Referral to Chest Clinics

Usually, by the time a patient is referred to a local chest clinic or outpatient department he has already begun to suffer some disability from shortness of breath, and therefore the consultant can do little more than to confirm the diagnosis and reinforce the family practitioner's advice to give up smoking, stay indoors during fogs, and take antibiotics at the onset of every exacerbation.

Some chest clinics have a more energetic policy towards chronic bronchitis. Not only do they arrange for patients to have instruction in physiotherapy so that they can carry out such simple procedures as postural drainage at home, but their social workers make a detailed assessment of the patient's disability in the light of the circumstances of his housing, family and occupation. Because of their close links with the local health authority, chest clinics are often more successful than the family practitioner in obtaining for patients all the help which the social services and other agencies can provide.

The Contribution of The Family Practice Team

The main objective is to help the patient to live his life as fully and happily as possible within the limitations of his disability. The family practitioner and his team can do a great deal to achieve this. Receptionists should remember the difficulties which patients with chronic bronchitis face in coming to the surgery and they should be allowed to use their discretion in offering visits by the doctor to the patients' homes. Regular visiting of chronic bronchitics might seem to be unrewarding from a strictly medical point of view. However it can have great supportive value for the patients and their families and tends to counteract the impression which bronchitics so frequently gain that nothing further can be done for them. If the family practitioner himself cannot manage to see all his disabled patients regularly, he can arrange for the district nurse or health visitor to do so, and she can report to him if she considers that any patient is deteriorating and also advise on patients' needs for social services.

A home help can be of great assistance to patients who are confined to their homes by doing shopping for them. Meals-on-wheels and convalescent holidays are further ways in which the local authority can help. Application for rehousing on medical grounds is justified if the patient lives in a damp house or if he has to climb many stairs. Unfortunately, it is often difficult to persuade the managers of housing departments that chronic bronchitis is a disabling disease.

Supportive Treatment

It is hardly surprising that the limitations which advanced chronic bronchitis impose upon a patient's whole mode of life results in some degree of emotional disturbance[3]. A recent study of the emotional effects of chronic bronchitis revealed how commonly emotional disturbances occurred, not only in the patients themselves, but often in their families. One of the findings in this interesting report from a medical social worker with special experience of chronic chest disease concerned the contribution which the family practitioner and his team could make towards maintaining a patient's morale in the face of steady physical deterioration.

Many bronchitics struggle along in isolation. Some do so bravely and uncomplainingly, but the majority exhibit some degree of resentment or despair. This may express itself either as increasing apathy and an unwillingness to do anything for themselves or as petulance and irritability. Bronchitics are usually 'difficult to live with'. Some of their moodiness, which may be exasperating for their relatives, can be attributed to chronic hypoxia, but long before this stage is reached the inability to work with its consequences of reduced income, loss of self-esteem and boredom are potent causes of depression.

Social Services for Chronic Bronchitis

An illuminating survey of the social circumstances of disabled chronic bronchitics carried out in Scotland revealed how much distress, hardship and loneliness was experienced by these patients and their relatives.

It is not difficult to discern some of the reasons for society's apathy over chronic bronchitis. In the UK it is so common that it is regarded as almost part of the national way of life. It does not touch our social conscience in the same way as pneumoconiosis calls attention to the working conditions and dangers which miners undergo. Usually, chronic bronchitis affects the older age groups and particularly the unskilled (and less articulate) social classes and its chronicity contrasts with the more dramatic course of tuberculosis which used to have a high mortality in young adults.

It is interesting to contrast society's attitude to chronic bronchitis with its concern for tuberculosis when that disease was still a major public health problem. A cynic might not unreasonably conclude that it was the fear induced by the infectious nature of tuberculosis which stimulated the community to make some provision for tuberculous patients and their families. Although the notification of tuberculosis was conceived as a measure to control the spread of infection by keeping patients under surveillance and enabling their contacts to be traced, it also had the effect of ensuring that patients received all the benefits to which they were entitled.

Because chronic bronchitis is not notifiable, no one has any true idea of the size of the problem. Whenever surveys are carried out they invariably disclose that many disabled patients have received no help whatever from the social services, apparently because nobody thought of informing the appropriate agencies.

Re-Employment and the Disablement Register

Most chronic bronchitics have reached 50 years of age when they become unable to continue working in their former jobs. The majority have no skills and therefore the difficulties of finding then suitably light and sheltered jobs are immense. The ideal form of employment is indoors, involving no physical exertion or stair climbing, or exposure to dust and fumes. Employment which even begins to approach this ideal is almost impossible to find. Jobs as lift attendants and messengers are often considered to be suitable for chronic bronchitics but there are insufficient of these and many firms are understandably reluctant to employ bronchitics who they know in advance are likely to have a bad sickness record.

The most satisfactory solution is to persuade the patient's present employers to find him some lighter work even if this involves a drop in income. If this is impossible, simply because a firm does not have sufficient light jobs to offer, the only course is to register the patient as disabled and to hope that the disablement register officer has a rare amount of imagination and skill in finding suitable employment for bronchitics.

A very few younger and more intelligent bronchitics may be able to take advantage of rehabilitation training schemes and be taught a new trade at a Government training centre. However, few of the skills that are taught at these centres are suitable for bronchitics. Another problem is the delay between a patient's completion of his retraining and his finding a job in which he can use it. The present situation is that a depressingly high proportion of bronchitics cannot be rehabilitated and have to be regarded as unemployable. Until the community recognizes that it has an obligation to these patients (many of whom have served it for many years by doing unpleasant jobs which others would avoid and which are often a contributory aetiological factor in their disablement) there is little more that the family practitioner can do than to convince them that he and his team have not forgotten them and that they understand and will try to ease the special physical and emotional problems which are imposed by chronic bronchitis.

References

1. Capel, L. H. and Caplin, M. (1964). *Chronic Bronchitis in Great Britain*, (London: Chest and Heart Association).
2. May, J. R. (1972). *Chemotherapy of Chronic Bronchitis and Allied Disorders*, 2nd edition, (London: English Universities Press).
3. Rubeck, M. F. (1971). *Social and Emotional Effects of Chronic Bronchitis*, (London: Chest and Heart Association).

7

Asthma

I. Gregg

INTRODUCTION

Asthma is a very common disease and one which every family practitioner is bound to see frequently in the course of his day to day work. Although it only rarely causes death, it is responsible for a great deal of disability and absence from school or work and it also gives rise to much anxiety on the part of patients and their relatives.

Asthma is a pre-eminent example of a serious disease whose management ought to be carried out mainly by the family practitioner rather than the hospital outpatient department or chest clinic[1]. Not only is the family practitioner more accessible for dealing with acute attacks of asthma whenever these occur, but he can provide greater continuity of care than is usually possible in an outpatient clinic, where a patient may encounter a succession of unfamiliar doctors. Following on from this, the family practitioner can instill greater self-confidence in his asthmatic patients and he has a better opportunity for educating them about the nature of the disease and the various forms of treatment which are prescribed to relieve or suppress it.

DEFINITIONS OF ASTHMA AND OF REVERSIBLE, REFRACTORY AND IRREVERSIBLE AIRWAYS OBSTRUCTION

Asthma has defied all attempts to define it on either an aetiological or a pathophysiological basis. So long as the fundamental abnormality which gives rise to asthma remains unknown, it is impossible to define the disease except in descriptive terms[2].

The most widely accepted definition of asthma is that proposed in 1959 by the Ciba Foundation Guest Symposium, which suggested that it should be defined in terms of a disorder of function as follows; 'a disease characterised by variable dyspnoea due to widespread narrowing of peripheral airways in the lungs, varying in severity over short periods of time, either spontaneously or as a result of treatment'. The definition deliberately avoided any reference to such aetiological factors as allergy and infection, because no single aetiological factor is common to all patients with asthma.

Twelve years later, a study group of experts convened by the Ciba Foundation concluded that on the information available in 1971 it was impossible to define asthma in such a way that it could be clearly differentiated from other conditions which closely resemble it. Nevertheless, there was general agreement that the cardinal criterion of asthma is an abnormal degree of resistance to airflow within the bronchi and that the processes which give rise to this are *reversible*.

Patients with asthma can be regarded as having bronchi which are hyperreactive and therefore tend to constrict when provoked by a wide variety of stimuli. It becomes clinically recognizable when obstruction to airflow becomes sufficiently great for the patient to perceive it as a disturbance of breathing. Reversible airways obstruction can be caused by three processes, acting either singly or in unison. These are:

1. bronchial muscle constriction,
2. oedema of the bronchial mucous membrane,
3. intraluminal obstruction by mucus or exudate.

The term 'bronchospasm' enjoys a wide but undeserved use. It implies that muscle constriction is the sole or predominant abnormality in asthma and thus tends to direct attention away from the other components of reversible airways obstruction which are often of much greater importance.

Airways obstruction may subside spontaneously or be reversed by treatment. However, a situation may arise when airways obstruction, although reversible, does not respond readily to simple treatment such as a bronchodilator and under these circumstances it may be described as *refractory*. This has to be distinguished from *irreversible* airways obstruction which occurs in some patients with asthma in whom there is permanent structural damage of the bronchi, due either to long-standing, unrelieved asthma or the co-existence of chronic obstructive bronchitis or emphysema.

No difficulty arises in identifying patients with 'typical' asthma, who have paroxysmal attacks of wheezing, often provoked by some readily recognisable factor. Difficulties arise mainly in patients who have reversible airways obstruction, associated with wheezing, which occurs only when they have a respiratory infection: some children are subject to recurrent wheezy bronchitis while some adults with chronic bronchitis have acute exacerbations during which wheezing is a prominent feature. Most clinicians draw a distinction between 'wheezy bronchitis' and asthma, and are probably justified in so doing in our present state of knowledge. Nevertheless, it must be emphasized that the physiological disorder which gives rise to wheezing is common to both conditions and the treatment called for is also the same in both.

PREVALENCE

The importance of our present inability to define asthma with any degree of precision is seen immediately when one attempts to give some estimate of its prevalence. Widely different figures have been quoted, varying between 1 per cent and 19 per cent in children and between 2 per cent and 9 per cent in adults. These differences can largely be explained by differences of opinion between investigators over whether recurrent wheezy bronchitis in children and recurrent bronchitis with wheeze in adults should be regarded as asthma or not.

The often quoted prevalence of asthma of between 1 and 2 per cent is undoubtedly an underestimate, because it includes only those patients in whom asthma is easily recognized by 'reason of the frequency or severity of typical attacks. It seems probable that at least 5 per cent of all persons have been subject to attacks of asthma at some time in their lives and about the same percentage have had episodes of acute wheezy bronchitis.

CLASSIFICATION OF ASTHMA

It has long been recognized that many patients with asthma are hypersensitive to certain substances which are inhaled, such as pollens and animal dander. As long ago as 1698 Floyer (himself an asthmatic) noted that house dust provoked asthma. Others are hypersensitive to foods, especially nuts and fish, or to certain drugs, such as aspirin. Many asthmatic patients have in addition other allergic conditions, particularly hay fever.

For many years it has been customary to classify asthma into *extrinsic* and *intrinsic* types, the former comprising patients in whom an allergic cause can be identified and the latter comprising those patients in whom no allergic causes can be found. Hypersensitivity to aspirin does not appear to be of an allergic nature and in all other respects aspirin-sensitive patients closely resemble those with intrinsic asthma.

The performance of skin tests confirms the presence of hypersensitivity in the *extrinsic* group of patients, whereas it is characteristic of patients with *intrinsic* asthma that skin tests are entirely negative. This has led to the belief that any patient with asthma who can be shown to have positive skin tests should be included within the *extrinsic* group, even if there is no circumstantial evidence that any of the allergens to which he is hypersensitive on skin testing has ever provoked in him an attack of asthma.

Only recently has it come to be realised that about 15 per cent of normal subjects who have never had asthma or allergic rhinitis give unequivocally positive reactions on skin testing, particularly to the house dust mite antigen. Therefore, the term *extrinsic* asthma should be restricted to those patients in whom there is a clear history of attacks being provoked by exposure to an allergen, hypersensitivity to which can be confirmed by skin tests. Other patients who give positive skin tests but in whom there is no such history of provocation should be referred to as being 'skin test-positive'.

The classification of asthma into extrinsic and intrinsic types has certainly been of value in clinical practice because there are several important differences between these polar groups, including their response to treatment. These differences are summarized in Table 7.1. For instance, sodium cromoglycate is usually highly effective in extrinsic asthma whereas it is generally disappointing in intrinsic asthma. Likewise, sympathomimetic drugs are usually much more effective in extrinsic than in intrinsic asthma. Although steroids are effective in both forms, the majority of patients with extrinsic asthma can be managed without them, whereas the majority of patients with intrinsic asthma require steroids either intermittently or on a long term basis.

Although there are true differences between these two polar groups of asthma, the validity of this type of classification has increasingly become open to doubt. As we have seen, there are many skin test-positive asthmatic patients who cannot be regarded as falling into the extrinsic group. Although it seems probable that the fundamental abnormality of the bronchi which gives rise to

Table 7.1 Contrasting features of the polar groups of asthma.

	Extrinsic	Intrinsic
History of provocation by allergens	Yes	No
Skin tests	Positive	Negative
Serum levels of IgE	Usually raised	Not raised
Coexistence with hay fever	Frequent	Infrequent
Past history of eczema	Frequent	Infrequent
Close relatives with:		
Asthma	Frequent	Frequent
Other allergic disorders	Frequent	Infrequent
Onset	Usually in early life	Any age, commonly after 30
Course	Usually intermittent	Usually persistent
Provocation by exercise	Frequent	Infrequent
Response to: Sympathomimetics	Good	Often poor
Sodium cromoglycate	Good	Usually disappointing
Steroids	Good	Good

airways obstruction is not the same in both forms of asthma, our present knowledge is too meagre to permit a classification of asthma to be made on a pathophysiological or pathopharmacological basis.

AETIOLOGICAL FACTORS

Allergy |

The realisation that many patients with asthma were hypersensitive led to a situation, particularly in continental Europe and in North America, in which allergy held a predominant place in both research and therapy of asthma. It was widely believed that patients with intrinsic asthma must be hypersensitive to some allergen which had yet to be discovered. Although it is highly probable that some, as yet undiscovered *immunological* mechanism is responsible for intrinsic asthma (this being suggested by the beneficial action of steroids), it is clear that factors other than immunological ones must be operative.

Host Factors

Inherited Predisposition
There is considerable evidence that predisposition to asthma is inherited. Studies of twins have shown there to be a much higher concordance of asthma in monozygotic than in dizygotic twins. Nevertheless, complete concordance is not found in monozygotic twins, suggesting that there is an interaction with environmental factors which may activate a latent, inherited predisposition.

A familial history of asthma is commonly given by patients with both extrinsic and intrinsic asthma. However, whereas patients in the former group frequently give a familial history of other allergic conditions as well, in patients with intrinsic asthma such a familial history is no more common than that given by control subjects. This suggests that the predisposition to bronchial hyper-reactivity and the predisposition to allergy are inherited separately.

Age
The most common age at which children begin to have recognisable attacks of asthma is between two and four years. Before that age many children who later become subject to typical attacks of asthma suffer either occasionally or repeatedly from episodes of 'wheezy bronchitis' when they have a respiratory infection.

There is a marked tendency for children to 'grow out' of asthma between the ages of 8 and 12 years. Although some may never have a further episode, it seems probable that latent hyperreactivity of their bronchi persists in all subjects who have had asthma or wheezy bronchitis in childhood. In an unknown proportion of them this latent tendency becomes reactivated later in life, presumably by environmental factors, leading to a recurrence of asthma.

In some patients asthma first begins in adolescence or early adulthood, this being particularly true of those who have developed hay fever a few years previously. In other patients asthma begins for the first time in middle age or even in old age: usually such patients are found to have the intrinsic form of asthma.

Sex

It has long been recognized that asthma and recurrent wheezy bronchitis is more than twice as common in male than in female children. On the other hand, it is widely believed that late onset asthma occurs more commonly in women. However, this may be because this form of asthma is more easily recognized in women, who usually smoke less heavily than men, and therefore are not so liable to be regarded as having chronic bronchitis.

Psychological Factors

Patients themselves often attribute an attack of asthma to some emotional disturbance and there is abundant evidence, much of it of a highly anecdotal nature, which is cited as evidence that asthma is a 'psychosomatic' disease. While no clinician would deny the great importance of psychological factors in the *management* of asthma, their role in its aetiology is much more questionable. Although some clinicians continue to believe that an asthmatic patient's personality and his reactions to emotional stress are primary aetiological factors, no study has shown that asthmatic patients have a higher incidence of neurotic traits than the general population. However, undoubtedly severe asthma itself may be a potent cause of emotional disturbance in both the patient and his family.

THE BASIS OF BRONCHIAL HYPERREACTIVITY

An enormous amount of knowledge about asthma has been accumulated from clinical studies and experimental research. Attempts have been made to explain bronchial hyperreactivity on the basis of a single fundamental abnormality.

Immunological Abnormalities

It has already been noted that a large group of patients with asthma (those with the extrinsic form) are hypersensitive to a variety of antigens and that many of their attacks of asthma can be directly ascribed to exposure to these antigens. It would appear that such patients have inherited not only bronchial hyper-reactivity but also the propensity to become sensitised to substances which are encountered commonly in the environment but to which normal subjects, despite an equal degree of exposure to them, do not become hypersensitive. At present it is impossible to explain why many subjects become sensitised but never have any symptoms of hypersensitivity, nor why in others hypersensitivity symptoms are confined to the upper respiratory tract (allergic rhinitis), while in yet others the lower respiratory tract is affected (as in asthma). The efficacy of steroid therapy in patients with intrinsic asthma suggests that some, as yet unknown immunological mechanism is operative in this form of asthma also. Nevertheless, in both forms of asthma there are features which are not readily explained on an immunological basis; for instance, the provocation of asthma by exercise, beta-blocking agents and other pharmacological agents such as methacholine.

Biochemical Abnormalities

In the final analysis, it is possible to account for the manifestations of asthma and of many other diseases on the basis of a biochemical abnormality at the cellular level. Neuro-transmitters, catecholamines, hormones, enzymes and — more recently — prostaglandins have all been shown to influence airway resistance. Furthermore, the response of the bronchi to an antigen-antibody reaction must depend in the last resort upon the release of chemical mediators.

While the importance of biochemical factors in asthma is undeniable, it has so far proved impossible to demonstrate the existence of a specific biochemical abnormality in asthmatic patients by which they can be distinguished from normal subjects. It has been postulated that asthmatics might have an inherited or acquired deficiency of adenylcyclase, an enzyme which is essential in the cycle of chemical processes involved in bronchial muscle relaxation, but actual proof of such deficiency is so far lacking.

One of the most interesting developments in the field of asthma research during the last ten years has been the discovery of sodium cromoglycate. It has proved to be of great value, particularly in patients with extrinsic asthma, and it is believed that its action is to stabilise mast cells and to prevent the release from them of bronchoconstrictor mediators. It has also been shown that sodium cromoglycate gives protection against exercise-induced asthma, but the mechanism by which it does so remains obscure.

DIAGNOSIS

In patients who are subject to typical, paroxysmal attacks of wheezing, diagnosis presents no problem. However, in other patients the diagnosis of asthma may be easily overlooked. It should be considered in any patient who has recurrent attacks of bronchitis during which wheeze is a prominent feature.

History

Enquiry should be made about the circumstances in which attacks of asthma have occurred and whether the patient has noticed any factors which might have provoked them, such as contact with dust, pollens, animals or after eating certain foods. Patients who are allergic to the housedust mite have often noticed that they wheeze when bedroom dust is disturbed or their bedding is shaken. Asthma occurring only during the late spring or summer is suggestive of hypersensitivity to the pollens of grass, flowers or trees, particularly if there is also a history of hay fever. Contact with house pets does not have to be direct to provoke an attack. Children may have asthma attacks associated with visiting a house where a dog or cat is owned even though the animal is not present at the time of the visit.

Hypersensitivity to aspirin or a closely related chemical, tartrazine – used for colouring foods and soft drinks, is common in patients with intrinsic asthma. Other foods and drinks may give rise to asthma in some patients, particularly nuts, chocolate, milk, sherry and other wines.

Enquiry about the patient's occupation is of importance. Workers in the plastic industry and in the electrical trade are liable to develop asthma due to the inhalation of isocyanates: these are formed in the fumes given off when plastic is heated – for instance, during the soldering of wires sheathed in plastic for insulation and in the use of polyurethane varnishes.

In asthma, dyspnoea is characteristically worse during the early hours of the morning or on awakening. A history of sleep being disturbed by cough and wheezing is highly suggestive of asthma but of course these symptoms may also be caused by left ventricular heart failure. Physical exertion, particularly running and jumping, can provoke attacks of wheeze in some asthmatics and is very common in children.

Many asthmatics give a history of 'colds always going down onto the chest and starting an attack of wheezing'. This is common in those with the symptoms of chronic bronchitis, – that is, intermittent or persistent expectoration of sputum. In this context it is essential to ask patients about their smoking habits.

Patients should also be asked whether they have been or still are subject to hay fever or eczema. A history of recurrent or persistent sinusitis and nasal polypi, which often have led to numerous consultations with and operations by ENT surgeons, is common in both the extrinsic and intrinsic forms of asthma.

A familial history of asthma or recurrent bronchitis with wheezing in a first degree relative or grandparent is commonly given by asthmatic patients.

Physical Examination

Inspection of the chest may give some indication of the degree of airways obstruction. Hyperinflation, poor expansion and use of the accessory muscles are all suggestive of severe obstruction. Structural changes in the chest, arising secondarily from longstanding airways obstruction, may be present. Children with severe asthma tend to develop kyphosis and rounding of the shoulders.

Auscultation

The chief value of ausculation is to exclude other conditions resembling asthma which also give rise to dyspnoea and/or wheeze. It should permit the identification of other diseases which also cause dyspnoea (see the section below on differential diagnosis). Dyspnoea may not be caused by airways obstruction at all. It should also be remembered that dyspnoea occurring in an asthmatic patient may be caused by some superimposed disease, such as pneumonia, spontaneous pneumothorax, or the collapse of a part or the whole of a lung by bronchial obstruction, as occurs in bronchopulmonary aspergillosis.

Measurement of Ventilatory Function

This should be regarded as a part of the clinical examination. Provided that the earlier parts of the examination have excluded other types of disordered function, it can be safely assumed that impairment of PEF is due to airways obstruction. The reversibility of airways obstruction is the cardinal clinical criterion of asthma. One of the most important principles in the management of the disease, to which reference will be made repeatedly in the course of this chapter, is the objective measurement of airways obstruction. While auscultation is of value in a *qualitative* sense, — it enables asthma to be distinguished from other diseases which also cause dyspnoea — it is of much less value in a *quantitative* sense, being an unreliable guide to the severity of airways obstruction.

The characteristic abnormality of asthma is the presence of *wheeze*. This can be defined as a high-pitched sound, present during at least the greater part of expiration, which is heard more or less uniformly throughout all regions of the chest. However, neither the pitch nor the loudness of wheeze is determined by the severity of airways obstruction.

Both the degree of airways obstruction and its reversibility are easily measured. Two instruments, the Vitalograph and the peak flow meter, are available for the purpose and both are eminently suitable for use in family practice. A description of their use and a discussion of their relative merits are given in Chapter 5. One of these instruments should be part of the diagnostic equipment of every family practice.

If airways obstruction is *reversible*, FEV_1 and PEF improve after an inhalation of isoprenaline. Failure to respond to isoprenaline indicates that the airways obstruction is either refractory or irreversible. *Refractory* airways obstruction responds to corticotrophin or steroids given in high dosage for several days. *Irreversible* airway's obstruction does not respond to steroids.

Evaluation of airways obstruction is fully described in Chapter 5.

DIFFERENTIAL DIAGNOSIS

One of the most famous quotations concerning asthma was that made by Chevalier Jackson — 'all that wheezes is not asthma'. Although there is no justification for invoking his aphorism to make a firm distinction between asthma and recurrent wheezy bronchitis, it serves to remind the clinician that wheeze can be caused by mechanisms other than those which are operative in asthma — notably, bronchostenosis, carcinoma or an inhaled foreign body.

In children a common source of confusion is the resemblance between asthma, croup and the whooping cough syndrome[3,4]. In young children one should bear in mind the possibility of cystic fibrosis, because early diagnosis of that disease is all-important in the prevention of lung damage.

Although wheeze sometimes occurs with left ventricular heart failure and pulmonary oedema ('cardiac asthma') (page 235), this condition can usually be distinguished by a history of a very sudden onset of dyspnoea, the presence of a raised jugular venous pressure and fine crepitations at the lung bases.

Farmer's lung and other forms of alveolitis, such as bird fancier's lung and cryptogenic fibrosing alveolitis, can usually be distinguished from asthma by physical examination, widespread crepitations being the characteristic abnormality found in this group of diseases.

Asthma and Bronchitis

Reference has been made already to difficulties which arise from the resemblance between what is considered by some doctors to be bronchitis and by others asthma. From long custom each of these terms carries a special connotation, although in neither case is there any justification for this. Thus, bronchitis is generally considered to be of infective origin while asthma is regarded as being due to non-infective causes. Although in large part this is a problem of semantics, it is possible to distinguish between two polar extremes.

In acute bronchitis, occurring in patients with no previous history of either asthma or chronic bronchitis, there is hypersecretion of mucus and an inflammatory reaction in the larger airways, the latter process being due to one of the many different types of respiratory viruses or to a pathogenic bacterium. In uncomplicated asthma two of the components of airways obstruction — the intraluminal exudation and mucosal oedema — could be justifiably regarded as constituting an inflammatory reaction but it is believed that this is different in kind and causation from that which occurs in acute bronchitis due to respiratory infection.

Several difficulties arise when one attempts to place most acute episodes of lower respiratory illness in either of these polar categories.

1. Asthmatics are no less prone than normal persons to respiratory infections — indeed it seems probable that some asthmatics are especially susceptible.

2. There are patients who have recurrent episodes of 'wheezy bronchitis' when they have a respiratory infection but who never wheeze under other circumstances, and so are not generally regarded as having asthma. Although it would seem that their wheeze is caused by narrowing of the small airways, at present we are ignorant of the pathological nature of 'wheezy bronchitis' and whether it arises as an extension of infection from the larger airways or is due to the same mechanisms which operate in asthma.

3. Most patients with chronic obstructive bronchitis tend · to have recurrent 'exacerbations', during which they may or may not have wheeze. Undoubtedly, many such episodes are due to viral infection and secondary bacterial infection, but other causes include chemical irritation, such as atmospheric pollution, and other non-specific irritants. Whatever pathological changes occur during exacerbations, they are superimposed upon those of chronic obstructive bronchitis which include hypertrophy and hyperplasia of mucus-secreting glands and goblet cells throughout the bronchial tree.

From the above it will be seen that it is often impossible to infer from either the history or physical signs whether an acute lower respiratory illness is 'bronchitis' or 'asthma'. Moreover, it is now clear that some episodes which appear to be typical attacks of asthma are in reality caused by viral infection, while conversely some episodes which appear to be acute bronchitis are in fact manifestations of asthma.

There is no doubt that respiratory viruses are the most common, primary causes of infection of the upper and lower respiratory tract. A very large number of respiratory viruses have now been identified and almost certainly there are others which remain to be discovered. Respiratory viruses constitute one of the most frequently encountered environmental hazards to which the respiratory tract is exposed in urban populations. Because the majority of patients who are infected by viruses do not wheeze, it would appear that the occurrence of wheezy bronchitis is determined by the host factor of bronchial hyperreactivity.

However, the mechanisms whereby viral infection provokes wheeze in suscep-tible persons remains obscure.

There is increasing evidence that rhinoviruses, which formerly were thought to cause nothing more serious than the common cold, are associated more than any other type of virus with episodes of acute bronchitis. Since there are about one hundred antigenically distinct types of rhinovirus to which apparently there is no cross-immunity, it clearly must take a long time before an individual can develop immunity to all the serotypes which he may encounter.

Secondary bacterial infection commonly occurs in patients with long-standing, unrelieved asthma and in those asthmatics who have co-existent chronic obstructive bronchitis. The most common organism which infects the lower respiratory tract is *Haemophilus influenzae*. It is not known whether *H. influenzae* causes an immunological reaction in the bronchi which conceivably might reinforce the factors which gave rise to asthma in the first place.

INVESTIGATIONS

Eosinophilia
Specimens of sputum should be sent to the laboratory for examination of their content of eosinophil cells. Estimation of eosinophils in the blood is of less value, because it is often the case that little or no excess is found in the blood whereas sputum expectorated at the same time shows a pronounced eosino-philia. If the sputum appears to be purulent or the history and physical examination suggest that the patient has co-existent chronic bronchitis, it should be sent for bacteriological investigation.

Skin Tests
Although skin tests are of no value in the diagnosis of asthma, they are important for two reasons. First, a patient in whom no test gives a positive reaction can be assigned to the intrinsic group of asthma and this has important implications for treatment. Secondly, positive reactions are of value in confirming a history of provocation of attacks by exposure to house dust, pollens, moulds, or pets. Such a demonstration of allergy adds greater conviction to the clinician's advice over measures which should be taken to eliminate or avoid exposure to the offending allergens. It should never be forgotten that a positive reaction to any allergen occurring in the absence of a history of wheeze being provoked by exposure to it is probably irrelevant as an aetiological factor in that patient's asthma: it does not justify a course of desensitising injec-tions.

ASSESSMENT

Careful assessment of every patient is essential if he is to be treated properly. The family practitioner should try to obtain answers to the following questions:

1. How severe is this patient's airways obstruction at this moment in time: is he in danger?
2. How much of his airways obstruction is readily reversible and how much is refractory?
3. How much, if any, of his total airways obstruction is irreversible, due to co-existent structural damage?
4. What provocative factors may be responsible for this patient's asthma and are they preventable?
5. What treatment does the patient require now?
6. What is the plan of treatment in the long term?
7. How good is the patient's psychological adjustment to his having asthma?
8. How intelligent is the patient and how reliable is he likely to be in taking treatment?

Assessment of the severity, reversibility and causes of airways obstruction can only be made by measurements of PEF or FEV_1. A full account of the measurement of PEF and FEV_1 and the assessment of the severity and reversibility of airways obstruction is given in Chapter 5.

GENERAL PRINCIPLES OF MANAGEMENT

The most important principles in the management of asthma are:

1. *Education* of the patient (or the parents of an asthmatic child) about the nature of asthma and the purpose, side-effects, and possible hazards of any treatment which is prescribed for it;
2. *Simplicity of treatment*, using as few drugs as possible at any one time;
3. *Objective assessment of response to treatment* and the control of drug dosage by means of regular measurements of the patient's PEF or FEV_1.

Education

It is important to educate asthmatics about their disease and the nature, purpose, and limitations of the various drugs prescribed to treat it. Not only will adherence to this principle of management result in patients using their drugs correctly and therefore effectively but also it will enable them to gain a greater measure of self-confidence than is the case if they feel dependent upon medical advice being available whenever they have an unexpected attack of asthma.

Clearly, the extent to which patients are capable or willing to 'conduct their own campaign' is determined by their intelligence and personality. Ideally, the doctor's aim should be to help them to become as expert as himself in the management of their asthma. Even the least intelligent patient can be helped to achieve some understanding of asthma. It can be described as a disease in which the bronchial tubes are over-sensitive and tend to become narrowed. Such an explanation of the pathophysiology of asthma in its simplest terms will help the patient to adopt a more confident attitude towards his disease, and will also help him to use whatever treatment he is prescribed for it sensibly and safely.

Psychological Adjustment

Because asthma can at times be an intensely distressing or even alarming experience and also because of recent publicity about its increased mortality, it is hardly surprising that the word has a deeply fearful significance for some patients. The more the family practitioner can help patients to understand asthma and the more he conveys a confident impression that it is not a mysterious disease, the easier will be his patients' acceptance of it. Even so, honesty compels us to admit that there are some aspects of the disease which are still far from understood and that often there is no satisfactory answer to the question which patients so often ask — 'why do I get asthma?'.

Sooner or later, most patients with asthma are told by a well-meaning friend or doctor that they could overcome their illness if only they could relax or come to terms with their emotional problems. Not surprisingly, some asthmatics feel that they are misunderstood and as a result are either resentful or given to self-reproach. It is probable that an asthmatic's attitudes to his illness and to his doctor is determined to a great extent by his past experience of medical treatment.

Children with asthma may come to regard themselves as inferior to normal children and if they are overprotected by their parents the seeds of neurotic invalidism are easily sown. Therefore, children with asthma must be encouraged to regard their tendency to wheezing attacks as a nuisance which temporarily they have to learn to live with. Restrictions should be kept to a minimum and should be imposed only if they are clearly justified. The greater the doctor's success in relieving a child's asthma, the easier will be the child's and his parents' psychological adjustment to the disease.

If asthma is treated effectively and with confidence it should seldom cause psychological problems. When it occurs in patients who already have anxiety neurosis or depression these should be evaluated and treated in their own right.

Explaining the Drug Treatment

If the large number of different types of treatment[5] which are now available for asthma are a source of confusion to many doctors, how much more difficult must it be for patients to understand their purpose and action? All too often one encounters patients who have no idea what the purpose is of the treatment which they are taking. The action of bronchodilators can be described as that of relaxing 'spasm' in the bronchi. If the patient is taking a bronchodilator in the form of an aerosol he should be shown the proper way of administering it to himself: the canister must be activated at the very beginning of a deep and prolonged inspiration. The possible danger of excessive use of a bronchodilator aerosol should be explained. The patient must understand that if he obtains no relief from his aerosol or if the relief is only short-lasting, it is dangerous to keep repeating it: the mere fact of his bronchodilator aerosol 'not working' is an indication that he should seek advice. At the same time the patient should be reassured very firmly that, so long as he does not use his aerosol repeatedly when it gives him no relief, this form of treatment carries no dangers.

When sodium cromoglycate is prescribed for the first time it should be explained to the patient that this treatment is for the *prevention* of asthma and not for the relief of wheeze. One still meets patients who are disappointed by finding that sodium cromoglycate does not relieve their attacks of asthma.

If it is decided that a patient needs to be treated with steroids it is essential that he understands the implications of this form of treatment. It must be emphasized that steroids are not for the relief of 'spasm' but to suppress the factors which give rise to persistent bronchial obstruction and to give long-term protection against them. Hence, the patient can he told that 'steroid tablets are not for relieving the asthma which you have now but they are to prevent the asthma which otherwise you would have tomorrow'. The necessity of adhering to a carefully planned course of treatment must be explained. This is particularly important when a reduction of dosage is contemplated or if an attempt is to be made to withdraw steroids.

Many patients have heard about the side-effects of steroids and reassurance should be given that these should be minimal provided that the doctor's instructions over dosage are carefully followed. However, he should be warned that weight gain is common, although to some extent this can be prevented by adherence to a strict diet.

The recent introduction of steroid aerosols provides another source of confusion for patients. Unfortunately, the metered canister in which the aerosol is supplied is identical in shape and mode of operation with those containing a bronchodilator. The patient must understand the distinction between the actions of these two different aerosols. As in the case of sodium cromoglycate, in some patients the inhalation of a steroid aerosol causes reflex broncho-constriction. Furthermore, it is all important that a steroid aerosol is inhaled as deeply as possible so that it reaches the smallest airways. To promote this it is desirable that the patient should take an inhalation of a bronchodilator aerosol to overcome any bronchial constriction about five minutes before he inhales the steroid aerosol.

Simplicity of Treatment

Treatment must be kept simple and as few drugs as possible should be taken at any one time. Moreover, these should not merely be different types or brands of drugs which have an identical action. Sometimes a situation arises in which a patient may previously have obtained satisfactory relief from asthma by bronchodilator tablets but then finds that these are no longer effective. What often follows is that on each visit to his doctor a new form of treatment is substituted or added and eventually the sum total of tablets, suppositories and aerosols which the patient is supposed to be taking reaches a remarkable number. In such a situation it is essential to review the whole position very carefully and to plan the patient's further treatment on a rational basis.

Objective Assessment of Response to Treatment

No family practitioner can treat asthma effectively unless he has a peak flow meter or a Vitalograph and is prepared to make regular measurements of PEF or FEV_1. This is of particular importance in the control of dosage in maintenance steroid therapy which is discussed in a later section of this chapter.

TREATMENT OF ASTHMA

There are two aims in the treatment of asthma:

1. Effective alleviation of symptoms due to airways obstruction;
2. Prevention of further attacks of asthma by attempts to counteract the effects of supposed aetiological factors, such as allergy, infection or psychological stress.

However, before these two aspects of treatment are considered some discussion of the importance of the route of administration of various drugs is appropriate.

Routes of Drug Administration

It must be realised that any drug used for the treatment of asthma can only act if an adequate dose of it reaches the bronchi. Clearly, a drug given by mouth, by injection or in suppository form has to be transported to the bronchi by the circulation and therefore a large dose of the drug is required and there is the likelihood of systemic side-effects occurring when these routes of administration are used.

One of the major advances in the treatment of asthma has been the achievement of greater selectivity of both the actions of drugs and their mode of administration. Thus, bronchodilators have been introduced which have a much greater effect upon the bronchi than upon the heart whilst their preparation in aerosol form permits them to be given in a small dose which is applied directly to the bronchi. Likewise, the introduction of steroid aerosols obviates the systemic side-effects of steroid therapy.

Any drug given in aerosol form is absorbed to some extent through the buccal mucosa or from the bronchi and may give rise to side effects. Steroid aerosols are also absorbed to some extent but it appears that a large proportion of steroid so absorbed is converted into an inactive form.

Adrenaline is inactive when taken orally and therefore has to be given by injection or as an aerosol. Similarly, sodium cromoglycate is very poorly absorbed if taken by mouth and therefore it has to be inhaled.

The value of xanthine derivatives (theophylline, aminophylline etc.) is limited by the irritation they cause to the gastric mucosa. Aminophylline is best given by intravenous injection: although it is also well absorbed through the rectum it may give rise to proctitis if used over a prolonged period.

Alleviation of Symptoms

Bronchodilators bring about relaxation of the bronchi by either a sympatho-mimetic or anticholinergic action. The former alters the biochemical processes which are involved in the relaxation of smooth muscle, these being the cyclic AMP system in which adenylcyclase plays a vital part (see page 82). Because their action is concerned with bronchial muscle relaxation, they can only confer benefit if bronchoconstriction is the major component of airways obstruction. If this is the case, improvement after the inhalation of a sympathomimetic aerosol occurs rapidly and is maximal within about five minutes, as can be shown by serial measurements of PEF. Anticholinergic bronchodilators, while they bring about some relaxation of smooth muscle, probably exert their main effect by counteracting the other components of airways obstruction: in any case, their action is much slower than that of sympathomimetic broncho-dilators.

Some sympathomimetic drugs, such as adrenaline and ephedrine, stimulate both alpha- and beta- receptors in the bronchi. Because it is the latter which are involved in bronchial muscle relaxation, the search was made for drugs that had an almost exclusively beta-receptor effect. Isoprenaline was the first of these to be developed: although it was far more powerful than its predecessors, it was found to stimulate beta-receptors in the heart and to cause tachycardia. Orciprenaline was among the first of the more specific bronchial beta-receptor stimulants to be developed and it has the advantage of a longer action than isoprenaline. More recently, salbutamol, isoetharine and terbutaline have all been introduced: these possess a still greater selective action on bronchial beta-receptors and their effect is more prolonged than that of orciprenaline.

Bronchodilator aerosols, especially isoprenaline, were incriminated as a cause of the recent rise in mortality from asthma. Sudden death in asthma is discussed more fully in a later section of this chapter but here it needs to be said that the evidence on which that view was based was almost entirely circumstantial. Nevertheless, so long as any doubt remains about the safety of bronchodilator aerosols, the family practitioner must emphasize that their excessive use may be dangerous. It is reasonable to allow patients to use an aerosol up to 10 times in 24 hours.

Bronchodilator tablets take longer to act than aerosols, are generally less effective and are more liable to cause side-effects. Often they consist of two or more constituents, such as ephedrine and a xanthine derivative, combined with either an antihistamine or a mild sedative such as phenobarbitone or amylo-barbitone. Xanthine derivatives act by inhibiting an enzyme which destroys endogenous and exogenous sympathomimetics. Theoretically, they should have a synergistic effect when combined with a sympathomimetic drug and this has been made use of in some preparations. The regular taking of a barbiturate which is incorporated in all these preparations is to be deprecated because of their effects on the respiratory centre, the risk of habituation and because there is evidence that barbiturates reduce the efficacy of steroids if these are being taken concurrently.

Bronchodilators for Children

The principal need for orally taken bronchodilators is for the treatment of asthma in children. Medicines containing either orciprenaline or sulbutamol are the most effective of those which are available.

Apart from their use as a mild sedative, antihistamines are of no value in the treatment of asthma. When asthma either starts or is worse at night they may be given to ensure sleep in a frightened or restless child.

PREVENTIVE TREATMENT

Avoidance of Specific Allergens

Only seldom is it possible to determine with certainty the immediate provocative factor causing an attack of asthma. However, in patients giving a history of asthma occurring in relationship to exposure to house dust, whose hyper-sensitivity is confirmed by skin tests, preventive measures should be taken to reduce exposure. House dust is allergenic because it contains the excreta or dead bodies of the housedust mite — *Dermatophagoides pteronyssinus*. This is a minute arthropod which feeds upon skin scales shed from the body and high concentrations of mites are found in old mattresses. The regular hoovering of mattresses or enclosing them in a plastic container is probably of value in removing mites and skin scales and depriving any mites which remain of access to skin scales. The replacement of feather filled pillows and quilts by washable foam filled ones may be of value. Similar benefit may be obtained by replacing bedroom carpets with some alternative floor covering such as vinyl.

Hyposensitization

In patients whose asthma is clearly provoked by pollens or moulds (such as *Cladosporium* and *Alternaria*), hyposensitization should be considered. Although it is more effective as preventive treatment for allergic rhinitis, a proportion of patients with asthma derive some benefit. As yet, there is no conclusive evidence that hyposensitization against housedust mite confers any benefit. In patients with multiple hypersensitivity the attempt to desensitize them by means of 'cocktails' containing numerous different antigens is to be deplored.

Sodium Cromoglycate

The most logical form of preventive treatment is sodium cromoglycate[6] which prevents the release of mediators from mast cells on allergic challenge and also during exercise. It is of special value in children and in those adults whose asthma is clearly of allergic origin. It generally confers much less protection in those adults who are skin test positive but in whom there is no clear history of allergic factors causing asthma and likewise it is usually disappointing in patients with intrinsic asthma.

Sodium cromoglycate should be prescribed as *plain* spincaps (which, unlike the *compound* spincaps do not contain isoprenaline). Because in some patients the inhalation of the powder causes reflex bronchoconstriction (this being the reason why the makers originally combined it with isoprenaline), all patients should be told to take an inhalation of their bronchodilator aerosol a few minutes before inhaling sodium cromoglycate.

Steroids and Corticotrophin

Although the exact mode of action of steroids is far from understood, they are the only form of therapy which supresses the inflammatory component of asthma — that is, mucosal oedema and intraluminal exudation.

Many family physicians have a deeply held prejudice against steroids and regard them as a last-resort treatment which at best causes disfiguring side-effects and at worst is highly dangerous, and whose use is therefore justified only when the severity of asthma is life-threatening. It cannot be emphasised too strongly that the danger of withholding steroids is often much greater than that of giving them. A striking finding of the enquiry of sudden death in asthma was that a very high proportion of patients were either not being treated with steroids at all or were receiving a dose which was so low as to have no value. So far from restricting the use of steroids to patients with severe, intractable asthma, a good case can be made for their use on a 'pre-emptive' basis, the object being to prevent permanent deterioration of function occurring as a result of prolonged, unrelieved asthma.

Once the decision is made to use steroids they should be given as part of a carefully planned programme.

Systemic Administration

Prednisone (or Prednisolone): This is the best corticosteroid for oral treatment, none of the others having any advantages and indeed some (notably triamcinolone) cause side effects which do not occur with prednisone.

Initially, a high dose (30—60 mg) of prednisone should be given daily. Marked clinical improvement usually occurs within twenty-four hours but is not maximal for several days. After four or five days the dose can be reduced abruptly to an intermediate range of 15—25 mg per day. When measurements of PEF show that no further improvement of function is occurring the dose should be reduced gradually to that which just suppresses the symptoms of asthma, this usually being between 5 and 12.5 mg per day. At this stage it may be necessary to supplement prednisone by regular bronchodilator therapy.

Once a maintenance dose has been achieved there is a choice of three possible future lines of treatment:

1. to continue prednisone indefinitely,
2. to attempt to withdraw it altogether, or
3. to replace it completely or at least partially by a steroid aerosol.

Before reaching a decision to continue prednisone indefinitely, it is mandatory to make at least one definitive attempt to withdraw it. This will ensure that the patient does not continue to take it unnecessarily while, if the attempt is unsuccessful, he will better appreciate the importance of taking it regularly and of co-operating in his follow-up supervision. The maintenance dose should be kept as low as possible and it is usually possible to find a critical dose of prednisone below which the patient invariably relapses.

Advantages have been claimed for intermittent treatment with prednisone, the patient taking it only on alternate days. It is believed that this causes less suppression of the adrenals and in children less suppression of growth. Patients taking prednisone on a maintenance basis should be encouraged to make adjustments to their dose on their own initiative. It should be explained to them that an abrupt increase in dose for a few days is necessary when they suffer a respiratory infection: they should be reassured that no dangers arise from large but short-lasting increases in dosage, nor is it usually necessary to make a gradual reduction of dose once the infection has subsided.

If it is decided to withdraw prednisone without replacing it by a steroid aerosol it is essential that reduction of dosage should occur gradually over several weeks, during which the patient should attend regularly for supervision and measurement of PEF. The use of tablets containing only 1 mg of prednisone enables a small reduction of dose to be made with ease, for instance, 1 mg per day every week. Once steroids have been completely withdrawn the patient should be warned that if he should have a relapse of asthma in the future he will almost certainly need to resume taking prednisone at least in the short term.

The complete or partial replacement of oral steroid therapy by a steroid aerosol will be discussed below.

Corticotrophin: A raised output of endogenous cortisol can be obtained by stimulating the adrenals with corticotrophin (ACTH). This form of steroid therapy has two advantages; first, it does not suppress the adrenals and secondly, it has been claimed that it does not suppress growth in children. Its disadvantages are that it must be given by injection and that it stimulates the adrenals to produce all its hormones, including aldosterone which is liable to give rise to oedema and hypertension. Moreover, the efficacy of corticotrophin depends upon the patient's adrenals being able to respond to stimulation. Hence, in a patient who has received prednisone over a prolonged period and whose adrenals have thereby become suppressed, it is pointless to give corticotrophin for an exacerbation of asthma.

Corticotrophin gel is derived from pigs and occasionally causes severe hypersensitivity reactions, including anaphylactic shock. A synthetic form of the hormone, tetracosactrin, has been developed. Because its action is very short-lasting its only use is for the detection and measurement of adrenal suppression. When combined with zinc, however, its action is considerably prolonged and enables it to be used therapeutically as a depot preparation.

Side-Effects: Almost every patient taking systemic corticosteroids or corticotrophin gains at least some weight and usually there is some degree of facial swelling. Indigestion is often complained of by patients taking high doses of oral steroids but the risks of peptic ulceration and perforation have been exaggerated. A severe degree of hypertension or overt diabetes probably occurs only in those persons with a latent tendency to these diseases. Osteoporosis, leading to collapse of vertebrae, is one of the most serious side-effects to which steroid therapy may give rise. Suppression of the adrenals by oral steroids is discussed below. In general, the risk of any of these side effects is directly proportional to the maintenance dose and the duration of treatment.

It is widely believed that steroids reduce the body's resistance to infection. While this is certainly true in the case of tuberculosis and of some systemic viral diseases e.g., chicken pox and vaccinia, there appears to be no danger of this occurring with respiratory viral infection; indeed, it is the experience of many patients who take long-term steroids that they have less frequent and less severe respiratory infections than they had previously. Likewise, steroids do not reduce the resistance of the respiratory tract to infection by bacteria. Therefore, it is unnecessary to give long-term antibiotics concurrently with steroids.

Adrenal Suppression: Opinions differ about the frequency with which significant adrenal suppression occurs in patients taking long-term corticosteroids. It is most likely to occur when they are taken in high dosage and for several years, whereas it occurs to a negligible extent after courses lasting only a few days. Abrupt withdrawal in a patient whose adrenals have been suppressed by oral steroids creates a dangerous situation in which he cannot respond to the stress of infection, trauma or surgical operation by an increased output of endogenous cortisol. This is also a hazard in patients in whom adrenal suppression has occurred and the maintenance dose of steroids is insufficient. An enquiry into the circumstances leading to the recent increase of sudden deaths from asthma revealed that in a large proportion of patients who had died suddenly steroids had either been stopped a short time before death or were being taken in a low maintenance dose which was not increased before the terminal illness. When possible, it is valuable to carry out an adrenal challenge test by measuring plasma cortisol levels before and after an injection of tetracosactrin. By this means it is possible to find out whether adrenal function has returned to normal or not.

Steroid Aerosols

For many years an intensive search was made for a topically acting steroid which could be inhaled without causing any systemic side-effects or adrenal suppression. All attempts to produce a satisfactory steroid aerosol which satisfied these requirements were failures until the development of beclomethasone dipropionate. This was introduced as Becotide Inhaler in 1972 and already it has been widely used in clinical practice and many studies of its use have been reported[7]. Recently, another steroid aerosol has been introduced — betamethasone 17 — valerate — but despite some of the claims made on its behalf, it does not appear to have any advantage over beclomethasone dipropionate.

It is now clear that steroid aerosols have an important place in the treatment of asthma, particularly as a substitute for orally taken maintenance steroid therapy. It should be realised that it is valueless for the treatment of a severe attack of asthma for two reasons. First, it has to be inhaled deeply and this is impossible in the presence of severe broncho constriction and secondly, its action, like that of oral steroids, is not immediate. Although it has been used successfully as primary treatment in some patients with chronic asthma it is preferable to give oral prednisone first in high dosage, so as to achieve as complete suppression of asthma as possible and then maintain this state by substituting beclomethasone dipropionate aerosol.

In the case of steroid aerosols, perhaps more than in any other form of treatment for asthma, it is essential that both doctor and patient have a thorough understanding of their purpose, their action, and their limitations. Every patient in whom long term oral steroids have been successfully withdrawn and replaced by beclomethasone dipropionate must be given a reserve supply of prednisone and should be told to take this in high dosage (at least 20 mg per day for 3 or 4 days) at the first onset of a lower respiratory infection.

Withdrawal of long-term oral steroid therapy under cover of a steroid aerosol must be carried out gradually and under careful supervision with regular measurement of PEF, because of the dangers from adrenal suppression already discussed. When possible, assessment of adrenal function by the method outlined above should be carried out.

The likelihood of being able to replace prednisone entirely by beclomethasone dipropionate aerosol is determined largely by the maintenance dose of the former. When this is less than 7.5 mg per day it should nearly always be possible to withdraw oral steroids completely. On the other hand, the usual dose of beclomethasone dipropionate (400 microgrammes daily) will seldom be sufficient to replace a dose of prednisone greater than 10 mg per day, although it may permit a valuable reduction to be made in the dose of prednisone and therewith reduce the likelihood of systemic side-effects. It is possible to increase the dose of steroid aerosol to 1000 microgrammes per day and this may enable a higher dose of prednisone to be replaced completely. Still higher doses of the aerosol have no advantage over oral steroid therapy because a sufficient amount of beclomethasone dipropionate is absorbed to cause adrenal suppression.

THE MANAGEMENT OF LIFE—THREATENING ASTHMA (STATUS ASTHMATICUS).

The term status asthmaticus is impossible to define and therefore the term life—threatening asthma is preferred to describe a situation in which there is a severe degree of refractory airways obstruction, leading to exhaustion and serious physiological disturbances which, if unrelieved, will cause death. Asthma which has become life—threatening can only be treated in hospital.

Accurate assessment of this situation is one of the most important emergency decisions which the family practitioner has to make. In many instances of sudden and unexpected death from asthma occurring between 1961 and 1967 a retrospective enquiry disclosed that there had clearly been a failure by the patients themselves, their relatives and their doctors to appreciate how dangerously ill.

Assessment

There are certain categories of asthmatic patients who are especially at risk of life-threatening asthma:

1. Those who have recently ceased taking long-term steroids;
2. Those who have ever been previously admitted to hospital for severe asthma, particularly if this has occurred within the previous two months;
3. Those whose asthma is thought to be due to psychological causes;
4. Those who are regarded as being a nuisance and making unwarrantable demands upon their doctors;
5. Those who are unco-operative and unreliable in taking treatment or who are reluctant to seek medical advice.

One of the most important points in the history given by patients with life—threatening asthma is that they are unable to obtain any relief from a bronchodilator aerosol. The principal guides which should be sought in assessment are exhaustion, cyanosis and tachycardia. Auscultation of the chest may be completely misleading because so little air is conducted in and out of the airways that it does not generate wheeze or rhonchi. The ultimate cause of death is hypoxia, due not only to intense bronchial muscle constriction but widespread plugging of small airways by exudate or mucus.

Treatment

If the patient has tachycardia the only bronchodilator drug which can be safely given is aminophylline: a dose of 0.25—0.5 g for an adult should be given by slow intravenous injection. Hydrocortisone (at least 200 mg) should also be given intravenously, although this cannot be expected to exert any effect for at least an hour. Arrangements should be made to admit the patient urgently to hospital. Oxygen is vital and the ambulance should be told to bring this to the house so that it can be given at the earliest possible moment and continuously on the way to hospital.

It cannot be emphasized too strongly that severe asthma is an emergency. Even if the patient is known to be neurotic or liable to anxiety tension, it is highly dangerous to proffer reassurance that the attack will subside spontaneously. One can only deplore statements such as that which appeared in a book written for a family practitioner readership on the psychopathological aspects of asthma — 'severely ill asthmatics who do not respond to routine treatment usually have grave emotional illness. . . . Successful resolution of the emotional difficulties leads to the virtual disappearance of the asthma. And failure to resolve the problem is associated with the persistence of the asthma. Those physicians who do not find emotional conflict in status asthmaticus are, so to speak, emotionally tone deaf'. Be that as it may, any physician who fails to recognize the very severe physical disturbances of 'status asthmaticus' or hopes to relieve these by attention to the patient's emotional problems is running the great risk of a situation in which the emotional problems of his late patient are of no more than academic interest.

SUDDEN DEATH IN ASTHMA

An alarming rise in mortality from asthma occurred in the UK between September 1961 and March 1967. Thereafter, mortality fell sharply and the trend continued until September 1969 by which time it had fallen to its previous level during 1959 and 1960. During this period of six and a half years more than 3500 deaths in patients of all ages occurred in excess of the number that would have been expected on the basis of experience in the years before 1961. The largest increase in mortality occurred in children aged 10 to 14 years, in whom there was a sevenfold rise in the number of deaths.

During 1966 and 1967 one after another report appeared of unexpected and sudden deaths occurring in asthmatic patients. In many cases patients were found to have an empty canister of a bronchodilator aerosol by their sides. In Britain this led the Committee on Safety of Drugs in 1967 to issue a warning about the possible dangers of bronchodilator aerosols.

As soon as it became clear that a real increase in mortality had occurred, the British Medical Research Council set up a special Committee to examine the problem. By this time it had been noted that the sales of bronchodilator aerosols in this country had also increased between 1961 and 1967, and that this rise in sales closely parallelled the rise in mortality. By this time both the sales of aerosols and the mortality from asthma had begun to decline. This seemed to provide strong circumstantial evidence that the two phenomena were causally related.

The view became widely accepted that the excessive use of sympatho-memetic aerosols in patients who were already hypoxic had caused fatal arrhythmias. However, it was difficult to explain why the largest increase in mortality occurred in young asthmatics in whom arrhythmias would be less likely to occur than in patients over 55 years of age, in whom there was hardly any increase in mortality.

Correlations over time can be notoriously unreliable as evidence of causal relationships. Proof that bronchodilator aerosols were a direct cause of death is lacking. An alternative explanation for the rise in mortality might be that the recent introduction of a form of treatment which usually was so effective had made patients dependent upon their aerosols and when their asthma failed to respond they did not appreciate the great danger of that situation. On this view patients died despite their excessive use of bronchodilator aerosols because their asthma was of such severity that it could not respond to that form of treatment.

Another remarkable finding of retrospective enquiries into the circumstances preceding sudden death in asthma was that in over 80 per cent of cases death was said to have been unexpected and in a quarter of all cases in which information was available the terminal episode was said to have lasted for less than an hour. Yet, almost invariably the autopsy findings were those of severe asthma with extensive plugging of the small airways and it seems improbable that such changes could have occurred within so short a space of time.

The most important lesson to be learned is that the failure to respond to a bronchodilator is an indication that airways obstruction has become refractory and is a warning that a serious situation may have arisen requiring careful assessment and treatment on the lines outlined in the previous section.

SPECIALIST SERVICES FOR ASTHMATIC PATIENTS

Asthma Clinics

It must be conceded that not all family practitioners have either the time or the inclination to carry out themselves the investigation of their asthmatic patients, while some consider that they lack the expertise necessary for treating asthma if it does not respond to simple lines of therapy. Because of this, some hospitals have established asthma clinics to which patients can be referred for investigation and assessment.

These clinics provide a valuable service, especially in the case of patients who present difficult problems of management. Ideally, once a full assessment has been completed, the patient should be referred back to his family practitioner with recommendations about treatment which thereafter should be controlled by the family practitioner. Should fresh problems arise, the patient can be reviewed by the clinic and further advice given. Unfortunately, such a close liaison between clinic and family practitioner is all too rare and patients tend to be followed up indefinitely by a clinic while the family practitioner seldom sees them except at times of crisis.

Physiotherapy

Two techniques of physiotherapy are widely used for asthma. The first aims to promote the removal of retained secretions from the bronchi by postural drainage and percussion. There is no doubt about the value of this form of physiotherapy but unfortunately it is usually carried out only when patients are admitted to hospital. The techniques are not difficult to adapt for use at home and the mother of an asthmatic child should receive instruction from a physiotherapist so that she can continue postural drainage and percussion at home.

The other technique of physiotherapy — 'breathing exercises' — is more controversial. The intention is to restore the normal mechanics of respiration when prolonged airways obstruction has induced abnormal patterns of breathing. Enthusiastic advocates of breathing exercises claim that asthma will be improved if only the patient is taught to breathe correctly. What is often not appreciated by those who make such claims is that the disturbed mechanics of respiration are the result, and not the cause, of airways obstruction.

Once deformity of the chest wall has arisen it is unlikely that breathing exercises can reverse this. However, while breathing exercises should never be regarded as a substitute for intensive efforts to abolish airways obstruction by therapeutic means, they are undoubtedly helpful to patients by teaching them to relax at times when they feel an attack of asthma to be impending.

Schools

Many children with severe asthma are sent to special open-air schools with other handicapped children. Whenever possible the child's asthma should be brought under control so that he can remain in an ordinary school and, as far as his disability allows, take part in all its activities. If there is severe emotional disharmony in the child's home, it may be desirable to send the child to a residential school. The chief value of residential schools lies in their provision of constant medical supervision. Claims are often made that 'parentectomy' leads to improvement of asthma, but unless the home situation is extremely bad one should be sceptical about such claims.

References

1. Gregg, I. (1975). Management of Asthma. *Practitioner*.
2. Porter, R. and Birch, J. (eds). (1971). *Identification of Asthma*. Report of a CIBA Foundation Study Group, (London: Churchill-Livingstone).
3. Williams, H. E. and Phelan, P. D. (1975). *Respiratory Illness in Children*, (Oxford: Blackwell Scientific Publications).
4. Godfrey, S. (1975). *Your Child with Asthma*, (London: Heinemann).
5. Rebuck, A.S. (1974). Focus on Antiasthmatic Drugs. II. Therapeutic Aspects. *Drugs*, 7, 370–390.
6. Brogden, R. N., Speight, T. M. and Avery, G. S. (1974). Focus On Sodium Cromoglycate. *Drugs*, 7, 164–282.
7. Gregg, I. (1976). The Place of Beclomethasone Dipropionate Aerosol in the Treatment of Asthma. *Drugs*, 10, 161.

8

Tuberculosis

S. Carne and J. Fry

NATURE

Tuberculosis (TB) is a chronic infection involving mainly the lungs but almost any organ may be affected.

It is spread by inhalation or ingestion of the causative bacillus *Mycobacterium tuberculosis*. The clinical pattern of events in tuberculosis is different from that in other infections. In those who have never before been infected with the organism or who have not had a BCG vaccination, the response to the first infection is a primary tuberculosis (Ghon) focus. In areas of the world where bovine TB is endemic, primary foci commonly occur in the gut. In those areas, such as Britain, where bovine TB has been eradicated the most common route of infection is the respiratory tract and the primary focus is usually in the lung, but sometimes it is in the tonsil. The initial invasion is soon followed by a spread to the regional lymph nodes: the hilar glands if the focus is in the lungs; the mesenteric glands if it is in the gut; and the anterior cervical glands if the focus is in a tonsil. The primary lesion and regional adenitis together constitute a primary complex.

Six weeks after the primary infection hypersensitivity to the protein of the tubercle bacillus develops. This can be demonstrated by any of the tuberculin skin tests (see below). Once it has converted to positive, a tuberculin test only reverts to negative in exceptional circumstances. The primary lesion will usually heal, leaving no trace of its presence except the converted tuberculin test. Sometimes it heals by calcification and the calcified focus can be seen on subsequent X-rays.

Spread of infection from the primary focus may occur. In the lungs a direct spread leads to miliary tuberculosis. The infection may also spread via the lymphatics or the blood stream, leading to a tuberculous infection in almost any organ. TB meningitis*, nephritis and arthritis, once relatively common, are now rare complications in Britain.

Dr. Carne saw a child with TB meningitis during his first week in practice 22 years ago. He has not seen a case since.

Subsequently, a second infection, usually several years later, gives rise to post-primary (adult) pulmonary tuberculosis with all the well known features of that disease. In 1971 there were 12 000 newly notified cases in England and Wales, and 1400 deaths — a fatality rate of over 10 per cent.

Up to 25 or 30 years ago a large proportion of children in Britain had a positive tuberculin reaction, indicating they had had a primary focus at some time. With the successful treatment of adult tuberculosis by chemotherapy, and the consequent reduction in the number of infected persons spreading the disease, coupled with the almost total elimination of TB infected milk, most children today have a negative tuberculin reaction. Every child now found to have a positive tuberculin test, unless he is known to have had a BCG vaccination, should be carefully investigated. If there is any doubt, the child should be seen by a paediatrician or chest physician. Nowadays it is usual to treat every child with a primary focus with a full 12-month course of anti-tuberculous chemotherapy.

TUBERCULIN TESTS

Hypersensitivity to TB proteins can be demonstrated by any of the standard tuberculin tests described below.

The Mantoux Test
The Mantoux test uses an intradermal injection of 0.1 ml 1 : 10 000 old tuberculin (OT). A positive response is an area of induration, at least 6 mm in diameter, within 48 to 72 hours of the test. The site for the injection is usually the forearm and a control solution is injected into the same site on the other arm. If there is no reaction the child is tested with a second injection of 1 : 1000 OT. Sometimes both control and active solutions induce an erythema; this is regarded as a negative response. Instead of OT, purified protein derivative (PPD) is occasionally used.

The Heaf Test
The Heaf multiple puncture test uses a spring-loaded gun with 6 to 12 needles on the end plate. PPD is usually used in preference to OT. In young children the gun is set for a 1 mm injection and in older children or adults it is set for 2 mm. A positive response is the appearance of an indurated ring at the site of inoculation or a series of indurated nodules corresponding to the needle points. The end plate must be carefully sterilised every time it is used, to avoid the risk of hepatitis.

The Tine Test
The Tine test is similar to the Heaf test. Disposable impregnated four-pronged steel discs are used. The test is more expensive to perform than the Heaf test but

it is safer. In family practice, where tuberculin tests are required relatively infrequently, the Tine test is probably the most convenient.

PREVENTION OF TUBERCULOSIS

The main factors in the reduction of both morbidity and mortality from tuberculosis have been the introduction of chemotherapy and the contact follow-up of all identified cases. Additional protection is offered to every child by means of BCG vaccination which provides a controlled primary focus for those who are negative to a tuberculin test. Where there is a family history of TB, the BCG should be given shortly after birth but in most other children it is usual to wait until the age of 11 to 13 years.

PULMONARY TUBERCULOSIS

Pulmonary tuberculosis is very much a social disease being associated with urbanisation and social deprivation. It is still a major problem in Asia, Africa and South America. Although pulmonary tuberculosis may be controlled in developed societies a high degree of alertness is required if we are to maintain this control and achieve early diagnosis when it does occur.

A number of vulnerable groups can be defined:

1. Men over 45 and in particular those over 65;
2. Asian immigrants — Indians have a twelve-fold greater risk of pulmonary tuberculosis than average, and Pakistanis have a twenty-six-fold greater risk;
3. Alcoholic-dropouts and vagrants;
4. Diabetics.

Clinical Features

The most common way of presentation now is by the unexpected abnormal chest radiograph often taken for routine purposes. The old-fashioned presentation with cough, haemoptysis, loss of weight and night sweats, is still possible but unusual. It is the chronic bronchitic old man who has a chest radiograph showing radiological suspicion of tuberculosis that is the more usual pattern.

The Asian immigrant who continues coughing after an apparent common respiratory infection should considered as a 'possible' case. Vagrants and alcoholics should be screened periodically, for amidst their productive coughers there will be some with tuberculosis.

Diagnosis and Investigation

Once the condition is considered to be even remotely possible a chest radiograph must be arranged, sputum bacteriologically examined and cultures for tubercle bacilli undertaken. Contacts should also be investigated.

Management

The treatment of tuberculosis is by effective chemotherapy and regular supervision to assess progress.

The management now is relatively simple providing that the physician knows and is familiar with the multi-drug regimes to be used and realises the importance of regular supervision of the patient to ensure his cooperation with the medication and to assess progress by chest radiography and sputum examination and culture.

If he is prepared to arrange the supervision there is no reason why the family practitioner should not treat his patient himself. Alternatively, he may consider that the experience and the organisation at the disposal of the local chest clinic are such that his patient will fare better under their care.

Chemotherapy

Unless two or three antituberculous drugs are given together, drug resistance in the tubercle bacilli will soon develop, Even now, about 4 per cent of new untreated cases of tuberculosis are infected by organisms resistant to one standard drug.

Initial therapy should be triple, using isoniazid, para-aminosalicylic (PAS) and streptomycin. Isoniazid (300 mg) and PAS (12 g), combined in a single medicament, should be given in two divided doses daily, and streptomycin injected daily (1 g daily in those under 45 and 0.75 g daily for those over 45). Triple therapy should continue for the first three months and then streptomycin can be stopped. Isoniazid and PAS should be continued for 18 months to 2 years.

As alternatives, newer drugs are now available as companions to Isoniazid. Thiacetazone (150 mg daily) is cheap and effective but is liable to cause allergic reactions. Ethambutol (25—15 mg/kilo daily) is expensive. It is effective but has risks of ocular toxicity. Rifampicin (450—600 mg daily) is also highly effective but expensive and there is some evidence of hepatotoxicity.

General Measures

Once chemotherapy has started there is little reason for restricting the patient's activities and once the sputum has been shown to be free of tubercle bacilli, then no restrictions of contact need be made.

Follow-up
It is essential to continue follow-up of tuberculous patients for some years after chemotherapy has stopped, since breakdown and recurrence may occur. Therefore, a once or twice yearly chest radiograph should be taken.

9

Bronchial Cancer

J. Fry

Cancer of the bronchus is now the most frequent single type of cancer in developed nations. The case mortality rate over 5 years is still over 90 per cent. Nevertheless the first role of the family practitioner is to make a diagnosis as early as possible to pick up those who may be treated successfully, and the second role is the care of terminal cases.

AETIOLOGY

There is no single cause. There is interaction between a number of causal factors. Tobacco smoking, particularly of cigarettes, has been shown to have a definite positive relationship. This is the probable explanation of the dramatic increase in numbers over the past 30—40 years in males, who have been smoking more and more, and in the more recent but progressive increase in deaths from bronchial cancer in women, whose habits of heavy cigarette smoking have been developed only in recent years.

Other sources of irritation are atmospheric pollution, which may account for the greater incidence in urban compared with rural communities, and industrial processes which may also exert some effect on the development of bronchial cancer.

CLINICAL FEATURES

There are no specific symptoms of bronchial cancer. Diagnosis will depend on the need to consider the condition as a possible cause of many symptoms, some associated with the chest and others apparently arising elsewhere in the body.

Any person over 40 with persistent respiratory symptoms should be considered as a possible case, especially if a smoker.

Cough, haemoptysis, breathlessness, chest pain or recurrent chest infections over a short period or slow resolution of a single infection all require urgent investigation to confirm or exclude the diagnosis.

In 10—15 per cent of cases the first features of a bronchial cancer may be quite unrelated to the chest. There may be general malaise, depression or loss of weight. It may present as a confusing neurological picture with features of a cerebellar or cortical disturbance, as a peripheral neuropathy, a myopathy or as myasthenic syndrome. Headache and other features of progressive raised intracranial pressure may be the first symptoms of an intracranial metastasis.

Odd endocrine syndromes may be the first presentations of a bronchial cancer with hypercalcaemia, the carcinoid syndrome and the effects of ectopic oversecretion of ACTH or ADH.

In the chest complications such as lung abscess or pleural effusion as well as pneumonia may be the first feature.

DIAGNOSIS AND INVESTIGATIONS

Once the possibility is raised the diagnosis has to be established by chest radiography followed in most cases by bronchoscopy, biopsy and pathological examination of the material obtained at biopsy.

Two-thirds of bronchial cancers can be visualised at bronchoscopy. In the others diagnosis may have to be based on sputum cytology or biopsy of enlarged cervical lymph glands (when present) or by waiting for some later signs.

The question of the benefits of routine screening by chest radiography is still unsettled. Survival is longer in those picked up early by screening but the ultimate 5-year survival rates are little different.

ASSESSMENT

All persons with a possible bronchial cancer must be radiographed and if suspicion remains they must be referred to a specialist for bronchoscopy and a decision on possible resection. At present only a quarter of all bronchial cancers are suitable for surgical removal, and the decision is that of the surgeon.

All persons with a possible bronchial cancer should be given the benefit of a specialist's opinion, not only for the good of the patient and his family but also to add weight and support to the family practitioner.

MANAGEMENT

The management of any individual case will depend on the site, extent and nature of the tumour as revealed by the investigations. It will depend also on the age and general state of the patient and on a reasoned humane balance of the likely benefits of the treatment against the discomfort and suffering that will be added by the treatment and investigations.

All this has to be considered in the face of the reality that at present the average survival rate is in months rather than in years.

Surgery

Surgical removal is the treatment of choice but the procedure carried out will depend on the stage and site of the lesion. A lobectomy results in less respiratory functional loss than a pneumonectomy. The effects of a pneumonectomy on heavy-smoking middle-aged or elderly men usually are disastrous and lead to a respiratory crippledom for the rest of their lives. A lobectomy in men under 65 should result in little loss of respiratory function.

Radiotherapy

A few dramatic and unexpected long-term cures can sometimes be achieved by external beam radiotherapy but the place of this form of treatment is mainly in palliation and in relief of certain special situations. As well as treating the primary tumour radiotherapy is specifically indicated for the following:

> *Pain* may be caused by infection from bronchial obstruction, and radiotherapy may lead to shrinkage of the primary tumour leading to aeration and drainage. Local spread to involve the mediastinum and chest wall causes severe pain which is only partially relieved by radiotherapy but is occasionally helped by cytotoxic drugs such as nitrogen mustard or radioisotopes instilled into the pleural cavity. Pain from bone involvement by primary spread or metastases should respond well to radiotherapy.
>
> *Cough and haemoptysis* caused by bronchial obstruction or irritation or ulceration often respond quickly to radiotherapy.
>
> *Superior vena caval obstruction* is an indication for radiotherapy in palliative doses and the immediate results are dramatically successful, although the ultimate outcome is hopeless.
>
> *Dysphagia* caused by displacement or distortion of the oesophagus by the tumour may respond to radiotherapy but not when ulceration has occurred.
>
> *Enlarged lymph nodes* and *secondary skin deposits* are responsive to radiotherapy
>
> *Cytotoxic drug therapy* at present has not been very helpful in the treatment of bronchial cancer.

GENERAL CARE AND FOLLOW-UP

The general care of the patient and his family with bronchial cancer is that of a patient with a progressive terminal condition. It follows the principles outlined in chapter 26. The family doctor is the key member of the team of hospital specialists and community generalists who are brought into action from the beginning and who all have their parts to play during the course of the disease.

Once the initial steps of referral to a specialist and investigation have been taken then time has to be allowed for the whole process to take place. During this time the patient and the family should be seen regularly and some explanation of the condition should be transmitted to both, perhaps with different degrees of seriousness to patient and family, but with constant hope for both.

Once the patient has received the hospital part of the care process then a plan should be organised for the future. The patient should follow his normal routine for as long as possible. Symptoms and problems should be dealt with as they arise but a flexible and optimistic attitude should be maintained. The patient should be seen regularly for general support and review.

FUTURE

It is the great failure of health education that knowing the direct association of tobacco smoking and bronchial cancer the amount smoked has not fallen. Some 70 per cent of men and 50 per cent of women still smoke. Bronchial cancer would become a rare condition if smoking became uncommon and this is a challenge for us all in the future.

The hopes for early diagnosis leading to better results are uncertain. Screening by chest radiography and sputum cytology will need to be done every 3–6 months if early cases in their early stages are to be picked up which is a major and costly national exercise.

10

Ear, Nose and Throat

G.W. Hickish

INTRODUCTION

A large proportion of patients in family practice come with complaints involving this region, and it must be faced at the outset that examination, and treatment, require rather special methods and equipment.

If a certain basic minimum of equipment is not available the practitioner will be frustrated in his efforts to reach a correct diagnosis, and to apply the appropriate treatment. The verb 'apply' is apt, for ear, nose and throat work has an essential manipulative component and frequently calls for more than a quick glance and the writing of a prescription.

Much of the examination and treatment of the ear, nose and throat, involves looking into obscure cavities. This requires:

1. a source of illumination,
2. devices (speculae and tongue depressors) for opening the entrance to the nose, ear and pharynx,
3. lenses for providing magnification in the inspection of the ear,
4. mirrors for revealing cavities otherwise hidden from view (post nasal space and lower pharynx and larynx).

Since both of the examiner's hands need to be as free as possible — particularly where any manipulative measures are needed — it is desirable that he should not have to use one hand purely for holding a light.

In deciding how best to provide suitable illumination in the consulting room, the choice lies between a fixed lamp (mounted on the wall or on a stand) used in conjunction with a head mirror, or a light strapped to the head. Both methods give good illumination. The fixed source of light requires a lens to provide a narrow concentrated beam of light which is reflected by the concave head mirror, to the site under examination. The examiner looks with one eye through the central hole in the mirror down the beam of reflected light. The focal length of most mirrors is about 25 cm.

A head lamp must have a focusing lens and is worn between the eyes. It is a more easily portable method of illumination but requires a transformer (or heavy battery), and once 'plugged in' the examiner is not free to walk about. A transformer with a rheostat is invaluable as a power supply for electrocautery — a facility with many applications in minor surgery. A headlamp, worn at the same time as lens spectacles, if of great value in searching for foreign bodies in eyes. On balance the doctor first equipping himself would probably be best advised to obtain a focusing headlamp and transformer equipped with rheostat controls for both light and electrocautery.

The electric auroscope is indispensible because of its convenience, portability and its magnification. Where the external meatus is clean an excellent magnified view of the inner meatus and tympanic membrane is obtained. An inflation-bulb should be fitted so that the mobility of the tympanic membrane may be assessed. Where wax, discharge or debris obscures the view this will have to be removed and here a headlamp or mirror are more practical.

The inspection of illuminated chambers is much easier if conducted in relative darkness, and the facility to darken the consulting room, or a portion of it, is important. Much of the difficulty in visualising what may be somewhat unfamiliar territory is due to attempting the examination in conditions of lighting which would daunt the specialist.

The Ear

DEAFNESS

The handicap of deafness is common and can have far reaching effects on the sufferer's enjoyment of life, educability, earning capacity, and integration in the family and community — not to mention personal safety. Whilst the prospect of a blind man with dark glasses and a white stick will evoke sympathy, pity, protective instincts, and often admiration, an encounter with a deaf person all too often engenders irritation, exasperation and even contempt.

The causes of deafness are divided into three groups according to the point at which the fault occurs along the route of transfer of sound stimulation from the atmosphere to the brain:

1. *conductive* deafness arises from faults in the external auditory meatus, tympanic membrane, or ossicles;

2. *sensory* deafness arises as a result of cochlear disease;
3. *neural* deafness results from abnormality in the acoustic nerve or its central connections.

Distinction is usually made between *conductive* and *sensori-neural* deafness.

Recognition of Deafness

Whilst the majority of patients experiencing deafness will come sooner or later for help, it behoves the doctor to be on the lookout for deafness which may be either unnoticed by the patient, or even deliberately concealed. There may be partial or total hearing loss in only one ear with normal hearing in the other and this may not be detected unless each ear is tested separately. There may be loss of hearing for only certain frequencies, especially the high tones from about 4000 Hertz.

Recently acquired deafness in young children is suggested by uncharacteristic inattentiveness, disobedience, and inappropriately loud speech – the child may not himself appreciate that he is not hearing normally. Mumps is of importance in this connection. In a survey of mumps in Islington in 1967 2 per cent of cases were found to develop severe unilateral deafness, predisposing them to traffic accidents[1].

During school years, deafness should be excluded where a child's poor scholastic performance cannot be otherwise explained. Deaf children may be slow to learn and may present with behaviour disorders.

One comes to recognise a characteristic form of speech with malpronounciation especially of consonants, monotony of tone, and inappropriate volume, accompanied by an attentive reading of one's own lips, which signifies the patient is 'hard of hearing'. Occasionally the patient himself may be remarkably unaware of his handicap and may become depressed, and almost paranoid, as a result of misunderstood deterioration of communication with his fellows.

It is of the utmost importance to detect deafness in early life as soon as possible, and preferably before one year of age, so that all possible steps can be taken to make the maximum use of such hearing as is present. By means of hearing aids and special training the child may then learn to appreciate the meaning of words and to speak, and may ultimately be capable of integration into an ordinary school. If the hearing defect goes unrecognised till after the age of two years, the best chance of helping the child effectively has been lost.

'At Risk' Groups
Certain infants form an *at risk* group who need careful follow-up:

1. offspring of families where hereditary congenital deafness has occurred, especially where there is consanguinity;

2. premature infants;
3. those who may have been damaged in utero by, for example, Rh incompatibility, postmaturity, anoxia, rubella, toxaemia, syphilis, and teratogenic drugs;
4. infants who suffered severe anoxia during labour;
5. infants who have suffered from such infections as meningitis, mumps or measles during the first year;
6. infants born with disability syndromes which are associated with deafness e.g., cleft palate;
7. any child whose parents suspect deafness is present.

In over 30 per cent of cases the cause of deafness can never be identified. Deafness tends to be suspected by the mother between the ages of 3 and 5 months, either because of lack of facial expression or general awareness, or failure to respond to sounds, especially her voice. Approximately 3 per 1000 children are born with a serious degree of deafness.

Screening for Deafness
It is highly desirable that a list of *at risk* children should be maintained. Under the 1974 National Health Service reorganisation this will be the duty of the Community Physician who should ensure that hearing is tested in these children at least 3 times, first between 8 and 12 months, then at 2—3 years, and finally about 6 months before school entrance, and that, where indicated, they are referred to a special Childrens' Hearing Clinic. These clinics are provided by the area Health Authorities and are normally staffed by a consultant otologist, a paediatrician, a speech therapist, an audimetrician, a peripatetic teacher of the deaf and an educational psychologist.

At the first screening, which may be carried out by the family practitioner, Health Visitor or at an infant welfare clinic, the baby sits on his mother's knee whilst the tester makes low pitched and high pitched sounds (e.g., using a low pitched rattle, then rustling paper or using a bell respectively) at the baby's ear level, one metre removed from each ear in succession and out of sight of the child. His capacity to respond is noted. A range of noise-makers are used which should be meaningful and interesting to the child. Great care must be taken to avoid visual clues. Accuracy at this first screening is crucial.

At 2—3 years the testing consists mainly of getting the child to play with toys, then asking him, at one metre from each ear successively, to perform some act with the toys e.g., 'put the ball in the box''. Above this age more sophisticated screening and testing techniques are used. An Audiotester* provides a useful screening technique in family practice, identifying those children who require a full audiometric examination.

* The Audiotester is available from Keeler, Marylbone Lane, London, W.1.

Children failing screening tests are further investigated at the Childrens Hearing Clinic, and where appropriate are provided with hearing aids. Special training is initiated in which parents play a leading part. Normal children learn speech and language as a result of coming to associate words spoken by their mother with particular objects. Then they imitate their mother's voice, and the foundation of verbal communication has been laid. Much of the work of special training for deaf children is based on an imitation of what has happened in earlier life in normally hearing infants.

Visual Examination of the Ear

When confronted with a patient complaining of deafness in one ear, especially if the patient is a nervous youngster, it is a good practice to look first at the good ear. This will serve to 'desensitise' the patient to the idea of having a speculum introduced to the external meatus, and will reveal to the examiner (provided this side is healthy) the normal appearance of the particular patient's external meatus and tympanic membrane.

The deaf side is then inspected. In many adult cases of recent onset of deafness the cause will be seen to be plugging of the external meatus by wax. Often the patient has been swimming. Removal of wax is considered on page 122.

A view of the tympanic membrane may not be obtained without a certain amount of trouble. The external auditory meati of children are small, and the narrow channel may be obstructed with wax and debris. This may be removed by mopping with pledgets of cotton wool mounted on a Jobson-Horne probe but this must be done with great gentleness or the young patient's confidence will be lost. It is far easier, and more comfortable for the patient, if it is done under direct vision using either a head mirror or head lamp. One hand of the examiner lifts and slightly rotates the pinna to straighten the meatus whilst the other holds the Jobson-Horne probe. Sometimes wax and debris is best removed by syringing, preferably after instilling sodium bicarbonate ear drops for a few days, but never when there is any suggestion of perforation of the tympanic membrane (see page 123).

Where the ear is found to be blocked with a thin purulent material, it will be necessary to mop this out with a Jobson-Horne probe as described above. It is desirable in such cases, particularly at the initial examination, to take a swab for bacteriological examination prior to performing the aural toilet.

When the ear has been thoroughly cleaned it may be possible to discern either that the discharge has exuded from the walls of the meatus as a result of otitis externa, or that it has emerged through a perforation in an inflamed tympanic membrane. Sometimes however it is difficult to be sure at the first inspection which is the case. In otitis externa the skin of the tympanic membrane may itself be inflamed and may have been further irritated by the actual toilet. In otitis media the perforation may be very small, concealed, or even healed, whilst the presence of pus in the ear may have produced an otitis externa. Some guide may be given by a history of an upper respiratory infection, followed by a severe earache which eased simultaneously with the development of actual discharge, indicating otitis media with perforation. Any doubt will usually be resolved at subsequent examination. Toilet, followed by local application of antibiotic and steroid, either as drops or by an impregnated wick, will usually produce improvement in otitis externa, with quick return of the tympanic membrane to a normal appearance.

Where a tympanic perforation is suspected but cannot at first be visualised, the application of negative pressure using the bulb on the electric auroscope or Seigle's speculum may result in a conclusive oozing of pus.

Where the external meatus is clean and dry, the tympanic membrane may be red and bulging as a result of otitis media which will usually have been anticipated where there has been much pain (see page 127), or the dull grey/bluish appearance of 'glue ear' may be seen. Detailed descriptions of the appearance of the tympanic membrane in various disorders are given in the sections which follow dealing with specific conditions. If the tympanic membrane is indrawn and immobile, indicating Eustachian obstruction, inflation of the electric auroscope or Seigle's speculum with the rubber bulbs will help to confirm the immobility.

The existence of Eustachian obstruction may be confirmed by Valsalva's manoeuvre or by Politzerisation.

Valsalva's manoeuvre: The patient is asked to pinch his nostrils with his fingers, blow out his cheeks, and swallow, in an attempt to inflate the Eustachian tube.

Politzerisation: A greater force of air is provided by blowing air into one nostril, (with the other closed) by means of a Politzer bag whilst the patient is asked either to say 'Key, Key, Key . . .' or, alternatively, to sip a glass of water. If the Eustachian tube is patent the tympanic membrane will be seen to move.

A tympanic perforation, dry or moist, will point to past inactive, or active otitis media respectively.

Finally, the tympanic membrane may be seen to be normal. Free mobility on inflation, and translucency so that the long process of the incus can just be made out are strong indications of normality of the tympanic membrane. If the tympanic membrane is completely healthy it is likely that the patient's deafness is either due to otosclerosis or is sensori-neural in type.

Hearing Tests

The Whispered Voice Test
The degree of deafness may be crudely assessed by testing the patients ability to repeat words spoken increasingly quietly at arms length range whilst the ear not

being tested is turned away and closed by the examiner. The words used should sound identical except for the initial consonant and several different groups should be used for each ear. The higher frequencies (which form the consonants) are the most likely ones to be affected.

Tuning Fork Tests

Tuning fork tests are not as reliable as the whispered voice test in detecting defects in hearing because it is very difficult to vary the volume of the sound produced. The value of tuning fork tests lies chiefly in distinguishing between conductive and sensori-neural deafness. A fork vibrating at 512 Hertz is the most commonly used. The doctor equipping himself for the first time with a tuning fork would be well advised to purchase a large one. Lighter tuning forks are cheaper, but their intensity of vibration falls off so quickly after striking that much confusion may result.

Rinne's Test: The fork is struck and the base firmly pressed on the patient's mastoid process. He is asked to lower his raised hand when he can no longer hear the sound. The fork is then transferred forwards and held 1 cm from the external auditory meatus. If he can now hear the fork again the test is said to be positive. If he cannot, the procedure is reversed. If the fork is heard longer by bone conduction the result is described as *Rinne negative.*

A positive result is obtained in the normal ear and in sensori-neural deafness and a negative result occurs in conductive deafness.

A falsely negative Rinne's test may occur in cases of severe unilateral sensori-neural deafness. No sound is heard by air conduction, but when bone conduction is tried sound is heard by conduction across the skull to the other ear. In such cases the better ear must be 'masked' — for example by crumpling a piece of stiff paper close to the ear — and the test repeated.

Weber's Test: This test is useful where there is a marked difference in hearing on the two sides. The base of the vibrating fork is placed on the skull in the midline. Reference of the sound to the deaf ear indicates conductive deafness, whilst reference to the good ear alone occurs in sensori-neural deafness. It has been postulated that extraneous sounds are excluded by the conductive lesion leaving the cochlea on that side free to 'concentrate' on the skull-born vibrations.

Audiometry

The place of audiometry in family practice depends to a large extent on local circumstances. There is no doubt that the availability of a graphic record of a patient's progress can be of great value — for example in determining whether mild 'catarrhal deafness' is responding to treatment, and whether presbycusis or acoustic trauma deafness is severe enough to warrant a hearing aid. The ready availability of audiometry will facilitate much greater selectivity in the referral of patients to hospital clinics for consideration of surgery or the provision of hearing aids.

In some areas doctors are fortunate enough to have the willing co-operation of an audiometrician employed by the Health Authority.

Where this is not possible, the purchase of an audiometer could well be considered. Suitable pure-tone audiometers cost rather less than an ECG machine. They are usually battery operated, and are simple to use, the only important requirement being a quiet cubicle in which to make the recordings. Sounds of a range of frequencies (e.g., 250, 500, 1000, 2000, 4000, 6000 and 8000 Hertz) are fed into the ear under examination at increasing volume starting at 5 decibels (dB) and rising in 5 dB steps until the patient signifies that he hears the note. The threshold is actually determined by an 'up 5, down 10' approach. From the results obtained a graph is plotted of threshold decibels against frequency. Where deafness is encountered on air conduction, bone conduction is then measured with the microphone applied to the mastoid process.

Where there is a marked difference in hearing on the two sides, and whenever testing bone conduction, it is essential to mask the ear not under test, otherwise the deaf ear may be credited with the hearing of the good ear. The audiometer has the facility to supply 'white sound' for this purpose, of a loudness a little greater than the threshold on that side.

Mention might be helpful at this point of a phenomenon known as *recruitment*, which occurs in deafness due to cochlear disease but not in neural deafness. In unilateral cochlear deafness, the difference in sensitivity of the two ears diminishes as the loudness of the 'test tone' increases[2]. A possible explanation for this is that, of the two groups of hair cells in the organ of Corti, the outer is concerned with threshold appreciation, while the inner group is stimulated only by louder sounds. The latter group is thought to be less vulnerable than the former. Presbycusis is a degenerative condition of the cochlea and thus exhibits *recruitment*. One practical result of this is that a slight increase in sound intensity may be heard by the sufferer as a considerable sudden noise. Hence elderly deaf patients may jump with alarm when they finally hear a noise which has been building up (e.g., a bus approaching from behind). Patients with presbycusis who exhibit much recruitment may have considerable problems with hearing aids.

For conversational purposes the most useful hearing occurs around 1000–2000 Hertz and a rough guide is that a hearing loss at this range greater than 40 dB is a serious social handicap. In the absence of other methods for improving hearing, such a hearing loss will usually call for the provision of a hearing aid.

The recording of audiograms is a simple matter which can well be performed by a suitably instructed nurse or other assistant. The procedure only takes a few minutes and the provision of this facility in a practice or medical centre can be of great convenience and benefit to the patients.

Acoustic Impedence Audiometry: For the sake of completeness mention should be made of this technique which is being used, amongst other applications, for screening large numbers of children for deafness. The method essentially measures the capacity of the ear to vibrate when presented with a test sound. It has the advantage of being a purely objective measurement, but is difficult to perform and would not be suitable for occasional use.

Specialist Referral

Having explored as fully as possible a patients' deafness, the decision will have to be made as to whether referral to a specialist is called for.

Conductive Deafness

In the conductive deafness group, referral will usually be with a view to surgical intervention, as in:

1. established 'glue ear';
2. catarrhal deafness, especially where there has not been a satisfactory response to a trial period of medical treatment;
3. deafness due to chronic middle ear disease (where active infection is present, examination under microscopy, suction clearance, snaring of aural polypi, or such active intervention as mastoid surgery may be required; where there is no longer evidence of infection, but appreciable deafness persists, operations to repair perforated tympanic membranes, and sometimes reconstruct the ossicular chain, are available);
4. where the diagnosis of otosclerosis is suspected (many highly successful stapes replacement operations have been performed in patients well over the age of 60).

Sensori-neural Deafness

Where deafness has been established as being of sensori-neural type, an effort must be made to determine the cause. In younger persons with sensori-neural deafness, help in identifying the likely cause may be obtained by careful enquiry into the history.

Acoustic trauma may have resulted from a sudden or continuous loud noise, (for example gunfire, or noisy occupations such as boilermaking).

Infections such as mumps, meningitis and syphilis, and head injuries, and space-occupying lesions such as acoustic neuroma, are other causes of sensori-neural deafness.

Drugs, such as streptomycin and kanamycin, can produce severe deafness whilst others, such as quinine and aspirin, are often responsible for mild sensori-neural deafness which is usually accompanied by marked tinnitis and is usually reversible.

Patients with unexplained unilateral sensori-neural deafness of recent onset require special investigations particularly with a view to excluding the possibility of acoustic neuroma. Caloric tests and sophisticated audiometry and radiology techniques may be required.

Sudden profound sensori-neural deafness constitutes an emergency. Some cases appear to be due to acute, but initially, reversible vascular disturbances, and may respond to stellate ganglion block, intravenous histamine infusion, or other vasodilatation methods. No time should be lost in getting the patient to an ENT Department before ischaemia results in irreversible cochlear damage.

The majority of cases, however, are idiopathic[3], and immediate steroid treatment (for example, prednisone 30 mg daily) has been shown to improve the prognosis dramatically. In one series 90% of cases of sudden idiopathic sensori-neural deafness improved when steroid treatment was initiated within a week of onset, whereas none improved if treatment was delayed for 1—3 months[4]. If geographical or other difficulties threaten more than a few hours' delay in admission to an ENT Department, there is a strong case for withdrawing a sufficient sample of blood for subsequent tests (such as for virus antibodies, syphilis, and auto-immune disease), then commencing treatment with prednisone. Full investigation can be completed later in hospital.

Sensori-neural deafness leaving the patient with a loss greater than 40 dB in his better ear almost always calls for a hearing aid.

WAX

Wax (cerumen) is a mixture of the secretory products of the sebaceous and ceruminous glands of the external auditory meatus. These glands are confined to the outer, cartilaginous, third of the meatus — as also are the hairs. The ceruminous glands are simple coiled tubes surrounded by a smooth muscle coat. Histologically they are identical to the apocrine glands of the axilla. This muscle coat contracts in response to adrenal stimulation (as in fear or pain), and as a result of mechanical manipulation (as in vigorous chewing). The expelled secretion is a white watery fluid which on drying becomes a sticky semi-solid. After a few days it darkens in colour.

The bony inner two-thirds of the external audiotory meatus is extremely sensitive and is normally immaculately clean — the result of epithelial migration. Growth occurs centrifugally from the umbo to the drum margin, then outwards along the meatus at a rate of about 0.05 millimetres per day. Wax is normally shed imperceptibly from the meatus as fast as it is produced, and only becomes troublesome when it accumulates excessively. This gradual jettisoning may be hindered by narrowing or pecularities of direction of the meatus, by a profusion of large hairs in men, or by undue application of soap and water which prevents drying of the wax. After prolonged retention the wax may harden to a rock-like consistency. The incidence of impacted wax in men has been put at 18 per cent[5].

Accumulations of wax may be harboured quite unconsciously in the outer third of the meatus. Discomfort results when excessive collections irritate the wall of the meatus, and particularly if contact is made with the very sensitive skin of the inner meatus or drum.

Deafness, tinnitus, and vertigo may result when wax occludes the meatus sufficiently. After swimming or washing, water may be trapped behind plugs of wax, paving the way for otitis externa. Even small amounts of wax may obscure a view of the tympanic membrane, hindering examination of the ear.

Removal of Wax

Two methods are available — syringing and 'dry-cleaning'. Syringing has the advantage that only limited skill and equipment are required and so the task can sometimes be delegated. It is a convenient way of removing wax in the majority of cases. However, syringing has some serious limitations:

1. it is contraindicated where there is any suggestion of perforation of the tympanic membrane;
2. it is too painful and dangerous in the presence of acute otitis media or myringitis;
3. it may precipitate an attack of otitis externa, especially in patients prone to this condition;
4. sometimes wax is too hard to be removed by syringing;
5. where examination of the tympanic membrane is the reason for wax removal, syringing is not always ideal, because a confusing hyperaemia of the membrane sometimes results.

Individual doctors will reach their own decision whether to confine their efforts to syringing, referring cases where this is contraindicated or unsuccessful to suitable colleagues (e.g., in the ENT out-patient department), or whether to acquire the equipment and expertise needed for 'dry-cleaning'.

Syringing

Two kinds of syringe are in general use — the metal 'cylinder and piston' (Wood's) type, and the Bacon type, incorporating a Higginson's syringe. Metal syringes are rather clumsy and can be troublesome. The piston is liable to seize in the cylinder even when diligently maintained and lubricated (e.g., with silicone fluid). The syringe may have to be recharged several times, making the operation tedious and time-consuming. The nozzle should be unscrewed and removed each time the syringe is refilled, partly to speed refilling and partly because otherwise infection contaminating the nozzle will be aspirated into the syringe, to the detriment of the next patient. The nozzle should be winged, and its thread should have a minimum number of turns, to ease this frequent removal and replacement. Two or three alternative sized nozzles should be available.

The Bacon type of syringe is more satisfactory, especially if about six extra feet of tubing are let into the tube. An easily controlled jet of water is obtained, speeding up the operation considerably. A vaginal douche-can makes a convenient reservoir.

Water for syringing should be at about $99°F$ ($37.3°C$), otherwise thermal currents may be set up in the labyrinth producing distressing vertigo. A disposable paper towel on the patient's shoulder, or a 'Valcron' fastened bib, will protect his clothing while he steadies the receiver to collect the washings. During syringing the pinna should be lifted upwards and backwards with the free hand helping to straighten the meatus as much as possible.

Ideally, at the end of the procedure, the meatus should be mopped dry with cotton wool mounted on a Jobson-Horne probe, to minimise the likelihood of subsequent otitis externa.

Wax Solvents: Wax is sometimes too hard to be removed by gentle syringing. Temptations to use excessive force, with the risk of damage to the tympanic membrane, must be resisted. An attempt may be made to soften the wax with various solvents.

In an experiment designed to compare the usefulness of Cerumol, olive oil, Waxsol, Xerumenex, sodium bicarbonate ear drops BPC, and Dioctyl ear capsules only one product, Cerumol, was found to be significantly more effective than sodium bicarbonate ear drops BPC, and even Cerumol was open to the theoretical objection that it contains turpentine and dicholorobenzene which are skin irritants[6].

Ideally the patient should lay with the blocked ear upper-most while the selected drops are instilled, and remain in this position for several minutes. Cotton wool plugs tend to attract the solvent away from the wax unless previously soaked in it.

Dry-Cleaning

The removal of wax with a hook can save a great deal of time and inconvenience. Good visibility is required and two free hands (one to manipulate the pinna to straighten the meatus and to steady the speculum and one to wield the hook). Therefore a head mirror and suitable light source (or a head lamp) are essential. The hook itself should be carefully selected — the St. Bartholomew's Hospital model is ideal.

The hook, held flush with the wall of the meatus, is worked medially past the collection of wax. It is then rotated inwards and gently withdrawn scooping out the wax. The procedure is usually best carried out through a speculum — the largest admissable to the external meatus. Sometimes it is helpful first to free wax adherent to the wall of the meatus and the looped end of a Jobson-Horne probe is ideal for this. The wax plug can often be hooked until it comes to rest against the inner end of the speculum, when wax, hook and speculum can be removed as one unit.

Adherent flakes of wax are often most easily removed with a pair of mosquito-type forceps. Quire's forceps are suitable and a fraction the price of other types. Soft wax is most conveniently wiped from the external meatus using pledgets of cotton wool twisted onto a Jobson-Horne probe.

Stimulation of the auricular branch of the vagus nerve (which supplies part of the external meatus) during these procedures often initiates the cough reflex. It is essential for the patient to keep his head still. Because of the sensitivity of the meatus, particularly along its inner two-thirds, extreme gentleness is vital to retain his co-operation.

OTITIS EXTERNA

The characteristic presenting symptom is intense irritation but deafness may occur as a result of blockage of the ear by exudate and debris.

Aetiology

The condition is essentially a reaction of the skin of the external ear to local or general factors, or both.

A seborrhoeic form occurs as an extension of seborrhoea of the scalp. The pinna and external meatus are greasy, with scaling and crusting.

Eczematous otitis externa may be part of generalised eczema or may arise from local factors such as nickel contact dermatitis set up by spectacle frames, or from excessive obsessional washing with soap and water, or (with increasing frequency) from sensitivity to hair lacquer sprayed without protecting the ears. Irritation, inflammation, and oedema may be followed by blistering, weeping, and crust formation, which may spread to the surrounding part of the head and neck.

Infection — bacterial, fungal or viral — may be present and it is sometimes difficult to discern whether its role is primary or secondary.

Bacillus pyocyaneus, *Bacillus proteus* and *Staphylococcus aureus* are frequent infecting bacteria, and *Escherichia coli* is remarkably common, with obvious poor hygiene implications.

In fungal infection of the ear the mycelial elements may be readily visible with the lens of the electric auroscope giving the skin a delicate velvet-like appearance. More often however the ear contains moist debris resembling wet blotting paper. If *Aspergillus niger* is present the black pigment from the conidiophores is evident.

Viral forms of otitis externa are characterised by blistering. In bullous myringitis inspection with the auroscope reveals spectacular bullae on the tympanic membrane, bright pink in colour due to distension with haemorrhagic exudate, subsequently darkening. *Herpes zoster* of the geniculate ganglion occasionally gives rise to a herpetic eruption in the external auditory meatus, occasionally without any other evidence of nerve involvement. *Herpes simplex* may also produce crops of vesicles.

Some of the most severe cases of acute otitis externa are iatrogenic and derive from the use of topical applications containing substances to which the patient has become sensitive, neomycin being a common culprit. Syringing the ears may also give rise to otitis externa.

Patients who wear hearing aids, those with active middle ear disease and discharge, and those with radical mastoid cavities are sometimes prone to very troublesome and persistent otitis externa.

Management of Otitis Externa

The management of this common condition is essentially 'manipulative'. The primary objective is a clean meatus free of debris, and the application of suitable remedies.

The Jobson-Horne probe is essential for the task of cleaning the meatus; an orange stick is too thick. Small pledgets of cotton wool are twisted onto the serrated end of the probe and debris is mopped away, the pledgets being frequently removed (e.g., with forceps) and replaced.

Where much oedema of the meatal wall is present, a wick impregnated with a steroid-antibacterial mixture is helpful. The wick is left in for a day or two then changed. Once the swelling has subsided, the meatus may be painted, after cleansing, with a steroid-antibacterial mixture. The patient is asked to return for toilet of the meatus at increasing intervals until the inflammation has subsided. Where the condition is recurrent he should be advised to keep the ears scrupulously dry, and return at the first sign of further trouble, when prompt cleaning and application of a little steroid-antibiotic cream should prevent flare-up of otitis externa.

In fungal otitis externa the principal requirement is again the removal of debris. Topical applications of a steroid-fungicide mixture (such as Tri-adcortyl Otic ointment (Squibb) or Remotic (Squibb) or a mixture of miconazole and betamethasone cream) are indicated where much inflammation is present. Where there is little inflammation a little fungicidal powder should be puffed into the meatus. Some preparations (e.g., Penotrane and Nystatin) may be obtained ready for use as powders in a plastic puffer.

Idoxuridine has been introduced for the treatment of herpes simplex and herpes zoster. The dimethylsulphoxide solvent, used in commercial preparations of this drug, promotes penetration of the 5 per cent idoxuridine solution.

In eczematous otitis externa the application of local antibiotics alone is contra-indicated and steroid drops or, better still a steroid impregnated wick should be applied.

Furunculosis

Furunculosis begins as a staphylococcal infection of a hair follide and is therefore confined to the outer cartilagenous third of the external auditory meatus. It is a very painful condition. Surrounding inflammation and oedema may block the meatus and displace the pinna forwards. Moving the pinna is extremely painful.

Treatment consists of the administration of one of the broad-spectrum antibiotics, analgesics, and local measures. A wick consisting of ribbon gauze soaked in a steroid/antibiotic mixture (such as Terra-Cortril, Pfizer) encourages oedema to subside, promoting drainage. Once the furuncle has burst it is of course desirable to mop the meatus clear of debris. In recurrent cases the urine should be tested for sugar, and a nasal swab may reveal a 'carrier state'.

KERATOSIS OBTURANS

Keratosis Obturans is a rare disorder of the inner bony two thirds of the external auditory meatus in which, instead of migrating outwards, desquamating squames build up into very hard masses blocking the meatus and even enlarging it by eroding bone. The material resembles cholesteatoma. Treatment consists of regular removal of the material with a wax hook every few months. The initial cleaning may be very difficult, even requiring an anesthetic, but thereafter management falls within the scope of the interested family practitioner.

EXOSTOSIS

In exostosis of the external auditory meatus smooth bosses are seen on the wall of the innermost part of the meatus, next to the tympanic membrane. They are covered with healthy skin, and feel rock-hard when touched with a probe. They are usually encountered in older patients who admit having done a lot of swimming in cold water in their youth, and are an incidental finding during examination of the ears. It is desirable that the doctor should be familiar with the condition. No treatment is indicated except in the very rare cases where the exostoses produce sufficient blockage to cause deafness.

FOREIGN BODIES IN THE EAR

The distress caused by intrusion of an insect into the external auditory meatus is quickly soothed by killing it with spirit or olive oil drops. Small foreign bodies are conveniently removed by syringing. Larger foreign bodies must be removed (under direct vision using a head lamp or mirror) with a wax hook or small forceps. Where the foreign body is impacted, and occasionally with very nervous children, it may be necessary to resort to a general anaesthetic.

ACUTE OTITIS MEDIA

Commonest in poorer and larger families, approximately one child in four in Great Britain suffers at least one attack of acute otitis media[7]. The distress of a child weeping with earache is harrowing to behold.

Aetiology

Acute otitis media is almost invariably the result of obstruction of the Eustachian tube. It typically follows an upper respiratory tract infection, with resultant inflammation and oedema of the mucosa of the Eustachian tube (a rigid structure in its posterior bony third) leading to imprisonment of infected material in the middle ear. Children, with their narrower Eustachian tubes, are much more prone to otitis media than adults, and this propensity is increased up to the age of 5 years by the natural growth curve of lymphoid tissue with its peak at that age. Enlarged peritubal lymphoid tissue results in narrowing of the Eustachian lumen and increased liability to complete obstruction in the presence of infection. In babies the Eustachian tube is relatively wide and straight and mucus, milk and vomit may readily pass into the middle ear.

Whereas in children acute otitis media tends to be bilateral, in adults it is usually unilateral. Recurring otitis media on the same side in an adult raises the possibility of a post-nasal space neoplasm and, in addition to inspection of the post-nasal space, further investigations (radiology, examination of the post-nasal space under general anaesthesia, and possibly biopsy) are called for.

The bacteriological findings of a study of otitis media[8] are shown in Table 10.1.

Table 10.1   The organisms cultured from 65 per cent of middle ear aspirates in otitis media (after Hoekelman, 1974[8]).

Organism	Percentage
Diplococcus pneumoniae	54
Haemophilus influenzae	32
Group A beta-haemolytic streptococcus	7
Staphylococcus aureus	<1
Various other organisms	6

(In 35 per cent of aspirates no organism could be cultured)

Clinical Features

Pain is the principal feature of most cases of otitis media, accompanied by varying degrees of pyrexia, malaise, deafness and tinnitus. Young children may be distressed, feverish and ill, but unable to indicate the site of their pain. Examination of the ears of young children who are feverish and irritable is therefore essential. Discharge from one or both ears may be a presenting symptom but this has usually been preceded by pain which ceased with the start of the discharge. The rest of the upper respiratory tract may also be inflamed.

In the earliest stages of acute otitis media there is dilatation of vessels on the drum, along the handle of the malleus and at the periphery.

Next the tympanic membrane becomes red and dull and indrawn owing to absorbtion of air from the sealed middle ear cavity. Later, outpouring of inflammatory exudate produces bulging of the drum and, in untreated cases, rupture may occur followed by bloodstained otorrhoea. Localised bulging of the drum may occur where there has been a previous perforation. Occasionally perforation may occur at an early stage without a prior history of pain.

In the pre-antibiotic era rupture of the drum, and disappearance of pain, was usually followed by discharge and ultimately by healing of the perforation with a variable amount of scarring and deafness. Infection progressed in less fortunate patients who, a week or more later, experienced a return of pain, fever, and toxaemia heralding acute mastoiditis.

Management of Acute Otitis Media

The approach to the treatment of acute otitis media varies remarkably from one author to another, and is largely personal. Fry[9] reserves penicillin (by injection or orally) for those cases where there is severity of pain and fever, discharge, recurrences, or no improvement after two to three days. He finds this represents less than half of all cases.

Taylor[10] states 'in the early stages of acute otitis media where the tympanic membrane is injected and retracted, antibiotics should be withheld for 24 hours'. Ephedrine nose drops and steam inhalations should be tried. If the drum becomes 'full and red' Taylor suggests that 'antibiotics must be started at once', 'the use of daily or twice daily injections of penicillin having much to recommend it'. The author goes on to advise 'when the patient is first seen with a painful red bulging drumhead there is no doubt that the treatment of choice is myringotomy under general anaesthesia'. Colman[11] also advocates daily penicillin injections, with a switch to tetracycline if the response after 48 hours is unsatisfactory.

Taylor and Colman see the problem in a hospital setting. Indeed, discussing the diagnosis of acute otitis media Taylor[12] states 'it is an advantage if both parents, as well as the family doctor, are present when a child is examined'. This would seem to imply that the family doctor might not even be capable of making the diagnosis by himself, whereas in fact of course the vast majority of cases of otitis media are cared for by family doctors.

In a controlled trial[13] of 89 children with upper respiratory tract infections, including 15 per cent with otitis media, some were given antibiotics and some a placebo and the results showed no difference in relief of symptoms or improvement of physical signs in the two groups.

Diamant and Diamant[14] have commented that in the literature available, there are very few articles concerned with the indications for the use and non use of antibiotics in the ENT diseases. They analyse some results of a 4 year survey in Sweden in which 1608 ears with acute otitis media were treated without antibiotics, and 1367 were treated with antibiotics. Out-patients were seen twice weekly. Antibiotics 'were never administered unless the symptoms displayed a direct threat or existence of complications'. They claim that 88 per cent of patients with otitis media never need antibiotics, and that recurrence of otitis media within a month is commoner if antibiotics are started on the first day of the illness than if they are not given until the 8th day. There was no difference in recurrence rate in the group given an antibiotic from the 8th day onwards and those given no antibiotics.

Unfortunately these observations do little to clarify the problem of management of otitis media in practice. It may well be that 88 per cent of patients with otitis media 'recover' without antibiotics, but there is no information regarding the hearing loss or development of 'glue ear' with or without antibiotics. Nor is there any guidance regarding the identification of the 12 per cent who will need antibiotics and no definition of the 'direct threat of complications'. It seems that a large proportion of their cases developed suppuration and otorrhoea — although precise figures are lacking.

The approach of Hoekelman, is more in keeping with family practice in the United Kingdom. He advises[8] that although a high percentage of children who present with symptoms and signs of acute otitis media will recover with no treatment, specific therapy should be given to decrease patient suffering and the incidence complications. On the basis of anticipated bacteriology he advocates the immediate administration of penicillin (by long acting injection) above the age of 3 months, and ampicillin below this age. In his opinion there is no place for myringotomy in the treatment of acute otitis media, and adenoidectomy does not affect the recurrence rate of acute otitis media. He finds allergy is a common underlying cause of recurrence of acute otitis media, and if this is so the apparent benefit conferred by such antihistamine/alpha-stimulator mixtures as 'Dimotapp' is explained.

It is the author's opinion, it is sound practice, in children with acute otitis media, to commence treatment with oral phenoxymethyl penicillin in generous doses, except where the child is vomiting or his mother is unable to coax him to take medicine, or there is severe pain and a bulging tympanic membrane – in which case intra-muscular penicillin is given. In the case of adults, oxytetracycline is the drug of first choice, but of course tetracyclines are avoided below the age of 12 years in view of the risk of permanent tooth staining. Antibiotic treatment is continued for at least five days.

Oral antihistamine/alpha-stimulator mixtures (such as Dimotapp, Eskornade, or Triominic elixirs) have a place in promoting Eustachian drainage by shrinking mucus membranes and reducing secretion. The profound drying effect that these preparations have will be appreciated by those who have sampled them. Children are usually happy to take them, and they appear more likely to improve Eustachian drainage by their blood borne arrival in the tubal mucosa than decongestant nose drops, though there is no harm in using these as well. A clinical trial to establish the place of oral decongestants is long overdue.

The severe pain of acute otitis media usually subsides promptly with analgesics, such as aspirin, paracetamol, or codeine compound.

In the last 15 years the author has not seen a single case of otitis media in family practice which, treated on these lines, required myringotomy, or failed to subside promptly. No cases of drum rupture after commencement of treatment have occurred.

Follow-Up

Follow-up of acute otitis media is essential until the condition has completely resolved. Depending on the severity of the case, it is wise to re-examine the ear after two days, by which time the patient should be free of pain and apyrexial and any previous bulging of the tympanic membrane should be subsiding, sometimes leaving a characteristic 'crinkly' appearance. Failure to see evidence of response to treatment (a very rare event) calls for change of antibiotic therapy; cephaloridine orally or by injection, or co-trimoxazole are suitable alternatives. Myringotomy must rarely be called for these days. A further examination a few days later should reveal progression of the appearance of the drum towards normal, although full normality may not be seen for two to three weeks.

The hearing should be checked around the 10th—14th day, a quiet whisper should be audible at 3 ft, and Rinne's test should by now have been restored to positive. Ideally an audiogram should be recorded a month or two later to confirm the resolution.

Sometimes the development of acute otitis media draws attention to a 'catarrhal-adenoidal' state of affairs in a child who was not hitherto thought ill enough by his parents to need medical attention. The condition of the upper respiratory tract must be assessed and if the nasal mucosa is seen to be wet and swollen, and there is mouth breathing and enlargement of the posterior triangle glands indicating adenoid infection, then the effect of a prolonged course of decongestant treatment (e.g., with Dimotapp) is well worth trying. If otitis media becomes recurrent, adenoidectomy may need to be considered. Adenoidectomy is discussed later in this chapter, (page 154).

GLUE EAR (NON-SUPPURATIVE, SECRETORY OR SEROUS OTITIS MEDIA)

Non suppurative otitis media and its management with the help of a Teflon ventilating tube (Shepard's grommet) inserted through a myringotomy has become a familiar phenomenon in the last decade. It is therefore interesting to note that 175 years ago Astley Cooper[15] was performing myringotomy for the condition, and over 100 years ago Politzer[16] who appreciated the desirability of maintaining the tympanotomy opening, was experimenting with a silver cannula, a forerunner of the modern grommet. In 1954 Armstrong[17] introduced a satisfactory plastic tube, revolutionising the management of the condition.

Nature and Incidence

Non-suppurative otitis media is a disorder in which the middle ear is filled with sterile fluid. In children (some 3 per cent of whom are affected) it is usually bilateral, commonest around the ages of 5 and 6 years, and the fluid tends to be thick mucoid material referred to as 'glue'. In adults (who form a small minority of cases) it is nearly always unilateral and the fluid is generally thin and serous.

Aetiology

The aetiology of non-suppurative otitis media remains uncertain, nor is it agreed to what extent the same factors are at work in children and in adults.

Recurrent viral upper respiratory tract infections are generally considered to be a predisposing factor, although Adlington[18] failed to isolate a virus from middle ear fluid or from biopsies of middle ear or upper respiratory tract mucosa. The role of allergic factors in the aetiology of glue ear is unclear[19]. A study of secretory immunoglobulin A in middle ear effusions[20] suggested that mucoid effusions are the result of enhanced epithelial secretory activity.

Whatever the mechanism involved, it has been shown[21] that there is a histological change in the middle ear mucosa, with development of abnormal columnar ciliated epithelium capable of filling the middle ear with secretion whether or not Eustachian obstruction is present. Chronic inflammatory changes in the epithelium have also been described.

The epidermis of the tympanic membrane and external auditory meatus is also affected[22]. The normal migration of epithelium from the umbo outwards is interfered with, presumably as a result of hyperaemia of the tympanic membrane. Epithelium builds up on the tympanic membrane, affecting its appearance, and debris collects in the meatus. Hence a good deal of cleaning is often necessary before a good view of the tympanic membrane can be obtained.

Furthermore, this faulty epithelial migration is thought to be at the root of cholesteatomatous destructive middle ear disease. Jordan[23] (who is credited with having introduced the term 'glue ear'), considered secretory otitis media to be a major cause of cholesteatoma of the middle ear and mastoid. It has been suggested[24] that the course of events is that a dry adherent crust of keratinous debris develops on a collapsed area of tympanic membrane. Owing to failure of epithelial migration the static crust produces irritation and eventually destruction of the underlying squamous epithelium and ulceration. Granulations develop, with destruction of the surrounding tympanic membrane and formation of a perforation, either of the pars flaccida or the posterior part of the membrana tensa. Squamous epithelium then passes inwards from the deep meatus with the formation of cholesteatoma. If epithelial crusts are recognised and removed at regular intervals this will prevent further trauma of soft tissues and progress of disease — a very important reason for examining the children at frequent intervals.

Clinical Features

The child with 'glue ear' is usually quite happy himself and is brought to the doctor because his parents, or perhaps his teacher, have begun to suspect deafness. He is often 'full of catarrh' with a snuffly nose, a juicy swollen boggy nasal mucosa, and often a mouth breathing tendency, enlarged tonsils, and perhaps enlarged lymph glands in the jugulo-digastric and posterior triangle regions.

A rough assessment of the hearing may be made by the whispered voice test (see page 117). Tuning fork testing may give a negative Rinne test indicating a conductive loss.

It may be necessary to clean the external auditory meatus before a view of the tympanic membrane can be obtained. A discussion of the most suitable ways of doing this is given on page 116. Once the meatus has been cleaned (and mopped dry if it has been syringed) the ear should be examined using either a Seigle's speculum or an electric auroscope fitted with an inflation bag. The tympanic membrane in 'glue ear' will be seen to lack its normal translucency. Prominent vessels are visible especially at the periphery. It is dull and may be bulging especially posteriorly due to accumulation of fluid, or may be indrawn so that the handle of the malleus is unduly prominent. Variation of pressure (having warned the child that one is about to blow air into his ear) reveals that the tympanic membrane has lost its normal mobility. When the fluid is thin and serous a fluid level may be visible and the tympanic membrane may be yellowish.

Management

The question now facing the family doctor is what to do next, and in particular, whether to refer the child to a specialist. To reach such a decision it is helpful to consider the natural history of 'glue ear' and the results of surgical treatment.

The dangers if nothing is done are that, in addition to the existing reversible hearing loss, fibrosis of the ossicles may develop leading to 'adhesive otitis media'. Cholesteatomatous middle ear disease may ultimately follow, as already described. It has been pointed out[25] that many cases of 'glue ear' are mild and recover without any disability, and that in mild cases it is worth observing the child for a month or two as many will recover spontaneously.

The family doctor seeing a case of 'glue ear' for the first time, depending on local circumstances, should be guided by the severity of the deafness, the appearance of the tympanic membrane, and the presence or absence of other features calling for consideration of surgery, such as recurrently infected tonsils or gross adenoidal enlargement.

If early surgical intervention is not called for, the position will need to be reviewed every few weeks until the hearing is normal, the tympanic membranes are healthy, and the tuning fork tests are normal. The availability of audiograms to judge progress is of course of inestimable value.

Antibiotics may be called for if there is evidence of infection. In the author's experience the administration of such decongestant preparations as Dimotapp (a mixture of brompheniramine (antihistamine) phenylephrine and phenyl-propanolamine (alpha—stimulators)) has a pronounced beneficial effect. The drying and shrinking effect on the nasal mucosa is obvious, and it seems reasonable to assume that the middle ear and Eustachian tube mucosa is responding in a comparable way.

The surgical treatment of 'glue ear' consists of myringotomy under general anaesthetic, aspiration of the 'glue', and the insertion of a plastic grommet. At the same time adenoids and tonsils may be removed where indicated. The grommet is usually retained for 6–9 months, and when it is finally extruded the tympanic membrane heals quickly. In most cases the hearing remains satisfactory and the glue does not reform; prolonged ventilation appears to cause the metaplasia of the middle ear mucosa to revert to normal. In a minority of cases grommets may have to be replaced, sometimes several times.

Intratympanic injection of 2 ml of a 50 per cent solution of urea (a powerful mucolytic agent) followed by suction at the puncture site some 4 minutes later when the glue dissolves and starts to seep out, is preferred by some specialists to myringotomy and the use of the grommet[26,27].

CHRONIC SUPPURATIVE OTITIS MEDIA

Chronic disease of the middle ear is almost always the end result of upper respiratory tract infections in childhood. Tumarkin's theory[28] is generally accepted and postulates that these recurrent infections lead to Eustachian obstruction, and ultimately to:

1. purely inflammatory complications (otitis media and central perforations);
2. purely mechanical complications (vacuum collapse of the tympanic membrane and cholesteatoma formation);
3. mixed inflammatory and mechanical complications – including 'glue ear'.

Inflammatory Complications

The inflammatory processes tend to result in so called 'tubo-tympanic' perforation which characteristically involves the anterior and central part of the drum, and spares the drum margin. Hearing is not usually seriously damaged.

After improving tubal drainage as much as possible, for example by washing out infected sinuses and removing unhealthy tonsils and adenoids, treatment is by toilet and instillation of combined antibiotic and steroid drops. Some physicians prefer to administer the antibiotic systemically to avoid the risk of local hypersensitivity. The patient can often helpfully perform the mopping himself between visits to the doctor.

Once the perforation has been dry for a few months, surgical repair may be considered.

Mechanical Complications

Mechanical processes typically originate from indrawing of Scarpa's fascia or the postero-superior part of the drum, and result in 'attico-antral' disease. The drum margin is usually involved. Cholesteatoma invades the attic region and proeeds to involve the mastoid cells. There may be bone destruction opening the way for suppuration to enter the labyrinth, causing giddiness, and the middle cranial fossa, causing meningitis or brain abscess. Facial palsy may result from VIIth nerve destruction.

The discharge in patients with cholesteatoma is typically evil smelling. A fistula sign may be present (sudden pressure on the tragus increases pressure within the ear and this, in the prescence of an erosion of the labyrinth, results in giddiness and nystagmus) provided the labyrinth is still functioning.

Whilst the family practitioner can help considerably in the management of patients with 'tubo-tympanic' infection if he is willing to see the patient regularly for toilet and general management, early referral to a specialist is highly desirable in 'attico-antral' disease, and is especially urgent where pain, headache, giddiness, facial palsy or a positive fistula sign denotes dangerous bony destruction. Where such serious signs and symptoms are absent toilet of the ear, the instillation of antibiotic/steroid drops and perhaps mastoid radiography, will be helpful whilst a specialist appointment is being set up. In the ENT department suction clearance of the ear, often under the operating microscope, will normally be the first step. In the absence of radiological evidence of bone erosion such conservative management may result in a dry troublefree ear which can safely be left.

The ears of all patients with Bell's palsy should be carefully examined, for evidence of chronic middle ear disease involving the facial nerve in the tympanic part of its course in the fallopian canal. Particular attention must be paid to the attic region for the rest of the tympanic membrane may look quite innocent.

OTOSCLEROSIS

Nature

This is a progressive disease most commonly producing deafness in early adult life. The pathological process involved is a disturbance of ossification of bone embryologically derived from the otic capsule whereby mature bone is removed by osteoclasts and replaced by thick vascular unorganised bone. The commonest manifestation is conductive deafness produced by fixation of the stapes footplate in the oval window, but the process may extend to (or be confined to) parts of the cochlea giving rise to tinnitus and vertigo, and even sensori-neural deafness. Indeed it has been suggested[29] that a combination of stapedial and cochlear otosclerosis is the commonest single cause of severe adult deafness.

Incidence

The incidence has been put at 0.3 per cent[30]. It has been thought in the past to be commoner in females but this now appears to be a misconception partly due to the greater readiness with which females seek medical advice. The mode of inheritance in most cases is autosomal and dominant. Thus if an otosclerotic patient marries a non-otosclerotic a quarter of their offspring may be expected to become deaf. However the degree of penetrance of the abnormal gene varies from one family to another, and one generation to another, as also does the severity and rate of progression of the deafness.

Clinical Features

Deafness, usually bilateral, is the chief symptom but many patients also complain of tinnitus, and some also suffer from vertigo. The patient usually speaks in a quiet voice for he can appreciate the volume of his own voice due to bone conduction. Paracusis is characteristic of otosclerosis (the patient manages conversation better in the presence of background noise). This is because the person speaking to him automatically raises his voice to overcome the background noise, which the otosclerotic patient cannot hear anyway.

Patients are sometimes encountered in family practice with increasing deafness who have worn a private hearing aid for years and who have tympanic membranes of normal appearance and a negative Rinne's test (p. 118). They are very likely to have otosclerosis and may then benefit enormously from surgical treatment which should therefore be offered if the patient is fit for an operation.

As already indicated the otosclerotic process tends to originate in the stapes and later involve to some extent the cochlea. In a well established case there is likely to be some sensori-neural deafness, with a greater degree of conductive deafness, giving a characteristic audiogram.

The interval between the lines on the graph is referred to as the 'air bone gap' and it is this which the surgeon seeks to 'close'. There is a marked tendency for the sensori-neural deafness itself to improve after successful surgery so that not only is the air bone gap closed, but the final air conduction audiogram is even better than the pre-operative bone conduction audiogram.

Management

The treatment advised for most cases of otosclerosis consists of removal of most of the stapes and its replacement by a prosthesis. A variety of plastic and metal prostheses are used. Results are excellent; in general it may be stated that well over 80 per cent of cases followed up for many years have lasting closure of the air bone gap and are delighted with their restored hearing. In rather less than 2 per cent of cases the operation is a failure. The failure may be apparent at the time of operation or may be delayed, in which case a perilymph fistula should be suspected and an attempt made at re-operation to close the fistula. The incidence of a 'dead ear' following stapedectomy has been reduced to less than one per cent with modern surgical techniques.

It is current policy to confine surgery to one ear only in otosclerosis. The rationale is that if the operation on one ear is successful it is unwise to tempt providence by interfering with the other ear. If, on the other hand, operation on one ear was unsuccessful, there is an increased likelihood that operation on the other ear would also fail, leaving the patient completely deaf and beyond help with a hearing aid.

Fenestration operations for otosclerosis were replaced many years ago by stapedectomy. Patients who underwent fenestration when it was in vogue tend to be unhappy; they are left with mastoid cavities which may be troublesome, and many are deaf, and wear a hearing aid. It is worth directing such patients back to a specialist since a modified stapedectomy procedure is sometimes feasible.

Where surgery is not to be undertaken, hearing aids are very helpful in otosclerosis. Air conduction aids are nearly always more satisfactory than bone conduction aids.

Advanced cases of otosclerosis who have failed surgical treatment and who may be left with discharging fenestration cavities and perhaps troublesome tinnitus and vertigo, present a serious problem. They may become gravely depressed and require treatment with anti-depressants and much general support.

PRESBYCUSIS

Nature

Throughout life there is a progressive hearing loss especially for high tones. Individuals in whom this loss has advanced particularly rapidly are said to suffer from presbycusis. The lesion is in the cochlea, and involves primarily the basal turn. The hearing loss is typically symmetrical in the two ears.

Five types of presbycusis, varying in their exact pathology and prognosis, have been described[31]. Epithelial atrophy, giving an abrupt hearing loss above 4000 Hertz, and 'neural' presbycusis with disproportionately severe loss of auditory discrimination, are the two main types.

In addition to the high tone hearing loss, many patients with presbycusis also complain of a continuous high pitched tinnitus. Some are also troubled by distortions of sound and some by vertigo.

Aetiology

The basal turn of the cochlea is stimulated by all frequencies whereas the higher turns are only stimulated by low frequencies. Presumably there is greater resultant 'wear and tear' on the basal turn with the passage of the years so that the hearing for high notes goes more quickly than that for low notes.

In support of such a 'wear and tear' hypothesis, presbycusis appears to be fostered by background noise exposure. For example, presbycusis has an earlier onset in Greater London residents than in rural populations[32], and an interesting case has been described of an 82 year old man who had worn a cotton wool ear plug in one ear for 32 years and had much less presbycusis in that ear[33]. Such observations add strength to the campaign for reduction in noise pollution.

A tendency to develop this type of deafness prematurely (so that it is severe by the age of 60) runs in some families. The condition often advances insidiously and only comes to light when aggravated by some other factor such as eustachian catarrh or wax.

Treatment

The only effective help is a hearing aid but because of the diversity of forms of presbycusis it is not always possible to predict which patients will benefit from a hearing aid. A trial with an instrument is the only real test.

There is of course no effective treatment for the tinnitus and it is best to explain this to the patient, reassuring him that it will become less troublesome with the passage of time, and that patients usually eventually cease to notice it just as a person who goes to live by a railway line comes not to notice the trains, only hearing them when deliberately listening for them.

MENIÈRE'S DISEASE

Nature and Aetiology

In 1861 Prosper Menière described a condition characterised by recurring sudden attacks of vertigo, often accompanied by nausea and vomiting, associated with deafness and tinnitus, and he asigned the symptoms to labyrinthine disease. The condition as encountered in family practice is almost invariably unilateral, although at one specialist centre 42.5 per cent of cases had become bilateral when followed up for 20 years[34].

The basic aetiology of Menière's disease remains elusive. It is known that the membranous labyrinth becomes enormously distended but whether this is primarily due to excessive production of endolymph, or reduced absorption, is not agreed, and the part played by vasodilatation, or vasoconstriction, ionic disturbances, accumulations of histamine, or other factors remains debatable.

It is also known that herniation and rupture of various parts of the endolymphatic chambers may occur, but whether rupture results in easing or exacerbation of symptoms is not clear. Such confusion over aetiology has frustrated attempts to plan any rational treatment, medical or surgical.

There is no evidence of a hereditary influence.

Incidence

Over half of all cases of vertigo referred to specialist departments prove to be suffering from Menières disease. The incidence of Menières disease is unknown and although the course followed by the selected and unrepresentative cases referred to specialist departments and subjected to a variety of treatments is profusely tabulated and documented, a true picture of the natural history of the disease is lacking.

Clinical Features

When a patient is seen in an attack of what is suspected to be Menière's disease he is likely to be in considerable distress, lying very still, with a basin near at hand and an aroma of vomit in the air. He may exhibit spontaneous nystagmus of variable direction. Examination of the ear may reveal a sensori-neural hearing loss, but no other abnormality, and neurological examination excludes central nervous system disease.

The attacks of giddiness tend to be accompanied by tinnitus and deafness which at first clear away after a day or two but later become more persistent. With successive attacks deafness tends to become more profound and eventually permanent, and the tinnitus may become very distressing, often likened to a dynamo.

Associated with attacks the patient may also complain of distortion of hearing and an uncomfortable 'full' feeling in the ear.

Probably as a result of distention of the saccule, so that it comes to lie in direct contact with the stapedial footplate without being cushioned by perilymph, loud sounds in Menière's disease may actually produce giddiness.

This is known as the *Tullio phenomenon*. Symptoms such as 'giddy feelings when lorries go by' are liable to be wrongly dismissed as hysterical if such a possibility is not appreciated.

There is a strong tendancy for the disease to 'burn itself out' after a few years, leaving the patient with varying degrees of permanent deafness in the affected ear or ears but free of attacks of vertigo and with little or no tinnitus.

Differential Diagnosis

It is difficult in the first attack to be sure that the patient is not suffering from a vestibular neuronitis — a condition often occurring in small epidemics and sometimes accompanied by upper respiratory tract infection. Similar disturbances are seen in older patients who have cardio-vascular disease. Time alone will reveal whether the attack is the first of a series.

Investigations

At what point, if at all, referral to a specialist department is desirable will depend on individual circumstances. If two or more attacks occur within a few months investigations are indicated. An audiogram will be helpful to serve as a base line for future reference. If deafness is present, audiometric recruitment tests (p. 119) will confirm that it is cochlear in origin. Caloric tests may signify normal vestibular function, or vestibular damage may be revealed. Normal internal auditory meati X-Rays will further help to support the diagnosis of Menière's disease, but it must be admitted that all these investigations are seldom of much practical help and are sometimes seriously misleading.

Management

The future course of the disease may be influenced by the manner in which the early attacks are handled. At the time of an attack an intramuscular injection of prochlorperazine (12.5—25 mg) or promazine (50 mg) usually helps to alleviate the vomiting and the vertigo. Everything should be done to reassure and encourage the patient.

In recurrent attacks the usefulness of medical or surgical treatment is difficult to judge. Diuretics, salt restriction, antihistamines, and vasodilator drugs have enjoyed phases of popularity but their value is questionable. There is no doubt that drugs such as prochlorperazine, cannarizine and thiethylperazine exert a beneficial effect on vertigo and vomiting and they are often given as a regular maintenance therapy in the hope of lessening the frequency as well as the severity of the attacks. More recently betahistine has come into vogue. It is claimed to lower endolymph pressure. It should not be administered at the same time as antihistamines. The dose is one or two 8 mg tablets three times daily.

Many patients not unnaturally become extremely apprehensive and this stress appears to be a factor in the precipitation of further attacks. Benzodiazepines such as oxazepam (10 mg twice daily) may therefore be useful. The atmosphere should be kept in a 'low key' and the patient reassured that he has a non-fatal, self limiting condition which can be helped by medical treatment and for which surgical help is available for the very small minority of cases who eventually need it.

As regards surgical treatment, one or two quite empirical measures have found support. For some unexplained reason the insertion of a grommet into the tympanic membrane appears to benefit some patients[35]. In others the application of salt to the round window may help[36].

If more conservative methods have failed and the hearing in a unilateral case is poor, the giddiness can be stopped by destruction of the labyrinth. If useful hearing is present, or if the other ear is abnormal, selective ultrasound destruction of the labyrinth may be tried, the vestibular branch of the VIIIth nerve may be divided, or decompression of the saccus endolymphaticus on the posterior surface of the petrous may be performed. This latter operation has been advocated in early cases to prevent subsequent hearing damage[37].

To put the place of surgical treatment in perspective, not one case of Menière's Disease has undergone surgery in the experience of one family practioner with an average sized list in 20 years, nor has any case of bilateral deafness due to Menière's Disease been encountered. Management has principally involved sympathetic listening to the patients problems, especially occupational, explanation, and firm reassurance.

The Nose

NASAL ALLERGIES

Clinical Features

The clinical picture of nasal allergy is of violent sneezing, profuse watery rhinorrhoea, conjunctival injection and lachrymation, sometimes proceeding to wheezing. It is most vividly encountered in the form of hay fever in which the nasal, pharyngeal, conjunctival and bronchial mucosae may be involved. Sufferers can be consoled by the observation that there is evidence that they are less likely than their non-atopic counterparts to develop tumours[38].

Aetiology

This type of allergy is an example of so called 'atopic allergy' which is also the basis of allergic asthma and urticarial reactions to ingested allergens. Atopic allergy shows a strong familial trait. It has been noted that West Indian immigrants to the UK are especially prone to hay fever[39].

A major milestone in the understanding of this condition was the discovery of the Prausnitz–Küstner phenomenon. Fifty years ago Prausnitz had a patient named Küstner who was allergic to fish. Prausnitz showed that transfer of Küstner's serum to another individual resulted in the recipient also becoming hypersensitive to fish. The factors responsible for the transfer of hypersensitivity were labelled 'reagins' and in recent years have been identified with a class of immunoglobulin known as IgE. (The E refers to a particular allergen in ragweed which was first suspected of stimulating production of this immunoglobulin class).

It seems that in hay fever allergens in pollen stimulate production of IgE which becomes attached to mast cells in the nasal mucosa (and skin generally). The sera of patients with hay fever have a mean IgE level 2–3 times greater than that of healthy controls[40]. Subsequent exposure to the allergen results in combination of this with the cell-bound IgE, leading to release of histamine and other vasoactive amines such as serotonin, and an acute attack of hay fever.

Seasonal Allergic Rhinitis

Seasonal allergic rhinitis involves allergy to a variety of pollens. In Northern Europe true hay fever (allergy to *grass* pollens) has its season centred on the month of June and in North America in late September and October (ragweed). Tree pollens are liberated earlier, in March, April and May. Pollens have been known to travel 400 miles so that avoidance of the countryside is no guarantee of impunity.

Non-Seasonal or 'Perennial' Allergic Rhinitis

Non-seasonal allergic rhinitis produces similar symptoms to the seasonal form but usually less dramatically. It also differs from the seasonal form from the practical point of view in that the identity of the allergen may not be obvious from the history and differential diagnosis from 'vaso-motor rhinitis' may not be easy – indeed both conditions may exist in the same patient. Allergens include: inhalents such as the house dust mite *Dermatophagoides pteronyssinus* and orris-root used in cosmetics; ingestants such as wheat, eggs or fish; and contactants such as nasal sprays. In addition, a state of allergy to bacteria is believed to occur and idiosyncratic side effects to drugs such as aspirin, may give the picture of nasal allergy. A discussion of the provocative factors in allergic asthma is given on page 83.

Differential Diagnosis

The likelihood that attacks of sneezing and rhinorrhoea are allergic in origin will be suggested by a history, or family history, of allergy. Inspection of the nasal mucosa may strengthen suspicion of allergy — it is wet and usually pale, and polypi may be present. A careful history may give a guide to the allergen (for example the patient may say the symptoms are particularly bad when making beds, suggesting the house dust mite).

Eosinophils

A reliable technique for identifying eosinophils in nasal secretion has been described and they were considered demonstrable in abnormal abundance in up to 90 per cent of cases of allergic rhinitis[41]. Unfortunately the same applied to up to 20 per cent of patients with common colds. This does not in itself deny a correlation between allergy and eosinphilia for infecting bacteria might themselves be allergens in some patients.

Skin Prick Tests

It is quick and simple to perform a batch of skin prick tests to common allergens in the consulting room. However, undue emphasis should not be placed upon the presence or absence of a skin response. The most important criterion for diagnosis is a good clinical history. A positive immediate weal-and-flare skin reaction on challenge with specific allergen is not always given by patients with a clear clinical history of allergic rhinitis. For example, patients can present with a history strongly suggestive of house-dust-mite allergy which is confirmed by provocation tests, yet fail to give a positive reaction on skin testing. In a study of a group of such patients local IgE antibodies were found in the nasal secretions whilst serum allergen-specific IgE tests remained negative, indicating if these interesting results are confirmed, that symptoms were due to local factors in the nasal mucosa and not to systemic production of IgE[42]. Some individuals give positive skin tests and have raised levels of allergen-specific IgE but have no suggestive history of response to the particular allergen and fail to give a positive provocation test.

Skin prick tests are useful, in that they may implicate a particular allergen, provided that their limitations in diagnosis are born in mind. Intradermal tests are less useful since apart from being more tedious to perform they are much less reliable, and are potentially dangerous.

Technique: The author's practice is to number the test bottles to be used (including the control), then with a ball point pen to write the numbers (for example 1—12) on the patient's forearm in a vertical column with a dash opposite each. A small blob from each test bottle is placed on the skin opposite each appropriate dash using the rod supplied attached to each stopper. It is then a simple matter to prick the skin through each blob with the needle supplied in the kit, rinsing it and drying it between pricks. The column of blobs can be 'blotted' with a paper towel (taking care to avoid contaminating one site with another) to prevent running, and the patient left for 20 minutes. The results are then read, and any strong reactions noted.

Management

The doctor confronted with a case of suspected allergy will have to decide whether to manage the problem himself or whether further help is needed. If nasal polypi large enough to cause symptoms are present the patient will need referral to a specialist department for their removal.

The Acute Attack

Treatment of the acute attack is principally a matter of administering antihistamines such as chlorpheniramine 4 mg four hourly. A beclomethasone dipropionate nasal spray is helpful in bringing an acute attack under control and does not suppress the hypothalamic/pituitary/adrenal axis.

Prophylaxis

'Slow Release' Anti-histamines: These are widely used to help ward off further attacks during the season, but unfortunately all antihistamines are liable to cause drowsiness and this should be explained when they are prescribed together with a warning against mixing them with alcohol. In the UK the Civil Aviation Authority will not grant Pilot Licences to persons suffering from hay fever.

Sodium Cromoglycate: This has proved of immense value in the management of asthma (see page 94) and now has a place in the prophylaxis of attacks of hay fever in both adults and children. It is inhaled into each nostril through a nasal insufflator or spray at regular intervals and acts locally by inhibiting the release of histamine and associated substances from mast cells. The treatment is expensive and tedious but has been greatly appreciated by some sufferers, particularly those for whom antihistamines in effective doses are too soporific.

Steroids: The place of systemic steroids in hay fever is controversial. Many feel there is no justification in a benign self limiting complaint for such potentially hazardous therapy. However intranasal drugs are costly and not always well tolerated and there is no doubt that one, or possibly two, injections of a long acting preparation (such as methylprednisolone acetate) when seasonal symptoms begin will often see a patient happily through the season without the need for any other measures. It has been shown that hay fever sufferers given two injections of methylprednisolone acetate failed to achieve adrenal responses as high as those seen before treatment 30 days and in some cases as long as 85 days, after the injections[43]. Oral prednisolone has the advantage that drug dose

may be more accurately gauged and the drug may be withdrawn if necessary[43].
Where depot corticosteroids are the treatment of choice the same precautions as
are taken with other patients given these drugs should be carried out. That is,
after a full explanation of the treatment the patient should be given a steroid
card to carry for 3 months[44].

Immunotherapy: Evidence from controlled clinical trials support the efficiency
of hyposensitisation injections in hay fever[45]. The allergen-neutralising capacity
of post-hyposensitisation serum has been demonstrated[46]. Serum was taken
from patients before a course of injections of Allphyral-G (Dome) which was
prepared from 5 common grass pollens. Two to three weeks after the last
injection a further serum sample was taken from each patient. The two sets of
serum were then separately incubated with some of the Allpyral and injected
into the skin. The post-hyposensitisation serum was able to 'neutralise' the
antigen preventing the development of a skin weal, at dilutions where the
pre-hyposensitisation serum mixture gave a positive skin reaction. In every case
the post-treatment serum possessed an increase in allergen-neutralising capacity.
This procedure was comparable with the Prausnitz-Küstner test (page 142) with
the great advantage that the risk of serum hepatitis was avoided.

It was thought that injections of antigen derived from grass pollens stimulate
production of immunoglobulin G (IgG) which acts as a 'blocking antibody'
diverting the allergen from contact with the IgE bound to the mast cell membrane
(page 142). However, the mechanism of successful hyposensitisation
is at present a controversial topic and 'blocking' IgG is not now regarded as an
adequate explanation. Following experiments in animals in which chemically
modified ragweed pollen has been shown to suppress IgE synthesis, possibly by
means of suppressor T cells[47], it is expected that future developments will lead
to more precise and acceptable forms of immunotherapy. Pre-seasonal immunotherapy may involve a course of up to 9 injections, which is usually repeated
annually for 2—3 years, and this is inconvenient to all concerned. Depot and
sustained-release pollen preparations are now available, reducing the number of
injections required to 3 but even with these preparations hyposensitisation is not
without its potential hazards.

VASO-MOTOR RHINITIS

This condition has already been referred to in the discussion of non-seasonal
allergic rhinitis.

Clinical Features

In some patients with vaso-motor rhinitis nasal obstruction is the principal
complaint, whilst in others the dominant feature is copious watery rhinorrhoea.

Patients often complain that their obstruction varies from one side to the other. It has been shown that there is a physiological alternating swelling and shrinking of the nasal mucosa of the two sides of the nose. In patients possessing an airway already narrowed by vaso-motor rhinitis this phenomenon becomes noticeable.

Aetiology

The underlying mechanism is presumably the same as that which produces rhinorrhoea in normal people experiencing exposure to severe cold, or suffering grief, but actuated with undue readiness.

In addition to provocation by cold, excessive dryness of the air, pollution (e.g., by tobacco smoke), and psychological factors such as anxiety and frustration, endocrine factors also play a part in some patients, for example 'honeymoon rhinitis' and the 'dew drop' on the tip of the nose of some elderly people. Many drugs used in the treatment of hypertension are liable to produce a similar disturbance.

Diagnosis and Investigation

Examination of the nose with Thudichum's speculum may reveal swollen turbinates. The mucosa may be dry or moist, red or pale. Spraying the nose with 5 per cent cocaine solution produces rapid shrinking of the mucosa so that the nasal cavities can be fully examined especially for the presence of polypi. In some patients the appearances anteriorly are within normal limits, but the posterior ends of the inferior turbinates, seen on posterior rhinoscopy, are greatly swollen ('Mulberry turbinates').

Posterior Rhinoscopy
Posterior rhinoscopy is sometimes impossible, as with children with enlarged tonsils. A post-nasal mirror is warmed in a spirit flame to prevent condensation, and the patient is asked to open his mouth and breathe through his nose. The examiner (wearing a head mirror or head lamp) depresses the patient's tongue with a spatula in one hand, whilst the mirror is passed behind the soft palate with the other. The posterior edge of the septum serves as a landmark in identifying the posterior ends of the turbinates, and Eustachian orifices. For practitioners not performing this examination very often, an adjustable post-nasal mirror (e.g., Michel's) is very helpful.

Radiography
Radiography of the nasal sinuses is desirable in any patient complaining of nasal obstruction or rhinorrhoea, but it must be said that the results seldom influence the treatment in vaso-motor rhinitis. Furthermore, some radiologists are prone

to give misleading reports, by wrongly interpreting radiological appearances in pathological terms. Possibly the chief benefit of sinus radiography lies in reassurance of over anxious patients. Films may reveal unsuspected antral infection, but infection will usually have been indicated by history of pain and fever, and by the noting of muco-pus, especially in the middle meatus, on anterior rhinoscopy.

Management

The severity of the symptoms tend to wax and wane over a period of years according to the stresses of life. Most patients are best helped by a combination of a little sympathy and the prescription of decongestant preparations. Many patients give themselves a superadded rhinitis medicamentosa as a result of excessive use of decongestant drops and the regular use of these must be condemned. A substantial proportion of patients are sufficiently depressed to warrant treatment with tricyclic antidepressants.

Elderly men with a persistent and annoying 'dew drop' on the ends of their nose are sometimes treated with a short course of androgen.

A relatively small percentage will require referral to a specialist as submucus diathermy under general anaesthesia is helpful in resistant cases with nasal obstruction.

NASAL POLYPI

Clinical Features

Nasal polypi are easily recognised on anterior rhinoscopy. Their colour is different from the rest of the nasal mucosa, they are soft and mobile on probing and they mostly lie either in the middle meatus or in the roof of the nose. Most polypi arise from the mucosa of the ethmoid sinuses whence they pass into the middle meatus. Occasionally they arise in the antrum and pass out through the antral ostium and extend backwards towards the post nasal space (antrochoanal polypi).

Aetiology

Polypi are the results of oedema of the nasal mucosa progressing to such an extent that an area of mucosa 'falls away' and becomes attached to its site of origin by a stalk. They are nearly always bilateral.

Polypi arise in association with allergy or with infection. Most of them originate as a result of allergy and the infective element is secondary to the obstruction they produce. Once the polyp-forming tendency has developed in a patient this may continue long after the allergy itself and any associated infection have been treated.

Management

Where nasal polypi are causing obstruction they must be removed, and although snaring in the clinic will often get the patient out of immediate trouble, admission to hospital for more thorough treatment under a general anaesthetic is sometimes necessary. It frequently turns out that the visible polypus is only one of a whole row of polypi. The sinuses should be radiographed to exclude underlying infection.

It is a wise rule that all polypi removed should be examined histologically as, rarely, malignant changes may have occurred with nothing to rouse suspicion to the naked eye.

SINUSITIS

The paranasal sinuses are cavities within the skull continuous via ostia with the nasal cavities, and comprise an anterior group (maxillary, frontal, and anterior ethmoidal) opening into the middle meatus, and a posterior group (sphenoidal and posterior ethmoidal) draining into the spheno-ethmoidal recess and superior meatus.

Any of these sinuses may become infected as a result of spread of acute upper respiratory infection. In addition, the maxillary sinuses ('antra') may become infected as the result of infection in teeth of the upper jaw (accounting for about 10 per cent of cases). In children over the age of 3 or 4, and in adults, the maxillary sinuses are the most frequently involved, but in children below this age acute ethmoiditis is just as common.

All the sinuses are lined by columnar ciliated epithelium secreting mucus which is constantly moved towards the drainage ostia by ciliary action. As a result of infection this ciliary action may be impaired resulting in stagnation and further infection.

Acute Sinusitis

Acute infection of sinuses is liable to complicate an upper respiratory infection if their drainage is impaired by obstruction due to such conditions as deflected nasal septum, polypi, or vaso-motor rhinitis.

Clinical Features

The development of acute sinusitis during an upper respiratory infection will be suggested by the complaint of pain, together with fever and constitutional upset.

Frequently all the sinuses are involved, one more than the others. The patient may indicate the frontal or maxillary sinuses as the site of maximum pain, and there may be tenderness on pressure over them. Pain from ethmoidal infection is deep-seated behind the eyes and may be accompanied by tenderness at the back of the bridge of the nose just below the inner canthus. Sphenoidal pain is said to be felt in the centre of the head radiating towards the back of the neck.

Anterior rhinoscopy may reveal swelling and inflammation of the walls of the middle meatus, with oozing of pus (unless ostial obstruction is complete).

Acute ethmoiditis may spread outwards to involve the orbital cavity and ominous first signs are swelling and redness above and below the inner canthus.

Acute frontal sinusitis may also extend through bone to the orbital cavity, usually in the medial part producing a similar picture.

Management

The treatment of acute sinusitis is medical and consists ideally of rest in bed, and the administration of antibiotics in adequate doses, decongestants both orally and as nasal drops, steam inhalations such as Menthol and Eucalyptus which seems to promote drainage, and analgesics as required. It is desirable to take a swab of any visible pus in the nose before starting antibiotics so that a change to a more suitable antibiotic may be made if the first choice proves ineffective. Surgical drainage is very rarely required.

With adequate treatment acute sinusitis in otherwise healthy individuals should resolve completely and does not tend to recur.

Chronic Sinusitis

Aetiology

Chronic sinusitis may follow acute sinusitis where treatment has been unsuccessful or where there are underlying abnormalities such as gross septal deviation, polypi, or severe vaso-motor rhinitis. It may be associated with chronic bronchitis and bronchiectasis, and it is often debatable whether chronic chest infection is producing recurrent sinusitis, or vice versa. As sinuses and bronchi are both lined with similar epithelium it is likely that a common fault in this is responsible for both conditions.

Clinical Features

Chronic sinus infection may give rise to a constant boring pain, but more typically the complaint is of recurrent 'colds', a bad taste in the mouth, or an offensive nasal discharge. Almost always the maxillary sinuses are principally involved, and serve as a reservoir for recurrent infections in other sinuses. Polypi frequently complicate the picture.

On anterior rhinoscopy unhealthy nasal mucosa is to be expected, often with flecks of muco-pus especially in the middle meatus. Transillumination using a bright pen torch within the mouth directed upwards may show opacity of the maxillary sinuses. The method however is of more value in excluding disease when both sides transilluminate well.

Radiography in chronic sinusitis may reveal loss of radio-translucency where chronic thickening of mucosa exists, or the sinus is full of pus. There may be a fluid level (demonstrable in any of the sinuses).

Management

Where such evidence of chronic sinusitis is present, treatment with antibiotics and decongestants may be tried, but surgical intervention will often be required. Antral washout with the drainage of purulent material, sometimes repeated on several occasions, frequently restores the mucosal lining to a healthier state, and allows ciliary action to be resumed. Where conservative measures have failed in chronic maxillary sinusitis, intranasal antrostomy is indicated (an opening is made between the antrum and the nose), or, where severe changes in the antral mucosa are suspected, a Caldwell—Luc operation is performed, the antrum being opened anteriorly through the mouth. It can be fully inspected, diseased mucosa removed, and a larger more durable opening from the antrum into the nose constructed for future free drainage.

In addition, other surgery such as submucus resection of a markedly deviated nasal septum may be required.

Complications

Orbital spread from ethmoidal and frontal sinus infection has already been mentioned. Spread upwards from these sinuses may result in meningitis, and osteomyelitis and brain abscess may complicate frontal sinus infection. Untreated ethmoid sinusitis may lead to cavernous sinus thrombosis.

EPISTAXIS

Aetiology

This is probably the commonest type of haemorrhage the family practitioner is called upon to treat. In the great majority it comes from Little's area where ethmoidal, greater palatine, sphenopalatine and superior labial vessels anastomose, in the anterior and inferior part of the septum. In this region some of the vessels may be poorly supported and the overlying epithelium frail. Blowing the nose, or breathing excessively dry air, or endulging in physical activity with a resultant rise in blood pressure, may then be sufficient to precipitate bleeding from this vulnerable area. Such activities as 'scuba' diving may have similar results. Very often however the immediate cause of the bleeding is a mystery.

Bleeding from the nose may also occur as a result of trauma from nose picking, foreign bodies, or fractures, from infection, from vicarious menstruation, and from neoplasms. One of the most dramatic and potentially disastrous causes is juvenile angio-fibroma, a condition affecting males between the ages of 10 and 20 years which though rare should be borne in mind particularly by doctors responsible for youngsters at schools or in the Forces.

Hypertension and atherosclerosis predispose to epistaxis, as of course do anticoagulent drugs, and such blood disorders as thrombocytopoenic purpura, leukaemia, and sickle-cell anaemia.

An important though rare cause is Hereditary Telangiectasia (Osler's Disease) which is transmitted as a Mendelian dominant. There is no evidence of this disease till adult life, when aggregations of minute vessels begin to appear scattered over the mucus membrane of the nose, mouth, pharynx, and skin of the face neck and arms. The patients usually present with epistaxis and the multiple lesions are noted.

Management

By the time medical aid is requested a patient with an epistaxis, and his relatives, have often become somewhat frantic. A physiologically insignificant volume of blood, distributed amongst numerous tissues and old rags, may appear to them to constitute a near lethal haemorrhage. The general alarm may elevate the patient's blood pressure thereby aggravating the bleeding. An important part of the doctor's task is therefore to introduce an atmosphere of calm and reassurance. The patient should be advised to sit upright, with the head tilted slightly forward so that he can drip and spit into a bowl, and the nose should be firmly pinched between thumb and fingers for 5—10 minutes. The patient is instructed to breathe through his mouth. As most bleeding is from Little's area, and this will be compressed when the nose is pinched, on releasing pressure the bleeding will usually have stopped.

The patient's blood pressure should be recorded and if elevated hypotensive treatment may be begun at once.

When compression is released the nose may be gently inspected, using a Thudichum's speculum in an effort to locate the bleeding point. If this can be identified, and the bleeding recurrs, it can be cauterised later. If, on the other hand, no bleeding point can be seen, and bleeding continues, it must be coming from further back. This is common in arteriosclerotic patients, and hospital admission is often advisable. However, an attempt should be made to compress the unseen bleeding point and this may be done either by packing the nose with gauze tape, or, more conveniently, with an inflatable bag such as Simpson's or Brighton's inflatable tampon.

ENT specialists are very insistent that unanointed gauze is traumatic to nasal mucosa and encourages early putrefaction, and strongly condemn its use. Down the ages it has become a tradition to impregnate the gauze with BIPP (Bismuth iodoform paraffin paste), and no better substitute has been found. An obliging pharmacist may be willing to make up supplies of such 'BIPP wick' ready for emergency use. Failing this, the gauze tape should at least be lubricated with paraffin. Simpson's and Brighton's tampons are very effective but often seem to be either unavailable or perished.

Whichever method is used, the nose should be sprayed with 10 per cent cocaine solution unless the rate of bleeding makes this useless. Tape packings are built up in layers inside the nose from below upwards. If a Simpson's tampon is used, after introduction it is taped in position with strapping then 6—10 ml of air are injected with a disposable syringe.

A pair of angled forceps (e.g., Pritchard's), a Thudichum's speculum, and good illumination are needed.

If despite such packing bleeding continues the patient will certainly require hospital admission where it may be necessary to introduce a pack or balloon into the post nasal space, and of course transfusion may become necessary. On rare occasions arterial ligation proves necessary. Bleeding from above the middle turbinate is usually from the anterior ethmoidal artery, a branch of the internal carotid which may be ligated on the medial wall of the orbit. Bleeding from below the middle turbinate originates from branches of the external carotid artery.

If a persistently or recurrently bleeding site can be visualised it may be cauterised (after local anaesthesia with 10 per cent cocaine spray) either with the electrocautery or with chromium trioxide, silver nitrate, or trichloroacetic acid applied on a small pledget of wool mounted on a Jobson—Horne probe. These caustic chemicals must of course be used with great care.

In cases of telangiectasia it is often difficult to determine which of the multiple lesions is the source of bleeding on any one occasion and the disease can constitute a difficult and dangerous problem. Multiple repeated blood transfusions are often required. Oestrogens have been claimed to be helpful, and skin grafting inside the nose has been advocated.

There is a tendency for the family practitioner to be expected to cope with an epistaxis at the patient's home, and to send the patient to the hospital clinic when his efforts are unsuccessful. It would appear more sensible, where possible, for the patient to be conveyed, pinching his nose, to the doctor's surgery where proper lighting and equipment and possibly nursing help may make a hospital journey unnecessary.

FOREIGN BODIES

Young children are liable to put foreign bodies into their noses and then find they cannot remove them. Pieces of paper, beads and buttons are common choices. They generally come to be lodged in the inferior meatus and are easily seen on looking into the nose. When seen early, it is often possible to get the child to blow the foreign body out by compressing the opposite nostril and getting him to 'snort'. Deliberate induction of sneezing with pepper has been recommended. Failing this, if the child can be persuaded to co-operate, 10 per cent cocaine may be gently sprayed into the nose and the foreign body may be hooked out or grasped with angled forceps — taking great care not to push it further backwards.

If the introduction of a foreign body is unknown to the parents the child may be brought to the doctor weeks or months later with unilateral nasal obstruction, and an offensive, possibly blood streaked discharge on that side. It is important to bear in mind the possibility of a foreign body in such cases. Typically, culture of the swab of the discharge reveals a mixed infection. It may be possible to see, and remove the offending object. Sometimes it is too far back to be seen, when radiology may help. Such cases will usually require referral to a specialist for examination and removal of the foreign body under general anaesthesia.

It is remarkable how long foreign bodies may be preserved in the nose. A case has been recorded of a patient aged 25 who complained of nasal obstruction and underwent an operation for correction of a badly displaced nasal septum[48]. Behind the septal deflection was found a piece of cardboard, encrusted with salty deposits, which had apparently been put up her nose 20 years previously. There was only shallow ulceration, no bleeding and no smell, at the time of its discovery. Such salt encrusted foreign bodies are known as 'rhinoliths'.

INJURIES TO THE NOSE

Family practitioners are frequently confronted with patients whose noses have been injured (e.g., on the football field) and a course of action has to be decided upon. The two main types of injury are from sideward blows, which may produce lateral displacements, and frontal blows which may result in broadening of the nasal bridge. Either may be accompanied by septal injuries.

It is sometimes difficult to appreciate the degree of deformity when face to face with the patient, and a better idea is obtained by standing behind the seated patient whose head is tilted backwards so that the examiner looks down along his nose with the forehead as a 'foreground'. Any deformity then becomes more obvious.

If the patient is seen immediately after the injury, before swelling has developed, and has obvious deformity, it is worth getting him quickly to a specialist department where the nose can be manipulated and the deformity corrected.

If, however, the injury is sufficiently long standing for much swelling to have developed, then accurate correction of the deformity will not be possible until the swelling has subsided, which may be expected to take some 6 days. Thereafter the displaced bones will be easily manipulable for a further two weeks or so.

Radiography is not of great help in the management of nasal injuries — they give little more information than clinical examination.

The Throat

TONSILLECTOMY AND ADENOIDECTOMY

The management of tonsillitis has been fully discussed in Chapter 4. Where tonsillitis becomes a recurrent problem the question of tonsillectomy and adenoidectomy arises. As a rule of thumb, three attacks of tonsillitis in a year are judged to warrant consideration of tonsillectomy. However, tonsillectomy will not be beneficial where the diagnosis of tonsillitis has been loosely applied to upper respiratory infections, especially those with an allergic element. Indeed, it may do harm: in some children the onset of asthma can be directly related to tonsillectomy. Assessment of the need for surgery can only be made by a person who sees the child regularly over a prolonged period of time, i.e. the family practitioner. Except in a few special circumstances this is not a decision which can be made at a single consultation on specialist referral.

Much emotional discussion of the merits and demerits of adenotonsillectomy has taken place, and still continues. Around 150 000 operations on tonsils and/or adenoids are performed each year in the UK and the most frequent age is seven years. Many consider that too many operations are being performed, and some lives unnecessarily lost. Post-operative haemorrhage accounts for most of the 15—20 deaths which occur each year in the UK. In a paper presented at a recent meeting of the US Society for Paediatric Research, Hurtado[49] re-emphasised the role of tonsils in providing local immune protection against viruses, almost all of which enter through the nose or mouth, and considered that surgeons should think long and hard before removing them.

There is less disagreement on the indication for adenoidectomy, where recurrent otitis media is associated with severe adenoidal enlargement. Nevertheless Hoekelman[8] states 'There is absolutely no evidence to indicate that adenoidal size influences the frequency of otitis media or that children who have had their adenoids removed have fewer recurrences of acute otitis media than those who are not adenoidectom'sed' (p. 1202). Adenoidectomy for the treatment of glue ear has now largely been superseded by drainage of the middle ear with the use of a grommet.

A ring (Waldeyer's) of lymphoid tissue, consisting of the tonsils and adenoids and other less celebrated structures including the lingual and tubal tonsils and lymphoid nodules on the posterior pharyngeal wall, surrounds the pharyngeal entrance. If any part of this ring is removed during the peak of the lymphoid tissue growth curve, between the ages of 4 and 8 years, there is a strong tendency for hypertrophy of the remaining components of the ring.

This has two practical bearings on the sequelae of surgical removal. Surgeons removing adenoids to improve middle ear drainage, and naturally reluctant to remove apparently healthy tonsils, may confine themselves to adenoidectomy. All too often the tonsils then undergo considerable compensatory hypertrophy and can become very troublesome. It is of course to the family practitioner that the child's parents now turn. There is a pressing need for a survey to see how often this happens, and the results might lead to a change in surgical custom towards more frequent removal of tonsils at adenoidectomy.

A second consequence of this compensatory Waldeyer ring hypertrophy is that after adenotonsillectomy there may be enlargement of lymphoid tissue in the region of the Eustachian orifice, resulting in middle ear problems for the first time. This is a perplexing predicament, for further surgery is seldom practicable, – the risk of cicatricial stenosis following attempts to remove this offending lymph tissue is prohibitive. Fortunately, the 'decay' of the lymphoid tissue growth curve means that improvement can be anticipated with the passage of time.

Gross adenoidal enlargement can block the post-nasal space and result in mouth breathing and ingress of unmoistened and undecontaminated air which may encourage the recurrence of throat infections. Tonsillectomy alone in such cases would be unsound. Lateral soft tissue X-rays of the post-nasal space gives a valuable indication of the degree of adenoid enlargement.

A series of patients has been described[50] in whom adenotonsillectomy was a life-saving operation. Respiratory obstruction from grossly enlarged tonsils and adenoids was producing potentially fatal anoxia and *cor pulmonale*. The author has also encountered a case where emergency tonsillectomy was called for on this account. An attempt to intubate the child for emergency tonsillectomy resulted in complete obstruction and emergency tracheostomy was necessary. The existence of this small but hazardous group of patients is insufficiently well known.

The importance to health of tonsils and adenoids, and the indication for their removal, remain undecided. Widespread family practice surveys to clarify this problem are long overdue.

GLANDULAR FEVER

Throat infections, and particularly tonsillitis, developing and typically recurring over a period of months in teenagers and young adults, suggest glandular fever. The cervical and axillary glands of such patients should be palpated, and an enlarged spleen sought. A blood examination for atypical mononuclear cells, and a Paul Bunnell test, should be requested where the findings are consistent with glandular fever. If the diagnosis is supported the patient and his family should be warned of what to expect in coming months in the way of relapses of sore throat, lassitude and depression, possible skin rashes and even jaundice, and of the lack of specific therapy. It is helpful to explain that in a minority of cases the tonsils will be so damaged by the infection that they will continue to give trouble in the future and their removal may be called for. Steroids have a small but useful place, in short courses, in patients greatly distressed by excessive tonsillar and lymph gland enlargement. Some physicians make a point of excluding splenomegaly, before allowing suspected glandular fever cases to indulge in sporting activities.

HOARSENESS

Hoarseness of recent onset and accompanied by evidence of respiratory infection is usually self limiting and little active treatment is required beyond sparing the voice and remaining in as equitable an atmosphere as possible. Steam inhalations with Friar's Balsam or Vap. Menthol are soothing.

Where hoarseness persists beyond two to three weeks and particularly where there has been no apparent upper respiratory infection, serious disease may be present and of course inspection of the larynx is called for.

Indirect Laryngoscopy

The larynx is examined using a head mirror or focussing head lamp and a laryngeal mirror. The examiner sits facing the patient who is asked to remove any dentures, open his mouth wide, stick out his tongue and breath quietly through his mouth. In the meantime a laryngeal mirror, the largest convenient, is warmed in a flame and the back touched on the back of the examiner's hand to check it is not too hot. The examiner then wraps a gauze swab over the end of the tongue, grips the tongue between his thumb and forefinger, and draws it forwards. The light beam is focused on the uvula. The mirror (held like a pencil) is introduced into the mouth with the back resting against the uvula and adjoining soft palate. Great care must be taken that the mirror does not touch the fauces, back of the tongue, or posterior pharyngeal wall, or the gag reflex will be stimulated. Extreme gentleness is essential. Some patients cannot tolerate the mirror without the help of a local anaesthetic, such as a benzocaine lozenge, or a spray with 5 per cent cocaine.

Manipulating the mirror, the oropharynx, laryngopharynx, and then the larynx are examined. The pink false cords, and beyond them the pale vocal cords are inspected, and their mobility on inspiration and phonation ascertained. Occasionally it is possible to see far down the trachea.

Patients vary considerably in the ease with which their larynges may be examined. Much depends on the examiner's success in getting them to co-operate and relax — nervous patients sometimes start to 'gag' as soon as the mirror approaches their incisor teeth. The individual anatomy of the patient may also defeat the examiner — as in the case of 'infantile' configuration of the epiglottis.

Aetiology

Causes of hoarseness include:

1. *Acute laryngitis* — often part of a generalised upper respiratory infection. The laryngeal mucosa and cords are likely to be infected, and hoarseness may persist for up to two weeks after the inflammation has resolved.

2. *Chronic laryngitis* — due to faulty use of the voice (e.g., in auctioneers, barrow boys), chronic infection of teeth, tonsils, or sinuses, excessive alcoholic consumption and smoking, prolonged breathing of irritant fumes and dust. The vocal cords may be hyperaemic, hypertrophic, or oedematous. The changes are typically bilateral and symmetrical.

If the condition is of appreciable duration, referral to a specialist will be called for, as, apart from avoidance of obvious aggravating factors, speech therapy, eradication of sepsis in the upper respiratory tract, and even operative stripping of hypertrophied cords may be called for.

The following conditions also require accurate diagnosis and treatment in the ENT Department.

3. *'Singers' Nodules'* are seen especially in those who use 'forced' voices or who sing above their normal range. The lesions are really local hyperkeratoses. In many cases voice rest is enough to cause disappearance of nodes, but they can be removed surgically if they persist. The attention of a speech therapist is usually desirable.

4. *Acute haemorrhagic laryngitis* may cause sudden hoarseness following coughing or shouting. Submucosal haemorrhages are visible on one or both cords. Treatment is chiefly voice rest.

5. *Contact ulcers* may occur in singers, the result of pressure of one arytenoid process against the other. The most important part of the treatment is voice rest.

6. *Keratosis of the cords* giving rise to raised white areas on the cords; atrophic laryngitis, with dryness and perhaps crusting of the cords, sometimes associated with atrophic rhinitis; tubercular laryngitis with variable appearances ranging from mere injection to ulceration and granulation; and acquired syphilis, may all cause hoarseness.

7. *Papillomata of the cords*, single or multiple, *fibromata* and *polyposis* typically present with hoarseness and require removal in the hospital department and histological examination.

8. *Myxoedema*. Hoarseness of the voice is often one of the presenting signs in myxoedema — the pale bulky appearance of the cords is virtually diagnostic.

9. *Intermittent oedema* of the cords may be a manifestation of allergy.

10. *Muscle fatigue* ('*myasthenia of the larynx*') may result in tensor weakness with 'bowing' of the cords on phonation, and consequent hoarseness.

11. *Squamous cell carcinoma* of the larynx may be supraglottic (i.e., above the vocal cords), glottic, arising from the cords themselves, or subglottic. Hoarseness is naturally an earlier feature in glottic carcinoma than in carcinoma in the other two sites. Subglottic carcinoma may be advancing unseen for many months before becoming big enough to be visible beyond the edges of vocal cords. Early treatment is vital.

12. *Cord paralysis* may cause hoarseness. The lesion may be anywhere along the pathway from the cortex to the terminal branches of the superior and recurrent laryngeal nerves. Because of its longer course, the left recurrent laryngeal nerve is the more frequently involved. Nerve conduction may be interfered with as a result of spread of local disease (such as bronchial carcinoma), trauma, peripheral neuritis due to poisoning or to viral disease, or to radiotherapy. A cord may be:

1. flabby due to paralysis of the cricothyroid muscle — the 'tensor' of the cord, supplied by the external branch of the superior laryngeal nerve;
2. fixed in the midline and fail to abduct when the patient is asked to take a deep breath;
3. lying in the 'cadaveric' or paramedian, position — neither abducting on deep inspiration nor adducting on phonation. In the case of a unilateral lesion the normal cord will cross the midline to meet its fellow on phonation.

Semon's law states that in a progressive recurrent laryngeal nerve lesion the abductors are paralysed before the adductors. Thus 2, above may be a stage in progress toward 3.

In the case of functional dysphonia the cords fail to adduct when the patient is asked to phonate, but movement is seen to be normal when she is asked to cough.

The place of indirect laryngoscopy in family practice is obviously limited, for most patients will require specialist referral either because a lesion requiring treatment is seen or strongly suspected, or because no abnormality can be visualised to account for persisting symptoms, and therefore more experienced attention, probably supported by radiology, direct laryngoscopy and microscopy, is needed. However even though a specialist consultation is decided upon, the patient can often be put at his ease whilst waiting for this, and the doctor may obtain guidance as to how much delay can be accepted at the hospital appointment department. It should be possible in group practices and medical centres for one member of the family practitioner staff to acquire some practice and competence in indirect laryngoscopy.

CANCER OF THE THROAT

Cancers occurring in the 3 divisions of the pharynx — nasopharynx, oropharynx and laryngopharynx, have individual characteristics. In all, squamous cell carcinoma is the most common variety.

Nasopharynx

Most tumours in the nasopharynx are anaplastic. They are particularly common in first generation immigrants from South East Asian countries, such as Chinese restaurant workers, and must be suspected in cases of high cervical lymph node enlargement, unexplained epistaxis, recent acquisition of a 'nasal' voice, or unilateral Eustachian obstruction. The tumours may be difficult to see and biopsy even of virtually normal looking mucosa is sometimes needed.

In every case of suspected neck cancer, palpation of the neck for the presence of lymph gland involvement is of course essential. This is best performed standing behind the seated patient. First the neck is lightly felt with the flat of the finger tips, then the deeper tissues beneath the sternomastoids are examined, gathering them up between finger and thumb.

Oropharynx

Malignant tumours of the oropharynx tend to be anaplastic if arising from the tonsil or base of the tongue, but are usually more highly differentiated on the soft palate and fauces.

They can become surprisingly large before symptoms, such as problems with swallowing, result in medical advice being sought, and in more than half of patients cervical gland enlargement is present at the first consultation. The tumours may be 'exophytic', producing a luxuriant growth, or ulcerative with more tendency to deep invasion.

Tumours of the oropharynx should be easy to see in good light. A laryngeal mirror will be required to look at the back of the tongue. It is very important to move each side of the tongue medially in turn with a spatula to inspect the tonsillo-lingual sulcus, where a tumour is easily missed.

Statistically men are five times more liable to oropharyngeal cancer than women. Tobacco and dental decay appears to be an important factor. Overall 5 year survival rates with treatment are in the region of 20–30 per cent.

Laryngopharynx

Cancer of the laryngopharynx, which in effect extends from the hyoid bone to the entrance to the oesophagus opposite the 6th cervical vertebral body, usually presents with discomfort on swallowing, initially of solids only. Pain on swallowing tends to be referred to the ear.

The pyriform fossa is much the commonest site of laryngopharyngeal cancer, and men are more often affected than women. However post-cricoid carcinoma is most frequently encountered in women (even as young as 30 years) in association with the Paterson–Brown Kelly syndrome (dysphagia, often associated with an upper oesophageal web or stricture, and iron-deficiency anaemia).

Tobacco again appears to be an important aetiological factor, but pipes and cigars seem to be more dangerous than cigarettes. Heavy spirit drinking is also suspect as a causative factor, but as heavy drinkers are usually heavy smokers the truth is difficult to disentangle.

On examining the laryngopharynx (see page 156) the lesion may be too far down to be visible, but its presence may be suspected by pooling of saliva in one pyriform fossa.

The complaint of a sensation of a 'lump in the throat' is common and where no abnormality can be detected on clinical examination, judgement is required in deciding which cases require urgent specialist referral. If food and drink go down easily on swallowing, and the symptoms are intermittent, the cause is unlikely to be cancer.

The 5 year survival rate following surgery for laryngopharyngeal cancer is 20–25 per cent. The figure following the radiotherapy alone is 10–15 per cent.

Oesophagus

Oesophageal carcinoma is much commoner in men than women. The cure rate by any form of treatment is poor, largely due to the difficulty of early diagnosis. Early symptoms may be vague 'indigestion', or a feeling of food 'sticking' on swallowing. Chronic oesophagitis appears to be one predisposing cause, and any alteration in symptoms following malignant change in these cases may be for a long time imperceptible. The only hope for early diagnosis is a constant awareness of the possibility of carcinoma in patients with the suggestive symptoms mentioned, and the early performance of a barium swallow X-ray. Where this is negative but the symptoms persist, referral to a specialist department with a view to oesophagoscopy is indicated. The majority of cases are inoperable but it is sometimes possible to relieve obstruction for long periods by the insertion of a flexible tube (Souttar's or Mousseau—Barbin) with a rim which sits above the growth.

Larynx

Laryngeal cancer accounts for 2 per cent of all cancers. Squamous cell carcinoma is the commonest form. Tobacco, spirits, and prolonged vocal strain, appear to be aetiological factors. Anatomically, laryngeal cancers are divided into supraglottic, glottic (arising on the vocal cord itself, usually the middle or anterior third) and subglottic.

Glottic Cancer
Glottic cancer is much the commonest, and is usually well differentiated. It produces hoarseness at an early stage, resulting in the opportunity for early diagnosis whilst still confined to one cord. Here the prognosis is exceptionally good, with a 5-year survival rate of about 95 per cent whether treatment is by radiotherapy or by surgery.

Supra- and Sub-glottic Cancer
These carry a much worse prognosis. They tend not to produce symptoms until well advanced, and are often difficult to see with a laryngeal mirror.

ACUTE LARYNGEAL OBSTRUCTION

Acute laryngeal obstruction constitutes a grave emergency in family practice.

The commonest cause of acute laryngeal obstruction is acute laryngo-tracheobronchitis in infants and children up to the age of 6 or 7 years. Viral and/or common respiratory bacterial pathogens may be responsible for what at first appears a minor upper respiratory infection with a hoarse cough, but which proceeds to stridulous breathing and severe respiratory distress. There is indrawing of the soft tissues of the thorax, and 'plunging' of the trachae on inspiration, and cyanosis. There may be a high fever and convulsions.

Acute inflammation of the mucosa of the larynx, trachea and bronchial tree, with exudation of tenacious, often haemorrhagic material, results in anoxia from occlusion of the lower bronchial tree as well as laryngeal obstruction.

Admission to hospital in good time is of course vital, for treatment with antibiotics, oxygen, humidification, steroids, and trachial intubation where necessary. Apart from overcoming laryngeal obstruction, intubation makes possible suction aspiration of secretions in the lower bronchial tree.

Inflammatory swelling of the epiglottis (acute epiglottitis) may also produce laryngeal obstruction severe enough to require intubation. Inflammatory oedema of the larynx sufficient to cause acute obstruction may complicate quinsy, Ludwig's angina and retropharyngeal abscess. Laryngeal diptheria is fortunately a rarity these days.

Acute laryngeal obstruction may also occur in angioneurotic oedema. External trauma may give rise to haemorrhage into the lax submucous layer of the laryngeal mucosa, causing acute obstruction (there may be actual fracture of the laryngeal cartilages), and internal trauma from inhalation of steam or irritating fumes, swallowing of corrosives, or aspiration of foreign bodies may have the same result. It is rare however for foreign bodies to stick in the larynx. They usually either pass into the oesophagus or pass down through the larynx to the tracheal bifurcation and right main bronchus. Sharp foreign bodies may impact themselves in the larynx. Pieces of partially chewed meat may pass into the larynx and be held there by reflex spasm, often with immediate fatal consequences. Children are the main victims of foreign bodies – such as coins – lodged in the larynx which can sometimes be released by turning the child upside down and slapping the back.

Rarely, bilateral recurrent laryngeal nerve palsy of viral origin may result in acute laryngeal obstruction, the paralysed vocal cords coming to lie in the median position (see page 158).

Any of these causes of acute laryngeal obstruction may of course prove fatal if not immediately relieved and since there may not always be time to get the patient to hospital, all family practitioners should be prepared to perform an emergency laryngotomy should the need arise. This is of course quicker and simpler than a tracheostomy or intubation, which can subsequently be performed under proper conditions if required.

Laryngotomy

In performing a laryngotomy the patients head is extended, the laryngeal cartilages are palpated and the gap between the thyroid and cricoid cartilage identified. A transverse incision is made over this gap using any knife or pair of scissors available, passing first through the skin and next through the cricothyroid membrane. The cartilages are prised apart (e.g., by rotating the knife blade) allowing the passage of air. If any suitable tube is available – such as the barrel of a ball point pen – it can be inserted to maintain the opening, otherwise the cartilages can be kept separated by the rotated knife blade (caution — disposable blades may snap).

A council of perfection would be for every doctor to have in his bag a combined knife and laryngotomy tube[51].

Acknowledgements

I am indebted to Mr. Alan P. Fuller and Dr. Geoffrey S. Udall for their help with the section on deafness in children, and to Mr. Lance N. Dowie for reading the proofs and giving much valuable advice.

References

1. Fuller, A. P. (1975). Personal communication.
2. Fowler, E. P. (1950). *The Laryngoscope* 60, 680.
3. Morrison, A. W. (1975). In *Management of Sensorineural Deafness*, p. 176, (London: Butterworths).
4. Morrison, A. W. (1975). In *Management of Sensorineural Deafness*, p. 207, (London: Butterworths).
5. Perry, E. T. (1957). In *The Human Ear Canal*, (Mass., USA: Thomas Springfield) p. 59.
6. Fraser, J. G. (1971). *J. Laryngol. Otol.* 10, 1055.
7. Taylor, L. (1971). In *Diseases of the Ear, Nose and Throat.* (Scott-Brown, 3rd ed.) vol. 2, p. 101.
8. Hoekelman, R. A. (1974). *Update* 9, 1199.
9. Fry, J. (1972). *International Handbook of Medical Science*, p. 629. (Lancaster: MTP Press).
10. Taylor, L. (1971). In *Diseases of the Ear, Nose and Throat*, (Scott-Brown, 3rd ed.) vol. 2, p. 106.
11. Colman, B. H. (1973). *Diseases of the Nose, Throat and Ear*, p. 344, (Edinburgh and London: Churchill Livingstone).
12. Taylor, L. (1971). In *Diseases of the Ear, Nose and Throat*, (Scott-Brown, 3rd ed.) vol. 2, p. 104.
13. Gordon, M., Lovell, S. and Dugdale, A. E. (1974). *Med. J. Austral.* 1, 304.
14. Diamant, M. and Diamant, B. (1974). *Arch. Otolaryngol.* 100, 3, 226.
15. Cooper, A. (1801). *Philos. Trans.* 91, 435.
16. Politzer, A. (1867). *Wien. med. Wschr.* 17, 244.
17. Armstrong, B. W. (1954). *Arch. Otolaryngol.* 59, 653.
18. Adlington, P. and Davies, J. R. (1969). *J. Laryngol.* 83, 161.
19. Senturia, B. H. (1963). *Proc. roy. Soc. Med.* 56, 687.
20. Mogi, G., Honjo, S., Maeda, S., Yoshida, T. and Watanabe, N. (1974). *Annals Otol. Rhinol. Laryngol.* 83, 239.
21. Friedmann, I. (1963). *Proc. roy. Soc. Med.* 56, 595.
22. Thomas, R. (1967). *J. Laryngol.* 81, 1071.
23. Jordan, R. E. (1963). *Arch. Otolaryngol.* 78, 261.
24. Harrison, K. (1971). In *Diseases of the Ear, Nose and Throat*, (Scott-Brown, 3rd ed.) vol. 2, p. 135.
25. McNab-Jones, R. F. (1973). *Update* 7, 829.
26. Editorial (1975). *Lancet* ii, 397.
27. Bauer, F. (1975). *Lancet* ii, 618.

28. Tumarkin, A. (1961)*J. Laryngol.* **75**, 487.
29. Morrison, A. W. (1969). *Proc. roy. Soc. Med.* **62**, 959.
30. Morrison, A. W. (1967). *Ann. roy. Coll. Surg, Eng.* **41**, 202.
31. Schuknecht, H. F. (1964). *Arch. Otolaryngol.* **80**, 369.
32. Weston, T. E. T. (1964). *J. Laryngol.* **78**, 273.
33. Philipzoon, A. J. (1962). *J. Laryngol.* **76**, 593.
34. Morrison, A. W. (1975). In *Management of Sensorineural Deafness*, p. 149, (London: Butterworths).
35. Tumarkin, A. (1966). *J. Laryngol.* **80**, 1041.
36. Arslan, M. (1972). *The Larynogoscope* **82**, 1736.
37. Morrison, A. W. (1975). In *Management of Sensorineural Deafness*, p. 165, (London: Butterworths).
38. Roitt, I. (1971). In *Essential Immunology*, p. 111, (Oxford: Blackwell).
39. Coffman, D. A. and Chalmers, C. P. (1974). *J. roy. Coll. gen. Pract.* **24**, 171.
40. Johansson, S. G. O. (1969). *Proc. roy. Soc. Med.* **62**, 975.
41. Manners, B. T. M. (1974). *J. roy. Coll. gen. Pract.* **24**, 143.
42. Huggins, K. G. and Brostoff, J. (1975). *Lancet* ii, 148.
43. Ganderton, M. A. and James, V. H. T. (1970). *Brit. med. J.* **1**, 267.
44. Brostoff, J. (1975). *Lancet* i, 1424.
45. Anon. (1975). *Lancet* i, 786.
46. Munto-Ashman, McEwen, H. and Feinberg, J. G. (1971). *Int. Arch. Allergy* **40**, 448.
47. Ishizaka, K., Okudaira, H. and King, T. P. (1975). *J. Immunol.* **114**, 110.
48. McNab-Jones, R. F. (1971). In *Diseases of the Ear, Nose and Throat*, (Scott-Brown, 3rd ed.) vol. 3, p. 39.
49. Hurtado, R. C. (1974). *Proc. US Soc. Paed. Res.* **00**, 0000.
50. Jaffee, P. S. (1974). *The Laryngoscope* **84**, 7.
51. Cawthorne, T. (1964). *Lancet* i, 1081.

11

The Alimentary Tract

J. S. Norell

INTRODUCTION

The chief function of the alimentary tract is to serve as the first stage in the nourishment and growth of the individual. The sequence of processes by which this is accomplished — ingestion, digestion, absorption and elimination — suggests a conveyor belt activity with a hopper at one end and provision for periodic expulsion at the other, but this mechanistic view of the alimentary tract would be incomplete for it ignores an essential function, namely, providing satisfaction. At the extremes of life, eating and to a lesser extent defaecation have no equal as sources of pleasure: the infant's existence is dominated by these events, and in the regressed elderly they again assume a significance of almost obsessional proportions. But at every age there is a close connection between an individual's sense of well-being and the functioning of his alimentary tract, a relationship to which folklore and ordinary language bear testimony.

This has two important clinical consequences. Firstly, disorders of the alimentary tract may be expressed in a wide variety of symptoms. Secondly, many of the symptoms are not exclusive to this particular body system. For instance, although haematemesis and melaena are straightforward indicators of gastro-intestinal pathology, dysphagia, sialorrhoea and vomiting are not necessarily so. Heartburn and flatulence may reflect alimentary disturbance, but abdominal pain and distension may have causes outside the tract, and so too may anorexia, nausea, constipation and loss of weight. Individual symptoms do no more than offer pointers to possible disorders; what really matters is the way symptoms are clustered together, time associations, and relationships to other factors.

Diagnostic Approach

Presentation

A feature of family practice is its closeness to events. Very often, only in retrospect is it possible to discern a beginning or an end to a 'medical episode'. The start of an illness can be expressed in only a limited number of ways and some of the presenting symptoms may be of a minor nature, scarcely noticed by the patient or not reported by him. The family practitioner has the additional difficulty therefore of operating against a background of 'normal ill-health' and matters are made worse when the onset is insidious or acute-on-chronic. But even where the presentation is obvious enough he still has a problem. Does he step in straight away or does he wait for the picture to clarify? In the first case he risks intervening unnecessarily in a self-limiting condition; in the second, he may regret procrastinating where early treatment may have cut short the illness.

Associated Symptoms, Time-relationships

A detailed history may be difficult to elicit in family practice. Only later, perhaps in hospital, may it be possible to piece the story together with the help of relatives. At this point the doctor's aim is to discern a pattern in what may be rather diffuse symptomatology.

Self-medication

It is unusual for patients not to have taken some patent medicine prior to seeking advice from their family practitioner, and this is especially true with gastro-intestinal symptoms; laxatives and antacids are the most popular preparations. A further problem for the doctor is that the patient may have been taking analgesics for a pre-existing condition and the gastric symptoms he is complaining of may be related to that medication.

Iatrogenic Factors

A significant proportion of ill-health in the community is directly attributable to preparations prescribed by doctors. The increasing complexity of medical teamwork, both inside and outside the hospital, leads to a situation where several doctors may be involved in the care of the same patient, each of them prescribing for him. Records may be incomplete and communication inadequate, so patients should always be asked what medicines they are taking. In patients' homes time spent scrutinising labels on medicine bottles and pill-boxes is well repaid.

Intercurrent Household or Family Illness

This may not be volunteered, and so should always be asked about. Where appropriate, enquiry should be made about school or the workplace.

Previous Illness
This is usually known to the family doctor and the necessary information should be capable of being retrieved from the records, particularly if a summary card has been properly utilised.

Key Symptoms
Most patients are indifferent historians and need to be taken over a check-list of important symptoms, such as melaena or change in bowel habit.

The Clinical Examination
This will take in the patient's demeanour, decubitus, presence of oral foetor, appearance of the tongue, state of teeth, appearance and feel of the abdomen. A more general examination may be necessary, and rectal and vaginal examinations may be needed.

The Patient's Personality
This again is usually familiar to the family practitioner who may have had a relationship with the patient spanning decades. The assessment of personality should embrace such factors as pain threshold – important in evaluating some symptoms – the patient's attitude to his present illness, and his general expectations of what medical services might provide.

The Family Atmosphere
It is important always to consider the patient in the context of his family circle. For one thing, the tensions there might be the cause of his symptoms or could certainly exacerbate them, but apart from this the general mood of the family will have a bearing on the way the doctor decides to manage the illness. He may not always have this previous knowledge in spite of being the 'family' doctor; the particular family may be the sort in which only one of its members is ever ill, or where the rest of the family get medical advice elsewhere. The emotional climate can be sensed, however, particularly during a home visit but also from the way relatives behave when they accompany patients in the consulting room.

Initial Assessment

No matter how brief the examination or scanty the data the family doctor has to come to an immediate decision on the urgency of the case. His first question therefore is not, 'What is the illness?', but 'How ill is this patient?' The answer to this will determine the pace of his subsequent actions.

The precise diagnosis may be unimportant at this stage; the broad diagnositic grouping may be sufficient to suggest a reasonable line of management and in this the doctor will employ the probabilistic approach, bearing in mind however that the probability (or improbability) of a clinical event must be weighted with its intrinsic seriousness and with the extent to which its course can be favourably altered by timely action. 'Common conditions commonly occur', but a relatively rare, serious illness in which early diagnosis could make a difference will loom large in the doctor's mind.

Management

Are the doctor's resources, and the facilities in the home adequate to cope with the illness? Can the family practitioner count on the co-operation of relatives or neighbours? What is the likelihood of a therapeutic regime being adhered to? A family doctor must weigh up these questions in addition to considering the purely clinical side of the situation.

He may decide that the case can be managed at home but that further investigations are necessary. He has a choice of actions. He can refer the patient to the appropriate specialist; or he might utilise the pathology or radiology departments. Some patients, though acutely ill, are reluctant to enter hospital even when advised to do so, and this may pose a problem for the doctor who may be unhappy at the prospect of managing a potentially serious condition at home. Here, he could decide to call on a domiciliary consultation with a specialist colleague, either to back up his original advice or perhaps to reassure him that it would be justifiable to continue treating the patient at home.

No family practitioner is truly single-handed: he can call on a wide range of para-medical and supportive services, statutory and voluntary, to help him in the optimum management of sickness in the home. To some extent community nursing, welfare and social work services can fill the gaps in care which some families are unable to bridge because of housing conditions or outside commitments. The deployment of nurses, home-helps and others is an important function of the family doctor: he is in a position to orchestrate the entire range of community health and welfare services for the care of his patient.

Opportunities for specific therapy are relatively few in family practice: most episodes of illness are self-limiting and call for supportive measures only while the doctor keeps a watching brief. It is watching, however, not gazing, and he will be continually reviewing the clinical course and considering treatment in its several perspectives: immediate action, therapy for the current illness, and long term plans.

Lack of progress may dictate the need for further tests, or this may be obvious from the outset. The simpler, readily available tests relevant to alimentary tract disorders include faecal occult blood, urinalysis and culture, blood counts and blood chemistry. Straight X-ray of the abdomen and contrast radiology may be indicated and is usually available to the family practitioner.

Proctoscopy can be performed in the surgery or home, but other instrumentation such as sigmoidoscopy or the use of fibre-optics will necessitate specialist
referral in most cases, and laparotomy certainly will.

Treatment in its widest sense will take account of the whole person in the
context of his family and social situation, and will range beyond the immediate
issue to considerations of aftercare and rehabilitation, and, paradoxically, to
prevention — the measures required to prevent recurrence or complications.

ACUTE GASTRO-ENTERITIS

This is a common condition in family practice and is frequently referred to as
diarrhoea and vomiting (D. & V.) or 'food poisoning'. In the UK there is an
incidence of newly diagnosed cases of between fifty and one hundred per
100 000 population at risk. Though nowhere as common as coughs and colds,
acute gastro-enteritis (including dysenteric forms) ranks as one of the
commonest communicable illnesses which the family doctor will face.

Aetiology and Pathogenesis

The precise cause is identified in only a small minority of cases but a food-borne
mechanism or otherwise accidental ingestion is assumed to be a factor. Among
the causes which have been established are bacteria (Shigellae, Vibrios, pathogenic
Escherichia Coli, Salmonellae, Clostridia, Staphylococci), viruses (especially
entero-viruses), protozoons (*Entamoeba histolytica, Giardia lamblia*), worms
(*Trichinella, Trichuris*), chemicals (used in the household, or in agricultural and
industrial processes), and medicines (through overdosage, hypersensitivity or
idiosyncracy).

Where contamination of food by an infective agent is responsible the
resulting illness may be due to the effects of pre-formed toxin, that is,
elaborated by the organism prior to ingestion, rather than to the growth and
spread of organisms in the alimentary tract. This is particularly the case in
staphylococcal food poisoning. Relatively few bacteria can survive passage
through the stomach, and amongst them are the organisms responsible for
dystentery, cholera and salmonella food poisoning.

The evidence for incriminating viruses as a common cause of gastro-
enteritis comes from electron microscopy studies of infected faeces and from the
demonstration of virus particles (parvoviruses, picornaviruses and rotaviruses) in
the intestinal mucosa of young children with the acute illness. Moreover,
symptoms of the illness have been produced by administering the agent to
volunteers, especially on serial passage[1].

Epidemiology

The outbreaks of gastro-enteritis experienced in the UK a century ago resemble the situation which is commonplace in underdeveloped countries today. High standards of public health, notably in sewerage and in clean water supplies, has completely altered the epidemiological picture, but sporadic outbreaks still occur and they are not confined to the warm weather when flies abound. Family practitioners see cases throughout the year.

The steady incidence of cases is favoured by the following factors:

1. Increased communal eating in restaurants and school and works canteens;
2. Growth in the packaging of cooked or partly-cooked food, especially of meat intended for consumption without further cooking;
3. The popularity of deep-frozen, 'oven-ready' foods, especially poultry which may be subjected to inadequate thawing so that organisms survive and multiply during cooking;
4. The increase in consumption of food from abroad which is prepared and packed in the country of origin; for example, canned meat from South America which was the source of an outbreak of Salmonella food-poisoning in Aberdeen[2];
5. The increased provision of nursery care for children, residential and day;
6. The increase in migration, in holiday and business travel to the tropics and sub-tropics, together with much shortened travelling times, (a traveller can complete his journey home within the incubation period of his illness).

When several people fall ill together the explanation is usually apparent, as for example when all the members of a family become affected simultaneously, or a coach party, or wedding guests, or even — as has happened — delegates attending a medical conference. But the chain of infection may be difficult to establish without considerable investigation. In the Aberdeen outbreak referred to above, the primary source of the infection was traced to contaminated water used in the cooling process of the meat canning plant. A fault in the metal seam allowed water to enter under the negative pressure created by the cooling. But it was not only those who ate this meat who were affected: in the shop in Aberdeen where the meat was sliced and served to customers the organisms were transferred to the counter and to knives used for preparing other meats, so that many more customers were affected than those who ate the South American product. Then, following the first cases, secondary and tertiary cases occurred.

Clinical Features

Most attacks are mild and short-lived. The patient vomits once or twice and experiences diarrhoea after a variable period, up to twelve hours later. There is no blood in the stools. The patient is not pyrexial and has no generalised symptoms. Pain, if present at all, is limited to waves of central abdominal colic immediately preceding another bowel evacuation. Physical examination reveals no abnormality; the abdomen is soft and not tender, though bowel sounds are increased and may be audible without a stethoscope. In such mild cases symptoms have abated in twenty-four to forty-eight hours.

Occasionally, severe cases are seen in family practice with an explosive onset; repeated vomiting and retching, intense cramp-like abdominal pains, profuse diarrhoea — thin, watery, and sometimes with blood — and rapid deterioration into a state of fluid and electrolyte depletion. These cholera-like symptoms may well be seen in a traveller recently returned from the tropics by air.

Or the onset may be insidious with low-grade pyrexia, lassitude, myalgia, headache, anorexia and nausea. Vomiting and diarrhoea are present but are not prominent and may not be what the patient complains about most. There are few, if any, abnormal physical signs apart from the slightly raised temperature and perhaps a mild pharyngitis. This is the condition often dubbed 'gastric 'flu' by the lay public, and — in the absence of a more plausible diagnosis — by many doctors also. The course of this illness is often protracted with lassitude and fatiguability persisting long after the gastro-intestinal symptoms have remitted.

In another variant of the illness symptoms may be virtually confined to the lower intestinal tract and the picture may merge into chronic or recurrent colitis.

In addition to the above features the patient's age may influence the clinical course, especially at the extremes of life. Infants tolerate fluid loss very poorly and may very easily pass into a state of irreversible peripheral circulatory failure. In the elderly in addition to the hazards of electrolyte depletion the mehanical effects of repeated vomiting and of diarrhoea may impose physical stresses on a myocardium already weakened by previous ischaemic disease; so possible sequels to gastro-enteritis in the aged include cardiac failure, as well as cerebral thrombosis and phlebo-thrombosis.

Diagnosis

In the mild case with typical symptoms a presumptive diagnosis of acute gastro-enteritis is justifiable provided examination excludes acute abdomen. In the young, appendicitis, especially where the appendix lies over the pelvic brim, may mimic the illness; and in the elderly or obese a strangulated hernia may be responsible and may be overlooked, particularly if femoral. Conditions outside the gastro-intestinal tract may need to be excluded, especially in the young and the old, and the cause may be found to lie outside the abdomen. Hence, where appropriate, peptic ulcer, gall-bladder disease, colonic and rectal neoplasm, pyelonephritis, pneumonia, myocardial infarction, and otitis media may have to be considered, as well as non-localised conditions such as diabetes and uraemia. Pregnancy hyperemesis may have to be excluded.

The actual cause of the gastro-enteritis may be guessed from the circumstances or revealed by enquiry. Patent or prescribed medicines, household chemicals, or toxic occupational hazards should be considered. Or a meal may be incriminated in the case of a family outbreak of illness. The shorter the interval between ingestion and the symptoms the more likely is it that the illness is due to pre-formed toxin, possibly staphylococcal. Infective cases such as from Salmonella may have generalised prodromal symptoms of up to twenty-four hours. The identification of the precise infective agent requires bacteriological investigation of samples of the suspect food and of vomit and faeces, the results of which are often negative so that a viral cause is presumed.

In regard to medication as a possible cause, digoxin overdosage in the elderly, aspirin in susceptible individuals, and wide-spectrum antibiotics, especially a prolonged course, should be excluded, as should oral contraceptives.

Management

The usual cases seen in family practice are mild, self-limiting, and leave no sequelae. An expectant attitude is therefore justified. It is sensible for the patient to remain in bed, though he rarely needs to be advised on this point. Once vomiting has ceased fluids should be encouraged: plain water or well-diluted fruit juice, little and often. Medicines are unnecessary for the short-lived case and patients should be discouraged from resorting to proprietary 'stomach mixtures' and the like, some of which contain aspirin and may well exacerbate their symptoms.

Special care must be exercised with the very young and the very old, even in apparently mild gastro-enteritis. The prevention of dehydration becomes a prime concern and may require the attention of a home nurse visiting twice a day. Her close liason with the family practitioner is obviously of great importance, and one of her functions will be to interpret and reinforce the doctor's instructions to the relatives.

Otherwise fit adults who have the moderately severe form of the illness may also be satisfactorily managed at home, provided family resources are available. Relief of pain, together with sedation, can be achieved with a single intramuscular injection of 100 mg pethedine. Persistent vomiting and nausea may be helped by the administration of metoclopramide 10 mg; again, when needed it will be required parenterally and may be given intravenously as a 2 ml injection. This preparation also helps to relieve intestinal spasm and the gastric stasis which is a prominent feature of gastro-enteritis.

Once oral medication can be tolerated, troublesome diarrhoea can be treated with diphenoxylate 5 mg four times daily, or kaolin and morphine mixture 15 ml four-hourly. Usually, however, diarrhoea ceases spontaneously and medication is unnecessary.

Hospitalisation should be considered for the following:

1. All those with the severe form of the illness;
2. Moderately ill young children and elderly patients, and adults with serious pre-existing medical conditions;
3. Any patient failing to improve, or deteriorating, after twenty-four hours;
4. Those in whom cholera, typhoid, or para-typhoid fever is suspected;
5. Patients in whom a surgical condition cannot confidently be excluded.

The question of antibiotics is a controversial one. Those with serious illness who are likely to benefit will very likely already be in hospital. There is some doubt about the value of antibiotics in clearing patients of *Salmonella typhimurium, Shigella sonnei*, or pathogenic *Escherichia coli*. There is evidence that the administration of antibiotics may actually delay the final excretion of these organisms[3] and they may aggravate diarrhoea.

The choice of antibiotic will be determined by bacterial sensitivities but while awaiting laboratory results it is reasonable to start the patient on neomycin 500 mg four times daily if dysenteric symptoms predominate, or co-trimoxazole 480 mg four times daily if *S. typhimurium* food-poisoning is suspected.

Trichuris and *Trichinella* may be treated with thiabendazole 25 mg per kg body-weight twice daily with fluids, to a maximum of 3 g daily. For *Giardia lamblia* infections in adults, furazolidone 100 mg four times daily may be given; children over five years, half this dosage.

A preparation widely taken for the prevention of 'traveller's diarrhoea' is clioquinol (Entero-vioform) but neomycin 500 mg four times daily is probably more effective for those patients requiring this form of prophylaxis.

Women on oral contraceptives should be warned not to rely on the 'Pill' in cycles during which acute gastro-enteritis has occurred.

Public Health and Preventive Aspects

Food poisoning and infective gastro-enteritis are notifiable conditions and the district community physician should be informed whenever these are suspected.

Where indicated the staff of the Public Health Inspector will arrange bacteriological tests of food, restaurant kitchens and food handlers. This is the only way in which sources of infection can be traced and may be necessary in order to limit the spread.

Schools, nurseries, and food establishments may require the submission of medical certificates testifying to freedom from infection and stipulating the number of negative stool cultures obtained.

Whatever the source of infection the family doctor can use the opportunity to reinforce health education on simple but effective hygiene measures including standards of food preparation and storage, the use of refrigerators, and the washing of hands.

Research

Any one doctor sees relatively few cases of gastro-enteritis each year but in total family practitioners can contribute an impressive amount of data to various research bodies. In the UK there is the Public Health Laboratory Service, the Research Unit of the Royal College of General Practitioners, the Committee on Safety of Drugs, and the Poisons Reference Centre*. These bodies, together with local virology laboratories and local public health departments put out a good deal of useful and topical information that is helpful to family practitioners but in turn they rely on input from the field.

The main gaps in knowledge to which research needs to be directed are:

1. The virology of gastro-enteritis.
2. Double-blind trials to decide whether antibiotics are of benefit in the less severe forms of bacterial gastro-enteritis.

PEPTIC ULCER

It is traditional to group together ulcers of the lower end of the oesophagus, the stomach, and the duodenum, because they share the feature of upper abdominal discomfort related to the taking of food. But the differences between them as regards aetiology, clinical presentation, prognosis and treatment are more striking than the similarities; and clinically they share many characteristics with the class of 'non-ulcer dyspepsia'. Taken together, they constitute one of the commonest reasons for an adult to consult his family practitioner.

---

* Poisons Reference Centre, New Cross, London, S.E. Epidemiological Bulletins, Central Public Health Laboratory, Colindale (weekly). Committee on Safety of Medicines (annual reports). Bulletin on Adverse Drug Reaction, Newcastle-on-Tyne.

Aetiology and Pathogenesis

The immediate cause of peptic ulcer is the chemical action of pepsin with hydrochloric acid of the gastric juice causing digestion of the mucosa. The ultimate cause is unknown, and clearly the factor of tissue resistance must be important. A number of associated factors have been elucidated, experimentally as well as from studies of patients and healthy individuals; but it cannot be assumed that a factor which causes peptic ulcer necessarily contributes to its chronicity.

Acid hypersecretion is the outstanding feature in duodenal ulcer, due most likely to hyperplasia of the gastric mucosa; but why this should occur is uncertain, though there may be a genetic basis. In gastric ulcer, acid production is usually diminished as a consequence of associated gastritis, and here the factor of diminished tissue resistance is probably crucial. Causes of the gastritis may include bile reflux, smoking, alcohol, and the habitual ingestion of hot drinks.

A family history is often prominent in cases of peptic ulcer, and it is likely that duodenal and gastric ulcers are inherited independently. In the rare instances when a child is affected the family history is particularly strong. Individuals of blood group O and non-secretor status are more liable to duodenal ulceration than are the rest of the population.

No consistent emotional make-up accompanies peptic ulceration but the incidence of anxiety neurosis is significantly higher in patients with duodenal ulcer than in a cross-section of family practice. Apart from the question of a causative effect, stressful anxiety is associated with relapse or exacerbation of ulcer symptoms.

Among exogenous factors cited are smoking, alcohol, curries, pickles, and certain drugs. The latter include corticosteroids, phenylbutazone, indomethacin, and salicylates. This last is especially significant in family practice because as aspirin it is a constituent of many proprietary medicines and may be bought 'over the counter.' It may even be present in so-called 'stomach mixtures.'

Epidemiology

In gastric ulcer, but not duodenal ulcer, there is a socio-economic gradient with disproportionately more cases occurring in the poorer groups. This may be related to the higher incidence of chronic gastritis in this section of the community. It used to be thought that the tension-ridden managerial and executive classes were particularly liable to develop duodenal ulcers, or vulnerable to perforation; there is no class basis however, though certain occupations have a higher than expected incidence. For instance bus drivers have more ulcers than bus conductors, but physical activity may be operative here.

World-wide, there are large variations in the incidence of peptic ulcer, even between neighbouring communities. For instance, the lower incidence of duodenal ulcer in Northern India is thought to be related to the high fibre content of the diet compared to the blander food of Southern India. Moreover migrants tend to experience the pattern of their hosts rather than that of their country of origin.

There are very pronounced sex differences, gastric ulcer occurring twice as often in men as in women, while duodenal ulcer occurs up to ten times as often. The mortality from complications is also higher in men, but the relative immunity that women enjoy becomes less after the menopause.

Clinical Features

The classical presentation of duodenal ulcer is of a youngish man complaining of localised epigastric pain coming on about half an hour after meals and temporarily relieved by food and antacids (most patients have already medicated themselves before resorting to the doctor). Some patients experience relief from vomiting, and this may be self-induced. They may complain of heartburn and waterbrash and nausea, but appetite is unimpaired or even enhanced. Intervals between meals may be accompanied by hunger pangs, and sleep may be broken. More attacks seem to occur in the spring and autumn than in the other seasons.

The patient is usually otherwise fit, there is no loss of weight, and the only finding on physical examination is tenderness in the epigastrium to the right of the midline. The individual may be anxiety-prone, and interpersonal or occupational stress factors may be elicited.

The course of duodenal ulcer is marked by remissions and exacerbations over the years, punctuated in a small minority by haemorrhage, perforation, or pyloric stenosis.

The patient with gastric ulcer tends to be older, poorer, and is more likely to have had an illness predisposing to chronic gastritis. He is more likely to be a smoker and to drink. A seasonal pattern is less evident. Relation to food is less clear than in cases of duodenal ulcer, but the pain is often reported to be worse after meals, and antacids to be unhelpful. A small proportion of gastric ulcers, fewer than five per cent, undergo malignant conversion.

Diagnosis

With characteristic symptoms the diagnosis of duodenal ulcer may be made on clinical grounds with a fair degree of confidence. Radiological confirmation is necessary in the following situations:

1. atypical symptomatology, including loss of weight.
2. patients over forty years of age.
3. women.
4. departure from usual pattern of pain; or failure to improve from a course of treatment.
5. suspected pyloric stenosis.

If symptomatic improvement has occurred, there is little point in seeking radiological proof of healing in the majority of cases of duodenal ulcer.

The position is different in gastric ulcer, and these patients should have repeated radiological checks until satisfactory healing has been demonstrated, in the absence of which specialist referral should be sought for gastroscopy. The interpretation of radiological abnormalities may be difficult and the family practitioner may need to make personal contact with his radiologist colleague over this.

The faecal occult blood test (on three consecutive samples) is a useful accessory investigation, and so is a blood count to pick up anaemias from chronic blood loss. Patients should be asked about self-medication, and about medicines prescribed for other conditions.

Alteration in the site of pain, especially radiation to the back, should be enquired for; haematemesis and melaena should be specifically asked about.

The most important differential diagnoses in peptic ulcer are from carcinoma of the stomach and carcinoma of the lower end of the oesophagus.

Management

Peptic Oesophagitis

Minor degrees of hiatus hernia are fairly easily demonstrated, perhaps too easily, with modern barium meal techniques, and it is doubtful whether all a patient's epigastric symptoms should be ascribed to this condition. Nevertheless reflux oesophagitis can be a distressing symptom even in the absence of an ulcer or of hiatus hernia. Postural factors are contributory so patients should be discouraged from prolonged stooping (as in housework, gardening), an extra pillow or two under the shoulders in bed should be tried, and finally the head of the bed raised on nine-inch blocks. Intra-abdominal distension is often a factor (as in pregnancy) and it is worth pursuing a weight-reducing regime in obese patients. Meals should be small and frequent, with a minimum of fluids so as to reduce gastric distension. Patients will generally already have discovered the wisdom of avoiding very hot (in both senses) food.

Medication plays only a subsidiary role in peptic oesophagitis, but can provide prompt symptomatic relief. Usually an antacid is all that is necessary; e.g., magnesium trisilicate with aluminium hydroxide, two tablets or 15 ml of the suspension as required. A suspension containing the local anaesthetic oxethazaine may be helpful, as may be tablets containing alginic acid which is said to act as a viscous neutralising gel coating the lower end of the oesophagus.

Gastric Ulcer

Most gastric ulcers will heal rapidly if patients are put to bed and their smoking cut right out. However this degree of co-operation ('patient compliance') is becoming rarer and it is more realistic to devise a satisfactory ambulant treatment in the first instance. Carbenoxolone sodium, 100 mg thrice daily after food has been found to increase the rate of healing of gastric ulcers, but it may raise the diastolic blood pressure, cause oedema from water retention, and lead to hypokalaemia. As the course of treatment may last up to twelve weeks these can be serious disadvantages, which a thiazide diuretic with potassium may help to mitigate. Deglycyrrhizinized liquorice extract also promotes healing of ulcers and is free from the drawbacks of carbenoxolone.

Patients should be followed up with serial barium meals until satisfactory healing has been demonstrated radiologically. Recurrence of symptoms, at any age, should be the occasion for renewed investigation, which may include gastroscopy.

Failure to achieve healing with ambulant treatment will necessitate bed rest, however reluctant the patient may be to lose time from work. The family practitioner must use his knowledge of the patient's personality, his family and his home in judging whether a hospital bed might be preferable. Nursing requirements for gastric ulcer are not high, but some homes may not provide the optimum conditions of rest and quiet and regular meals. For that matter neither do some hospital wards under today's staffing conditions, and the family practitioner may have to weigh this factor too. In either case the patient should be helped to accept that a period off work of about six weeks will be necessary, with a very good chance of complete healing at the end of it.

Specialist referral should be considered for those patients whose ulcers fail to heal steadily, for those who relapse frequently, where the character of the symptoms changes, and for frank gastro-intestinal bleeding.

Duodenal Ulcer

The successful management of duodenal ulcer turns more on establishing a better life-style for the patient than the prescribing of medication or subjecting the patient to surgery. Meals, which should contain a normal amount of fat, should be evenly spaced, and snacks taken between the main meals. The occupations followed by many patients may make this difficult but it should be possible to take a sandwich and a glass of milk to work. A similar snack should be taken immediately before going to bed, and some milk should be available at the bedside in case of night pain.

The aim of this regime is to ensure that food is present in the stomach to buffer the high amounts of acid that are being secreted. 'Nulacin' tablets (so-called 'milk-alkali drip'), placed in the buccal sulcus and allowed to dissolve, also achieve this neutralisation. Larger amounts of antacid may be necessary and this is conveniently given as a powder of magnesium trisilicate compound, or as a ready-made mixture (many patients prefer this). The amount and frequency of the doses should be determined by the patient himself as a result of experience: it is pointless to instruct him to take a fixed amount three or four times a day. Present antacids do not carry the dangers of alkalosis which sodium bicarbonate for instance has.

Where night pain is a persistent problem poldine methylsulphate 4 mg at night may succeed in cutting down acid production sufficiently to allow a night's undisturbed rest. The place for spasmolytics in duodenal ulcer is controversial. They do not hasten healing: the only question is, do they bring symptomatic relief? Belladonna is a traditional constituent of ulcer remedies; a suitable synthetic analogue would be propantheline bromide 15 mg four times a day. It should be borne in mind that reduction in stomach motility may make matters worse for patients with some degree of pyloric stenosis; and the anticholinergic drugs may precipitate symptoms of glaucoma or prostatic obstruction.

Carbenoxolone does not give the same reliable results in duodenal ulcer as it does in the gastric variety but 'position-release' capsules are available and a two or three month trial of these would be justifiable.

There is no place for the routine prescribing of sedatives in duodenal ulcer, notwithstanding the frequent accompaniment of anxiety states. It is preferable to explore the sources of possible stress with the patient and his family, and so help the patient to identify and adjust to difficulties of an interpersonal nature, or in his marriage, his job, or his housing situation. If medication is required for overt tension state it is better to use a preparation such as meprobomate, rather than chlordiazepoxide or diazepam (which are habit-forming) or barbiturates (which the profession seems to be moving away from). This need not be a signal for the doctor to withdraw: the patient still stands in need of his family practitioner's support and encouragement and understanding.

Surgery and Aftercare

The family practitioner's counselling role will also need to be employed should the question of surgery be raised. Apart from the clear-cut indications such as onset of complications, most decisions are reached on the basis of balancing the operative risks against the discomfort of the ulcer and the disruption of normal life brought about by relapses. After operation the patient will need to be helped over the short term sequelae and perhaps the persistent distressing symptoms. In addition he will require surveillance if a gastrectomy has rendered him at risk for nutritional deficiencies; as well as an annual haemoglobin estimation he may need a blood film and estimations of serum B12, folate, iron, and calcium.

Preventive Aspects

Since the aetiology of peptic ulcer is unknown and the mechanism far from clear, opportunities for prevention are not promising. Even tertiary prevention, forestalling recurrences, seems to be beyond our reach, and there is certainly no evidence that the continued administration of antacids or anticholinergics can achieve this. The relative freedom from side-effects of deglycyrrhizinized liquorice would justify a trial of this preparation in the long term managment of gastric ulcer.

For the rest, the family practitioner's advice must be the usual sensible, if not always popular, measures for promoting good health; namely regular wholesome meals, adequate rest and recreation, and avoiding smoking, alcohol and aspirin. Most patients will need positive encouragment to allow their diets to be as full and varied as possible, while in the UK old age pensioners and the impecunious may require certification by the family practitioner to enable them to obtain supplementary social benefits.

NON-ULCER DYSPEPSIA

This is a syndrome rather than a defined disease state, but is real enough to family practitioners who are consulted more on account of this than for all the proven organic causes of chronic alimentary tract disorder put together. It contains an assortment of conditions, and since the diagnosis is made largely on exclusion of other conditions it may also embrace 'organic' states which are too subtle to be picked up by current diagnostic techniques. Hence there will be some cases of chronic cholecystitis and duodenal ulcers which cannot be visualised. Hyperacidity may exist, and there may be oesophagitis and minor degrees of hiatus hernia. Other cases may be accounted for by alcoholic gastritis or mild liver dysfunction. Angina may be responsible.

For a few it is possible to postulate rare causes, such as atherosclerosis producing upper intestinal 'intermittent claudication'. For others, dubious entities such as 'chronic appendicitis', 'duodenitis', or fleeting, superficial erosion of the gastric and duodenal mucosa; or epigastric fibro-fatty herniae.

Clinical Features

The feature they share in common is upper abdominal discomfort related to the taking of meals. The pain is variously described as boring, burning, cutting, and so on, but the vividness of the description is of little help diagnostically. Neither is the precise site of the pain, though the more localised it is the more significant it is likely to prove. One exception is the peculiar tightness reported by patients with chronic gall-bladder disease, 'like a pyjama cord, too tight'.

Discomfort tends to be diffuse and lacks clear radiation. It may be accompanied by flatulence, waterbrash, nausea, anorexia or vomiting; in fact any of the ulcer symptoms. An obvious anxiety state may be noted; depression may be masked. It would be going too far to suggest a characteristic personality type, but many patients do evince a sourness which reflects some sort of bitterness or resentment in their lives. The syndrome picks the 'tender' rather than the 'tough'; inability to cope and a readiness to give up explains the requests for sickness certification, both for private and for national insurance purposes. This is a chronic condition in which repeat prescriptions as well as repeat certificates are a feature.

Diagnosis

Many patients will have had a barium meal, with negative result, and some a cholecystogram. If serious symptoms persist a few may have to be submitted to gastroscopy, fibre-optic endoscopy, or even laparotomy. Faecal occult blood tests should be performed; a blood count, urinalysis and liver function tests may throw further light.

The family practitioner must exercise discretion over the extent to which he will subject an otherwise fit patient to a battery of investigations. The search for the cause of a symptom may be very worthwhile but it may not always be appropriate to 'leave no stone unturned' in its pursuit. Very often the family practitioner will employ 'the test of cure'; if an antacid provides adequate relief of symptoms and the patient is not especially at risk for a more sinister condition, this may be regarded as sufficient. Of course this entails a watchfulness in order to pick up any change in the pattern of symptoms; in this event fresh investigations may be necessary.

Management

Advice on meals and general life-style applies with equal force in non-ulcer dyspepsia as it does for peptic ulcers, and it is sensible to test the effect of restricting tobacco and alcohol.

Antacids will almost certainly have been tried and should be continued if there is any benefit, even if marginal. It has been noted that dyspeptic patients have a great faith in their medicines, and come into the class of 'positive placebo reactors'. Spasmolytics may also provide some relief. A useful preparation, especially if nausea is a feature, is metoclopramide in a dosage of 10 mg thrice daily. For flatulence a traditional remedy is aromatic cardamom tincture in a dose of 0.5 ml; a modern alternative is methylpolysiloxane, 125 mg.

For some patients repeated prescribing may itself become an essential feature of the syndrome and when this happens the family practitioner should consider whether the benefit the patient is getting derives more from the 'doctor' as a drug than from the ingredients in the medicine. Not that he should necessarily alter the regime — patients may misunderstand this — but armed with this understanding the doctor might be able to explore tactfully personal areas of the patient's life, the aim being to help him achieve a better adaptation even if it does not wholly succeed in eliminating the dyspepsia.

Research

There are wide gaps in our understanding of peptic ulceration and in non-ulcer dyspepsia. More research is needed on the aetiology of ulcers at different sites, and on the natural history of dyspepsias with no proven cause. What is their outcome? Can they be assumed to carry a good prognosis?

A reliable medical treatment for duodenal ulcer is required, matching the success of carbenoxolone in gastric ulcer, and an effective regime for ulcer-prone individuals to follow so that they may remain free from recurrence.

CHRONIC NON-MALIGNANT DISORDERS OF THE LARGE BOWEL

This group comprises diverticulosis, ulcerative colitis, spastic colon, and other states of chronic constipation or diarrhoea. For the most part the aetiology of these conditions is obscure but in some instances the physio-pathological mechanisms have been worked out.

Diverticular Disease

This is a more apt title than 'diverticulosis' since the presence of diverticula can be demonstrated in the colons of a large proportion of elderly people and does not correlate with states of ill-health.

Aetiology and Pathogenesis
It is a disease of the elderly, affecting one in three of people over the age of 60, and over forty per cent aged more than 70. It appears to be another of those disorders afflicting western industrialised countries as opposed to under-developed nations and this has led to the presumption that dietary factors are important, notably the relative deficiency in our refined foods of adequate cellulose-fibre roughage. The condition is commoner in the descending and sigmoid colon and is thought to result from increased muscular contractions which in turn generate high intra-luminal pressures and thus mucosal herniation.

Clinical Features
The presenting symptom is usually left-sided abdominal pain, and there may be constipation; bleeding per rectum is not common. Physical examination may

elicit only vague tenderness in the left iliac fossa, but occasionally a painful inflammatory mass may be palpated. Abscess formation and adhesions may lead to a fistula into the bladder, with characteristic pneumaturia, but generalised constitutional symptoms are not prominent, especially in the very old. Pyrexia may be slight, but there is usually a leucocytosis.

Diagnosis is confirmed by barium enema, which also excludes malignant disease of the colon. This procedure is probably best done in the course of an overnight stay in a hospital ward so that the elderly patient can be suitably prepared and receive adequate rest afterwards.

Management

The acute inflammatory episode will require an antibiotic, e.g., ampicillin 250 mg four times a day for ten days. The patient should remain in bed until the acute symptoms have subsided, perhaps five or six days, and then be mobilised. Long term management should encourage as much physical activity as possible. Bran should be added to each meal to provide the necessary roughage. When successful this obviates the need for laxatives in the elderly, who should in addition be encouraged to keep to a high-residue diet (thus reversing our earlier advice).

Ulcerative Colitis

Aetiology and Pathogenesis

The aetiology and the pathogenesis are both unknown. It affects young adults without pre-existing illness. A characteristic personality type has been described, namely, immaturity and dependency with obsessive-compulsive traits and suppression of hostile feelings. It is not clear how this mediates the immunological fault which is thought to underlie the condition. Colonic segmentary wave activity is reduced, and so is intra-luminal pressure.

Clinical Features

The onset may be explosive with fulminating diarrhoea and profuse bleeding per rectum, leading rapidly to a dire clinical state. More often the onset is insidious, some bowel looseness at intervals, then bouts of bloody diarrhoea which gradually merge into a continuous affliction. Colonic motility is reduced, the contents of the bowel literally falling out for want of muscular activity. There is progressive anaemia, weight loss, and weakness.

Pain is not a feature, and physical examination of the abdomen contributes little. Proctoscopy however usually reveals a deep red, granular mucosa, bleeding readily; the rectum is said to be involved in 95 per cent of cases of ulcerative colitis, the diagnosis of which may be confirmed by sigmoidoscopy. Characteristic radiological changes are seen on barium enema.

Management

General measures include bed rest for acute episodes, and a high protein diet with vitamin and iron supplements. The mainstay of treatment is salicylozosulphapyridine in a dosage of 1 g four times a day; a high fluid intake should be encouraged. Rectal and left-sided disease is benefited by the administration of rectal corticosteroid, either as hydrocortisone suppositories or prednisone in disposable plastic enemas.

Hospitalisation will be required for correction of electrolyte disturbance, for blood transfusion, and for the treatment of other serious complications such as perforation. Surgery will be contemplated when medical measures fail, and the patient will need to have the possibility of an ileostomy discussed with him. It would be helpful to put him in touch with the Ileostomy Association but the family practitioner must expect to be very much involved in the often stormy phase during which the patient has to adapt to life with an ileostomy.

In the quiescent phase of ulcerative colitis specialist surveillance is needed to detect pre-malignant changes in the mucosa: six-monthly rectal biopsy may achieve this, and total procto-colectomy advised only in those patients who show sinister changes, the remainder continuing with follow-up. With this proviso, there is a normal life expectancy for patients who are still well a year after their operation.

Spastic Colon

Aetiology

This condition, also referred to as Mucous Colitis or Irritable Colon, affects adults of all ages but more particularly younger adults, and a first occurrence over the age of 50 is unusual. There is a marked sex difference in the incidence, women being two or three times more commonly affected.

The cause is unknown but emotional features are prominent, especially depression, inappropriate handling of hostility, and marital disharmony. Patients seem to be particularly vulnerable to everyday stress factors, and these may precipitate relapses even though they are not the cause.

Dietary factors have been implicated, mainly by patients themselves: fruit, especially oranges, have a bad reputation. Specific food sensitivities like gluten and lactose, though they occur, are rare; and lactase deficiency can be demonstrated in normal subjects who have no bowel disturbance. An alternative view traces the trouble to the deficiency of food-fibre in modern refined diets. Bowel infection is not a cause, though again it may be a precipitant, and recovery from amoebic or bacillary dysentery may be very protracted.

Physio-pathology

The immediate pre-condition is disordered motility of the large bowel. It is necessary to distinguish between the segmental contractions, which may be painful if they are excessive, from the propulsive action, peristalsis, which is usually not painful. With hypersegmentation, high intra-luminal pressures are caused, transit time is lengthened, and residues further dehydrated. In turn this reduced bulk encourages increased contraction of the colon musculature. In diarrhoeal states muscular tone is lower than normal, and intra-luminal pressures are correspondingly reduced so that the bowel contents are allowed to flow on, unhampered apart from the anal sphincter. The lack of segmentation activity in the colon reduces opportunity for the re-absorption of fluid.

Clinical Features

The principal features are irregular and disturbed bowel habit associated with abdominal pain, in the absence of any organic disease of the large bowel. Pain is generally experienced in the left iliac fossa but may also occur along the line of the colon, and even in the epigastrium. Pain is often exacerbated by eating, may be intermittent or continue for hours, and is sometimes relieved by a bowel action. Colicky in nature, it may build up very gradually, and may be described as stabbing.

Characteristically, periods of constipation alternate with diarrhoea. Incomplete rectal emptying is often complained of, the faeces being thin and ribbon-like, or hard and the size of peas. Perhaps after a fortnight of this diarrhoea ensues, with the passage of much mucus. Blood is not passed in this syndrome.

In ten per cent of cases pain is not prominent and constipation does not occur, but the stools may be very copious, watery, and passed up to a dozen times a day. Even so, sleep is usually not interrupted.

There is usually no abnormality on physical examination, patients appearing thin and wiry. Abdominal distension is not marked, but the descending colon is usually palpable and may be tender. Rectal examination may reveal hard motions, and proctoscopy a mild proctitis only.

Diagnosis

When presented with this sort of story the first thing the family practitioner will want to establish is the pattern of laxative-taking. It may be safely assumed that some aperient has been taken at some time or other, and even ritual purgation may be indulged in by the very patients who are seeking advice for diarrhoea. Exploration of this area may need to be tactful and persistent.

Bleeding per rectum, apart from spots of fresh blood obviously related to anal tears, should prompt further investigations including sigmoidoscopy and barium enema to exclude neoplasm, ulcerative colitis and diverticulitis. In women genito-urinary conditions will need to be ruled out by pelvic examination. Where the pain is predominantly right-sided, appendicitis, Crohn's disease, and gall-bladder disease may need to be excluded.

The condition is a chronic and relapsing one, but any departure from the patient's usual pattern of experience should lead to consideration of the need for fresh investigations, even in young patients. Stool cultures should be done on patients with persistent diarrhoea, and on those who have had dysentery.

Management

Patent laxatives should be withdrawn. The importance of this should be stressed to patients, and in the home a joint exploration of the medicine chest will usually prove acceptable and can lead to the turning out of accumulated aperients − often of the phenolphthalein type. Repeated catharsis can induce a state of hypokalemia, which may aggravate constipation. If the family practitioner suspects this has been happening it is justifiable to try the effect of giving potassium supplements while awaiting the results of serum electrolytes; effervescent potassium chloride, 1 g four times a day.

A full, varied diet should be advised, high in residues, and with bran supplements to increase the fibre content, 5 g sprinkled on food, thrice daily. Proprietary preparations which act as bulk additives include methyl-cellulose, 1 g night and morning with half a pint of fluid, and Ispaghula husk 3.5 g night and morning with fluid.

Antispasmodics may be necessary for the relief of the continuing abdominal pain; mebeverine hydrochloride 100 mg four times a day half an hour before meals; mepenzolate bromide 25 mg thrice daily.

The control of watery diarrhoea may be difficult; diphenoxylate hydrochloride and atropine should be tried. There is no point in combining this with neomycin unless bacterial infection has been demonstrated. Kaolin and morphine mixtures are generally ineffective in this chronic condition.

Morale is very easily reduced in this affliction and the family practitioner will always be required in a supportive role. Apart from this however, he may be able to help by exploring with the patient the interpersonal difficulties which are often present, or ventilating the resentments or aggression that may be locked up in the patient. If psychotropic drugs are used to overcome undue tension, the choice should be of a non-habit forming preparation, such as meprobomate 400 mg thrice daily. Antidepressants have been advised even in the absence of overt depression, with relief of abdominal symptoms in some cases. The tricyclic compounds are probably best; amitriptyline 25 mg three or four times daily.

Very occasionally in the early phase of treatment of spastic colon laxatives may be necessary until normal bowel function is restored by the action of bulk additives. Stimulant laxatives are best avoided. Liquid paraffin is a lubricant, 10 ml thrice daily, but may seep out from the rectum. Dioctyl preparations act by lowering surface tension and hence softening the faeces.

Research

More studies are needed on the natural history of spastic colon. How do these patients fare in the long run? It is worthwhile excluding specific foods such as wheat or milk? What is the contribution of the patient's personality in the causation of his illness?

MALIGNANT DISEASE OF THE ALIMENTARY TRACT

With the exception of a few sarcomata and lymphomata, the overwhelming majority of cancers of the alimentary tract are carcinomata, accounting, in Western countries, for a third of all malignant disease. Twenty per cent of all primary cancers are to be found in the oesophagus, the stomach, and the large bowel, including the rectum.

Cancer of the Stomach and Lower End of the Oesophagus

These cancers, which share clinical features, together comprise 5 per cent of malignant neoplasms.

Aetiology

There are world-wide differences in the incidence of stomach cancer, but whether this reflects racial, i.e., genetic susceptibility, or is a cultural determinant and therefore presumably dietary, is not known. Factors which have been investigated include tobacco, dietary deficiencies, soil content of trace metals, and air pollution. It is the commonest male cancer in countries as diverse as Japan, Finland and Chile; males are twice as commonly affected as females (four times for the oesophagus). Socio-economic factors are undoubtedly important and probably explain the threefold decrease amongst White patients in the USA in the past forty years. The reduction in incidence has been nowhere as steep in the UK.

Clinical Features

Onset is insidious and the initial symptoms of malignant diseases may be indistinguishable from 'everyday' flatulence, heartburn, epigastric discomfort, anorexia, or nausea. As a result the significance of the symptoms may not be appreciated by the patient; nor, when translated into 'complaints', by the family practitioner. It may be possible in retrospect to discern the presentation of the disease, but extremely difficult for the practitioner at the time.

Yet, because the results of surgery for stomach cancer are so poor the problem becomes one of early diagnosis. Dysphagia and unexplained anaemia are two features which should alert the practitioner to the possibility of malignant disease, especially in a middle-aged patient. He will not expect to find signs such as enlarged lymph nodes or loss of weight, recalling the aphorism: 'Patients with loss of weight are not suffering from cancer, they are dying from it.'

Faecal occult blood tests can be done, but once the suspicion is raised a barium swallow and meal should be arranged, followed by referral for appropriate endoscopy. The urgent need is for a diagnostic procedure which can detect cancer while it is still limited to the mucosa; air contrast barium studies, and the cytological examination of gastric washings are two promising lines, but are as yet limited to certain centres.

Patients with known gastric ulcers should be regarded as at risk until their lesions are known to have healed, and the family practitioner has a role in ensuring that patients do understand the need for adequate follow-up and do not default from surveillance.

Management

The surgery and chemotherapy of malignant disease are necessarily specialist procedures but the family practitioner will need to be conversant with the techniques so as to outline them to the patient and relatives. While fully knowing the poor prognosis he is justified in emphasising the hopefulness of achieving a worthwhile remission. Total gastrectomy, or gastrostomy, will bring problems of aftercare, and so will courses of chemotherapeutic agents such as fluorouracil and mitomycin C.

In later stages the family will need the family practitioner's support, both emotionally, and in practical measures such as arranging for the services of the district nurse, invalid equipment, home meals, and social services and voluntary agencies as required. When the time comes for terminal care (see Chapter 26) the decision whether to admit to hospital or not can be a difficult one. The family may have conflicting feelings on the matter, and the need of the patient to remain in his accustomed surroundings will have to be balanced against the drain on the family's emotional and practical resources. From his personal knowledge, and with his close involvement with all the parties, the practitioner is in a position to shift the weight in one direction or the other, either sanctioning hospital admission or encouraging a further week or two at home.

Pain relief will require the administration of analgesics in ample amounts. Nausea and vomiting may necessitate the intramuscular or rectal route at first. Pethidine 50–100 mg, and methadone 5–10 mg, can be given by mouth; so may dipipanone combined with cyclizine. In the face of severer pain a mixture of diamorphine and cocaine may be necessary and is best given in frequent small doses to anticipate distress rather than in larger amounts to attempt to relieve it; this regime has the advantage of allowing the patient to remain lucid.

Emotional distress can be alleviated by diazepam 5 mg four times a day, or by chlorpromazine 25 mg four times a day. The latter preparation may also help the nausea. An antidepressant may be helpful; imipramine 25 mg four times a day. The practitioner will have to judge whether the patient wants to talk about his coming end or whether the subject is to be avoided.

Cancer of the Colon and Rectum

Cancer at these sites accounts for one in eight of all malignant disease; skin cancer is commoner when the sexes are considered together, but in females breast cancer is commoner, while in males lung cancer is commoner.

Aetiology

More males are affected than females in rectal cancer, while the reverse holds true for the colon. There are geographical differences which seem to be the inverse of stomach cancer. Incidence is higher in Europe and the USA than in Africa, Asia or Japan. However Japanese migrants to the United States acquire the same incidence, after a generation, as their American hosts, so a dietary factor is probably implicated. Presumably the bulky high-residue diet of primitive peoples is protective in a way that the highly refined diet in our country is not. There is evidence that colon cancer is increasing in the developing countries as they adopt Western eating habits.

The longer stool transit times and the particular bacterial flora encountered amongst Europeans compared with Africans suggests the possibility that the bacterial degradation of bile salts may be a factor in producing carcinogens.

Familial polyposis and ulcerative colitis are predisposing conditions. Unlike stomach cancer there has been no reduction in incidence in the last generation; and with improvement in the five-year survival rate its prevalence in this country may soon be greater than that of cancer of the bronchus.

Clinical Features

A change in bowel habit may be the earliest clue to the presence of malignant disease in the large bowel, particularly the rectum and descending colon. In the latter site obstructive features occur relatively early in the disease and by drawing attention to the tumour in an unmistakable way contribute to the rather better prognosis. Tumours of the caecum and ascending colon do not generally declare themselves through any mechanical effect but tend to bleed readily so that blood is evident per rectum and anaemia is often present. Abdominal pain may be colicky or persistent. In the rectum growths may give rise to local discomfort, a sense of incomplete emptying, and spurious diarrhoea. Alternating constipation and diarrhoea is characteristic of growths of the rectum and colon. So is the passage of blood and mucus.

On physical examination anaemia and loss of weight may be evident, and a tumour mass may be palpable. A high proportion of rectal cancers can be felt on digital examination of the rectum or seen through the proctoscope. It should be remembered that haemorrhoids may co-exist with cancer of the large bowel and so bleeding should not be attributed to them without excluding neoplasm higher up by sigmoidoscopy, and by barium enema. Generally these latter tests require specialist referral.

A patient who has blood and mucus originating from beyond the reach of the sigmoidoscope but in whom barium enema is negative may be a candidate for endoscopy through a fibre-optic colonoscope. With this instrument it is possible to visualise the whole of the colon and caecum, and polyps and suspicious areas can be biopsied without the need for laparotomy.

A semi-specific antigen test is being developed for colon cancers, relying on the detection of carcino-embyonic antigen in the serum of patients. Though of no value as a screening test at present it can signal recurrence of cancer after an apparently successful operation for removal.

Management

The most important factor in prognosis is the degree of local spread, the involvement of lymph nodes, and the completeness of excision. The trend in surgery is towards conservation of the anal sphincter so obviating the need for colostomy. Chemotherapy may be used as well as endocavity radiation. Overall prognosis is still poor however, 20 per cent surviving five years, though specialist centres can claim up to 70 per cent five year survival.

Important preventive measures are the prompt eradication of polyps and benign tumours of the rectum and colon, and the adequate follow-up of patients who have recovered from ulcerative colitis.

Research

Primary prevention: Will diets of high fibre-content eventually reduce the incidence of colon cancers?

Secondary prevention: Can a satisfactory screening test be developed, suitable for application to patients in family practice, and administered by practitioners to detect patients in the pre-malignant phase?

Tertiary prevention. Can diagnostic techniques be improved sufficiently to detect the earliest structural changes, i.e., while the cancer is still limited to the mucosa?

References

1. Editorial: More about D & V (Diarrhoea and Vomiting). (1974). *Brit. med. J.* 4, 1.
2. The Aberdeen Typhoid Outbreak: report of a departmental committee of enquiry. (1964). *Brit. med. J.* 2, 1652.
3. Ramsay, A. M. (1968). Acute infective diarrhoea. *Brit. med. J.* 2, 347.

12

Rheumatic Diseases

J. D. E. Knox

INTRODUCTION

A clinician attempting to give a family practitioner's eye-view of rheumatic diseases is faced with a series of challenges and opportunities. The challenges are posed by the lack of clear definitions, not only of the boundaries of this group of conditions (is gout primarily a rheumatic disorder, or a metabolic disease?), but also of many of the conditions themselves (what is 'fibrositis'?). The opportunities relate to helping to close a gap in information from family practice in the published literature, most of which is based on highly specialised experience of hospital clinics complemented by epidemiological studies of random samples of the community or studies from industry, or official government reports.

A Working Definition of 'Rheumatism'

The main feature linking different conditions commonly regarded as rheumatic is a complaint of pain and/or stiffness apparently related to the locomotor system and for which no cause is obvious. Such a definition has several shortcomings. A patient may have evidence of gross rheumatological pathology and yet be symptom free, for example radiological changes of osteoarthrosis in an otherwise apparently healthy person. Again, all that aches is not 'rheumatism', thus a patient may have musculo-skeletal pains from, say, metastatic carcinoma. Furthermore, pain and stiffness are not the only characteristic features of rheumatic conditions; many other symptoms can be important components, e.g., the urethral discharge of Reiter's syndrome, the nodules of rheumatoid disease, the wrist-drop (or other evidence of peripheral neuropathy) of mono-neuritis multiplex. Some of these 'other' symptoms may be of special importance to the primary care physician because they can be early pointers (the Raynaud phenomenon in rheumatoid disease, for instance). However, pain and stiffness in muscles, bones or joints are associated especially in the lay mind with 'rheumatism'.

Problem Definition and the Family Practitioner

In addition to the more obvious potential difficulties in differential diagnosis posed by conditions, many ill-defined, which may give rise to symptoms in virtually any part of the body, several other hazards face the doctor of first contact working outside the rheumatic clinic. Important factors determining any doctor's diagnostic strategy include the range of possible morbidities with which he has to deal and his awareness of the range and the prognostic significance of each of its components[1]. Pain is a common presenting symptom in primary care: analysis of presenting complaints in 1000 consecutive new contacts in my urban practice in 1969 showed pain was the prime motivating factor in over 300 such consultations. While much of this symptomatology was clearly 'non-rheumatic', the possibility of 'rheumatism' was considered in 100. Hull[2] recorded 8.6 per cent skeletal pain complaints in a similar study from rural practice. Analysis of 17 124 consultations of all kinds by 32 Dundee family practitioners during a 3 week sample in 1972 showed that 1121 (6.5 per cent) were allotted to the group 'musculo-skeletal disorders'. The UK second National Morbidity Survey[3], based on a population of about ¼ million studied over 1 year, showed that episodes of rheumatic diseases comprise just over 7 per cent of all morbidity brought to the family doctor. Patients presenting with possible 'rheumatism' in primary medical care have to be viewed against a wide range of diagnostic probabilities before the diagnostic process can progress as far as 'rheumatic—non rheumatic'. When a patient's complaint has been allotted to the rheumatic group, the need for the diagnostic process to continue to operate is apparent from the second National Morbidity Study[3]. Over 10 per cent of 5546 diagnostic amendments in that study concerned the rheumatic diseases (Table 12.1). While most of the amendments were within that group (393/550 remained in diagnostic category XIII) there were significant shifts to and from most of the other 17 broad categories of diseases. Furthermore, many complaints encountered in family practice are short-lived or are regarded by both patient and doctor to be insufficiently incapacitating to warrant inconveniences inherent in specialist referral. In the Dundee study[2] quoted above, of the 1121 consultations concerning musculo-skeletal disorders only 44 resulted in referral to hospital as in-patient or out-patient. Such a high degree of selection inevitably alters the perception of morbidity patterns by the hospital-based clinician. The pattern of rheumatic morbidity encountered by the family doctor differs from that seen by the rheumatologist in several respects, chief of which is the very much higher proportion of non-articular rheumatism seen in family practice[4,5] and the illness behaviour component of the clinical rheumatology. Hitherto, undergraduate medical education has been based almost exclusively on teaching-hospital practice. In the absence of wider postgraduate training, many doctors have thus acquired distorted appreciations of patterns of disease and its management[6].

Table 12.1 Numbers of diagnostic amendments by the eighteen main diagnostic categories of classification. (from Second National Morbidity Study 1970–71[3]).

Amended diagnosis	Original diagnosis																		All causes
	I	II	III	IV	V	VI	VII	VIII	IX	X	XI	XII	XIII	XIV	XV	XVI	XVII	XVIII	
I. Infective and parasitic diseases	97	4	11	1	7	6	1	63	27	18	3	55	7	1	0	3	5	0	309
II. Neoplasms	1	51	0	1	3	1	1	4	12	3	0	5	3	2	0	1	1	1	90
III. Endocrine, nutritional and metabolic diseases	16	3	38	3	12	4	7	11	1	1	1	8	8	0	0	0	2	3	118
IV. Diseases of blood and blood-forming organs	5	4	4	31	21	1	3	3	1	3	0	4	2	0	0	2	0	2	86
V. Mental disorders	11	4	7	7	275	17	9	15	9	12	7	3	5	0	0	4	4	0	389
VI. Diseases of the nervous system and sense organs	10	9	6	1	32	185	11	11	4	1	0	3	22	0	0	0	6	0	301
VII. Diseases of the circulatory system	1	4	6	4	18	20	181	13	21	5	2	8	17	1	0	0	6	0	307
VIII. Diseases of respiratory system	289	35	40	6	36	20	28	381	30	8	2	4	13	0	0	1	1	0	894
IX. Diseases of the digestive system	59	64	7	9	60	9	14	13	360	45	19	6	12	4	0	3	6	3	693
X. Diseases of the genito-urinary system	28	50	5	1	29	0	3	3	39	263	311	9	22	0	0	3	5	10	781
XI. Complications of pregnancy, childbirth and the puerperium	1	1	0	0	4	0	1	0	2	35	153	0	0	0	0	1	0	3	201
XII. Diseases of the skin and subcutaneous tissue	76	12	14	1	11	4	8	2	3	6	2	190	6	0	0	0	3	0	338
XIII. Diseases of the musculoskeletal system and connective tissue	7	10	22	0	12	19	19	6	8	8	0	9	393	2	0	1	32	2	550
XIV. Congenital anomalies	0	1	0	0	0	1	0	0	0	0	0	0	3	0	0	0	0	1	6
XV. Certain causes of perinatal morbidity and mortality	0	0	0	0	0	0	0	0	0	0	0	0	0	0	1	0	0	0	1
XVI. Symptoms and ill-defined conditions	12	3	7	11	32	5	7	10	10	5	1	2	7	0	0	1	4	0	117
XVII. Accidents, poisonings and violence	4	2	2	0	16	10	2	2	4	1	0	7	68	0	0	0	206	4	328
XVIII. Prophylactic procedures and other medical examinations	2	1	0	4	2	1	0	1	2	0	3	2	2	0	0	0	2	15	37
ALL CAUSES	619	258	169	80	570	303	295	538	533	414	504	315	590	10	1	20	283	44	5546

Some Consequences of Insufficient Knowledge

With such an incomplete frame of reference, we may be all too ready to accept at face value the patient's diagnosis or his version of the cause of minor morbidity. While there may be some substance in the folk-lore of rheumatology, a critical re-appraisal of some of the commoner myths is overdue: is there a cause-and-effect relationship between draughts and stiff-necks, or between variations in the weather and non-specific myalgias? At the same time, against such a background of insecurely based knowledge and despite his own uncertainties about his particular patient, the family doctor must be prepared to offer an acceptable — even if irrational — explanation of the presenting complaint. An important part of family practice management consists of knowing how far one can communicate one's ignorance to the patient. While one patient might accept unquestioningly the doctor's statement: "Yes, I think it is just a touch of 'rheumatism' ", another might be terror-stricken because the term conjures up a vision of a helpless crippled friend or relative. It is in these circumstances that terms such as 'fibrositis' and 'myalgia' have their uses, but they must not be allowed to blind the doctor's vision: these terms are not diagnoses in the sense of conveying clearly ideas concerning specific pathologies, aetiologies or even prognoses.

Some pharmaceutical commercial advertising has deliberately exploited the uncertainties of the diagnostic situation, promoting more powerful (and more toxic) analgesics not only for rheumatoid arthritis but also for non-articular rheumatism, when simple aspirin in appropriate doses would be as effective. The individual family doctor, anxious to do his best for his patient, and not usually in a position to review critically such evidence as may be incorporated in drug advertisements, has often succumbed to the blandishments: and patients, too, may occasionally put pressure on their doctor to prescribe inappropriately. Such factors are among possible reasons for disquieting results of surveys[7] of prescribing for rheumatoid disease by family practitioners. A further influence exerted by our lack of knowledge is to be seen in attempts to classify rheumatic morbidity. Table 12.2 taken from the second National Morbidity Study[3] from UK family practice may at first sight inspire confidence in our ability to cope with problems.

A more critical appraisal, however, raises several issues. In this classification, does 'lumbago not attributed to disc lesion' (category 407) differ from 'back pain alone' (category 425) in any significant pathological way apart possibly from localisation and radiation of pain? Is there any merit in separating 'back pain with sciatica' (category 423) from other backpain? What difference exists between 'Other non-articular rheumatism' (category 408) and 'other symptoms . . .' (category 427)? The reader is forced to the conclusion that there is a spurious accuracy about many of the categories in group XIII (Diseases of the musculo-skeletal system and connective tissue, Table 12.1).

Table 12.2   Rheumatic diseases in general practice, 1970–71. Episode rate per 1000 population (from Second National Morbidity Study, 1970–71[3]).

ICD No.	Condition	Rate	RCGP No.
713	Osteo-arthritis and allied conditions	20.3	406
728.9 (pt)	Back pain alone	13.5	425
720–738	Other diseases of musculo-skeletal and connective tissue	12.1	415
717.9	Other non-articular rheumatism	9.9	408
717.6	Lumbago (not disc lesion)	9.1	407
713.1	Spondylitis osteo-arthritica (including cervical spondylosis)	7.6	404
725	Displacement of intervertebral disc	6.4	412
712	Rheumatoid arthritis and allied conditions	5.9	405
710.718	Other forms of arthritis and rheumatism	5.9	409
787.3	Pain in joint	4.8	428
728.8	Backpain with sciatica	3.9	423
731 (pt)	Tenosynovitis	3.4	421
731 (pt)	Bursitis	2.6	420
724.1	Other forms of internal derangement of knee joint	2.1	411
717.1	Frozen shoulder	1.8	426
731 (pt)	Synovitis	1.6	422
728.9 (pt)	Back pain with other neuritis	1.5	424
724.1	Torn meniscus of knee	1.2	410
736	Flat foot	1.1	413
737	Hallux valgus and varus	0.9	414

ICD: International Classification of Disease.
RCGP: Royal College of General Practitioners.

A Simple Classification

For most practical purposes, the diverse conditions embraced by rheumatology can be classified into four groups:

1. *articular*, i.e., diseases acute, chronic or sometimes acute on chronic which afflict joints;
2. *non-articular*, conditions affecting primarily other structures of the locomotor system;
3. *back troubles*;
4. *other diseases of musculo-skeletal system.*

Despite its apparent loss of definition, such a re-classification serves to draw attention to the less easily defined non-articular and back conditions and the relatively high frequency with which they occur.

BACK TROUBLES

One of the commoner conditions encountered in family practice presents with the familiar 'It's my back, doctor'. Most family practitioners encounter such patients on average 2–3 times each week, and in my experience there does not appear to be any marked seasonal variation in this incidence. Backache of all kinds is almost universal in the elderly, though they may not always consult with this complaint.

Towards Diagnosis

Many factors, among them the clinical findings and severity of the pain, influence the diagnostic process. Sometimes the muscle spasm with associated abnormalities of gait or posture and limitation of movement tell the patient's story more eloquently than this words; back pain is a not infrequent reason for a housecall. In a series of 148 patients who presented to me with a complaint of pain in the back, the initial consultation took place in the patient's home in 37: in just under two thirds of these 37 it was possible to make a firmer diagnosis than 'fibrositis–lumbago'. By contrast, of the remaining 111 patients seen initially in the consulting room, only a quarter were more firmly diagnosed. The range of probabilities encountered in each setting differs, and it is likely that this in turn influences the diagnostic process at primary care level.

History

The history is usually short — from a few hours to several days. Approximately one third of the 148 patients mentioned above gave a history of 2 days or less. With back pain the odds are that the episode is a completely new one. A study[3] of the distribution of types of episode demonstrates that a previous history of a similar condition is found more frequently in patients allotted to category 'disc lesion' (about $\frac{1}{3}$) than to lumbago or 'other back troubles' (about $\frac{1}{7}$): perhaps, in the absence of other clear clinical features, a previous history of backache influences the diagnostic process.

Site

In many clinicians' minds, backache is virtually equated with low back pain. Yet, experience in family practice reveals that between one half and one third of our patients complaining of back pain experience *upper* backache. Comparison between the patients grouped by site of back pain reveals a significant excess of women over men where upper backache is concerned[3]. Although this phenomenon has been recorded before[8] its significance is still not clear.

Back Pain other than Lumbago

Backache refers to pain felt anywhere from the neck to the coccyx, and the site is not necessarily restricted to the midline. Upper back pain is a relatively frequent presentation in family practice, especially in women. While back pains of all kinds are uncommon in children, among such children as consult with this symptom, the upper part of the back is affected more frequently than the lower[3]. Both the intensity of pain and the associated disability may be marked, but in general they both tend to be less than that experienced in the low back.

Physical findings are usually tenderness, muscle spasm, limitation of movements and hyperaesthesia. Evidence of radiculopathy or myelopathy and other signs suggest that the patient may not be suffering from the common 'myalgia' or 'fibrositis' of family practice; the simple conditions are usually associated with rather meagre clinical features. Back pain, both upper and lower, may be a presenting symptom of many diseases prominant among which is depressive illness: Watts[9] ranked backache as fifth in a list of 71 presenting symptoms. Some aspects of differential diagnosis are discussed briefly at the end of this section.

Lumbago

The common findings associated with low back pain are local tenderness, hyperaesthesia and limitation of spinal movements, especially forward flexion: there is often a characteristic exacerbation of pain on straightening up. The difference between limitation of forward flexion when the patient is standing and sitting forward has been used as an index of the degree to which symptoms are exagerated by the patient. This sign may be valid in the orthopaedic clinic but I have not found it helpful in family practice. Other objective findings are not usually elicited although limitation of straight-leg-raising may be present (it was observed as a transient phenomenon in 8 of 62 patients with apparently straightforward 'lumbago'). The presence of various neurological deficits suggests that the presenting backache is not the common lumbago of family practice. A further useful diagnostic characteristic is the short natural history of the acute episode. With simple measures such as rest, adequate analgesics and local application of heat, most episodes subside within 10—14 days. Persistence of symptoms beyond this time calls for a reappraisal of the situation. Many episodes are of a relatively minor nature and require only one consultation in contrast to the backache associated with the disc lesion.

Radiology and Backache

While X-ray examinations of patients with back pain in family practice rarely yield positive diagnostic evidence, radiology is helpful in a variety of ways. Obviously, the use which individual family practitioners make of X-rays will be dependent, among other things, upon accessability of the service to their patients and availability to the doctor. A recent study in Scotland of radiological facilities built into an urban Health Centre[10] showed that there has been in the past an under-estimation by planners (and the profession) of the value of this on-the-spot service, especially for the diagnosis and management of back troubles. Broadly, X-rays can help in the following ways of which the first is particularly relevant to the family practitioner:

Diagnostic: 1. to 'clear the decks' — exclusion by negative findings is not absolute, but it can assist the diagnostic process at primary care level.
    2. to confirm a suspected pathology — this is the main use from the hospital clinician's point of view, in cases which have already been through the primary diagnostic process;

Therapeutic: this indication is occasionally a legitimate one in the managment of the anxious patient, relative or sometimes an employer. This use can also be therapeutic for the insecure doctor, and is relevant in the context of rheumatic diseases;

Medico-legal: this indication probably carries more weight in the casualty department than with the family practitioner.

Some Myths Concerning Aetiology

Carne (1963) summarises the situation thus: 'Many patients who consult their doctor because of backache have already made their own diagnosis and probably tried one of the commercially advertised remedies. The less knowledgeable attribute their pain to disease of the kidneys and will have gone to the chemist for some "pills to flush out the kidneys". The more sophisticated think of a slipped disc, while many women assume their pain is due to something gynaecological. Occasionally, patients may not present with the complaint of backache, but will describe an associated symptom, such as vaginal discharge, which they think is more representative of the disease they or their friends have diagnosed. It is always wise first to determine what the patient means by the symptom and also to ask what that symptom implies to the patient'. Other factors commonly cited as causes of lumbago include the interior sprung mattress, physical stress, the long narrow back, and obesity: yet, a careful study of such factors in my practice, of patients with backache and of a comparison group, yielded no firm evidence to support these theories.

Differential Diagnosis

In theory, a wide spectrum of clinical medicine may present with the complaint of back pain. The list of final diagnoses in Table 12.3 was compiled retrospectively in connection with 148 consecutive patients who presented with back pain over six months. While such a table indicates broadly something of the probabilities involved in the diagnosis of back pain in one family practice, the value of such information is limited because it is based on the experience of only one observer. Many possibilities are not listed (e.g., visceral conditions such as cholecystitis, pancreatic diseases, or obliterative and other vascular diseases). Broadening the base by more observations from different practices could help to form a reference for monitoring the ways in which we work. Yet, this *quantitative* approach also needs to be supplemented by a consideration of

Table 12.3   148 consecutive patients presenting over six months with back pain.

Condition	No. of patients	Comment
Vague: 'fibrositis', 'lumbago', etc.	100	32 upper back pain mainly women
Trauma, sprain, bruise etc.	15	$\frac{2}{3}$ men: violence mainly indirect
Osteoarthrosis, osteoporosis multiple disc degeneration	10	Mainly elderly: includes 2 cervical spondylosis
Acute disc lesion	8	Only 1 new case
Renal lesions	5	2 renal colic
Vertebral epiphysitis	1	
Paget's disease	1	
Polymyalgia rheumatica	1	Gross elevation of ESR helpful
Painful spacticity: old MS	1	
Systemic reaction to oral penicillin	1	
Herpes zoster	1	Seen before rash appeared
Posterior duodenal ulcer	1	
Pregnancy and gastric upset	1	
Uterine prolapse	1	Symptom relief following operation
Pulmonary infarction	1	

influences acting on the primary diagnostician other than simply the frequencies with which diseases may occur. A *qualitative* approach involves an indication of awareness of, for example, early, possibly minor, signs of major illness which may be managed by appropriate treatment. Thus, although spinal metastatic carcinoma or spinal cord tumour are not common causes of back pain in family practice, the family practitioner needs to be alive to these and other possibilities. Keeping constantly on the alert for such eventualities inevitably dulls our receptivity and may not be the most effective or efficient way in which to operate. Most of us learn to 'switch on' at the appropriate cues, and we need to learn a great deal more about this process, which has been developed to a very high degree by some family practitioners. There is a need for recording and sharing this information much of which has in the past been labelled (wrongly, in my view) as 'intuition'.

NON-ARTICULAR RHEUMATISM

Most family practitioners encounter each week one or two patients whose complaints might be placed in this category, conditions often labelled 'fibrositis'. Copeman[11] points out that such terminology is inaccurate because the soft tissues apparently affected may not consist primarily of fibrous tissue and because it is not certain that inflammatory changes are necessarily involved. In addition to connective tissues such as tendon sheaths, aponeuroses and ligaments, fibrous *fatty* tissue in certain parts of the body may also be sites of pain and tenderness.

Attempts to assess frequencies with which these conditions may occur in family practice are rendered less accurate by our traditional classification system. Many conditions of this nature are grouped under several different categories (e.g., lumbago, and certain other trunk pains), so that what is left is probably a heterogeneous collection of disease states characterised in the main by pain, stiffness and limitation of movement affecting predominately the limbs and limb girdles, but not the joints. Despite such a negative definition, several more or less clear-cut entities can be identified clinically.

Limb Girdle Afflictions

A family practitioner in the UK with a list of 2500 patients may expect in the course of one year to see some 15–20 patients presenting with pain in and around the shoulder and hip regions. In at least half of such patients the clinical features are largely subjective, with little to show beyond slight limitation in the range of many movements because of pain, some tenderness and no evidence of constitutional disturbance. The disability is relatively minor, though such complaints can impair the working capacity of the heavy manual and outdoor worker to a greater extent than that of the clerical worker who is apparently afflicted to the same degree. The condition usually resolves spontaneously over the usual 2–3 weeks, though it can persist very much longer. The over-all ratio of consultations/episodes in this group of conditions in the second National Morbidity Study[3] was 1.4/1. Waves of such conditions may be encountered in a practice, but the hypothesis that an infectious agent is always responsible is not substantiated. The distribution of episode rates by age and sex shows a peak among women in the menopausal and post-menopausal ages.

More Specific Clinical Entities

From among this group of patients with aches and pains around the limb girdles, several clinical entities can be discerned, usually because of characteristic clusters of features or because the condition does not follow the usual relatively short self-limiting course.

Frozen Shoulder   This painful condition has a gradual onset and runs a longer course than other soft tissue rheumatism, before the 'thaw' sets in. This is reflected in a rather higher consultation/episode ratio — 1.8/1 — compared with limb girdle pains generally in the second National Morbidity Study[3]. Children rarely suffer from this condition, which is seen most frequently in women aged

45–65 and men over 65 years of age. The pain, which may interfere with sleep, is usually associated with immobility of the shoulder joint, and such movement as occurs in the shoulder girdle is achieved largely by scapular rotation. Some wasting may occur in muscles around the shoulder, with flattening of contours and increase in prominence of the point of the shoulder. The condition may resemble the early stages of brachial neuritis or 'shoulder-hand syndrome'. In this latter chronic painful and disabling state, the trophic changes are more marked, with shiny skin of the fingers, poor peripheral circulation and even flexion deformities of most joints in the upper limb. There may be a preceding history of hemiparesis (usually from a cerebro-vascular accident) or myocardial infarction: either arm may be affected.

The differential diagnosis of 'capsulitis' (frozen shoulder) is usually straightforward. Supraspinatus tendinitis gives rise to a painful arc on abduction beyond 45°, and passive movements are not usually painful: in long-standing cases, there may be radiological evidence of calcification in the region of the tendon. Most family practitioners will have encountered the patient (usually male) whose apparent frozen shoulder has been the earliest indication of carcinoma – usually bronchogenic carcinoma. The pathogenesis of carcinomatous neuromyopathy is not clear[1][2] and the phenomenon does not depend on mechanical infiltration of the nerves and vessels of the shoulder (though this may occur). It is therefore worthwhile estimating the ESR and possibly also arranging for a chest X-ray in patients with shoulder pain persisting for more than 3–4 weeks.

Limb girdle pain of more gradual onset, marked chronicity and a grossly elevated ESR are features which should raise suspicions concerning polymyalgia rheumatica in the elderly. Although it is rare in family practice (the average family practitioner may expect to encounter one new case in about 5 years) that condition is important because of the prompt relief which can be afforded by steroid therapy – or aspirin in high dose.

Vague limb girdle and other somatic pains are sometimes the presenting complaint of depressive illness. The associated features of depression of mood, altered sleep rhythm, anorexia, loss of drive, loss of libido and a normal ESR will usually serve to alert the doctor to the true nature of the underlying illness. The response to appropriate antidepressant drug therapy (and resistance to common analgesics) are further helpful diagnostic pointers.

Sciatica and Brachial Neuritis

Although these painful conditions are considered elsewhere (pages 280, 281), they are mentioned here because the borderline between rheumatic diseases and neurological conditions is not always as clear cut as textbooks would suggest.

Back Pain with Sciatica

In the second National Morbidity Study[3] 'sciatica' alone is grouped under 'Diseases of the Nervous System'. The frequency of episodes is 1.7 per 1000 population. Sciatica in association with back pain, grouped under rheumatic diseases, is recorded with an episode frequency of 3.9 per 1000 population. The distribution by age and sex is remarkably similar in both conditions apart from an increase in the over 75 years age group with sciatica. The obscure nature of many of these conditions is reflected in the relatively low episode rate for 'disc lesion' recorded in a group of conditions widely held to be due in the main to prolapsed intervertebral disc.

Brachial Neuritis, Back and Neck Pain

The aetiological factors and the possible inter-relation of the painful back, neck and upper limb conditions are equally obscure. 'Pure' brachial neuritis, grouped under nervous system afflictions, is encountered with an over-all episode frequency of 0.8 per 1000 population, while 'back pain and other neuritis', grouped under rheumatic conditions, is recorded with an episode frequency of 1.5 per 1000 population. The situation is further obscured by the fact that a proportion of episodes are buried in 'spondylitis osteo-arthritica' which includes cervical spondylosis. The clinical features of these less ill-defined conditions will not be detailed because they are already fully documented in standard works, but some of the diagnostic problems they may present in first contact medicine are worth considering.

It is the radiation of the pain and its persistence which, in the absence of other clinical findings, alert the doctor to the probability that the condition is more than a simple localised 'rheumatic' complaint. In the upper limb, difficulty is occasionally experienced in clearly identifying the carpal tunnel syndrome in which the pain sometimes is felt widely *up and down* the arm: the other local features of median nerve involvement (tingling and pain felt in the middle fingers, etc.) will usually help to differentiate that condition from brachial neuralgia. Rheumatoid arthritis may occasionally present with any one of a variety of limb non-articular rheumatic complaints (e.g., carpal tunnel syndrome and capsulitis of the shoulder) and the nature of the underlying condition emerges more clearly only with the passage of time.

Painful Fibro-fatty Pads

This form of soft tissue rheumatism is encountered some two or three times in a year in a family practice of average size. The patients are usually post menopausal women, whose general health is good, though they are usually obese. The region most commonly affected is the inner aspect of the knees; occasionally both limbs are affected. Often there is no more than localised tenderness to be made out, but occasionally there is thickening of the skin and subcutaneous tissue. This is the commonest form of 'panniculitis', a condition which may affect the back and other parts of the body. It usually runs a self-limiting course over several weeks, and may be associated with other evidence of osteo-arthrosis.

Polymyalgias

Generalised aches and pains are a common enough experience in every-day living — as a result of strenuous or unaccustomed exercise, or as part of the malaise of almost any febrile illness. It is likely that most 'patients' with such symptoms do not bring them to the doctor. In the minority who do, the nature of such complaints will be clear from the history. This section deals briefly with some of the less common conditions but is not concerned with the varieties and oddities like the 'stiff man syndrome'.

Acute Polymyalgias

The acute infections of virus type seem to be associated more frequently with such symptoms, e.g., influenza and other virus respiratory diseases: one virus disease (dengue) even carries the soubriquet of 'break-bone fever'. Often pain is felt especially in the low back, and this has been noted as a feature of the early phase of smallpox. The acute myalgia of Bornholm disease (usually associated with Coxsackie B types 1—5 infection) is characterised by much more localised and even dramatic pictures (the synonym 'Devil's grip' is indeed an apt one). It is possible that in addition to the commonly recognised pleurodynia, such infection is in fact the cause of at least a proportion of cases of acute lumbago, or interscapular fibrositis, but insufficient evidence exists. Here is an enigma which the family practitioner is well placed to explore.

Chronic Polymyalgias

As with acute myalgias, long continued, usually low grade, generalised aches and pains are associated with infection — though the organisms are more often bacterial than virus in nature, e.g., brucellosis and tuberculosis. Coxsackie B virus infection may also be associated with a chronic intermittent condition characterised by periods of malaise, fatigue, and muscle aches, especially in the limb girdles: widespread muscle fasciculation may also be a feature. This condition may resemble motor neurone disease but muscle wasting is not a feature and the prognosis is better.

In addition to infection, low grade generalised pains are encountered as part of the clinical picture of many other diseases — neoplasia (including leukaemia, in which the locomotor involvement may appear to dominate the picture), hypothyroidism, and depressive illness.

Although the 'myalgia' may be the presenting complaint usually such symptoms will be seen in the wider context of the disease process. The uncommon condition polymyalgia rheumatica has already been mentioned. The relationship between cranial arteritis and polymyalgia rheumatica is discussed in Chapter 24, page 607.

The ill-defined bone pains of osteomalacia, osteoporosis and osteitis deformans are readily interpreted as 'myalgic rheumatism' The true nature may be revealed belatedly by X-ray or by the development of various complications.

It has already been pointed out that soft tissue rheumatism may be the early presenting feature of subsequent rheumatoid disease. In addition to the localised syndromes, such as carpal tunnel syndrome and frozen shoulder, generalised muscle aches and stiffness — especially marked on rising in the morning — may precede by months (or even a year or two) the more definite features of rheumatoid arthritis.

ARTHRITIS

Osteo-arthritis

Among the many possible conditions, acute or chronic, which make up this substantial component of rheumatic diseases, far and away the commonest are those articular affections labelled 'osteo-arthritis'. Because degeneration, rather than inflammation, is believed to be the underlying pathogenesis, perhaps the term 'osteo-arthrosis' is less inaccurate. Some radiological characteristics of the condition (especially osteophytosis) occur in most people over the age of 65 years[13], so that the relationship between symptoms and pathology is unclear. The overlap between this group and others (especially neck and back pain) of the rheumatic diseases has been noted. The episode rate is age-related, with a peak occurring in women over 75 years of age. This accords with other experience from family practice, where osteoarthrosis of hip and knee of elderly women were the main clinical components[14]. The classical clinical features of osteo-arthrosis as it affects major joints are too well known to need recapitulation here. Yet, diagnostic difficulties continue to arise in primary care.

Referred Pain from the Hip
While osteo-arthrosis of the hip usually conforms to the classical text-book descriptions, it may present with pain, apparent stiffness, and even limitation of movement of *the knee*. Occasionally the knee is also the seat of osteo-arthrosis as well as the hip, and in such cases the hip disease may readily be missed in the therapeutic activity focused on the knee.

The Knee: Acute on Chronic
The crepitus, pain and tenderness of the knee and the associated wasting of the quadriceps muscles are all familiar features of chronic osteo-arthrosis. Occasion-

ally, however, a much more acute picture may be presented, usually super-imposed on the chronic condition. The pain is more severe, there is an effusion, and the overlying skin is warm, with dilated veins. The condition usually responds in a week or 10 days, with rest and supporting pressure bandage, and phenylbutazone. The quadriceps muscles should continue to be exercised by static quadriceps exercises.

Generalised Osteo-arthrosis

Some doctors experience difficulty in recognising the form of arthritis known as 'generalised osteo-arthrosis'. Such a presentation may occur less than once a year in a practice with an average size list, but prompt recognition can allay the patient's anxiety about possible rheumatoid arthritis. The patient is commonly a post-menopausal woman who presents with pain, swelling and even redness in the distal inter-phalangeal joints of one or more fingers; both hands may be affected. There may be associated pain and tenderness at the base of the thumb, and occasionally painful juxta-articular pads of fat are found in relation to the knees. Tiredness, irritability and interference with sleep are additional complaints, and the ESR may be moderately elevated (in the range 20—40 mm in the first hour). There is no radiological evidence of erosive arthritis, and tests for the so-called rheumatoid factor are likely to be negative.

While many of the rheumatic conditions considered so far run a relatively short course, osteo-arthrosis has a much more chronic natural history, characterised by 'ups and downs'. The intensity of the exacerbations tends to be much less than that encountered in other types of arthritis, and patients do not as a rule have to contend with the effects of constitutional disturbance which characterise those other diseases. Nevertheless, the chronicity of degenerative arthritis and the relative inefficiency of available measures tax the morale of the patient and test the initiative and other abilities of the doctor concerned with continuing care — the family practitioner. In my view, although this continuing care is a task which we may sometimes thankfully share with other clinical colleagues in, say the rheumatic clinic, that contribution to over-all management has to be carefully monitored and controlled: such a degree of co-operation will prevent an over-enthusiastic hospital team acting, with the best of intentions, to the ultimate detriment of the patient and family because of inadequate information about the wider circumstances. We can assume a more active role than that of dispenser of the newest so-called anti-rheumatic at the behest of the follow-up clinic, though the family practitioner may have to take the initiative in communicating with his hospital colleague.

Rheumatoid Arthritis

Perhaps this disease, of all the rheumatic conditions, has received more than its due share of attention. It is the main focus of attention in rheumatic clinics and textbooks are full of minute descriptions of the classical condition and its many variants — yet much of its nature still remains shrouded in obscurity. Fry[15] gives a neat profile of the disease: 'Rheumatoid arthritis is an uncommon disease of family practice. The incidence rate during 10 years was 7 per 1000. This implies that a family practitioner with an average population of 2500 will have the clinical care of some 15—20 patients with rheumatoid disease over 10 years. The rates were higher in females than in males (by 1.5). In females the disease tended to start in middle age (30—60) but in males the most usual periods of onset were in young adults (20—30) and in elderly men aged 70 and over. The outcome was worse in females, 48 per cent being severely disabled compared with 18 per cent of males so disabled'.

Some of the problems, clinical and psycho-social, associated with the illness have recently been discussed from the family practitioner point of view[16]: they include difficulties in recognition, problems in illness — behaviour of patients and relatives, communications and drug therapy.

Although established rheumatoid disease is classically an articular affection, it occasionally presents for the first time as non-articular rheumatism. The context of the mass of soft tissue rheumatism makes the early recognition of such presentations all the more difficult, and it is usually only the further developments which clarify the picture. Because most other 'rheumatic' complaints in family practice are likely to be associated with a normal ESR, an elevated result is of considerable value to the first contact physician in directing his search strategy in moves towards the early diagnosis of rheumatoid arthritis. The term 'rheumatism' is sometimes equated by some patients with 'rheumatoid arthritis' and considerable anxiety is attached to both. Management of this anxiety, as well as pain or stiffness is often the key issue in helping the rheumatic patient.

Rheumatoid disease usually runs a chronic course, punctuated by exacerbations and remissions; the local impairment of function is compounded by malaise and other features of constitutional disturbance. Striking and maintaining an appropriate balance between necessary adjustments in living to accommodate the illness and too ready capitulation in the face of a chronic disease is a difficult business for patient, relatives and family doctor. This aspect of management calls for much tact and professional skill in deploying the many resources available — support from within the patient's immediate circle, from the primary health care team and from specialist colleagues in hospital.

An important aspect of management in such a long-term and painful condition is the physician's willingness to review any and every advance in treatment and to be prepared to discuss this with patient and relatives, often at their instigation. The need to temper enthusiasms with a critical approach and yet not to destroy hope is an important aspect of management. Perhaps we are too willing to sacrifice this professional role in our drug therapy, and it is worthwhile emphasising the fact that a least in family practice there is insufficient evidence to support some of the claims made for the superiority of many new drugs over aspirin administered appropriately.

Polyarthritis

Several conditions, widely differing in pathogenesis, course and management, are associated with both acute and chronic polyarthritis. In family practice all such conditions, other than osteo-arthrosis and rheumatoid disease are uncommon if not rare. Little useful purpose is served merely by cataloguing them and their clinical features are very much the concern of specialist rheumatologist. They may present some problems to the family practitioner, including recognition and the difficulties of management of a condition during the phase when no firm label can be attached to the disease.

Acute Polyarthritis

In adults, gonococcal arthritis and Reiter's syndrome (polyarthritis, conjunctivitis and urethral discharge) may enter the differential diagnosis, especially in polyarthritis involving the lower limbs, hence a history of possible venereal infections should be sought. The child who has had a recent respiratory infection may be developing rheumatic fever or Henoch—Schönlein purpura. Patients at any age might be exhibiting manifestations of a drug hypersensitivity. The early clinical phase of some virus infections, notably rubella, may also be characterised by pains in several peripheral joints. Much rarer diseases include sarcoidosis, polyarteritis nodosa and systemic lupus erythematosus.

Chronic Polyarthritis

By the time a polyarthritic disease process has become sufficiently established to be labelled 'chronic' it is unlikely that patient care will have remained solely at primary level, especially if there is doubt about the diagnosis. Recognition and details of the rarer syndromes are more commonly a matter for hospital specialists, and the reader is referred to appropriate textbooks for clinical descriptions. Perhaps one disease worth passing mention is gout, because it is easily overlooked and management, though theoretically straightforward, presents problems for the family practitioner.

Gout

The classical onset of acute gout is not always recognised at the first attack. This may be due in part to the probability approach to diagnosis — skin infections, even of the foot, are much commoner than podagra which can mimic cellulitis very closely. We need to maintain a higher 'index of suspicion' for gout when we deal with *any* apparent cellulitis of the foot, especially when the patient is male, and the condition flares up after a 'night out' or some surgical operation.

Similarly, because chronic gout is a relative rarity (less than 1.8 episodes per 1000 population) it is fairly easily confused with other forms of chronic polyarthritis, especially rheumatoid disease. The presence of tophi (characteristically around the helix of the ear or on the eyelids) and elevation of the serum uric acid are attributes worth seeking. The management of the acute phase is probably best achieved by bed rest, and phenylbutazone: colchicine is still an effective drug, and has the additional advantage of assisting in the diagnosis because of its specificity, but its side effects, especially the diarrhoea and nausea, make it a second choice. The main problem in long term management of gout in family practice is one of patient compliance. Patients stop taking medicines when they feel well, and those on uricosuric drugs or allopurinol are no exception: they sometimes need prompting. Some family practitioners have a system of calling up certain 'at risk' patients periodically to help them with problems of compliance. This can also be combined with enlisting the co-operation of the patient in daily self-recording of his medication.

TRAUMA

By definition, in which 'rheumatism' is a group of painful conditions of unknown causation, trauma is apparently excluded. Yet, the subject cannot be ignored in this context, if only because we all feel a need to find something to blame for unpleasant experiences. In the UK this natural desire has, in the past, been encouraged by a State insurance scheme which 'rewards' conditions ascribed to industrial injury at a rate higher than that applicable to 'natural' illness. Patients, especially those with acute back troubles, will occasionally put pressure upon their doctor to issue a sickness absence certificate specifying a traumatic cause for their condition. When there is such a huge gap in our professional knowledge concerning the aetiology of rheumatic conditions, we will usually give the patient the benefit of the doubt: yet, this can sometimes open the door to a lengthy process of litigation which in the long run is so often against the patient's interests.

Trauma is more directly implicated as an important factor in the causation of some instances of osteo-arthrosis: the classical traumatic Heberden's node in the male, following a stub-injury of the finger is one example: another is the osteoarthrosis so commonly the sequal to the torn meniscus, or the congenital dislocation of the hip. Clearly, however, this is only one of many factors operating.

Trauma is more readily implicated in certain forms of soft tissue rheumatism. A classical instance is 'tennis-elbow'. The repeated and especially unaccustomed exercising of a limb may be associated with localised pain, stiffness and swelling, yet, this condition is usually unrelated to injury. The causative relationship of trauma to locomotor tissue conditions is usually obvious from the history and from the circumstances. Occasionally, however, the patient may not be aware of the significance of the injury — or, as in the case of young children, be unable to communicate it. This may be the explanation of some cases of acute painful hip, where a child is noted to have a transient limp lasting usually less than a week. The older child may present with a limp and a painful tender area at the lower edge of the patella: this traumatic osteitis usually subsides in a period of a few weeks.

Trauma is occasionally invoked as a cause of chronic pain and tenderness under the anterior part of the heel: this plantar fasciitis may be associated with calcaneal spur: it is not very common in family practice — an estimated episode frequency per 1000 population is 0.5[17]. Because this condition may sometimes be associated with ankylosing spondylitis the diagnosis of plantar fasciitis, especially in a man in his late teens or early twenties, may alert the physician to seek the appropriate confirmatory evidence including oblique X-rays of sacro-iliac joints.

Trauma may sometimes appear to be the precipitating factor in the onset of the shoulder-hand syndrome, or even in its extreme form, Sudeck's atrophy, in which a chronic painful osteoporosis follows some minor injury. The more overt traumatic lesions of the musculo-skeletal system, including fractures, sprains, traumatic arthritis, and bursitis are dealt with in appropriate textbooks.

MANAGEMENT OF DISEASES OF THE LOCOMOTOR SYSTEM

While there are obviously individual differences in the detailed management of each of the conditions outlined in this chapter, certain broad underlying principles exist to guide us in our approach.

1. *Rehabilitation*: This starts with the first contact. Unfortunately too much lip service is paid to this vital principle, especially by those responsible for planning the service. The supreme example of this is to be encountered in the management of back troubles. The importance to both patient and doctor of firm diagnosis (even if this is an 'exclusion' diagnosis) has been highlighted. Thus, the doctor faced with a patient with an acute back will have his hand strengthened enormously by the ready availability of specialist out-patient consultation backed up with an X-ray. In too many areas, the waiting time before such an orthopaedic appointment is made and kept is of the order of 6—8 weeks. By this time many conditions have resolved, yet it is not possible to rehabilitate the patient until this assessment has been completed. There is a need for a clear national policy on this numerically large and important problem.

2. *Symptomatic treatment*: In most rheumatic conditions the cause is not fully

known. Specific treatment in the sense of effective therapy rationally applied is not possible. The most that can be offered is symptomatic treatment. Much is made of anti-inflammatory properties of drugs by commercial drug firms. Aspirin possesses this property and in so far as it is relevant, possesses it to the same extent as many more toxic preparations except possibly steroids.

3. *Morale*: Pain relief is not simply a matter of prescribing analgesics, morale is important. There is evidence of a relationship between pain relief and morale. Understanding of the patient and communicating that understanding are as important as prescribing analgesics.

4. *Domiciliary physiotherapy*: Pain relief can also be achieved by physical measures. Rest both to the part and to the patient, is helpful. Warmth and massage judiciously applied as part of a planned regime are important. Much can be done by the patient and his family — but more can be achieved by readily available and accessible professional help. The case for domiciliary physiotherapy as part of the health care team's joint effort is, in my view, solidly based.

5. *Local application of drugs*: The local application of steroids and local anaesthesia should be an integral part of family practice management in appropriate cases of tennis elbow, frozen shoulder, arthritis of the knee, among other conditions.

6. *The patient's views*: The patient's views on management should be taken into account: failure to pay sufficient attention to this has allowed such practices as manipulation to pass largely out of trained medical hands. I am not personally totally convinced of its value, but most of us are aware of its potential dangers.

7. *The social worker*: The social implications of the more chronic rheumatic complaints are sufficiently numerous and complex to warrant a closer link being forged between social work departments and the primary care team. Ideally, social workers should work with both the family practitioner and the rheumatic clinic. At present, the emphasis appears to be on the association with the hospital at the expense of the primary care team.

8. *Communications between family practitioner and rheumatic clinic*: More attention needs to be paid to improving communications between family practitioner and rheumatic clinic — and *vice versa*. The family practitioner could assume a greater responsibility for follow-up of the patient referred to hospital: the regular communication of progress reports to hospital colleagues would make for more efficient long term care, relieving the clinic of a snow-balling commitment and the patient of unnecessarily tedious and time-consuming journeys.

9. *The nursing sister and health visitor*: The routine follow-up and home visiting of patients with chronic rheumatic diseases can and should be shared by appropriate members of the primary health care team: especially the nursing sister and health visitor.

10. *The patient's role*: Patients should be encouraged to assume as much responsibility for the management and prevention of disease as they can. It is true that in the absence of knowledge of causation specific prevention is not possible, but the link between obesity and osteo-arthrosis is clear, and failure to maintain efficient quadriceps muscle action can lead to problems with the unstable knee. Aspirin is an appropriate analgesic in most instances, in the absence of specific contraindications, and it is readily available. The infra-red and ordinary heat rays are produced as effectively by a domestic electric fire as by sophisticated equipment in a physiotherapy department.

By the application of such principles, even in our imperfect state of knowledge, we can help to improve the lot of our patients with this painful and enigmatic group of conditions.

Acknowledgements

My thanks are due to Dr. A. G. Reid for sharing ideas and to Mrs. Carole Kent-Robinson for secretarial support.

References

1. McWhinney, I. R. (1972). *Proc. roy. Soc. Med.* **65**, 34.
2. Hull, F. M. (1969). *J. roy. Coll. gen. Pract.* **18**, 65.
3. Office of Population Censuses and Survey (1974). *Morbidity Statistics from General Practice* Second National Study, 1970–71. Studies on Medical and Population Subjects, No. 26. H.M.S.O. London.
4. Knox, J. D. E. (1966). *J. roy. Coll. gen. Pract.* **12**, 81.
5. Wood, P. H. N. (1971). *Brit. med. Bull.* **27**, 82.
6. Gardner, W. S. (1970). *J. roy. Coll. gen. Pract.* **19**, 319.
7. Lee, P., Ahola, S. J., Grennan, D., Brooks, P. and Buchanan, W. W. (1974). *Brit. med J.* **1**, 424.
8. Blair, W. (1963). *J. roy. Coll. gen. Pract.* **6**, 355.
9. Watts, C. A. H. (1966). In *Depressive Disorders in the Community*. (Bristol: John Wright and Sons.
10. Howie, V. (1974). *Evaluation of an X-ray Unit in a Health Centre* Scottish Health Service Studies, no. 30, Scottish Home and Health Department, Edinburgh.
11. Copeman, W. S. C. (1969). In *Textbook of the Rheumatic Diseases* 4th edition, (Edinburgh and London: E. and S. Livingstone).
12. Lancet Annotation (1974). *Lancet* ii, 448.
13. Lawrence, J. S., Bremner, J. M. & Bier, F. (1966). *Ann. rheum. Dis.* **25**, 1.
14. Partridge, R. E. H. and Knox, J. D. E. (1962). *J. roy. Coll. gen. Pract.* **17**, 144.
15. Fry, J. (1966). In *Profiles of Disease*, (Edinburgh and London: E. and S. Livingstone).
16. Knox, J. D. E. (1974). *Update* **8**, 635.
17. Hodgkin, G. K. H. (1973). In *Towards Earlier Diagnosis* 3rd edition, (Edinburgh and London: Churchill Livingstone).

13

Cardiovascular Disease

H. T. N. Sears

INTRODUCTION

Cardiovascular diseases form a very large part of the work of a family practitioner, and more especially in the older age group of patients. In the future, with the increase of longevity, one might reasonably expect even more work in this field of disorders. Certainly, the older the patient, the more likely he is to develop some pathological state of the cardiovascular system.

In family practice, arteriosclerosis and ischaemic heart disease are met most often, followed close on the heels by congestive failure and hypertension. Peripheral vascular disorders are on the increase, and more women are now affected by claudication than thirty years ago, when it was almost entirely confined to men. It is certainly very tempting to attribute this to the change in smoking habits.

The nature of arteriosclerosis, atheroma and ischaemic heart disease is still little understood. How is it that atheroma of the aorta is often found in children and young adults who die of other causes, such as in road accidents? Much work has now been done[1] on the response of the ECG to stress. In car drivers it has been shown that provoking situations resulted in a noradrenaline response, and was associated with mobilization of lipids from adipose tissue, with successive peaks of free fatty acids and triglycerides in the plasma[2].

In family practice, there are many ways in which one may possibly lower the morbidity risk. Perhaps, as a family practitioner, one can advise better than the consultant, because of full appreciation of the patient's make-up, environment, and other associated family factors.

It seems to me that no one can better assess the full picture and act accordingly, consistently and regularly. Weight and smoking are the two primary problems with which the family practitioner can help by seeing the patient frequently for encouragement, explanation and general assessment. More exercise and less reliance on the car are major items to advocate. I have several company directors who, for instance, following myocardial infarcts, walk up the first two floors by the staircase, before going into the elevator to reach the upper storeys of the building in which they work.

Diet is mainly directed at keeping a reasonable weight – height ratio for age, but I think there is enough work now available to suggest the benefit of restriction of saturated fat and sugar intake. For instance, there is considerable evidence to show that there is an increase of cardiac arrhythmias after myocardial infarction if the plasma free fatty acids are elevated[3].

Other positive help may now be given with the adequate treatment of hypertension. Until recently, the production of a normotensive situation has only been believed to protect against stroke and renal failure. Now, there is work to suggest that the use of beta-blockers may in itself protect against myocardial infarction[4], and therefore it may be that we shall see protection of hypertensives treated with the beta-blockers. The situation is constantly changing as we learn more of the complexities of causation of the various diseases of the cardiovascular system.

The family practitioner is the first one to be on the scene in many of these conditions, and even with all the modern advances and diagnostic aids, it is still the carefully taken history that is essential. Very often, the history is the only clue as to the diagnosis. This is particularly so of chest pain, and it is necessary to spend adequate time going over this ground again and again, with as little resort to leading questions as possible.

It should be followed by a careful clinical examination, remembering that inspection usually yields far more information than the laying on of hands or the stethoscope: these should be the last on the list. Ultimately of course, there is the whole armamentarium of investigations including ECG, serum electrolytes, cholesterol, triglycerides, urea, catecholamines and possibly, nowadays, the renin level. An intravenous pyelogram can be arranged by the family practitioner, as well as an examination of a mid-stream specimen of urine. For more complicated investigations such as arteriography of the coronary arteries, renal and femoral arteries, it is necessary to refer the patient to specialist departments, at the nearest centre.

There is little doubt that the family practitioner is the best collator of facts and assessor of the situation, and it is my belief that he is the best person to manage events to the maximum benefit of the patient – which is, after all, the only thing that matters, and which, unfortunately, is often overlooked in modern times.

CORONARY ARTERY DISEASE

Nature and Condition

Occlusive disease of the coronary arteries has become one of the foremost killers of mankind, and it is therefore one of the diseases which has, of recent years, become of particular interest to doctor, layman, and research worker alike. At the moment, coronary artery disease accounts for about forty per cent of middle-aged male deaths, and it is little wonder that so much work and so many projects have been initiated to investigate and probe the numerous ramifications of the disease process.

One of the earliest records of angina was described in the Earl of Clarendon, who eventually died with it in 1674 in Rouen. The original description of the heavy chest pain associated with pain in the left arm is graphically described by his son in a book published in 1759[5].

William Heberden, born in 1710, published an account of angina pectoris in the Medical Transactions of the College of Physicians in 1768[6], and it was this detailed account that first led to its recognition as a disease entity. His description of the substernal gripping pain, more inclined to the left than the right, and radiating down the left arm and sometimes both, details vividly the symptoms as we know them to-day.

The symptoms are caused by diminution of the lumen of the coronary arteries by the disease process of atherosclerosis. This starts in early age, and it is little understood why it progresses so rapidly in some people and not in others, and more particularly why premenopausal women are so comparatively little affected. In Western countries, coronary artery disease is occurring in younger and younger men, and it is nowadays not uncommon to have patients in their twenties or thirties. There seem definite links to hypertension, cigarette-smoking, obesity, lack of exercise and familial traits. The obsessionally perfectionist business executive is especially open to this hazardous disease process. It is interesting to note the relative infrequency of the condition in the poorer areas of the world, and it is because of this that there is considerable speculation as to the role of dietary factors, especially the level of sugar intake.

The pathology is one of diminished blood supply to the myocardium. This is usually directly proportional to the degree of narrowing of the lumen of the coronary arteries by atheroma, but there may be a relative lack of oxygenation of the myocardium by, for instance, a severe anaemia. In January 1974 one of my eighty-year-old female patients had severe angina of exertion. She looked pale, and the haemoglobin estimation revealed a level of 8.3 g per cent. The other features of the blood examination showed evidence of an iron-deficiency anaemia. Two months later, after appropriate iron therapy, she was completely free of symptoms, and the haemoglobin had risen to 13.0 g per cent.

The pain itself is thought to be caused by the production and retention of toxic pain-producing metabolites, and this mechanism was originally described by Sir Thomas Lewis in 1934[7], and no-one has since been able to refute this hypothesis.

Clinical Features

The discomfort and pain associated with myocardial ischaemia is essentially a constricting, band-type of pain, mostly associated with exertion, and often radiating to the neck or jaw, or into the left and sometimes both, arms. It may stop short at the elbows, but more often it extends down to the fingers. Occasionally it can be bizarre in its pattern, and it is not unusual to find its manifestation solely as pain in the thighs or in the jaw, unassociated with chest discomfort.

The pain can vary from a mere suggestion of discomfort, often thought to be indigestion, to a very severe crushing pain that brings the patient to a halt, and if experienced for the first time severely, and particularly if it comes on at rest, is accompanied by extreme fear and anguish, and a sense of impending dissolution.

Diagnosis

The diagnosis is usually clear-cut. Substernal pain or discomfort, often associated with pain in the jaw or radiating down one or both arms, and brought on by exertion or change of atmospheric temperature, such as going outside into the cold air from a warm room. These symptoms are especially produced after a meal.

In the acute case of an actual infarction of course, the clinical picture is different. One minute the patient is quite well and the next, he is seized with a severe retrosternal pain and rapidly assumes a shocked, pale and sweating countenance. This is often associated with a drop in blood pressure and a bradycardia.

Electrocardiography usually reveals diagnostic changes, including ST elevation, or depression, T wave inversion and the appearance of Q waves. There may be a leucocytosis, and serial enzyme estimations may show an increase over the first few days.

The early symptoms of myocardial ischaemia are easily missed. One must be particularly aware of the tense and obsessional business man who complains merely of tiredness. This is a symptom that is now recognized as being one of the several criteria for suspecting a pre-coronary situation. The other factors in this early-warning system are where there is a family history of the disease, obesity, lack of exercise, cigarette smoking, other organic diseases such as hyperlipidaemia, diabetes mellitus, or hypertension. The latter is said to promote the development of obstructive coronary disease by accelerating atherosclerosis. Also, in this direction a hypertrophied left ventricle may be less capable of adapting to an acute infarction.

Many advances have been made over the past decade with the increasing use of coronary cine-radiography[8,9]. Lord Brock, in his assessment of the present position of cardiac surgery[10], pointed out that in Mason Sones' department at Cleveland, 13 602 cases had this investigation performed between April 1959 and December 1968.

Research is also being undertaken into the vessel wall changes. It is thought that some of these may be caused by an increase in carbon monoxide level, which is in turn, related to cigarette smoking.

Assessment

When a patient presents with a history of chest pain of gradual onset over a few months, it is important at that stage to make up one's mind as to whether his symptoms represent ischaemic heart disease or not. Very often, close attention to the history will give the necessary clue as to the diagnosis. Sometimes, however, it is very difficult to differentiate between for instance, lower oesophageal symptoms, or those caused by hiatus hernia or gall bladder dysfunction.

It is at this early stage of seeing the patient that it is most important to elucidate the situation. Certainly, one should arrange for a chest X-ray, an electrocardiogram at rest and after exertion, and an estimation of serum lipids. It is also wise to do a haemoglobin estimation, as it is remarkably easy to fall into this pitfall of a missed diagnosis of anaemia.

Lesions of the lower oesophagus can often mimic anginal pain and if there is any doubt about this, barium studies with tilt are advisable. The gall-bladder can be a problem because it is now well documented that there is a close relationship between its disease and symptoms from coronary insufficiency. In fact, there may often be a double diagnosis, the one not excluding the other.

At this stage, one must remark on the increasing number of women with ischaemic heart disease. Whereas thirty years ago it was comparatively uncommon to see females with a coronary thrombosis, not only is it now relatively common but, as with males, the age at which infarction occurs seems to be getting younger and younger. It is easy to relate this to cigarette smoking habits before and after World War II, but it is unlikely that this is more than just one factor in aetiological events, and for example, the role of oestrogen in 'protecting' the premenopausal woman is not yet clearly understood.

Management

Having established that one is dealing with a case of angina of effort, it is important to explain the cause and nature of the pain to the patient. His mode of life may have to be altered, more regular exercise advised, smaller meals taken and with an adequate time afterwards before resuming work, reduction of weight and, if possible, total cessation of cigarette smoking. I always tell such people that I have actually recorded gross electrocardiographic changes of ischaemia in some patients who have only had a few puffs of a cigarette. Also, that it may take as long as half an hour before the tracings return to normal. I am pleased to find that the vast majority of patients respond to clear cut examples like this, and usually stop smoking altogether.

Sometimes, I think a short rest from work is advisable when one first sees a patient with angina. However, I try to let them continue as near to normal a life as possible, but to be moderate in all things and, if possible, to increase their physical activities, such as walking to the office or to the pillar-box, rather than going by car.

Diet sheets are issued to the overweight, who are seen monthly for encouragement and support. Patients are advised to reduce the animal fat intake and sugar consumption. The question of diet is still an open problem, but I think most authorities are agreed that undue intake of saturated fats is best avoided. The previously held views that replacing butter with polyunsaturates protects the coronary arteries from atheroma are no longer entirely supported.

In a report of an Advisory Panel of the Committee on Medical Aspects of Food Policy, published by the UK Department of Health and Social Security in 1974[11], the panel was asked to evaluate evidence on the relation between diet and cardiovascular disease.

The report made five recommendations. First, obesity should be avoided and treated. Second, the amount of fat in the diet — especially saturated fat should be reduced. Third, the panel unanimously agreed that there was no reason to increase the intake of polyunsaturates to reduce the incidence of ischaemic heart disease. Fourth, the intake of sugar should be reduced 'if only to reduce the risk of obesity', and finally, caution was advised in any proposals to soften the water supply in any part of the country.

The Report on Prevention of Coronary Disease by the Royal College of Physicians of London and the British Cardiac Society has more recently been published[12]. As well as alluding to the 5 items above, it concludes that the prevention of coronary heart disease in the community is predominantly the role of the family practitioner, and that the continuation and extension of good family practice should provide the main means of identifying high-risk subjects.

After general attention to the mode of living, various drugs may then have to be employed. Possibly a small dose of sedative is all that is needed in the tense and anxious patient. If the blood lipids are raised, there is a large school of thought that believes that clofibrate should be taken routinely. Certainly, I would prescribe this drug if the serum cholesterol was 350 mg per 100 ml (9.25 mmol/l) or over. In one of my patients with a level of 450 mg per 100 ml (11.75 mmol/l) I have seen not only his angina lessen, but the periorbital xanthomata gradually disappear completely, and this had a remarkably beneficial change in the whole outlook and manner of the patient.

Of the other drugs, glyceryl trinitrate 0.5 mg sublingually is still the best treatment for relieving anginal pain, and apart from the occasionally fierce headache that it produces, patients may take these tablets in a fairly unrestricted way. In severe effort angina, I think it is entirely justifiable to let a patient take a tablet prophylactically prior to a procedure that he knows will bring on the pain; for example, before having a bath or climbing the stairs. Long-acting preparations are sometimes very useful to take at bedtime, if the patient is otherwise awakened several times during the night with pain. Tablets of Sustac 6.4 mg can completely change the otherwise troubled nights of some patients.

Of recent years, the beta-blockers have assumed a large place in ischaemic heart disease. Angina is often associated with a tachycardia, so the antagonism of the cardiac sympathetic receptors thereby producing a slowing of heart rate, may in itself be the major beneficial effect. Other haemodynamic effects are also probably involved in easing the myocardial oxygen requirements, such as decrease of systemic arterial pressure, and counteraction of the direct cardiac effects of increase of circulating catecholamines associated with muscular exertion. This reduction in cardiac activity by the beta-blockers one must assume, means that there is a considerable decrease in the left ventricular myocardial oxygen requirement, and hence, less likelihood of developing anginal pain.

There are many beta-blockers in current use. They should not be used in cases of bronchial asthma, nor where there is overt failure. One can build up the dose of, for instance, oxprenolol to really big levels in order to relieve the pain of angina, and yet it does not drop the blood pressure below 'normal' levels. Certainly doses of up to 160 mg qds., can be used where angina is severe, and some physicians use even higher doses.

For the acute episode of infarction, the symptoms of which have already been described, the most important decision comes right at the beginning. Should one immediately send the patient into hospital, or should one treat the case at home?

At the moment, experience suggests that the results of hospital as opposed to home treatment are more or less identical. The mortality rates are about equal, and there is less likelihood of arrhythmias developing in those cases treated at home[13,14].

The advantages of home treatment are legion. Not only is it nearly always less stressful, but the attention of a wife, the older members of the family, the trusted district nurse and the family practitioner is far more natural to an ill patient than the fearsome array of impedimenta associated with an intensive care unit. There are, of course, other situations which may dictate in the opposite direction, quite apart from clinical considerations. One example of this might well be in the household of a busy family practitioner whose work is carried on at his home. The continuous ringing of the front door bell and telephone (especially the frustration if either are not answered promptly), might make it essential to hospitalize such an unfortunate victim of myocardial infarction.

The young person, or the patient where failure is a feature should probably be sent to hospital. Otherwise, my own feeling is that all other cases are best treated at home by the home team. Patients with infarction do not travel well in an ambulance (unlike head injuries), and the distance from hospital and degree of initial shock may influence the decision.

The diagnosis is often associated (but not invariably) with electrocardiographical changes. However, in my opinion, clinical judgment must always override the diagnostic aids. The possible exception to this, may be the help one might get from changing enzyme levels over the first three or four days.

The most important initial treatment is the giving of morphia. The dose depends on the size and build of the patient, and the severity of the pain, but is usually 15–30 mg. Half the dose may be given slowly intravenously, and the rest of the dose intramuscularly. There is much to be said for using a preparation containing an anti-emetic as well, as both the infarction as well as the morphia may cause vomiting, which leads to an added strain on the myocardium.

Morphia acts in many ways. It allays pain and anxiety and relaxes muscle. It decreases heart rate, dilates peripheral and coronary vessels, constricts abdominal visceral vessels, and may also mobilize blood from the pulmonary circulation to the venous system.

In acute myocardial infarction, death from ventricular fibrillation is most likely during the first hour of symptoms. This may be preceded by frequent ventricular extra systoles, and lignocaine can safely be given intravenously in the dosage 1–2 mg per kg body weight as a bolus, or else 120 mg intramuscularly without any deleterious side-effects, should extra systoles be noted.

A close watch must be kept for minimal signs of failure by observing the jugular venous pressure, or positive hepato-jugular reflux, and diuretics given accordingly. Frusemide 40 mg is now the drug most often used under these conditions. A marked bradycardia may necessitate the use of intravenous atropine sulphate 300–600 micrograms.

There seems little doubt now, that the main role of the hospital coronary-care unit is to prevent deaths due to ventricular fibrillation, 80 per cent of early deaths being due to electrical failure rather than pump failure. I think, however, that a vigilant family practitioner may be able to assess which case is most likely to develop this fatal phenomenon, and with the judicious use of lignocaine, prevent its occurrence. Oral phenytoin (100 mg b.d.) is used by some physicians to lessen the likelihood of arrhythmias developing.

Follow-up and Continuing Care

There is still no agreement on the question of either short-term or long-term anticoagulant therapy, but the current view appears to be that poor-risk patients and the younger patients should receive anticoagulants in the acute stage. Certainly, this is not embarked upon to prevent further thrombosis in the coronary artery, but only to prevent the embolic phenomena that occur after the initial stage is passed. Long-term anticoagulant therapy beyond two months after the infarction, has not been conclusively proved to be of value, and there seem to be real risks of haemorrhage if anything like useful prothrombin levels are to be achieved.

After some days in bed, and providing no appreciable degree of failure has developed, patients should be activated gradually. The period of bed-rest will depend on the general state of the patient. Some could be allowed up within a few days, others may require some weeks before full ambulation is possible. Needless to say, the day of the bed-pan is over, and right from the start, patients should be allowed to sit on a commode for their bowel movements. Also to this end care must be taken to see that constipation does not occur, with the consequent straining at stool.

Gradually increasing activity should be allowed, each case being judged on the cardiac reserve and degree of severity of the original illness. Climbing up and down the stairs once in the day should be the first achievement, and ultimately, depending on circumstances and progress, walking and more extended exercise be permitted.

Evaluation, Assessment and Future Needs

Cardinal in all considerations should be the aim not to produce a cardiac cripple. Sir Maurice Cassidy, one of the foremost pre-war British cardiologists, made this dictum quite clear to his students. The treatment should never be worse than the disease, and the quality of life was paramount in one's aim of management. He so rightly pointed out that it was achieving little to have an extra three months of life by sitting permanently in a bathchair waiting for death to strike. It has also recently been stated by other authorities that older people should live life to the full, and indeed, 'live dangerously'. How right they are! All these thoughts should be considered carefully when rehabilitating the case of myocardial infarction and, as usual, moderation in everything should be the rule of the day, with no extremes of thought.

The future of the man or woman after an infarct depends entirely on the individual case and circumstances. With a minor episode, it is quite usual for a patient to resume his business activities. He should pay careful attention to details such as regular exercise, regular meals, regular holidays, and delegation of responsibility. A man can often return to full work, and continue for many years in his previous capacity, providing he pays a little attention to details such as weight, exercise and general mode of life.

The most difficult case is the severe angina, with crippling limitation of activity. With the advent of cineradiography, much information has been gained about the coronary blood flow and its impairment, and it is now considered an essential part of the evaluation of all such patients. There is little doubt that a new area of management has now been introduced, and that operative techniques offer a new lease of life to some people either by endarterectomy with patch graft reconstruction of the affected coronary artery, or by using vein by-passes. The status of 100 patients after coronary artery by-pass surgery[15] and the survival and angiographic results of 1000 patients[16] have been described.

Summary

Ischaemic heart disease is now the most important cause of male deaths. Its recognition is vital in the early stages so that evasive action can be taken, such as giving up cigarette smoking, losing weight, taking more regular exercise, or by taking drugs, either to lower the blood lipids, or else to spare the heart of sympathetic overaction by the use of beta-blockers.

Overt infarcts are probably best treated at home, providing the family practitioner can try to foretell those patients most likely to develop arrhythmias. Whilst it is quite possible for the family practitioner to anticoagulate his patients at home, providing the family can take blood daily to the laboratory, the efficacy of this treatment has not yet been conclusively proved. All efforts must be geared to achieving a good quality of life, and above all, to avoid producing cardiac cripples.

There is an increasing place for surgery.

HYPERTENSION

Nature and Condition

Since the description of the circulation by William Harvey in 1628, dedicated to King Charles I, it has been known that blood is forced round the body through arteries, and that a pressure effect is sustained by contractions of the heart. Because of this pressure, blood is transported to all areas of the body, and oxygen and other vital materials are conveyed to the organs, thus sustaining life.

It is difficult, if not impossible, to define what a normal blood pressure might be. The so-called normal varies with race, sex, age, time of day, position and temperature to mention but a few things. The blood pressure can vary in the same person by wide margins depending on a host of circumstances.

The actual figure above which hypertension is diagnosed is still entirely arbitrary, but for the majority of doctors, levels of over 150/90 mmHg, would be considered as being above normal. Age of course, plays a part. A baby of ten days has an average pressure of 70/40 mmHg, a child of ten years about 100/65 mmHg, and an 18 year old has a pressure of 125/75 mmHg.

At this point it is necessary to stress various obligatory details in the technique of taking the blood pressure, which should be uniform and consistent. A standard-sized sphygmomanometer cuff must be used, with a rubber bag at least 12 cm wide. It must be applied smoothly to the arm, and the stethoscope should be placed over the brachial artery close to the lower border of the cuff. During the first inflation of the cuff, a finger should be placed on the radial artery, and a rough estimate of the systolic pressure recorded. Then, at least two further readings of systolic and diastolic pressures should be recorded on auscultation, and the lowest readings obtained used for the records. The first sound to be heard is the systolic pressure, and the diastolic pressure is usually accepted as being that pressure at which there is an abrupt change from loud to muffled beats.

By feeling the radial pulse at the first inflation of the cuff, one can be certain of not missing the 'silent gap', which may otherwise be overlooked in hypertensive patients, and when the sounds heard by the stethoscope may fade twice during the decline in cuff pressure.

Hypertension is a very common condition, and about 35 per cent of people of 55 years and over, are found to have diastolic pressures of 95 mmHg, or over[17]. More evidence is now being produced suggesting that the older conception, of only the diastolic pressure being important, is not true. The level of systolic pressure is as important from the point of view of both morbidity and mortality[18,19], and figures have been produced by the Society of Actuaries[20] showing that for every age group, the higher the level of systolic pressure, the higher the mortality rate.

The incidence of stroke and renal failure can be markedly reduced by adequate control of hypertension[21], and recently, evidence has also been produced that the use of beta-blockers may protect against myocardial infarction[4]. Perhaps the control of hypertension with beta-blockers may improve the mortality rate caused by infarction.

Hypertension can be conveniently divided into primary essential and secondary types, only 15 per cent being of the latter variety, and caused by such conditions as coarctation of the aorta, phaeochromocytoma, renal artery stenosis, kidney disease, Cushing's syndrome or toxaemia of pregnancy.

Much work has been done trying to find the cause of primary essential hypertension, but at the moment it is little understood. Various exciting facts are currently being discovered, and the renin-angiotensin-aldosterone systems are receiving much attention[22,23,24]. It is known that an enzyme called renin, which is released from the renal cortex passes into the blood stream and acts upon the plasma substrate angiotensinogen converting it to angiotensin I. Angiotensin I, an inactive precursor, is converted to angiotensin II, and this has an aldosterone-stimulating effect, in addition to its pressor action. A loss of sodium from the body leads to an increased release of renin by the kidney, and this in turn, produces a rise in angiotensin concentration. This stimulates aldosterone secretion, elevates the blood pressure, causes renal sodium conservation, and restores sodium balance. This normal cycle, some authorities think, becomes upset in a variety of ways in hypertensive disease.

Not only are these theories interesting, but they may well thrown light on the possible treatment likely to be effective in any given case, and the hitherto empirical treatments may shortly be outmoded.

Whatever the cause of the condition, there is much evidence that environmental factors play a large part, probably through psychological factors[25]. This aspect has been well documented by Brod[26], who showed the effect of mental arithmetic on the blood pressure as well as the mere thought of bicycling up a hill. After two minutes of each of these stresses, it took an average of seven minutes for the readings to drop to their previous normal levels in normotensive patients, and longer in those with hypertension.

Inheritance would seem to play a part, but it is not clear exactly what one inherits: whether it is the temperament or the actual hypertension. Much work still remains to be done in the elucidation of this common condition, and it is still not understood why all studies show that women are able to stand a high blood pressure better than men. Recent work by Zinner et al. at Harvard seems to show that high blood pressure tendencies can be well established before the age of 2 years[27,28].

Clinical Features

Most frequently there are no symptoms at all, and the only feature — the consistently raised blood pressure — is found on a chance reading at an insurance examination, by an optician, a blood transfusion unit, a medical examination for a new job or superannuation purposes.

Hypertension has usually to be severe before it produces symptoms, such as breathlessness, lassitude, headache or epistaxis. Sometimes the first clue as to its existence is the advent of a complication, such as a stroke, deterioration of vision, or atrial fibrillation.

It is however, far more likely to produce few symptoms. Most throbbing headaches, or headaches described as being 'like a tight band' are caused by anxiety or tension states. In the majority of instances, it is diagnosed on routine examination for some disconnected purpose or symptom, and it is on this score that family practitioners can best help with their screening efforts, and initiate treatment before symptoms or irreversible changes have occurred.

Diagnosis

This is usually made when the blood pressure is in excess of 150/90 mm Hg. There may be evidence of outward displacement of the apex beat, a left ventricular thrust, an accentuated second heart sound in the aortic area or retinal changes.

A chest X-ray will show the presence or not of cardiac enlargement, and an electrocardiogram may confirm left ventricular strain. Serum electrolytes should be estimated, and also a urea and creatinine level.

If there is any suggestion of a phaeochromocytoma, a 24 hour urine estimation of catecholamines and vanillomandelic acid (VMA) should be made. It may well be however, that new horizons are opening that may demand the estimation of the blood renin level in all cases to give a clue as to possible treatment. Between the ages of 20 and 40 an intravenous pyelogram should probably be done, and also an examination of mid-stream specimen of urine.

The question of secondary hypertension must be considered. It is always wise to listen for a bruit over the renal arteries suggesting a renal artery stenosis. The diagnosis of coarctation of the aorta is usually easy by feeling the femoral and radial pulses simultaneously, and the X-ray may show rib notching. On one occasion I have actually palpated, as well as auscultated, the intercostal arteries on the posterior chest wall that are so enlarged in this condition. Phaeochromocytomata are usually indicated by the paroxysms that occur. The question of aortography to outline the renal arteries is rather open to doubt at the present time, as are renal scans with radioactive isotopes. The end-results on the hypertension after corrective surgical procedures are disappointingly poor. They may seem hardly good enough to warrant these rather sophisticated and difficult procedures of investigation.

Assessment

All grades of hypertension have to be considered. From the mildest grades of primary essential, to the other extreme of accelerated hypertension, or what used to be called 'malignant hypertension,' characterized by a high blood pressure, grade IV retinopathy and albuminuria. Much depends on the length of history, symptoms and physical findings. These vary from an asymptomatic hypertension found accidentally, to the accelerated variety with a speedy end.

The latter patient develops a considerable retinitis and renal involvement, and usually dies in renal failure. In 1958 figures were published from Hammersmith Hospital[29] showing an 80 per cent mortality within six months of the diagnosis of accelerated hypertension having been made, and a 90 per cent mortality after one year.

In recent years, the incidence of the accelerated form seems to have receded, and this would seem most probably to be due to the earlier detection and treatment of the milder grades of hypertension by family practitioners.

Management

There are many general procedures to be observed. The mode of life may have to be adjusted. The dynamic managing director may have to be encouraged to shed more responsibility. The weight must be kept in check, and regular exercise encouraged. In many cities there are now, for instance, lunch-time gymnastic classes. Smoking should be discouraged. Excesses of animal fats, sugar and salt should be avoided.

In the tense and anxious, advice about relaxation should be given, with positive instructions as to how this can be achieved. Probably, lying on the floor with a pillow under the head, and consciously relaxing all groups of muscles in turn from the toes up to the scalp, and finally concentrating on the hands, is the best method of helping in this direction. It may be necessary to employ sedatives, tranquillizers, anti-depressants or hypnotics.

Of the drugs now available in the active reduction of blood pressure, much change of thought may be needed in their selection in view of the rapidly changing climate of opinion as to causative mechanisms of hypertension.

Until 1950, there was no actual drug specifically used for treatment. In the 1950 edition of Price's Textbook of Medicine[30] for instance, nothing specific was recommended, and the benefit of mistletoe was doubted! Since the advent of the ganglion-blockers, great strides have been made. The drugs in current use can be conveniently divided into six groups: the first having a salt-depleting effect, for example, the thiazides; the second having a direct CNS action, like clonidine and methyldopa, and the third being adrenergic-blocking drugs such as reserpine, guanethidine, bethanidine and debrisoquine. The fourth group has now largely gone out of favour, the ganglion blockers, such as pentolinium and mecamylamine, and the fifth group consists of the direct vaso-dilators such as hydrallazine and diazoxide. Lastly, is the latest addition to the armamentarium, the beta-blockers, which mainly reduce cardiac output and slow the pulse.

It is too early yet to say, but in the future, estimation of the blood renin level may be obligatory to decide on the best form of treatment. Low levels of renin suggest that a drug such as spironolactone may have good effect, and this may also be decided if there is only a small rise of renin level after frusemide stimulation[31,32]. Beta-blockers would seem to be of most use where the renin level is elevated. The situation is rapidly changing, and it is prudent to do no more than hazard a guess at this juncture, but the present research is certainly exciting and gives a possible direction of future management.

The mainstay of treatment is the use of a diuretic such as chlorothiazide. This not only lowers the blood pressure as such, but also usually means that a lower dose of some of the more potent anti-hypertensive drugs will be required. Potassium supplements are necessary if a high dose is used, or in any patient over 50 years of age who is given a thiazide.

Methyldopa in a dose starting at 250 mg twice daily and increasing slowly to a maximum of 3 g daily may be effective, when combined with a thiazide. The same applies to guanethidine, which should be given once daily, starting at 10 mg and building up to 125 mg daily if necessary. It is of course, essential in both these drugs to take the blood pressure in the sitting and standing position. If, in the case of guanethidine, there is any suggestion of exertional hypotension (which occurs in about one-third of cases) the blood pressure should be recorded after climbing some stairs. It is important in both these drugs, to warn patients of holidaying in hot climates. The dose of the drug may have to be halved in temperatures of 25°C and over.

Beta-blockers are now much in vogue, either used alone, with thiazides, or in addition to the beta-adrenergic-blocking drugs such as reserpine, guanethidine, bethanidine or debrisoquine, or an alpha-blocking drug such as hydrallazine. Large doses may be required to produce the desired effect, and with oxprenolol for example, starting at 40 mg twice a day, the dose may gradually be increased to 320 mg twice a day. These drugs should not be used where there is any evidence of cardiac failure or bronchial asthma.

Much work has been done in recent years to show the 'heart-sparing' effects of the beta-blockers, including the reduction in pulse rate of racing drivers, after-dinner speakers, and even normal people during travel by air[33]. However, little is known about the long term effects of beta-blocker therapy on the central nervous system. Side-effects such as nightmares and constipation are frequently met, and more serious adverse reactions such as psoriatic skin lesions, ocular lesions and sclerosing peritonitis have led to the withdrawal of practolol from therapeutic use.

Small doses of 0.025 mg clonidine have been used for several years in the treatment of migraine, and more recently, larger tablets of 0.1 mg and 0.3 mg have been manufactured for use in the treatment of hypertension. Whilst a clonidine-thiazide regime sometimes works by itself, it is more useful as an adjunct to some other regime which is not quite controlling the situation. Often, the addition of clonidine saves having to increase one of the more potent drugs, with the ensuing tiresome side-effects.

Certainly, the side-effects have to be weighed up very carefully when planning treatment. It is no good making a healthy, asymptomatic young man impotent, when his blood pressure elevation has been found accidentally at a life insurance examination for a house mortgage. It is in such a case as this, that hydrallazine, a potent vaso-dilator and an alpha-blocker, may be of use either by itself, or in combination with another drug, such as a beta-blocker. The earlier anxieties in the 1950's about hydrallazine producing a diffuse LE-type of illness, seem less relevant, now that we know it is in fact a reversible state of affairs.

All in all, one should aim at achieving a situation of having a blood pressure as near to normal for age as one can get, combined with a patient who is happy, free of too many side-effects, and more particularly, one with a good quality of life.

In a series of 80 patients[34] with a mean blood pressure of 240/150 mmHg, the treated mean pressure dropped to 140/90 mmHg, and some of these have survived twenty years. About one-third were originally diagnosed as suffering from accelerated, or 'malignant' hypertension. Very few are on similar therapy, and it has taken in some instances, a long time to find the treatment that best suited any particular patient. Maybe we are on the threshold of being able to save a lot of time previously spent in trial and error methods. By estimating the renin level, we may be able to forecast what treatment is likely to be most suitable in any given case.

It cannot be over-stressed that very energetic anti-hypertensive treatment in the elderly is not only unncessary, but may be disastrous. In a 70-year-old with a blood pressure of 190/100 mmHg, only very gentle treatment is indicated. Possibly a small dose of thiazide, especially if there is any evidence of mild congestive failure or nocturnal left ventricular attacks, combined with a small dose of reserpine, clonidine or methyldopa will be necessary. Treatment must be introduced slowly, and with care.

In all treatment, and at all ages, clinical judgment must override all other considerations, and particularly the sphygmomanometer readings. It is now well recognized that hospital or surgery readings are often elevated to a considerable degree, due to external factors.

A careful history may well reveal symptoms suggesting hypotension occurring at home, and it would be mischievous and indeed meddlesome, to increase the dose of a drug only by avidly reading the pressures on a scientific instrument. It is the patient who must be treated, and never the machine.

Follow-up and Continuing Care

It is important, having established that hypertension exists, to make several points to the patient: first, to explain the need for keeping the pressure as near to normal as can be managed, and second, to make it clear that, as in a diabetic, the treatment having been deemed necessary, it is a life-sentence. Only rarely does it occur that (myocardial infarction excluded) the treatment can be gradually lowered or even discontinued.

Patients should be seen at the same time of day and by the same doctor. If they have rushed to the surgery or omitted their tablets, the readings should be discounted. With the adrenergic-blockers, the interval between the taking of the tablets and the recording of the blood pressure should always be noted, and as far as possible, should be the same at each surgery attendance.

It is often necessary to re-arrange the scheme of treatment: perhaps increasing the thiazide, or lowering the dose of an adrenergic-blocker to lessen side effects, or adding another drug such as a beta-blocker. If diarrhoea is a problem, tablets of codeine phosphate 30 mg are invaluable.

Evaluation, Assessment and Future Needs

The patient must be seen regularly — certainly weekly, at the start of treatment. Not only to see how the therapy is working, but also to get used to the routine. As mentioned earlier, the psyche plays a large part in sustaining an elevated blood pressure. Once an even keel has been achieved, and this may mean much experimenting with different doses or combinations of drugs, one's discretion must be used. It is important not to see patients so frequently as to alarm them or make them introspective. Some patients can well be left for six months between visits. Those with accelerated hypertension or renal failure are best referred to hospital for assessment and for establishing the optimum treatment required.

For the future, Miall's work[35,36] shows the importance of screening. He suggests that significant hypertension is unlikely to develop if the diastolic pressure in the early twenties is less than 90 mmHg. On this basis therefore, one may be able to assume that a single recording of blood pressure in early life is enough to indicate which persons should be screened regularly, and which could be safely ignored.

The prevention and treatment of hypertension is fairly and squarely in the court of the family practitioner. Many more cases would be found, and much morbidity prevented, if every male patient between the ages of 20 and 40 years had their blood pressures recorded whenever they attended the surgery. Equally important, is to record the pressure even when it is normal.

One must await the outcome of the present fascinating work on the renin-angiotensin system, as it may influence the methods of treatment strongly, and work is now being done on the angiotensin II antagonist — saralasin, with results suggesting its potential use in the future[37].

Summary

Hypertension is a common disease. Women stand it better than men. It is often asymptomatic. Once hypertension has been confirmed, it is important to treat it to avoid stroke and renal failure, and to maintain a blood pressure as near to normal as possible, and above all, to ensure a high quality of life for the patient. To this end, and to avoid side-effects, multiple drug therapy is often necessary.

There is a likelihood of more definitive treatment being used from the outset, if the renin-angiotensin saga develops in the way it seems to be doing.

VALVULAR HEART DISEASE

Nature and Condition

There are four valves in the heart: the mitral and tricuspid separating the left and right ventricles from their respective atria, and the aortic and pulmonary valves separating the aorta from the left ventricle, and the pulmonary artery from the right ventricle. The mitral and tricuspid valves therefore open during diastole, and the aortic and pulmonary valves close during diastole and open during systole.

Disease of these valves can be divided into congenital and acquired. The latter can be caused by arteriosclerosis, rheumatic fever, syphilis and bacterial invasion, or may be produced relatively. For instance, tricuspid incompetence may be caused by enlargement of the tricuspid ring, as part of the process of some other cardiac condition causing enlargement of the heart.

The congenital abnormalities are often multiple, as in the case of the tetralogy of Fallot[38]. In this, pulmonary stenosis and right ventricular hypertrophy is associated with the aorta arising from the right, communicating with both right and left ventricles, and over-riding the intra-ventricular septum which is not fully developed.

Disease of the mitral valve is the commonest, and is nearly always rheumatic. If the valve is affected to any extent by acute inflammation, the two cusps may become fused together at their edges with resultant narrowing (stenosis) of the orifice. If the valves in addition become rigid, they may be held open, and blood may leak backwards during systole (incompetence).

Another feature in the rheumatic process is the scarring and shortening of the chordae tendinae, which can hold the mitral valve more open than ever. Stenosis and incompetence of the mitral valve are nearly always present together, but one usually predominates over the other, to give rise to the diagnosis of mitral stenosis or incompetence.

Aortic valvular disease, unless it presents as congenital stenosis, is caused by rheumatic fever in about 70 per cent of cases. The other 30 per cent of cases are caused by syphilis, arteriosclerosis or endocarditis. There is one considerable difference between the aortic and mitral valves in the acute rheumatic process. In the case of the aortic valves, these lesions usually develop during the active phase of the disease, whereas with the mitral valve, the deformities, signs and symptoms develop up to many years later. The oldest case of rheumatic mitral stenosis that I have seen was a female of over ninety years of age.

Clinical Features

In congenital valvular disease, the first symptom is usually cyanosis, especially on crying, exertion, or with an intercurrent infection. Other types of valvular disease usually exhibit breathlessness on exertion, going through the various stages to gross congestive failure, with moist lungs, enlargement of the liver and oedema.

The malar flush of the patient with mitral stenosis is well recognized, and is due to chronic venous stasis and back-pressure. In all cases of valvular disease, it is important to obtain an accurate history, especially about the question of rheumatic fever.

In some patients, a gradual onset of malaise, fever and anaemia must make one vigilant to the possibility of subacute bacterial endocarditis, especially if there is a history of sepsis or of a recent tooth extraction.

Diagnosis

Aortic valvular lesions resulting in stenosis, usually present a pallid patient, with a small or 'plateau' pulse, and a diminished pulse pressure. There is often a systolic thrill over the upper sternum, and a harsh systolic murmur over the same area, propagated upwards into the great vessels of the neck. Angina or syncopal attacks are frequent accompaniments of aortic stenosis.

Aortic incompetence is characterized by a bounding pulse with a big pulse pressure. It was first described as a 'waterhammer' pulse by Sir Dominic Corrigan in 1832[39]. There is a blowing aortic diastolic murmur. Some authorities say that with syphilitic valvular lesions, the murmur is best heard at the right sternal edge, and in rheumatic disease, it is best heard at the left sternal edge, and conducted downwards towards the apex.

Sometimes, in aortic incompetence, there is an associated mitral diastolic murmur, first described by Austin Flint in 1862[40], suggesting a co-existing relative mitral stenosis. Aortic incompetence, as well as showing a bounding pulse, produces such a considerable ventricular contraction as to cause pulsation of the whole patient, who may be very aware of each systole. Capillary pulsation may also be seen in the nail-beds.

Occasionally, it is difficult to hear a mild degree of aortic incompetence, and a soft diastolic 'whiff' is only audible on auscultation with the patient leaning forward and at the end of deep expiration. The eventual outcome of aortic incompetence is left ventricular failure and attacks of acute and distressing dyspnoea. In aortic stenosis, calcification may be visible in and around the cusps in both rheumatic and arteriosclerotic types on X-ray screening.

Mitral stenosis presents with breathlessness, and perhaps symptoms of chronic heart failure, with cyanosis, raised jugular venous pressure, moist bases, hepatomegaly and oedema. It accounts for over 50 per cent of all cases of chronic rheumatic heart disease. It is one of the common causes of atrial fibrillation.

In early cases, the left atrial pressure increases and overcomes the narrowing of the orifice, but eventually, the back-pressure is conveyed to the lungs, with resultant exertional dyspnoea, and maybe attacks of acute pulmonary oedema and haemoptysis.

The murmur is a diastolic rumble, which crescendoes up to and eventually replaces, the first heart sound at the apex. If there is any difficulty in hearing it, exercise, and resultant tachycardia, will often make it more audible, or else, it can sometimes be heard better by turning the patient half on to the left side whilst auscultating at the apex. There may be an 'opening snap' which is the high-pitched noise after the second heart sound, and immediately preceding the mid-diastolic rumbling murmur.

Pulmonary stenosis is often associated with other congenital defects, and is characterized by a harsh systolic murmur and thrill, maximal at the second left interspace, and with a diminished second pulmonary sound. Incompetence is usually functional and associated with a high pulmonary artery pressure, such as occurs in mitral stenosis.

Tricuspid incompetence is nearly always of functional origin, caused by stretching of the ring due to right ventricular dilatation. It is caused by pulmonary hypertension, especially when caused by mitral stenosis, but it can follow right ventricular failure from any cause. There is a pansystolic murmur over the right ventricle which increases greatly with inspiration, and a big visible fluctuation in the jugular venous pressure. The liver is usually considerably enlarged and can be felt to be pulsating with each heart beat.

The congenital diseases (see page 579) often present with cyanosis, due to mixing of venous and arterial blood, and there may be other signs of arterio-venous shunt such as clubbing of the fingers and toes, and polycythaemia.

Assessment

Congenital valvular disease calls for specialist review, and necessitates the full investigation of a modern paediatric cardiological team to try and determine the nature and the extent of the disease, and to decide whether any operative treatment is likely to be of help.

With aortic and mitral valvular disease, many years of life are possible with advice, care and treatment, but several factors help in the assessment. For instance, much angina and many syncopal attacks are of bad significance in the case of aortic stenosis. A patient with regular rhythm with mitral stenosis and no evidence of failure, may, on the other hand, last for many years before breakdown occurs.

Electrocardiography may help elucidate an abnormal rhythm, and confirm the presence of atrial fibrillation, and chest radiography may help by showing the size of the heart, any increase in size of the left auricle or left ventricle, and evidence of hilar congestion or pulmonary oedema.

Management

The congenital valvular lesions occurring alone, by and large, do not call for treatment. A congenital aortic stenosis, for instance, can do very well throughout life with no treatment at all, but should receive antibiotic cover for any dental extraction to prevent the chance of developing subacute bacterial endocarditis.

The more complicated and multiple congenital lesions require sophisticated investigation, and treatment by operation if deemed possible, such as Blalock's operation in the tetralogy of Fallot[41].

With acquired aortic and mitral valvular disease, much depends on the extent and degree of the symptoms and signs. It is surprising how long some people can exist without any major symptoms developing at all. With aortic lesions, angina may necessitate the use of glyceryl trinitrate, and if there are syncopal attacks, there may have to be restriction of activity (car driving, climbing ladders, etc.). With left ventricular failure, the use of more pillows at night and oral thiazides with potassium supplements may tide over many months or even years. Surgery of aortic valvular lesions is now being done more frequently in selected cases, and a ball-valve prosthesis or an aortic valve from a pig can be implanted. The main disadvantage of the former being the tiresome audible clicking with each heart beat.

Mitral stenosis patients may go on for years. Moderation in all things is the order of the day. Infection may tip the scales into failure, but more often, chronic failure sets in insidiously. Usually a small dose of digitalis and a thiazide will keep things in balance for a while, but eventually, and depending on circumstances, an operation of either splitting of the valve, or valve replacement may have to be considered[42,43].

Ultimately, one sometimes sees the final stage of rheumatic valvular disease, with atrial fibrillation and gross congestive failure, the patient being bed-ridden, and having ascites and considerable sacral and leg oedema unresponsive to diuretics. However, the changing face of disease, and the relative infrequency of rheumatic fever since the advent of penicillin, will make the incidence of mitral stenosis gradually decline, and future generations may hardly know what it is.

Follow-up and Continuing Care

The management of a child with congenital valvular heart disease in family practice is straightforward, if conducted properly. It is a condition where everyone must be fully aware of the situation — especially the parents. The health visitor, school medical officer, dentist, and the school teachers should know of the condition and its significance, and especially if there has to be some imposed limitation of activity.

The family practitioner often has to act as the interpreter between the patient and the hospital. It is important for the parents to have explained to them the kind of defect from which their child is suffering. I often find one or two pencilled diagrams invaluable to convey the type of defect, and hence the type of investigation necessary, and ultimately the type of operation most likely to help.

It is only by this type of approach, which seems to be the family practitioner's responsibility, that parents realize the necessity to tide over a year or two until the child is bigger and hence, the operation is safer to perform. They also understand why all infections and teeth extractions need antibiotic cover. It is my firm belief that even fifteen minutes of explanation at the onset, makes for a far easier and smoother life for the parents, child and doctor in ensuing months or years.

With acquired valvular disease, the family practitioner is also by far and away the best person to organize the medication and general mode of living. It is sometimes, for instance, very difficult to find the optimum dose of digitalis, and it may involve daily visits to do so. Too much can produce undue slowing of the pulse and even multiple alternate extra systoles (pulsus bigeminus), nausea and vomiting. This may especially be precipitated by the addition of a diuretic to the regime. Many times, I find I have to give a much smaller dose of digitalis under these circumstances, and prescribe 0.25 mg of Lanoxin on alternate days, or even a smaller dose by giving the paediatric 0.0625 mg tablets.

By close attention to detail, and judicious advice about mode of life and careful adjustment of medication, one can keep a middle-aged mitral stenotic patient going for years. I suppose one of the most important things is advice about getting over-tired, consistency of medication, and the prompt use of antibiotics for intercurrent infections.

Evaluation, Assessment and Future Needs

Naturally, the type of valvular lesion, degree of its severity, age and condition of the patient must influence the prognosis. It is a bleak outlook for the young blue baby with a multiplicity of defects. On the other hand, a healthy young adult with a chance finding of a harsh systolic aortic murmur suggesting aortic stenosis, is probably going to enjoy a normal life.

The incidence of rheumatic endocarditis is obviously going to decrease, and since the advent of penicillin, both rheumatic fever and acute nephritis have become increasingly rare. One may thus expect mitral stenosis and rheumatic aortic valve disease to decrease gradually over the years.

However, the proportion of aortic to mitral valvular lesions will probably increase, as the incidence of rheumatic heart disease lessens. More cases of atherosclerotic aortic valvular disease will appear evident. These can result in severe damage to and calcification of the aortic valves, and may warrant surgery.

The future of surgery of aortic valvular disease is still in the balance. In some cases it certainly seems worthwhile. As mentioned earlier, the audible clicking of the ball-valve type of prosthesis may make life difficult for some people if they are of anxious disposition or are musicians.

Much work remains to be done on the question of operative help to patients with aortic lesions. Already, many thousands of people with a tight mitral stenosis have been helped with a simple splitting operation.

The future of congenital valvular lesions seems to depend on the complexity of the associated defects. Even with all the modern pre-operative aids to diagnosis, operation often reveals a quite different situation, and because of this, only minor palliative procedures may then be possible.

Summary

Congenital valvular disease usually occurs in conjunction with other defects. The commonest acquired valvular disease, mitral stenosis, would seem to be becoming less, with the decreased incidence of rheumatic fever.

With general measures of advice, and the judicious use of digitalis and diuretics, the family practitioner can keep other patients with valvular lesions alive for many years. Surgery is playing an increasingly important part in the management.

Antibiotics must be used promptly for any chest infection, or to cover any dental manoeuvres.

ACUTE HEART FAILURE

Nature and Condition

As the title implies, this is a state of sudden onset, and is a common medical emergency. Acute left ventricular failure is caused by the sudden inability of the ventricle to pump efficiently. This may be caused by hypertension, myocardial infarction, a sudden change of rhythm such as paroxysmal tachycardia or atrial fibrillation, or an infection or fever suddenly posing an additional load on a heart with little or no reserve capacity.

Clinical Features

The main symptoms are shortness of breath, inability to lie flat, wheezing, and extreme apprehension. The feature of acute failure, is the suddenness of onset, most frequently being at night, when the patient is awakened with breathlessness, and has to sit bolt upright gasping for air, and may struggle to a window to try and relieve his distress. This is often referred to as cardiac asthma.

Examination shows an anxious patient, usually pale and possibly sweating, sitting upright and with extreme dyspnoea and wheezing. The pulse may be rapid, and sometimes the rhythm may be disturbed. A paroxysmal tachycardia, atrial flutter or fibrillation, or pulsus alternans may be evident.

Auscultation often reveals a triple or gallop rhythm, and there is usually associated wheezing with basal crepitations. If severe, moist sounds may be heard throughout the whole lung fields. An elevated blood pressure may give a clue as to the cause of the condition. If the condition has been present for a while, the patient may be coughing up a blood-tinged fluid, sometimes referred to as a 'salmon-pink' froth.

Diagnosis

The diagnosis of acute heart failure is not usually difficult. It may occur in a patient with known hypertension or known valvular disease. In myocardial infarction, there may be a previous history of angina, or in an acute episode, there may be all the features of pain and shock.

In cases of massive pulmonary embolism there is a sudden development of right ventricular failure, with breathlessness, cyanosis, tachycardia, increased jugular venous pressure, haemoptysis, and abdominal pain or vomiting due to hepatic engorgement.

The diagnosis can sometimes be difficult in the presence of underlying bronchial asthma, and it is as well to remember that both conditions may coexist.

Assessment

The underlying condition causing the acute episode must be assessed accurately in order to set in motion the correct lines of treatment.

In a profoundly shocked patient with evidence of failure, the most likely diagnosis is that of myocardial infarction or pulmonary embolus. A shocked patient never travels well in an ambulance, and it is important at this stage to make an overall assessment of the condition, cause and probable outcome of any given underlying state. The most important initial assessment, is to decide whether one can best deal with the situation at home, or whether the case should be transferred at once to an intensive care unit, or perhaps, be transferred after some initial treatment has been instituted at home.

Management

The patient should be made to sit upright in bed. Morphine is the immediate drug of choice, — 10 mg intravenously in the normal-sized adult will bring prompt relief to the anxiety and bronchospasm. Because of the possibility of vomiting, a preparation of morphia combined with an anti-emetic such as cyclizine may be a better choice. This may be administered half intravenously, and half intramuscularly.

To relieve the pulmonary oedema, frusemide 20 mg intravenously produces an almost immediate diuresis. If there is any uncontrolled supraventricular arrhythmia, digoxin may also be given intravenously, starting with 0.5 mg. It is probably wise not to embark on this procedure right at the start, and particularly if an acute myocardial infarction is suspected. It is better, under those circumstances, to think in terms of an intravenous injection of lignocaine.

By the following morning, the situation will have clarified. An electrocardiogram can be done, and a more detailed appraisal of the situation can be made. Oral treatment with frusemide and digitalis may be started to maintain the benefits already achieved with intravenous methods. Potassium supplements should be given, and it sometimes proves of help and comfort to tell the patient of the high potassium content of pineapple juice and burgundy. Treatment of a pre-existing hypertension can be started, or the routine treatment of bed-rest for a myocardial infarction can be initiated.

The majority of patients can be treated at home, and with the alerting of the 'home team', unnecessary hospital admissions can be avoided. The patient and family are much better pleased, and the patient usually fares better than being transferred hurriedly into a hospital environment.

In the majority of cases, the family practitioner is able to cope quite adequately at home, and only rarely need seek the help of a consultant on a domiciliary visit or have occasion to admit to hospital.

Certainly, in my experience, the patient is profoundly grateful if one can manage treatment at home, and apart possibly from the administration of high-concentration oxygen, I can see no real benefit of hospital admission in these instances, providing the home team can cope. This is, of course, the classical situation where relatives, the district nurse, health visitor and home-helps can show their mettle. In country districts too, it is often possible for isolated people to get their prescriptions collected by various organizations such as the W.R.V.S. or Ladies Circle, and telephone numbers are often available at the local Post Office to obtain this kind of help.

Follow-up and Continuing Care

Much will depend on the cause of the acute failure. The underlying causal hypertension should be treated, the underlying atrial fibrillation controlled, and the general management of the patient's life should be considered. Weight may have to be lost, the general mode of living restricted, and routine medication with a thiazide and digitalis instituted. The acute attack will have given the patient a fright. Although treatment may be immediately effective, and lull patients into a state of false security, it is important in some cases, to remind the patient of his original plight in order to persuade him to undertake some sort of continued regimen.

Frequently, with a restriction of extremes of activity, a small dose of frusemide and digitalis, and supplements of potassium, patients can lead normal lives for years after the initial event.

Evaluation, Assessment and Future Needs

The outcome of a case of acute heart failure must obviously depend entirely on its underlying cause. When the acute phase is over, an electrocardiogram may help elucidate the state of the myocardium, or distinguish certain disorders of rhythm.

The assessment becomes clear with the progress of time. It is surprising how minimal administration of thiazides and a small dose of digitalis can prevent these episodes of acute failure, and how a patient can adapt himself by keeping within bounds of physical activity.

For the future of course, it is important to try and highlight any precipitating cause, so that the same situation may not arise again.

Summary

Acute heart failure is caused when the heart is suddenly unable to compete with its load. Usually it is caused by hypertension, myocardial insufficiency, a valvular lesion, a change of rhythm or infection.

Treatment consists of morphia, diuretics, digitalis if indicated, sitting upright, and attention to the underlying cause. Infection should be treated with the appropriate antibiotic.

CHRONIC HEART FAILURE

Nature and Condition

This is a state that is more insidious in its onset, and indeed, may take so long in coming on that the patient is hardly aware of his plight, and accepts his various symptoms as part of his daily life. It results in the heart being unable to maintain an adequate function due to a number of conditions. Valvular disease, hypertension, atrial fibrillation, chronic bronchitis and emphysema, anaemia and ischaemic heart disease are the most frequent causes of this insidious condition.

As mentioned in the section on acute heart failure, infection also plays a major part. It is not at all unusual for an older patient to be able to hold his own under normal day-to-day activities, and for an infection to supervene, and tip the scales into failure because of lack of cardiac reserve.

Clinical Features

Breathlessness is the main feature. At first this may be only exertional, but gradually comes on with less and less effort, and ultimately the patient will be breathless at rest, and orthopnoeic. He will find that he needs more and more pillows at night.

He may suffer from a cough related to exertion, and notice that his urine volume is diminishing. Epigastric discomfort due to hepatic enlargement is common, and eventually, he will complain of swollen ankles.

Diagnosis

Chronic heart failure can easily be overlooked. There are many older people walking around with a minor degree of failure, whose lives would be improved immeasurably with a small dose of diuretic or digitalis. It is very easy to miss such a case, as indeed, it is to miss a case of myxoedema.

In addition to breathlessness and ankle oedema, one may find a raised blood pressure, a rapid or irregular pulse, cyanosis or evidence of anaemia. There may be evidence of coronary artery disease or valvular disease of the heart, a raised jugular venous pressure, a sacral pad, basal crepitations and an enlarged liver with positive hepatojugular reflux. All these signs can range from minimal to gross, in which case the patient may well have ascites and bilateral pleural effusions, and be very incapacitated.

Electrocardiography, a blood count, serum cholesterol, PBI and T4 estimation, and X-ray of the chest may or may not be required. There should be no rigid rule-of-thumb series of investigations, as the family practitioner's judgment should usually decide whether such investigations are necessary, or whether they may in fact be actively harmful.

Assessment

The degree of failure, cause of the failure and length of time of the failure must all be considered. The age of the patient, his circumstances, and also any other pathological coexisting conditions must be taken into account.

It is always difficult to be sure of a prognosis, but it is relatively straightforward for instance, to forecast a good recovery in the mild chronic failure due to ischaemic atrial fibrillation. At the other end of the scale, the final stages of *cor pulmonale* can be hopeless, and one realizes that no amount of treatment — even continuous oxygen therapy in the home — is likely to be of any avail.

Management

Bed-rest is not necessary in the mild to moderate case of chronic failure. In fact, it would seem to be contra-indicated for fear of pulmonary embolism. Patients with low-output cardiac failure are particularly liable to venous thrombosis. However, the patients should be asked to undertake less strenuous activity. They should have more pillows at night, or may even be more comfortable in an armchair, with their legs elevated on a foot-stool.

Underlying conditions such as anaemia, infection or myxoedema must be treated. Many a case of mild chronic failure has been helped solely by the administration of an antibiotic. Diuretics should be given: either chlorothiazide 0.5 g each morning, frusemide 40 mg, or bendrofluazide 5 mg. Potassium supplements in the form of effervescent tablets or Slow K should be given in addition.

Digitalis should be initiated where there is atrial fibrillation at a fast rate, but it is important to remember that the use of thiazides can dramatically reduce the amount of digitalis required. It often leads to digitalis over-dosage when thiazides are added to a digitalized patient's regime of treatment. The digitalis requirement may need to be reduced to avoid nausea, vomiting and undue slowing of the pulse, and particular care must be taken in the older patient[44,45]. Research is being done on digitalis regulation by estimating serum levels[46]. A scheme of dosage has recently been devised by use of a nomogram, wherein one can plot the creatinine level, the age and weight of the patient, and predict the loading and maintenance doses required[46]. It is often necessary to use the paediatric tablets of Lanoxin of 0.0625 mg strength to avoid overdosage.

It still intrigues me to realize that the foxglove that grows so abundantly in my garden, and whose medicinal properties have been known for centuries, but were first described by Withering in 1785[47], has proved as big an advance in medical treatment as many of the twentieth century discoveries such as insulin and penicillin.

The loading dose of Lanoxin in a patient with failure and who is fibrillating may need to be 1 mg. Thereafter, a daily review is necessary, and a maintenance dose evolved to keep the pulse rate in the seventies.

Should the oedema not resolve, with the commonly used diuretics, and after their doses have been doubled, then one may have to add an aldosterone-antagonist such as spironolactone 25 mg q.d.s. One should always bear in mind in the elderly patient, that some drugs induce fluid retention, such as oestrogens, indomethacin, phenylbutazone and steroids.

With care, one can transform the life of a patient with chronic cardiac failure. As in all things, however, it is important not to be over-enthusiastic, and to approach the scene with caution and care.

Follow-up and Continuing Care

It is necessary to work out the specific treatment for each individual case. As I have already mentioned, patients with failure caused by atrial fibrillation for instance, fare very well with small doses of diuretics and digitalis. Close supervision is required at first, but eventually, long periods may be allowed to elapse between medical attendances.

The more difficult problem is the intractable failure due to severe ischaemic heart disease, multiple valvular disease, or *cor pulmonale*. These more serious forms of chronic failure may throw a great strain on the home team. I have no doubt, however, that if possible, all cases will be happier if treated at home. It is always more difficult if the wife is the patient, but even under these circumstances, I have managed to nurse the patient at home until death supervened.

Evaluation, Assessment and Future Needs

There is no doubt that the incidence of disease processes is changing. Rheumatic fever is much less common now than forty years ago — possibly due to the advent of sulphonamides and penicillin. Therefore, one is seeing much less acquired valvular disease of the heart. On the other hand, the incidence of ischaemic disease seems to be increasing, and at the moment, ischaemic disease and hypertension would seem to be the prime causes of chronic heart failure.

The underlying cause of the failure must be all important from the point of view of assessment. Where the degree of anaemia is remediable, or the rate of atrial fibrillation can be controlled easily, then the outlook is good. There is little doubt that anyone who deals with old people living alone, should be aware of the ease with which chronic cardiac failure can be overlooked and be vigilant to its diagnosis.

Summary

Chronic heart failure is common, especially in old people. It can easily be missed unless one is on the watch. Minimal treatment with the thiazides and digitalis may make a great difference to the quality of life of the sufferer, so it is most important to be constantly on guard, especially for any patient complaining of even mild breathlessness.

VARICOSE VEINS

Nature and Condition

Varicose veins are encountered almost daily by most family practitioners. In the United Kingdom it is estimated that about 16 per cent of women and 8 per cent of men suffer from the condition. There is a strong inheritance factor, and about 50 per cent of sufferers have a family history.

It is necessary to have an idea of the anatomy and physiology of the venous circulation of the legs in order to appreciate fully the problem of varicose veins, and more particularly, to understand the purpose of treatment.

There are two systems of veins in the legs. A superficial system and a deep system. Of the superficial veins, the long saphenous empties into the femoral vein and has up to twenty valves, and the short saphenous vein empties into the popliteal vein, and has up to thirteen valves in it. There are many variations or duplications in this superficial system.

The deep system, as well as having the two main connexions at the femoral and popliteal veins, connect with the superficial system with many small, valved, perforating veins.

Blood is returned from the legs to the heart by various means. The diaphragmatic movement and negative pressure in the thorax causes a sucking effect upwards, and the direct pumping action of the leg muscles, especially the soleus and gastrocnemius muscles, (sometimes referred to as the 'calf pump'), causes a positive pressure in the veins.

Depending on the degree of muscular activity, the pressure in the main veins may reach 50–130 mmHg. Whilst the deep veins have such a pressure, the superficial veins have only a very small pressure. Because of the presence of valves, blood is sucked into the deeper system of veins and thence forced upwards towards the heart. The connexion between the superficial veins and the deep veins is by small perforating veins, and the whole scheme of events, due to the valves and the muscular pump action, is for the venous flow to be inwards and upwards.

When the muscles contract, the blood in the deep veins is forced upwards.

During a phase of non-contraction, the blood does not leak backwards, either in the bigger veins, nor in the small perforating veins, because of the presence of valves which snap shut and prevent reflux.

It is only when these valves become faulty, and the blood can be pumped backwards into the superficial veins on every muscular contraction that engorgement of the superficial veins — or varicose veins — results.

At this point it is of interest to note why soldiers standing at attention for long periods of time at the Queen's birthday parade so rarely faint. They are instructed to stand at attention with their heels an inch off the ground. It is impossible to keep absolutely still, at attention, and holding a heavy rifle, without a great deal of leg muscle activity which of course, pumps the blood back to the right side of the heart. This works so well in practice, that a soldier is put on a charge if he faints.

Clinical Features

Varicose veins can be trivial, when there may be only one or two slightly enlarged veins in the calf. There may be every gradation from this, to gross varicosities, where there are varicose enlargements from the dorsum of the foot, right up the leg to the saphenous vein at its point of entry into the femoral vein in the groin.

Not only are they unsightly, but they can give rise to symptoms, especially in hot weather. The legs may feel heavy, and may be painful and swollen. Long periods of standing may be very wearisome because of the continuous discomfort.

Due to the interference with the normal drainage mechanism of the skin, the nutrition of the skin may suffer. Pigmentation, varicose eczema, and poor response to minimal trauma may occur. The blood supply to the skin between the knee and the ankle is one of the poorest in the body, and compared with scalp wounds, for instance, stitches have to be left in the lower leg for 10—14 days for any laceration instead of 3 or 4 days in the scalp. If there is a condition making this nutrition any worse, it is clear that minimal skin damage can produce lesions that may take a long time to heal. Hence, the fear of production of varicose ulcers, which may take months or even years to heal.

Trauma in another way, such as the direct puncture of a varicose vein, is fraught with danger. A minimal injury can produce catastrophic bleeding, and there has been more than one death of a farmer's wife who has been pecked by a cockerel and on whom a well-meaning neighbour or farm-hand has misguidedly applied a tourniquet on the thigh, rather than applying direct pressure to the bleeding point.

Diagnosis

Varicose veins are usually straightforward to diagnose. The patient should always be examined in the standing position, and the legs observed from foot to thigh in a good light. Valvular incompetence can often be demonstrated by emptying the vein by pushing upwards with one finger, whilst closing the lower part of the vein with another finger. When the upper finger is removed, blood descends, through the incompetent valves to the finger on the vein below.

Similarly, it is possible to detect the competence or otherwise of the small perforating veins at the ankle, the three on the inner aspect, and one on the outer aspect being the most important. These short perforating veins open directly into the main deep veins, and constitute the main venous drainage of the ankle region. It is in this region that varicose ulcers occur, so it is important to pay particular attention to these small perforators. The long and short saphenous veins, if involved, are so obvious as to need no comment.

Assessment

As in most things, the degree of the condition varies from localized and minimal, to widespread and gross. It is obvious from the purely physical danger of rupture that some patients must be advised to seek immediate treatment. In others, the varicosities in the lower leg may appear minimal, but the tell-tale signs of pigmentation will warn the family practitioner that treatment is required to avoid a worsening of nutrition to the skin of that area, and above all, to prevent a minor injury producing a varicose ulcer.

It is important to assess the situation well before advising the patient. Often they seek advice for cosmetic reasons with a few dilated superficial venules — so commonly seen in women in their forties. Their 'symptoms' of leg aching and so forth, can usually be ignored, and are used as a lever to precipitate one into a mood of avid interest and action. These women as a rule, do not take kindly to being told that nothing can be done bar covering up the blemishes with a cosmetic preparation.

Management

There are four methods of treatment: the wearing of elastic support stockings; multiple ligature and stripping, multiple ligature with simultaneous use of sclerosing agents, and injection/compression sclerotherapy.

The first method — the use of support stockings — is confined to the older or unfit patient, the patient with minor varicosities who is making up her mind, or the patient whose varicose veins worsen in pregnancy. There is a great place for support stockings when one is trying to improve the state of the skin prior to surgery. Many patients with pigmentation and varicose eczema, will improve with the application of hydrocortisone cream and some method of elastic support, and this will render the skin healthier for ultimate operation or sclerotherapy.

The surgical approach is based on the original operation of Trendelenburg — the tying of the long saphenous vein in the groin. Nowadays, in addition, the superficial vessels are stripped, and multiple incisions are made to tie off the incompetent perforating veins, especially in the region of the ankle. Frequently the surgical method is combined with sclerotherapy, as it may be evident that some small varicosities remain in spite of multiple ligation.

The fourth method, and one that is much in vogue to-day, is the injection/compression technique. It was first described by Linser[48] and more recently by Fegan[49] in Dublin and Dejode[50], and is now practised throughout the world and probably accounts for about half of the procedures for the treatment of varicose veins. The object of this method is to inject a substance into the empty vein to produce a rapid chemical endovenitis. If localized and compressed, the resulting thrombus will become organized and form a thin, solid cord. The injection has to be made over the mouth of the incompetent perforating vein, and the end result should be a local thrombosis and a T-shaped block. Each injection is made with the patient recumbent, and 0.5 ml to 1.0 ml of the sclerosant is injected at each site — not more than five injections being done at any one time on each leg. Compression locally is applied after each injection with a rubber compression pad, and ultimately an elastic support stocking is rolled up over the bandaged leg.

After the treatment, the patient is encouraged to walk up to three miles a day, and it is important to maintain the constant pressure effect on the leg. In a severe case, as many as two or three sessions of treatment may be required. This technique has the advantage of not having to be admitted to hospital, rarely requiring any time off work, and having few complications. In a series of 2230 patients treated by the injection/compression technique since 1964, Rhodes and Hadfield[51] recorded only two cases of pulmonary embolism, neither of which was fatal.

Follow-up and Continuing Care

In about 20 per cent of patients treated by operative or sclerosing techniques, further varicose veins develop subsequently. Patients should always be warned of this fact before any sort of treatment is undertaken, so that they do not regard the treatment as a failure.

They should be seen frequently after the injection/compression technique. Pain is usually present to a mild degree, but is usually only severe if some of the sclerosant has escaped extravenously. The legs should remain bandaged from four to six weeks.

Evaluation, Assessment and Future Needs

At the moment, approximately one half of patients requiring active treatment have multiple ligations combined with stripping, and the other have sclerotherapy. There is still some debate as to which method is best. Success rates for the multiple ligature technique are reported as varying from 40 per cent to 98.6 per cent[52,53], and for the sclerosing technique 21 per cent to 99 per cent[54,55].

Recent work[56] shows no difference between the two methods of treatment, but some workers[57] disagree with this and stress the correct selection of the case, and proceeding with the most appropriate method suited to the particular circumstances. They claim good results with stripping procedures on an ambulatory basis.

From these facts therefore, it seems that each case must be weighed up individually before treatment is decided upon. There is little doubt that, from the point of view of the family practitioner, certain surgical colleagues seem to achieve excellent results in one or other of the techniques. It is difficult to decide easily about the intermediate cases.

Summary

Varicose veins are common, being twice as common in women than men. It is dangerous to leave the more severe varicosities for fear of haemorrhage. It is wise in most instances, except in pregnancy and the aged, to advise some sort of treatment to prevent pigmentation, eczema or ulceration. Multiple ligation and stripping is now being done about equally with the injection/compression technique. The current situation and techniques are well described in a recent book[58].

PERIPHERAL ARTERY DISEASE

Nature and Condition

Whilst the vast majority of symptoms are referable to the legs, one must remember that other arteries are also affected by both occlusive disease and conditions such as arteritis. Cerebral vascular disease is discussed in Chapter 14, page 265.

It is a mere thirty years ago that I was taught as a medical student about Buerger's Disease[59] and how it affected mainly cigarette-smoking male Polish or Russian Jews. There is a changing face of peripheral vascular disease affecting the legs, not least, being the considerable increase in females suffering from the condition, when prior to World War II it was mainly a disease of men. There are many theories about this, the most popular being the change in cigarette-smoking habits of the population as a whole.

In the limbs, and mainly the legs, the arterial pathology can be divided into an insidious arteriosclerotic obliterating arteritis, or an embolic phenomenon of sudden and dramatic onset. The other transient condition affecting arms and legs is Raynaud's syndrome[60], which can be either primary (and often familial), or secondary to a general disease such as a collagen disorder.

Of the other areas of the body, a giant cell temporal arteritis is very common in the older patient and is often associated with a central retinal artery thrombosis — hence the importance of an early and accurate diagnosis, so that treatment with steroids can be initiated quickly.

Although technically, lesions of the coeliac plexus may be included in this group of diseases, I do not propose to consider them except to note their existence, and to remark on the modern methods of investigation which can make their diagnosis possible.

From the practical point of view, it is the disease of the arteries of the legs that must occupy most of this section.

Diagnosis

If we can dispose of the chronic temporal headache of the middle-aged or older patient, denoting a possible giant-cell temporal arteritis, then, the attention must be drawn to either Raynaud's phenomenon or obliterative arterial disease of the legs.

In Raynaud's disease[60], a condition which is often strongly familial, there is a history of deadness of the hands or feet on exposure to cold temperatures. The patients complain of pallor and numbness of the fingers brought on by contact of the hands with anything cold, and particularly if they are in a tense or apprehensive state. Many people experience it when sea-bathing. Often, in such cases, migraine may also be precipitated, and for this reason, some people refrain from bathing in the sea around the shores of Britain.

The attack can vary from one finger becoming pale and dead, to the involvement and numbness of the whole hand. It starts at the fingertips and spreads proximally to the bases of the fingers. When the attack passes off, the fingers become blue and blotchy, and eventually become scarlet in colour before resuming their normal colour. Investigations, including X-ray for cervical ribs, liver function tests, anti-nuclear and rheumatoid factors and LE cell tests are usually all negative.

In the lower limbs, arterial disease can present in two ways. A sudden cessation of arterial flow due to an embolus is dramatic. Pain is the first feature, rapidly followed by other evidence of stoppage of blood supply, with lack of function, cyanosis and swelling.

The most common form of vascular disorder of the legs is the slower onset of obliterative arterial disease. This is characterized by pain in the calf muscles on walking or intermittent claudication. The pain comes on gradually, and brings the patient to a halt. After a few minutes, the pain wears off, and the subject is able to set forth again — but usually at a slower pace. The pain is thought to be caused by the accumulation of pain-producing toxic metabolites.

The cause of these symptoms is usually atherosclerosis, and gradual diminution of blood supply to the limb below the narrowing or blockage. It is often part of a generalized condition of arteriosclerosis, but is frequently the first symptom that brings one's attention to this state of affairs.

Diagnosis

Pain is the cardinal feature. Either in the temporal region, if it is referrable to a temporal arteritis, or in the calf muscles if due to intermittant claudication.

Sometimes it may be months before one realizes that the vague leg pains are part and parcel of a more specific syndrome. In the latter stages however, the diagnosis is usually straightforward, with the patient complaining of being able to walk only a certain distance before being brought to a halt by the cramp-like pain in the calves.

With an embolus in the leg, the symptoms are instant and dramatic. There is a sudden onset of lack of function, pain, and change in colour of the limb. The pulses are absent, and the diagnosis is not usually difficult. Frequently of course in these cases, some cardiac condition, such as atrial fibrillation, is present.

Assessment

There are all degrees of leg involvement, from sudden catastrophic symptoms caused by an embolus, to the slower and more insidious onset of gradual diminution of blood supply. Obviously, much depends on the diagnosis, speed of onset, and general condition of the patient. Age, and the presence or otherwise of allied conditions (for example, diabetis mellitus) have to be taken into consideration.

With certain leg symptoms, it may be necessary to perform arteriography to establish where a blockage exists, in order to estimate the degree of obliteration, and also, to help in planning possible methods of treatment.

In men with intermittent claudication, it is very useful for gauging degree (and possibly response to therapy), to ask them how many lamp-posts they can pass in the street before being forced to stop because of pain.

Management

Temporal giant-cell arteritis should be treated promptly with steroids. It is only rarely necessary to substantiate the diagnosis beforehand with an arterial biopsy.

Prompt treatment is essential, not only to bring relief to the patient, but also, to avoid the serious complication of a central retinal artery thrombosis. Doses of prednisolone 60 mg daily in divided amounts should be given at the outset, and gradually diminished over a four week period to a maintenance dose of about 5–7.5 mg daily. It may have to be continued for up to two years.

Intermittent claudication due to arterial obstruction, should be treated by stopping cigarette smoking, and by exercises to promote a collateral circulation. This is the only condition in medicine of which I know, where there should be absolute insistence on altering the mode of life of the patient. In all other conditions, the treatment should never be worse than the disease, but with claudication, I insist on the patient stopping cigarette smoking completely. Needless to say, a full explanation should be given, and facts supplied to give credence to this advice.

Buerger's exercises are very useful to promote a collateral circulation, and it may be helpful to send a patient to the local Physiotherapy Department to be taught these. There is no doubt that spontaneous improvement occurs in a large number of people. This is why it is so difficult to assess the value of any of the plethora of vasodilator drugs on the market. It seems unlikely that any of them are of any help at all, except possibly the original one – tolazoline. They are certainly very expensive, and it is easy to prescribe the 'latest' vasodilator, but useless to evaluate the subjective improvements without objective evidence such as estimation of calf blood flow.

In some instances an arterial blockage may be demonstrable, and it is here, and in younger patients, that surgery has made great strides. Angiography may show quite definite reasons for undertaking vascular reconstruction with endarterectomy and patch grafts, or by a Dacron prosthesis[61,62,63].

A sudden incident caused by an embolus calls for surgical interference. A sympathetic block may cause the embolus to proceed further down the artery, and then an embolectomy may be performed. In the occasional patient, where this is not possible, streptokinase may prove effective. Quite a large proportion of thromboses will resolve if treated early with this fibrinolysin reactivator.

By and large, the older patient with gradually increasing claudication should be encouraged to undertake routine exercise, and pay attention to the care and hygiene of the feet. The urine should be tested for sugar, and it is also wise to send blood to the laboratory for a lipid profile.

Raynaud's phenomenon is difficult to treat. Patients usually respond to a sedative, and simple instructions as to the avoidance of precipitating factors. Help has been reported with reserpine and clonidine.

Follow-up and Continuing Care

As already mentioned, it is a good plan to have some kind of yardstick to assess intermittent claudication. The old method of counting lamp-posts is extremely useful, and I still use this measure as a guide to improvement of patients with angina or claudication.

Care of the skin and toe-nails is essential, and as in a diabetic, I encourage the patient to see a chiropodist regularly. Any sepsis must be vigorously countered with systemic antibiotics, and the smallest traumatic graze treated with great seriousness.

If the disease process continues in spite of all efforts, then an above-knee amputation may be unavoidable (see page 599).

Evaluation, Assessment and Future Needs

Uncomplicated claudication is a much less grave condition than the more advanced stages of ischaemia which eventually lead to gangrene.

Few cases of claudication come to surgery, but if the symptoms are severe, then full investigation by arteriography is justified, and reconstructive arterial surgery may be advisable. Because of the uncertain long-term results of surgery, there seems little reason to subject patients with minor degrees of claudication to the panoply of a full arterial investigation. Age also plays a part, and it is as a rule unwise, and indeed unjustifiable, to subject an elderly patient to the rigours of full investigation. Naturally, associated diseases such as chronic bronchitis, asthma and emphysema, or severe ischaemic heart disease and hypertension will also contra-indicate any over-enthusiastic investigation.

For the future, every day seems to produce more evidence of the dangers of cigarette smoking. Even for those who have taken refuge in cigar smoking, the warning cones have also been hoisted, and it seems evident that smoking in any form is a potentially lethal addiction and should be avoided or stopped at all costs.

Summary

Peripheral artery disease, whilst including such diseases as giant-cell temporal arteritis and Raynaud's disease, mainly concerns ischaemic disease of the legs.

Acute deprivation of blood supply may require urgent surgery or the use of streptokinase. The more chronic form usually responds to general methods, especially Buerger's exercises, and all cases demand the cessation of smoking.

References

1. Taggert, P., Carruthers, M. and Somerville, W. (1973). *Lancet* ii, 341.
2. Taggert, P. and Carruthers, M. (1971). *Lancet* i, 363.
3. Rowe, M. J., Neilson, J. M. M. and Oliver, M. F. (1975). *Lancet* i, 295.
4. Fox, K. M., Chopra, M. P., Portal, R. W. and Aber, C. P. (1975). *Brit. med. J.* 1, 117.
5. Clarendon, Earl of (1759). *The Life of Edward Clarendon*, Oxford.

6. Heberden, W. (1818). *Commentaries on the History and Cure of Diseases*,(Boston: Wells and Lilly).
7. Lewis, T. (1943). *Diseases of the Heart*, 42, (London: Macmillan).
8. Sones, F. M. and Sturey, E. K. (1962). *Mod. Concepts Cardiovasc. Dis.* **31**, 735.
9. Sones, F. M. (1972). *Circulation* **46**, 1155.
10. Brock, Lord (1972). *Med. Soc. Trans. (Lond.)* **88**, 214.
11. Department of Health and Social Security (1974). *Diet and Coronary Heart Disease Health and Social Subjects*, 7, (London: HMSO).
12. Report of a Joint Working Party of the Royal College of Physicians of London and the British Cardiac Society (1976) *J. roy. Coll. Phys.* **10**, 3.
13. Mather, H. G., Pearson, N. G., Read, K. L. Q., Shaw, D. B., Steed, G. R., Thorne, M. G., Jones, S., Guerrier, C. J. Eraut, C. D., McHugh, P. M., Chowdhury, N. R., Jafary, M. H. and Wallace, T. J. (1971). *Brit. med. J.* **3**, 334.
14. Mather, H. G. (1974). Paper read at British Medical Association Clinical Meeting, Jamaica.
15. Lawrence, G. H., Riggins, R. C. K., Hipp, R. and Johnston, R. R. (1973). *Amer. J. Surg.* **126**, 277.
16. Sheldon, W. C., Rincon, G., Effler, D. B., Proudfit, W. L. and Sones, F. M. (1973). *Circulation* **48**, suppl. 3, 184.
17. Hamilton, M., Thompson, E. N. and Wisniewski, T. K. M. (1964). *Lancet* i, 235.
18. Framingham Monograph (1974). No. 30.
19. Kannel, W. B. and Dawber, T. R. (1974). *Brit. J. Hosp. Med.* **2**, 508.
20. Society of Actuaries (1959). *Build and Blood Pressure Study*, vol. 1, Chicago, Illinois.
21. Breckenridge, A., Dollery, C. T. and Parry, E. H. O. (1970). *Quart. J. Med. NS*, **39**, 411.
22. Brown, J. J., Fraser, R., Lever, A. F. and Robertson, J. I. S. (1972). In *Clinics in Endocrinology Metabolism*, vol. 1 (A. Stuart-Mason, ed.), p. 397, (London: Saunders).
23. Brown, J. J., Fraser, R., Lever, A. F., Morton, J. J., Oelkers, W., Robertson, J. I. S. and Young, J. (1973). *International Workshop on Mechanisms of Hypertension*, p. 148, (Amsterdam: Excerpta Medica).
24. Laragh, J. H., Baer, L., Brunner, H. R., Bühler, F. R., Sealey, J. E. and Vaughan, E. D. (1972). *Amer. J. Med.* **52**, 633.
25. Pickering, G. (1968). *High Blood Pressure*, (Edinburgh and London: Churchill Livingstone).
26. Brod, J., Fech, V., Hejl, Z. and Jirka, J., (1959). *Clin. Sci.* **18**, 269.
27. Zinner, S. H., Levy, P. S. and Kass, E. H. (1971). *New Engl. J. Med.* **8**, 401.
28. Zinner, S. H., Martin, L. F., Sacks, F., Rösner, B. and Kass, E. H. (1975). *Amer. J. Epidem.* **100**, 6, 437.
29. Kincaid-Smith, P., McMichael, J. and Murphy, E. A. (1958). *Quart. J. Med.* **27**, 117.
30. Price, F. (1950). *A Textbook of the Practice of Medicine* p. 1143, (Oxford: Oxford University Press).
31. Burdon, R. P., Booth, L. J. and Aber, G. M. (1973). *Nephron.* **9**, 171.
32. Adlin, E. V., Marks, A. D. and Channick, B. J., (1972). *Arch. Int. Med.* **130**, 855.
33. Somerville, W., Taggert, P. and Carruthers, M. (1972). International Symposium, Scanticon, Aarhus, Denmark.
34. Sears, H. T. N. (1974). Symposium on Hypertension, Section of Medicine, Manchester Medical Society.
35. Miall, W. E. (1974). *Brit. J. Hosp. Med.* **2**, 141.
36. Miall, W. E. (1974). *Scot. med. J.* **19**, 41.
37. Streeton, D. H. P., Anderson, G. H., Freiberg, J. M. and Dalakos, T. G. (1975). *New Eng. J. Med.* **292**, 657.
38. Fallot, A. (1888).*Marseille Med.* **25**, 77.
39. Corrigan, D. J. C. (1832). *Edin. med. sci. J.* **37**, 225.
40. Flint, A. (1862). *Amer. J. med. Sci.* **44**, 29.
41. Blalock, A. and Taussing, H. B. (1945). *J. Amer. med. Assoc.* **128**, 189.
42. Cooley, D. A., Okies, J. E., Wukasch, D. C., Sandiford, F. M. and Hallman, G. L. (1973). *Ann. Surg.* **177**, 818.

43.. Ross, B. A., Housseini, H., Clement, A. J., Ersoz, A. and Braimbridge, M. V. (1973). *Brit. Heart J.* **35**, 556.
44. Kirsten, E., Rodstein, M. and Iuster, Z. (1973). *Geriatrics* **28**, 95.
45. Wedgwood, J. (1972). *Postgrad. Med.* **52** 179.
46. Mawer, G. E. (1974). Personal communication.
47. Withering, W. (1785). *An Account of the Foxglove and some of its Medical Uses*, (Birmingham: Swinney).
48. Linser, P. (1916). *Medizin. Klin.* **12**, 897.
49. Fegan, W. G. (1963). *Lancet* ii, 109.
50. Dejode, L. R. (1970). *Brit. J. Surg.* **57**, 4.
51. Rhodes, D. J. and Hadfield, G. J. (1972). *Practitioner*, **209**, 809.
52. Lofgren, K. A., Ribisi, A. P. and Myers, T. T. (1958). *Arch. Surg. Chicago*, **76**, 310.
53. Sherman, R. S. (1949). *Ann. Surg.* **130**, 218.
54. Orbach, E. J. (1944). *Amer. J. Surg.* **66**, 362.
55. Cooper, W. M. (1946). *Surg. Gyn. Obstet.* **83**, 647.
56. Chant, A. D. B., Jones, H. O. and Weddell, J. M. (1972). *Lancet* ii, 1188.
57. Nabatoff, R. A. and Stark, D. C. C. (1973). *Lancet* i, 201.
58. Dodd, H. and Cockett, F. B. (1976). *The Pathology and Surgery of the Veins of the Lower Limb.* (Edinburgh and London: Churchill-Livingstone).
59. Buerger, L. (1908). *Amer. J. Med. Sci.* **136**, 319.
60. Raynaud, M. (1862). *De l'Asphyxie Locale et de la Gangrène Symétrique des Extrémités.* (Paris: Rignoux).
    Mather, H. G., Morgan, D. C., Pearson, N. G., Read, K. L. Q., Shaw, D. B., Steed, G. R., Thorne, M. G., Lawrence, C. J. and Riley, I. S. (1976). *Brit. med. J.* **1**, 925.
61. Bevan, P. G. (1972). *Ann. roy. Coll. Surg. Eng.* **51**, 103.
62. Gillespie, J. A. (1972). *Practitioner*, **209**, 519.
63. Reichle, F. A. and Tyson, R. R. (1972). *Ann. Surg.* **176**, 315.

14

The Nervous System

H. W. K. Acheson

INTRODUCTION

In neurology, as in all clinical medicine, diagnosis is dependent upon a careful history and a thorough examination of the patient. Many of the diseases of the nervous system which carry a poor prognosis may present with symptoms and signs which are also found in minor illness. Therefore careful assessment is important. The first essential is to record the events of the history in chronological order and to note all abnormal physical signs and investigation results. Abnormal signs are *always* significant, even if they are minimal in degree. Enquiries must also be made into the patient's past medical history and the family history.

The choice of laboratory and other investigation procedures will obviously depend upon the differential diagnosis, but it is advisable always to include a full blood count, a Wasserman reaction, a test for glycosuria and a chest X-ray.

In the sections which follow emphasis has been given to the diseases which commonly occur in family practice. Diseases which occur less commonly have been mentioned briefly and very rare conditions have been omitted.

The technique of examination of the nervous system has not been described, and for this the reader is advised to consult a standard textbook on the subject.

MIGRAINE

After the passage of more than 80 years it is difficult to improve upon Gower's[1] description of migraine:

'Migraine is an affection characterised by paroxysmal nervous disturbance, of which headache is the most constant element. The pain is seldom absent and may exist alone, but it is commonly accompanied by nausea and vomiting, and it is often preceded by some sensory disturbance, especially by some disorder of the sense of sight. The symptoms are frequently one-sided, and from this character of the headache the name is derived. . . .'.

Aetiology

Migraine is a disease of multiple aetiology. A family history is common and some people may have a genetic predisposition to develop the disease. It is sometimes said to occur more frequently in people who have an obsessional type of personality or who are of rigid or perfectionist outlook. But opinion is divided about this and it may only be that such people are more likely to complain.

Attacks may be precipitated by a number of factors including: depression, stress, fatigue, exposure to bright lights, watching television or the cinema, high humidity and eating certain foods. Common food precipitants are: chocolate, cheese, alcohol, and especially sherry and red wine.

In women attacks may occur in association with menstruation or the taking of the oral contraceptive pill.

Pathology

The symptoms of migraine result from changes in the calibre of the intra- and extra-cranial arteries. Initial vasoconstriction, which may be responsible for the prodromal symptoms, is followed by vasodilation. Vasodilation leads to increased amplitude of arterial pulsation which gives rise to a headache of throbbing quality.

Thermographic studies have provided some evidence to suggest that migraine subjects may have an underlying abnormality in the vascular system on the side of the head on which they normally experience headache, and that this abnormality may be associated with an increased sensitivity to certain biochemical influences.

More than one type of biochemical influence may be responsible. The association of attacks with menstruation and the contraceptive pill suggest an endocrine factor. The common food precipitants all contain tyramine, a sympathetic amine which has been shown to induce headache in a proportion of migraine sufferers. In normal subjects tyramine is inactivated in the gut and conjugated in the liver. There is some evidence that in migraine subjects the conjugation of tyramine may be impaired. Tyramine can induce the release of noradrenaline from peripheral stores, thus leading to vasoconstriction. The resulting ischaemia may invoke a local increase in 5-hydroxytryptamine (serotonin) and bradykinin which in turn leads to vasodilation.

Epidemiology

Migraine often begins in childhood, and certainly the majority of patients will have had their first attack before the age of 40. Women are affected twice as commonly as men. There is a tendency for the condition to be self-limiting and for the frequency and severity of attacks to reduce after reaching a peak 5—10 years from the onset.

The prevalence of migraine is not known precisely; estimates have varied from five to 200 per 1000 patients at risk.

Clinical Features

Two phases may occur, the prodromal phase and the headache phase. In the majority of patients headache occurs without prodromata. Some patients may experience the prodromal symptoms without the development of headache. Attacks of migraine are paroxysmal, usually lasting a few hours, but may be as long as 3—4 days.

Prodromal Phase

The symptoms of the prodromal phase are transient, and generally last less than 30 minutes. The most common symptoms are: general malaise, a feeling of depression, blurring of vision and fortification spectra (flashes of light, zig-zags). Abdominal pain may also occur but is less frequent. Less common symptoms include: hemianopia, speech disturbance, paresis and paraesthesiae.

Similar symptoms may be present during the headache phase.

Headache Phase

The headache of migraine is characteristically throbbing and usually unilateral. As an attack develops the headache may become more generalised. It commonly begins in the frontal or temporal region, occasionally in the parietal or occipital area. It is unusual for a migraine headache to begin on the top of the head.

Nausea, vomiting, pallor and sweating may accompany the headache phase. Dilatation of the conjunctival vessels may also be observed.

Complications are extremely rare, and when they occur are more likely to be iatrogenic, from drug toxicity.

Variants of Migraine

Periodic Syndrome (Cyclical Vomiting)

In early childhood migraine may take an atypical form characterised by vomiting, with or without associated abdominal pain, in which headache is absent or only slight. On occasions the constitutional disturbance may be so severe that the child is literally prostrate.

Ophthalmoplegic Migraine
This may occur at any age. The headache is usually peri-orbital and more severe than in common migraine, of which there is usually a history. Diplopia or blurred vision will occur. The possibility of an underlying intracerebral vascular defect or neoplasm must always be excluded.

Hemiplegic Migraine
This is a rare condition in which transient hemiparesis occurs, with or without associated paraesthesiae. It is usually familial. A history of common migraine will often be obtained. The onset of hemiplegic migraine often gives rise to alarm in patients or relatives, with fears of epilepsy or stroke. The symptoms usually last for less than an hour.

Basilar Artery Migraine
Vasomotor changes affecting the basilar artery produce brain stem dysfunction leading to visual symptoms, which may be accompanied by circumoral paraesthesiae, paraesthesiae of the tongue, vertigo, ataxia, dysarthria or tinnitus. The associated headache is usually located in the occipital region and is usually throbbing in character.

Cluster Headache (Horton's Syndrome)
Attacks of unilateral periorbital pain of short duration, often more severe than in common migraine, which tend to occur in clusters with periods of freedom.
Attacks have a striking tendency always to occur at the same time, often at night causing the patient to wake from sleep. Symptoms include redness and watering of the eye, stuffiness of the nostril and tenderness in the paranasal area.

Week-end Migraine (Sunday-Morning Headache)
This is a rare form of migraine characterised by a generalised throbbing headache and sometimes vomiting which occurs at the weekend or at the beginning of a holiday. The syndrome appears to be associated with the relaxation that follows a period of tension.

Diagnosis

History
Except in the presence of the rarer variants of migraine the physical signs are nil. The diagnosis depends upon a careful and accurate history. The diagnosis is established on:—

> the site, frequency and duration of attacks,
> the character of the headache,
> precipitating or ameliorating factors,

associated prodromal symptoms,

gastro-intestinal symptoms and

whether there is a family history of migraine.

The pattern of symptoms experienced by a migraine subject tends to be constant, one attack being similar to another, varying only in severity. Any change in the pattern of symptoms must always lead to a search for another cause for the headache.

Migraine may sometimes be confused with a headache of psychogenic origin, e.g., tension or depression. Differentiation depends upon a careful history. Intra-cranial lesions, vascular or neoplastic, are seldom a cause of common migraine but must be excluded if paresis, paraesthesiae, speech disturbance or hemianopia is present. Infection in the ear or paranasal sinuses must always be borne in mind. Accelerated hypertension may cause a severe generalised headache but benign essential hypertension rarely causes any type of headache.

Migraine should never be diagnosed when symptoms occur for the first time in a patient over 40 without first excluding all other possible causes.

Examination

A general physical examination, including examination of the central nervous system should be carried out. The fundi must be examined to exclude papilloedema. The blood pressure should be taken. The paranasal sinuses should be palpated and if tenderness is present infection must be considered. The eyes and ears should be examined to exclude infection.

Investigations

There are no special investigations relevant to the diagnosis of migraine, but investigations may be required if there is evidence that the symptoms may be due to another cause, e.g., ear infection or an intra-cranial lesion.

Management

The Disease

Although there is no 'cure' for migraine, the frequency and severity of attacks can be reduced in most patients. Treatment is directed towards the prevention of attacks and the alleviation of the acute attack.

Prevention Frequent attacks, i.e., attacks occurring more often than once every 2—3 weeks, may be prevented by regular medication. Sometimes mild sedation is all that is required and may be achieved by promethazine 25 mg at bedtime and 10 mg on rising, prochlorperazine up to 10 mg t.d.s., or phenobarbitone 30 mg night and morning. If phenobarbitone alone is ineffective it may be combined with ergotamine tartrate 1 mg given at bedtime. If a more specific drug is required clonidine (0.025 mg b.d.s. or t.d.s.) can be prescribed. Methysergide 1 mg t.d.s., which can be increased up to 2 mg t.d.s. may be used instead of clonidine. Methysergide causes more side-effects than clonidine and its use must not continue for more than 6 months without a break of at least 4 weeks. Patients given methysergide must be warned to report any untoward effect, e.g., leg or chest pains, ill-defined dizziness, oedema or urinary symptoms. Clonidine or methysergide must never be prescribed concurrently with ergotamine.

The Acute Attack   Many attacks are relatively mild and can be controlled by the avoidance of precipitating factors and simple analgesics. If simple analgesics are insufficient ergotamine tartrate should be prescribed. This drug counteracts the vasodilation of cerebral blood vessels that occurs during the headache phase by causing vasoconstriction. However, it should never be prescribed when crisp focal ischaemic signs are part of the migraine. Ergotamine tartrate should be administered at the onset of an attack and the minimum effective dose should be given. The required dose may vary from one individual to another and will have to be determined by experiment. Always begin with a low dose; because of the danger of ergot poisoning patients must be warned never to exceed 6 mg of ergotamine in any one day and never to exceed 12 mg in any one week.

Ergotamine tartrate may be administered by various routes, though most patients prefer the oral route. Available routes, in order of effectiveness, and the appropriate dose are:—

Intra-muscular or sub-cutaneous injection 0.25 mg;
Rectal suppository 2 mg;
Inhalation 0.36 mg;
Sublingually 2 mg;
Orally 1—2 mg

Pethidine, opiates, or any drug of addiction, must not be given.

The Patient

Migraine subjects should be encouraged to lead a normal life, with the obvious avoidance of precipitating factors. The patient should be told that the natural history of migraine is that it is a self-limiting disease and that the attacks will become less frequent and less severe, and will ultimately cease. The patient should be helped to identify precipitating factors and advised how to avoid them. His life-style and environment may need to be modified in order to avoid undue stress or fatigue.

The Family

Occasionally the threat of inducing a migraine attack is used by patients to influence the behaviour of family members and necessitates appropriate counselling. Close family members should be instructed in the natural history of migraine, its prevention and treatment.

Parents who are themselves subject to migraine may seek advice regarding how the onset may be avoided in their child. Advice should be circumspect, taking into account that a family history is frequently found but avoiding any indication that the child needs to be protected from the normal stresses of life.

The Role of the Health Team

Health visitors or social workers may identify migraine in an individual with whom they have contact. General advice may be given if it is within their competence to do so but they should also advise the patient to consult his family practitioner for assessment and therapeutic advice. The support of the health visitor may be required to assist in the management of a child with the periodic syndrome.

Social and Other Agencies

Migraine clinics are available in some hospitals but the management of a patient is usually within the competence of a family practitioner.

Follow Up and Continuing Care

During the initial period, when an effective therapeutic regime is being established, frequent consultations with the family practitioner may be required. The physician must be alert to the onset of side effects and the need for the patient to adhere to the prescribed dosage schedule. Once an effective regime has been established repeat prescriptions may be allowed, but the patient must be seen by the practitioner personally at least once every 3 months.

The frequency and severity of attacks, and the frequency and dosage of medication, should be recorded by the patient in diary form and presented to the physician when he attends for review.

Further Research

Accurate information on the incidence and prevalence of migraine is lacking and there is little information regarding the frequency with which the various precipitating factors and prodromal symptoms occur. There is a need to attempt a more precise definition of the disease. Research must include study of the epidemiology and natural history of migraine and can best be prosecuted in family practice.

EPILEPSY

Epilepsy presents a vast human problem. The incidence is about 3 per 1000 of the population and it is likely that there are more than 150 000 epileptics in the

United Kingdom. Males and females are equally affected. There is a great deal of ignorance about epilepsy. It is regarded by some people as a disease which carries a social stigma akin to that given to leprosy in the middle ages; as a result some patients are forced into social isolation. Such attitudes must be dispelled by careful explanation.

Epilepsy is not a disease, but a symptom with multiple aetiology. The predominant characteristic is a fit or seizure, either focal or generalised, usually accompanied by a disturbance of consciousness. The mechanism producing the fit is not known precisely but EEG studies have shown that it is always associated with a brief excessive electrical discharge from cerebral neurones. There is considerable variation between individuals in the degree of stimulus required to produce a fit. Patients may suffer from epilepsy because they experience excessively high discharges or because they have a low threshold of excitability. In theory, even a normal person may experience an attack if a sufficiently large stimulus is applied.

Aetiology

Epilepsy may be idiopathic or acquired. Apart from the possibility of genetic inheritance the cause of idiopathic epilepsy is unknown. Acquired epilepsy may result from trauma to the brain at birth or in a subsequent accident, or from a cerebral tumour, cerebral vascular disease, metabolic disorder, or infection of the brain or its coverings.

The probability that epilepsy will follow trauma is approximately proportional to the severity of the head injury. Cerebral vascular disease is a common cause when fits first occur at or beyond middle age, but it is important to exclude the possibility of an intra-cerebral neoplasm.

Metabolic disturbances include hypoglycaemia, uraemia, and cerebral anoxia due to any cause. Occasionally drug withdrawal is responsible, particularly after long continued use of barbiturates or alcohol. In some patients epileptic attacks may be precipitated by repetitive extraneous noise or lights.

Clinical Features

An epileptic fit may be generalised or focal. Generalised fits are usually associated with loss of consciousness but focal fits are not.

Generalised Epilepsy

There are two types of generalised epilepsy, *grand mal* and *petit mal*.
1. *Grand mal* may occur during the day or at night, involving the sudden loss of consciousness accompanied by a generalised and sustained muscle contraction lasting about 30 seconds. The contraction phase is followed by a clonic phase of similar duration characterised by spasmodic jerking movements which may

include the whole body but is more commonly confined to the limbs. The clonic phase is followed by a relaxation phase, which may last several minutes, during which the patient lies flaccid and begins to rouse. The attack may be followed by a period of mild confusion. The muscle spasm may cause the patient to bite the tongue and the generalised muscle contracture may lead to cyanosis, because the respiratory muscles are involved, and result in raised intra-abdominal pressure causing evacuation of the bladder, bowel or stomach. Death from asphyxia may occur if the stomach contents are inhaled. Rarely, post-epileptic automatism may occur in which the patient proceeds with purposeful activity but later has no recollection of what he has been doing.

2. *Petit mal* begins in childhood, so much so that the diagnosis should be regarded as suspect if it is made for the first time in an adult. The characteristic occurrence is a short period of unconsciousness lasting only a few seconds during which the patient is unresponsive and unaware of events around him. The attacks may occur repeatedly over a short period of time. The duration of each is so short that the patient does not fall to the ground.

Focal Epilepsy

An epileptogenic discharge may occur in any part of the brain. The symptoms that result depend upon the area of the brain involved. Therefore there are many varities of focal epilepsy. Attacks may be followed by a generalised convulsion.

Temporal lobe epilepsy is the commonest variety. An aura generally preceeds the fit. Attacks may be limited to the aura alone. The aura may take various forms but is usually constant for any individual patient. Frequently focal discharges arise in the uncinate gyrus and give rise to an aura consisting of a hallucination of smell, often unpleasant, which may be associated with masticatory movements of the jaw. Sometimes the aura may involve abnormal patterns of behaviour or sudden changes of mood, such as feelings of panic or depression, or sudden outbursts of laughter at inappropriate moments. A transient disturbance of memory may occur in which there is a sensation of reliving a previous experience (*déjà vu* phenomenon) or a sensation of unfamiliarity when in a normally familiar environment (*jamais vu* phenomenon). Hallucinatory voices or visions may be experienced and sometimes the patient may utter repetitive and often incongruous phrases.

Jacksonian epilepsy is a variety of focal epilepsy in which jerks begin in either the thumb and index finger, the corner of the mouth or the great toe, followed by rapid spread and *grand mal.*

Diagnosis

Epilepsy is frequently misdiagnosed. The history is crucial and should be supplemented by the account of a witness. Without a witness's description the diagnosis must be regarded as tentative.

In idiopathic epilepsy there will be no abnormal physical signs if the patient is examined between attacks. If signs of a focal neurological disorder are found, epilepsy secondary to a brain lesion must be considered.

The patient should be questioned about events immediately prior to the attack, particularly for precipitating factors and whether or not an aura was present. The pattern and type of aura should be defined. Enquiries should be made about the frequency of attacks and whether they were diurnal or nocturnal, or both. Specific enquiries should be made about the patient's past medical history, particularly for evidence of previous meningitis, encephalitis, head trauma and birth injury.

The witness should be asked to describe the patient's actions immediately before the attack, the order of events during the attack, whether there was any change in the patient's complexion before, during or after the attack, and whether there was any evidence of vomiting or incontinence. Enquiries should also be made regarding the presence of any extraneous noise or flashing lights in the vicinity of the patient immediately before the attack.

In children suspected of having *petit mal* an attack may be precipitated by requesting them to breath deeply for 3 minutes.

It is desirable that any patient presenting with epilepsy should be referred to a consultant neurologist, for full assessment and confirmation of the diagnosis, because of the social and economic consequences that may follow an erroneous label of 'epilepsy'. It should be routine to refer to a neurologist all patients who present with epilepsy for the first time in adult life so that an organic neurological disease which may be remediable, e.g., meningioma, can be excluded.

The differential diagnosis of epilepsy includes:—

1. *Syncope* Prodromal symptoms of sweating or of subjective temperature changes are common. Complaints of breaking out into a 'cold sweat' are typical. The patient usually sinks to the ground, rather than falls to the ground, and after a moment's stillness begins to recover. A witness may describe facial pallor immediately before the faint. If the pulse is felt during the attack it will be noticed to be of reduced volume.

2. *Cough syncope* which may occur associated with bouts of coughing.

3. *Micturation syncope* is a rare type of faint occurring in males at or beyond middle age. The characteristic history is that the patient got up during the night to empty his bladder and collapsed in the lavatory.

4. *Drop attacks* True drop attacks are characterised by sudden weakness of the legs while walking, causing the patient to 'fold at the knees'. Their aetiology is uncertain, but they occur most commonly in females over the age of 35 and may be due to basilar artery insufficiency. Consciousness is not lost.

5. *Cerebral neoplasm* Epileptiform attacks may occur in the presence of a cerebral neoplasm, whether benign or malignant. The presence of abnormal

physical signs will usually provide objective evidence when the patient is examined between attacks.

6. *Narcolepsy*   Narcolepsy is characterised by an irresistable desire to fall asleep, often at inappropriate moments. It rarely occurs when the patient is undertaking purposeful physical activity.

7. *Cataplexy*   Characterised by a sudden feeling of muscular weakness. Falls are extremely rare. Consciousness is not lost.

8. *Hysterical attacks*   The history of events is often bizarre. Few, if any, of the features of *grand mal* or *petit mal* are present. The eyes are often closed during an 'attack' and the pupils react to light. Hysterical 'fits' never occur in the absence of an audience. Frequently a history of 'struggling' and of the need 'to be held down' will be obtained. However it is important to bear in mind that some epileptics may also have hysterical attacks. The diagnosis is often difficult and should never be made until organic disease has been excluded.

9. *Metabolic Disorders*   The commonest metabolic disorder with which confusion may arise is hypoglycaemia. Sixty-five per cent of daily glucose intake is utilised by the brain and is rapidly metabolised. Lack of glucose may be due to deficient intake (e.g., going for a long period without food) or to an excessive blood insulin level (e.g., diabetics on insulin, insulinoma).

Management

Once the diagnosis of epilepsy is confirmed it is important to impress upon the patient that treatment must be continuous and prolonged.

General Measures

The patient should be advised to avoid any precipitating cause, e.g., photic or audic stimulation. Circumstances where injury may occur should also be avoided, e.g., moving machinery, work at heights, fire, swimming unaccompanied, driving a car and cycling. The mechanisms of attacks should be explained to the patient and fear and superstition dispelled. Advice may be required in choosing a suitable occupation and the assistance of welfare agencies may be valuable.

During an attack apply commonsense. The patient should be protected from injury. A firm gag should be inserted between the teeth to prevent tongue biting, but this is rarely possible during the contraction phase. A hard object should never be forced between the teeth; it is more likely to cause injury than to prevent it. The patient should be rolled onto the side to aid drainage of fluid from the mouth and to prevent the tongue from falling back into the pharynx during relaxation. Wait for the attack to subside.

Drugs

Anti-convulsant drugs should be prescribed in a dosage sufficient to control attacks, a combination of drugs may be used. Because of the variation that may occur in the degree of stimulation required to precipitate an attack it may not always be possible to prevent them entirely. Should isolated or infrequent attacks occur while on treatment it is unwise automatically to increase dosage whenever an attack occurs.

Anti-convulsant drugs are usually given in divided doses two or three times a day. The commonly used drugs are:

Grand mal;

1. Phenobarbitone, the most useful drug, may be given in a dose of 30 mg–300 mg daily in divided doses. It should not be used in combination with primidone about 20 per cent of which is converted to phenobarbitone *in vivo*.
2. Phenytoin. The daily dosage may vary between 100 mg and 600 mg.
3. Primidone, in a dose of 250 mg up to 1.5 g daily. It should not be prescribed with phenobarbitone. If primidone is being substituted for phenobarbitone, or vice versa, the change should be gradual, increasing the dose of one drug and decreasing the other concomitantly.
4. Diazepam, 2–15 mg daily may be used in combination with another anti-convulsant.

Petit mal;

1. Troxidone, 600–1200 mg daily
2. Ethosuximide, 500–1500 mg daily.

Social Aspects

The patient should be encouraged to lead as normal a life as possible. The treatment and possible dangers to which the patient may be exposed at work or elsewhere should be discussed frankly. Because of the possibility of admission to hospital while unconscious, the patient should be advised to carry a card bearing his name and address and that of his family practitioner, together with the information that he suffers from epilepsy. In the UK the patient should be informed about the Medic-Alert organisation and advised to inform someone at his place of work whom he trusts that he has epilepsy.

Epilepsy is no bar to marriage but the patient should be advised not to conceal the fact. It may be helpful to offer a joint consultation between patient, fiancée and doctor so that the problem can be discussed freely. The question of inheritance will be raised. If one parent has idiopathic epilepsy there is a 1 in 40 chance that children of the marriage will be affected. If both parents have idiopathic epilepsy the chances are approximately 1 in 4, and these risks should be clearly explained. Of course, epilepsy secondary to brain trauma can never be inherited.

Complications of Epilepsy

Status Epilepticus

When one attack of *grand mal* follows another at short intervals status epilepticus is present. The condition must be regarded as an emergency, since permanent brain damage or death may result from cerebral anoxia. Treatment must be prompt and adequate. Initial treatment should be the intra-muscular administration of sodium phenobarbitone 200 mg (for children 5 mg/kg) or paraldehyde 5—10 ml (for children 0.15 ml/kg). Beware of using disposable syringes with paraldehyde. Either drug may be repeated if the patient has not begun to rouse within 5 minutes. If following initial treatment the fits continue or consciousness does not return within 15—20 minutes, the patient should be admitted to hospital where there are facilities for providing assisted respiration. Other drugs which are respiratory depressants may then be used, i.e., phenytoin, thiopentone or diazepam which can be given intra-muscularly or intra-venously.

Personality Changes

Psychotic features may be noted in epileptic patients, especially those subject to *grand mal*, but are not invariably present. Their cause is uncertain. They may be due to a summation of the effects of repeated episodes of cerebral anoxia, or they may be a secondary result of the feeling of insecurity and loss of socio-economic status that is so often the experience of epileptic patients. There appears to be a relationship between the frequency of fits and the presence of psychosis; patients who have few fits do not usually show evidence of psychosis.

Patients who are psychotic often have difficulty in maintaining consistent employment. Long or repeated periods of unemployment may destroy morale and lead to social deterioration. The situation may be aggravated if the patient is socially isolated, or if there is no relative willing to assist with care. In the presence of these and similar problems the Social Services Department should be informed and invited to give constructive assistance.

Follow-Up and Continuing Care

The continued surveillance of an epileptic patient includes monitoring his physical state, the social and occupational environment, and watching for any psychological effects of the illness. The patient should be seen regularly. At each attendance enquiries should be made about the frequency and type of attacks and whether there have been any employment or social problems. The need to maintain continuous therapy should be re-emphasised as often as necessary. Repeat prescriptions should be allowed for only limited periods.

In the UK an introduction to the British Epilepsy Association, 3—6 Alfred Place, London, WC1E 7ED may prove useful to the patient.

DISORDERS OF THE CEREBRAL CIRCULATION

Disorders of the cerebral circulation are an important cause of morbidity and mortality, especially in the elderly. Effects vary from the minor disturbance caused by transient cerebral vascular ischaemia to the major disablement that may follow the onset of a stroke.

Cerebral Circulation

The blood supply to the brain is derived from four main arteries: the left and right internal carotid arteries and the two vertebral arteries. The vertebral arteries combine to form the basilar artery which is linked to the two internal carotid arteries by the circle of Willis. The circle of Willis provides a collateral circulation which mitigates the effect of interruption of the supply of blood from any one of the four main arteries. The arteries which arise from the circle of Willis are end-arteries and a block of any one of them may lead to cerebral infarction.

Approximately 20 per cent of the cardiac output enters the carotid and vertebral arterial system. The maintenance of cerebral circulation is dependent upon an adequate level of systemic arterial pressure. The cerebral blood supply contains a considerable safety margin so that a reduction to about 60 per cent of the normal blood flow is required before symptoms of cerebral ischaemia appear. Partial or complete obstruction of the blood supply to the brain may occur in either the extra-cranial arteries (e.g., common carotid) or the intra-cranial arteries. There may be an interruption of the blood supply to a local area of the brain causing focal ischaemia or infarction, for example by an embolus, without reduction in the overall blood supply.

Pathogenesis

Cerebral Ischaemia
A block occurring in an artery or an arteriole will cause ischaemia of cerebral tissue and cell death unless an adequate collateral circulation develops rapidly. The commonest cause of cerebral ischaemia is an embolus. Emboli may originate from the heart or from the main arteries. Emboli of cardiac origin are commonly associated with myocardial infarction, subacute bacterial endocarditis or mitral stenosis. Emboli arising from a main artery usually result from thrombus formation on the ulcerated surface of an atheromatous plaque, e.g., in the arch of the aorta or at the origin of the internal carotid artery.

Intra-cerebral Haemorrhage
An intra-cerebral haemorrhage may be large or small and can occur in any part of the brain. A large haemorrhage may cause considerable destruction of cerebral

tissue with widespread effects, but a small haemorrhage may result in focal damage only.

Russell[2] indicated that there may be a relationship between the micro-aneurysms demonstrated by Charcot and Bouchard[3], and cerebral haemorrhage. Although the cause of Charcot—Bouchard aneurysms is not known, they are associated with the presence of systemic hypertension. Clinical[4] and pathological studies[5] have shown that intra-cerebral haemorrhage is also associated with hypertension and it may be inferred that Charcot—Bouchard aneurysms play a part in the pathogenesis of cerebral haemorrhage.

It is accepted that the level of blood pressure rises with age and therefore it is not surprising that intra-cerebral haemorrhage is more common in the elderly.

Sub-arachnoid Haemorrhage

A sub-arachnoid haemorrhage implies that there has been extravasation of blood into the sub-arachnoid space. The origin of the haemorrhage may be arterial or venous, and may come from single or multiple sites. Sub-arachnoid haemorrhage most commonly originates from rupture of an intra-cranial aneurysm, but it can arise from birth injury, head trauma, or from an intra-cerebral angioma.

Arteritis

Polyarteritis, cranial arteritis (giant-cell arteritis) and the arteritis associated with lupus erythematosus may affect intra-cerebral vessels and lead to cerebral ischaemia. Arteritis of the intra-cerebral vessels may also occur in association with systemic infection, especially tuberculosis and syphilis.

Aetiology

A study of the epidemiology of cerebral vascular disease in family practice revealed an incidence of 7.6 per 1000 of the population and a mean age at onset of 65.02 years for males and 70.88 years for females[6]. Cerebral ischaemia was found to be twice as common as all other forms of cerebral vascular disease, including haemorrhage (Table 14.1).

Clinical Features

Cerebral vascular disorders occur most frequently in patients over the age of 55. The symptoms and signs are of rapid onset. A neurological deficit which is slow to develop is more likely to be due to non-vascular disease, e.g., a cerebral neoplasm. The diagnosis of stroke is usually self-evident although the precise manifestations will depend upon the area of the brain affected.

Drop attacks occur in females over the age of 35. Typically the patient

Table 14.1   Cerebral vascular disease. Incidence and mean age at onset (Adapted, with permission, from Acheson et. al.[6])

Disease	Incidence rate per 100 000 of population			Mean age at onset	
	Male	Female	Total	Male	Female
Focal cerebral vascular ischaemia					
First stroke	235.6	196.1	215.2	65.3	75.6
Second or subsequent stroke	113.1	160.5	137.4	65.2	69.7
Transient cerebral ischaemia	169.7	196.1	183.2	64.2	68.3
Group total	518.4	552.7	535.8	64.9	71.3
Other types of cerebral vascular disease					
Cerebral haemorrhage	46.9	17.7	32.0	67.6	80.0
Sub-arachnoid haemorrhage	*	17.7	9.1	*	68.0
Miscellaneous group	103.5	267.5	187.7	64.5	69.6
Total	668.8	855.6	764.6	65.02	70.88

* insufficient data

falls suddenly to the ground without losing consciousness whilst walking, and injury may result. The attacks were at one time thought to be due to a temporary interruption of the vertebro-basilar blood supply. However it is now believed that other factors are involved and the cause is not established.

The Territory Supplied by the Carotid Artery   Motor disturbances may occur and commonly take the form of a hemiplegia or monoplegia. The affected limbs are usually flaccid to start with, later becoming spastic. Sensory disturbances generally follow the same distribution as the motor loss. Speech disturbances take the form of aphasia or dysphasia. Visual symptoms include homonymous hemianopia and monocular visual loss. The onset of monocular visual loss is characteristic and is likened by the patient to a shutter closing before the eye.

The Territory Supplied by the Vertebro-basilar System   Visual symptoms commonly occur, blurring of vision and diplopia are frequently the presenting features. Vertigo and unsteadiness of gait are also common. The patient may present with a speech defect in the form of a dysarthria. Although motor weakness is not so common a mono- or hemi-paresis or a mono- or hemi-plegia may occur. Sensory disturbances may be present in the limbs and characteristically the patient may complain of circumoral paraesthesiae.

Transient Cerebral Vascular Ischaemia
Transient cerebral vascular ischaemia is characterised by repeated attacks of neurological dysfunction which last for less than 1 hour and are followed by

complete recovery[7]. Therefore, typically, the patient is symptom free and has no physical signs at the time of consultation. Diagnosis will depend upon a careful assessment of historical data.

The attacks are caused by short periods of cerebral ischaemia thought to be secondary to either an embolus or a small focal cerebral haemorrhage. They may occur singly or in clusters spread over a period of time varying from a few hours to several months. They may or may not be followed by a stroke. In any case they have a tendency to cease after a period of time.

Stroke

A stroke is an episode of neurological dysfunction of cerebral vascular origin lasting for more than one hour[7]. It may be produced by an infract or intra-cerebral haemorrhage and is the commonest presentation of cerebral vascular disease. It may occur at any time of the day or night. In the majority of patients the onset is rapid. Unconsciousness, if it occurs, indicates a poor prognosis. The patient will usually be hypertensive.

Repeated small strokes, each of which causes infarction and cell death in a small area of the brain, may in summation lead to considerable damage and to intellectual deterioration.

Sub-arachnoid Haemorrhage

A sub-arachnoid haemorrhage is characterised by the sudden onset of a severe intractible headache which may be associated with vomiting. Signs of meningeal irritation will be found, i.e., nuchal rigidity and a positive Kernig's sign. Focal symptoms may occur. The finding of sub-hyaloid haemorrhages is pathogonomic. A large sub-arachnoid haemorrhage will result in unconsciousness and deepening coma and death may result.

The diagnosis can be substantiated by lumbar puncture and the demonstration of blood-stained cerebro-spinal fluid.

Cranial Arteritis (Giant-cell Arteritis)

Although any extra-cranial artery may be the site of arteritis, the temporal artery is the one most commonly involved and the occipital artery is the next most common site. The patient complains of a pain or a throbbing headache over the site of the affected artery. Presentation in elderly patients is described in Chapter 24, page 606.

If the temporal artery is involved it is likely that all ipsilateral branches of the carotid system will be affected, including the ophthalmic artery and the central artery of the retina. Sometimes blurring or loss of vision is the presenting symptom.

The suspected artery must be palpated for evidence of tenderness. The ESR will usually be elevated. Arterial biopsy may be required to confirm the diagnosis.

Management

Transient Cerebral Vascular Ischaemia

The effects of transient cerebral vascular ischaemia are of short duration and are not severe or disabling. There is no specific treatment. An expectant attitude should be preserved and the patient should be encouraged to maintain his normal activities. Attacks of transient cerebral vascular ischaemia may be due to the lodgement of emboli originating from the left side of the heart or from thrombi forming on atheromatous plaques in the main arteries, and this possibility should be investigated, especially in patients under 60 years of age.

Hypertension if present should be considered for treatment.

The management of patients who develop a stroke following transient cerebral vascular ischaemia is as described below.

Stroke

The diagnosis must be established. Investigation may be required to exclude causes other than cerebral vascular disease, especially in younger patients, and may entail hospital admission. The skull should always be examined carefully to exclude head injury, e.g., sub-dural haematoma, especially in the infirm or confused elderly patient who may not remember that a fall has occurred.

The degree of neurological deficit resulting from a stroke is maximal at the onset in about 50 per cent of patients. In the remainder the full picture takes some hours to develop. If the social circumstances permit and there is no doubt about the diagnosis, the patient should be nursed at home. He should be confined to bed for the first 24 hours and a mild sedative may be prescribed (e.g., diazepam 5—10 mg every 6 hours). After the first 24 hours progressive mobility should be encouraged and the patient should be allowed to undertake such exercise as he is able to perform. Relatives and other attendants should be shown how to put paralysed joints passively through their whole range of movement. If available, the skills of a physiotherapist will be invaluable. An adequate state of hydration and nutrition must be maintained. If the patient is unable to swallow hospital admission may be necessary on this ground alone.

If the patient is unconscious when first seen, priority must be given to the maintenance of an adequate airway and removal from a dangerous situation.

Subsequent management will depend upon the rate of progress towards recovery and the degree of permanent neurological deficit. A rehabilitation programme should be arranged. The first requirement is to pay particular attention to the maintenance of mobility and good muscle tone. Active and passive exercises at home should be supplemented as soon as possible by regular attendance at a physiotherapy department. The morale of the patient should be observed and will be helped if an attitude of confidence concerning the future is maintained by all attendants. Most patients of working age will be able to return to gainful employment, though it may be necessary to consider a change of occupation. The special problems of management in elderly patients are discussed in Chapter 24, page 602.

Sub-arachnoid Haemorrhage
Following discharge from hospital the patient should be encouraged to resume normal activity after a short convalescence.

Cranial arteritis (Giant-cell Arteritis)
Cranial arteritis should be treated with prednisolone in high dosage, commencing with 60 mg a day in divided doses and reducing to a maintenance dose of 5—10 mg a day. Treatment should be monitored by the ESR and may need to continue for 6—12 months. Analgesics may be prescribed in addition.

Involvement of the temporal artery must be regarded as a medical emergency because of the danger of blindness and treatment must be commenced immediately, even if the diagnosis cannot be confirmed.

The Patient
Attacks of transient cerebral vascular insufficiency may be isolated or occur in clusters, and in many patients the attacks cease after a time. In a proportion of patients the attacks may be followed by a stroke. In these patients the prognosis should be guarded but in general a confident attitude is justifiable.

A patient who has experienced a stroke will often be apprehensive about the future. Studies of the natural history have shown that when a patient has had one stroke a subsequent stroke, if it is going to occur will usually do so within 2 years. If a second stroke does not occur within this period the possibility of a further stroke becomes progressively less likely as time passes.

The Family
Relatives frequently express a high degree of anxiety, especially about the future care of the patient and the extent to which dependency will develop. The prognosis should be fully explained and anxiety may be alleviated to some extent by discussing the resources that are available in the community to assist with domiciliary care, i.e., from the health team, Social Services Departments and voluntary agencies.

The Role of the Health Team
The district nurse should be asked to assist in the care of the patient if he is likely to remain in bed for more than 24 hours. Domiciliary physiotherapy, if available, should be commenced as soon as possible. If there is a significant degree of permanent functional deficit the services of the health visitor may be required to assist with the mobilisation of welfare services and the provision of mechanical aids.

Follow-Up and Continuing Care

The patient should remain under medical care until maximal functional recovery has occurred and may need longer supervision if there is a major permanent deficit. He should be encouraged to retain his independence and to be as active as possible. If hypertension is present treatment should continue. The progress of the rehabilitation programme should be reviewed constantly, and an occupational retraining programme arranged if appropriate.

Further Research

Cerebral vascular disorders are usually the result of degenerative processes, especially the development of atheroma. There is a continuing need for research into the aetiology of vascular degeneration and into methods for their prevention. The medical, and other, resources that are required for the domiciliary care of stroke patients is another area requiring investigation.

DISSEMINATED SCLEROSIS

Disseminated sclerosis is a chronic disease with a prevalence of about one per 1000 of the population. Most family practitioners are likely to have at least one patient in their practice. It is more common in women than men, though men tend to be more severely affected. The disease usually makes its first appearance in early adult life but occasionally the onset may be delayed until late middle age. The course of the disease is usually protracted, interspersed with remissions, and may finally result in considerable disability.

Aetiology

The basic lesion is demyelination which may affect any part of the central nervous system. The cause of the demyelination remains uncertain. Mechanisms that have been suggested include immunological disorders, virus infection, trace element deficiency and nutritional factors.

Clinical Features

The clinical features of disseminated sclerosis are extremely variable, almost any combination of neurological signs and symptoms may be found. Early symptoms, which may be temporary, include diplopia, blurring of vision, ataxia, paraesthesiae, sphincter disturbance and weakness of one limb. The blurring of vision is due to retro-bulbar neuritis which may also cause pain in the affected eye and lead to optic atrophy. The initial symptoms often go into remission after a few weeks with apparent complete recovery. Remission may last for a variable period and can be as long as 20 years.

In some patients there is no early remission, the inital disability persists and further symptoms and signs may develop later. Occasionally the degree of remission is incomplete, the patient continuing to experience some disability though less than previously.

The physical signs depend upon the site, or sites, of demyelination. Evidence of motor dysfunction is common, especially pyramidal signs. Diplopia is due to palsy of one or more of the ocular muscles. Cerebellar signs are common, including ataxia and 'scanning speech'. Horizontal and vertical nystagmus is frequently found. In the late stages painful flexor spasms may occur.

Psychiatric features are common, especially changes in mood; the patient may swing between euphoria and depression within the space of a few weeks. As the disease progresses intellectual impairment becomes apparent.

Diagnosis

The diagnosis is based on clinical grounds. An essential characteristic of the disease is that the neurological disturbances are disseminated in time and in space, i.e., they vary with time and any part of the central nervous system may be affected. A careful history is of the greatest importance and specific enquiries should be made regarding visual, sensory or motor disturbances that might have occurred at an earlier period. Laboratory investigations are of limited assistance. Syphilis should always be excluded.

Because of the long term disability and poor prognosis which may be associated with disseminated sclerosis, it is advisable that the diagnosis should be confirmed by a consultant neurologist.

Management

The prognosis in disseminated sclerosis is variable. In many patients the disease remains relatively benign for long periods, even in the absence of a remission. In a few patients the disease may be rapidly progressive leading to death within a few years. Rapid and early increasing disability in the first 2–3 years usually indicates a poor prognosis.

Drug Treatment

There is no specific drug treatment. During periods of exacerbation the administration of ACTH may hasten the onset of a remission. It is best given twice weekly, as ACTH gel by intramuscular injection, in a dose of 120 units initially and reducing gradually over a period of about four weeks. Anti-depressant drugs may be helpful during periods of depression. Flexor spasms may be helped by diazepam 5 mg three or four times daily; occasionally intraspinal phenol injections may be necessary to destroy the affected nerves.

General Measures

The Patient

Because of the protracted nature of the disease and the lack of specific medical treatment, the maintenance of the patient's morale is of the utmost importance. Regular medical supervision is essential and the practitioner should always demonstrate his continuing interest in the patient's problems. Routine surveillance should include the physical, psychological and social aspects of the disease. Physical aspects include the need to maintain general health and the prompt treatment of intercurrent disease. The physician should be alert for evidence of lower urinary tract infection which is common.

Long periods of bedrest should be avoided. Physiotherapy will often be required in order to maintain muscle tone and to assist the patient to remain mobile and independent for as long as possible. There is no justification for withholding any necessary surgical or dental treatment. Mechanical and other aids should be used wherever needed, including wheelchairs, ramps instead of steps, additional grab-handles and handrails in the bathroom and additional handrails on the stairs. Home nursing assistance and domestic help should be provided wherever required.

At a suitable opportunity the natural history of the disease should be discussed frankly with the patient in terms that can be easily understood. The patient should be encouraged to continue with normal employment as long as possible. In the UK an introduction to the Multiple Sclerosis Society may be beneficial.

A female patient may seek advice regarding pregnancy. Occasionally pregnancy may initiate an exacerbation of the disease but this is impossible to predict. The advisability of pregnancy should be dependent upon the patient's wishes and the degree of physical handicap, rather than upon any possible effect on the disease process.

The Family

Members of the patient's family will usually express their concern and should be included in discussions about the disease. Ways in which relatives and friends may assist the patient should be suggested. In particular they should be asked to assist in mitigating the social isolation that may result from restricted mobility. Visits to friends, theatre, holidays, extra-mural education, and general social activity should be encouraged. Practitioners may be called upon for advice regarding special measures needed to fulfil such activities and ingenuity is often necessary.

INFECTIONS OF THE NERVOUS SYSTEM

Infection of the nervous system may involve the coverings of the brain (leptomeningitis), the substance of the brain (encephalitis), the spinal cord (myelitis), or any of the peripheral nerves.

Herpes Zoster (Shingles)

Herpes zoster (shingles) results from infection of the posterior horn cells of the spinal cord with the varicella-zoster virus. It is characterised by localised pain followed by the appearance of a cutaneous vesicular eruption confined to the area of distribution of the nerve roots affected. A full account of the diagnosis and management of herpes zoster is given in Chapter 18, page 427.

Poliomyelitis

Poliomyelitis is an acute viral infection of the anterior horn cells of the spinal cord. Following a widespread immunisation programme the disease is now rare in the United Kingdom (see page 558).

The poliomyelitis virus is an enterovirus, which enters by the mouth and multiplies in the oropharynx and lower intestinal tract. It is excreted in the faeces. Attention to hygiene will therefore limit the spread of the infection.

Clinical Features

Poliomyelitis may occur in paralytic or non-paralytic form.

Non-paralytic poliomyelitis is often a minor illness with little or no constitutional disturbance. An ache in one or more muscle groups may be the only symptom. Occasionally features similar to those found in leptomeningitis may be observed.

In the paralytic form the clinical features are the same as in the non-paralytic form but the constitutional disturbance is greater and muscular paralysis occurs. Any muscle group may be involved but the lower limbs are most frequently affected. Often a history of having recently undertaken exercise of a strenuous nature will be obtained.

Diagnosis

Non-paralytic poliomyelitis frequently remains undiagnosed unless the presence of an epidemic has alerted the physician to the possibility. In the paralytic stage the diagnosis is made initially on clinical grounds.

Management
The Patient   There is no specific treatment for poliomyelitis. Hospital admission is advisable. Rest is important and patients should be confined to bed. Physiotherapy is important, especially in the paralytic form, but should be confined to gentle passive exercise in the early stages. Symptomatic therapy may be prescribed but intramuscular injections should always be avoided. If the muscles of respiration become involved hospital admission must be arranged because assisted respiration may be required.

The Family   Because of the well-known danger that permanent paresis may result, relatives will be anxious regarding the outcome. The prognosis should be guarded until the full extent of the disease has become manifest. The ultimate prognosis will be dependent upon the degree of recovery, which may be considerable.

Leptomeningitis

Leptomeningitis may be bacterial or viral. Bacteria commonly involved include, in order of frequency, *Neisseria meningitidis* (meningococcus), haemophilus, pneumococcus, and coliform organisms. *Mycobacterium tuberculosis* is no longer a common causal agent in developed countries. Culprit viruses are usually either polio viruses, coxsackie viruses or echo viruses. The disease may occur occasionally as a complication of mumps, herpes simplex and infectious mononucleosis.

Leptomeningitis occurs mainly in children, especially those under the age of five, and in young adults. The majority of cases occur from January to April.

N. meningitidis (meningococcus) is the most common causal agent and the incidence of meningococcal meningitis is increasing. In 1967, 358 cases were reported in the United Kingdom where the disease is notifiable. By 1973 the incidence had doubled to 842.

N. meningitidis is endemic in the population and can be isolated from the nasopharynx of many normal people. It is transmitted by droplet, and therefore infection is more likely to spread in crowded communities, e.g., schools and army camps. Many strains of *N. meningitidis* are of low virulence and do not cause clinical leptomeningitis, but their transmission from one host to another leads to the development of naturally acquired immunity. The disease develops only when infection involves a more virulent strain or when the host has a low or absent natural immunity.

Clinical Features and Diagnosis
The diagnosis of leptomeningitis depends upon the clinical features which are the same whether the causal agent is a bacterium or a virus.

The disease develops insidiously over a few days with pyrexia and headache and may be difficult to diagnose in the early stages, unless the physician has been alerted by the presence of a local epidemic or by evidence that the patient has been exposed to infection. Within a short time the headache worsens and nausea and vomiting occur. In the baby the earliest sign may be the development of restlessness and a high-pitched cry. Photophobia is nearly always present. As the disease develops nuchal spasm appears and may be sufficient to cause opisthotonos. A positive Kernig's sign may be found. In meningococcal meningitis a roseola papular rash commonly occurs and may appear early in the illness before constitutional symptoms appear. It later becomes haemorrhagic.

In tuberculous leptomeningitis the typical picture of meningeal infection develops late. It is preceded by a prodromal phase lasting 2 or 3 weeks in which lethargy, a poor appetite and mood changes are prominent.

The differential diagnosis of leptomeningitis includes encephalitis, cerebral tumour, cerebral vascular disease (especially sub-arachnoid haemorrhage), and conditions in which meningism may occur, such as acute tonsillitis, cervical adenitis, pneumonia, bacillary dysentery and hypernatraemic acidosis.

Management

Any patient suspected of having leptomeningitis must be admitted to hospital. If fits occur anti-convulsant therapy may be required, even prior to hospital admission. Treatment will be with an antibiotic to which the infecting organism is sensitive or by antiviral chemotherapy.

Children who have had meningitis should be followed-up carefully, especially regarding their mental development and scholastic attainment. They should be included in the practice 'at risk' register.

Complications   Leptomeningitis of viral origin has a low mortality and complications are uncommon. Bacterial leptomeningitis has an appreciable mortality and is most dangerous in the very young and in the aged. Residual damage to the central nervous system may occur, especially in tuberculous leptomeningitis, and includes obstructive hydrocephalus and impairment of intellect.

The Family   Contacts of patients with leptomeningitis due to *N. meningitidis* should be traced and nasopharyngal swabs obtained. Infected carriers should be treated with sulphadiazine until negative swabs are obtained.

A guarded prognosis should be given to relatives until the extent of the disease becomes manifest. If complications do not occur a favourable prognosis may be given and the patient's return to normal life after convalescence may be expected.

Encephalitis and Myelitis

Encephalitis is a diffuse infection of the brain tissue. Myelitis is a local or diffuse infection of the tissue of the spinal cord. Neither condition occurs commonly.

The most frequent cause is a viral infection and it may occur as a complication of mumps, herpes simplex, herpes zoster, measles and infectious mononucleosis. Encephalitis and myelitis sometimes occur together in the same patient, though encephalitis alone is more common.

Clinical Features
The natural history of encephalitis is similar to that of leptomeningitis and the border line between them is blurred. The illness usually has an abrupt onset with fever, headache and confusion. Sometimes nausea, vomiting and a disturbance of sleep rhythm may be present. Signs of meningeal irritation are not uncommon.

Myelitis may be local or diffuse. The symptoms and signs may involve both upper and lower motor neurones.

Diagnosis and Management
If the diagnosis of encephalitis or myelitis is suspected hospital admission is required. There is no specific treatment. Most patients recover, though a few patients may show evidence of a permanent neurological deficit.

Neurosyphilis

Neurosyphilis can be prevented by effective early treatment of the acute infection. Spirochaetal invasion of the central nervous system may occur within the first few weeks of infection but symptoms of neurosyphilis develop in less than 10 per cent of all untreated cases. Neurological manifestations of syphilis are rare in the primary stage and are more commonly found in the secondary or tertiary stages.

In neurosyphilis an arteritis may develop and lead to focal cerebral infarction. Therefore syphilis must be considered in any young person who develops symptoms of cerebral vascular disease.

Late manifestations, which may occur up to 30 years after the initial infection, include general paralysis of the insane and tabes dorsalis. Less dramatic disturbances are not uncommon and it is a sensible practice to arrange for a Wasserman reaction to be carried out in any patient with a suspected neurological reaction.

THE PARKINSONIAN SYNDROME

The Parkinsonian syndrome is a disturbance of motor function due to a progressive degenerative disorder affecting the extrapyramidal system. Estimates of prevalence have varied between 60 and 180 per 100 000 of the population. The earliest symptoms usually appear between the ages of 50 and 60 years.

Aetiology

Commonly no cause can be determined, most cases being idiopathic. Other causes include repeated trauma (especially in professional boxers and wrestlers), viral encephalitis, and various drugs, e.g., reserpine, methyldopa and the phenothiazines.

Clinical Features

The Parkinsonian syndrome is a progressive disorder characterised by tremor, rigidity and hypokinesia.

The tremor is usually the first symptom to appear and in the early stages is usually intermittent. It is of slow rate and initially affects one or both hands (pin-rolling movements) but later involves other limbs and the lower jaw. It is usually most prominent when the patient is fatigued or under emotional stress.

Rigidity may be either 'lead-pipe' or 'cog-wheel' in type and is felt by the physician as a resistance to passive movement. With the gradual progression of the disease the rigidity causes the patient to assume a generally flexed posture.

Hypokinesia is manifest by slowness in initiating movement and a lack of precision in movement, such as when doing-up buttons. The facial expression becomes fixed, blinking is reduced and the patient may dribble from the mouth. Normal arm swinging movements when walking are reduced and the patient tends to walk with short shuffling steps.

Diagnosis

The diagnosis is made on clinical grounds. The fully developed picture of Parkinsonism is easy to recognise. The differential diagnosis includes other conditions causing tremor, e.g., hyperthyroidism, alcoholism, anxiety state and drug toxicity.

Management

The Patient

In drug-induced cases cure will usually follow withdrawal of the drug. In other cases cure is not possible, but medical or surgical intervention may alleviate the condition considerably.

Activity should be encouraged and intensive physiotherapy will often be helpful.

The most useful drugs are anticholinergic drugs and L-Dopa. Benzhexol hydrochloride, procyclidine hydrochloride or orphenadrine hydrochloride may be used. The dose should be increased progressively until the symptoms are relieved or side effects ensue. L-Dopa will often prove valuable but should not be given in conjunction with monoamine oxidase inhibitors. The drug should be introduced gradually commencing with 250 mg daily. Side effects include hypotension, nausea, muscular dyskinesia, cardiac arrythmias and psychiatric symptoms, any of which may limit the level to which dosage can be increased.

Stereotactic surgery should be considered for patients who fail to respond to drug therapy provided the disease is not rapidly progressive and they are otherwise in good health.

The Family
The natural history of the disease entails a gradual reduction in mobility and a danger that social isolation may result. Relatives should be warned of this possibility and encouraged to assist the patient to lead as normal a life as possible. Simple mechanical aids may be helpful and the Social Services Department should be asked to assist where required.

NEURALGIA

Neuralgia is not a disease but a symptom. It usually consists of a dull persistent ache or pain which may be burning, stabbing or lancinating in character. The discomfort, which is always of neural origin, may occur at various sites depending upon the nerve involved.

Trigeminal Neuralgia

The incidence of trigeminal neuralgia is approximately 0.1 per 1000 of the population. It is uncommon in patients under 50 years of age and rare below the age of 40. The cause is unknown and no lesion of the nerve is demonstrable. When trigeminal neuralgia is suspected in a patient under 50 a structural lesion should be assumed until proved otherwise.

Clinical Features
Trigeminal neuralgia is characterised by the appearance of an episodic paroxysmal lancinating pain of short duration which is unilateral and confined to the distribution area of the 5th cranial nerve. The maxillary division is most often concerned. Occasionally the mandibular or ophthalmic divisions may be affected. The pain occurs typically in short bouts of varying frequency which may be followed by a dull burning sensation. The normal motor and sensory functions of the nerve are preserved. The bouts of pain may be accompanied by spasm of the facial muscles (tic douloureux). Remissions are common and may last 2 years or more. Attacks may be precipitated by washing the face, touch,

wind blowing on the cheek and by chewing; so much so that patients may sometimes be afraid to eat, speak, wash or shave. Specific trigger spots may sometimes be identified. Attacks of trigeminal neuralgia seldom occur during sleep.

Treatment should be with carbamezapine 200 mg t.d.s., which may be combined with phenytoin 100 mg t.d.s. and should be continued for 3 months. Occasionally phenol or alcohol injection of the trigeminal ganglion or surgical division of the nerve may be required.

Diagnosis

The differential diagnosis of trigeminal neuralgia includes:

> dental pain,
> infection of the paranasal sinuses,
> tempero-mandibular arthrosis,
> cancer of the oro-pharynx,
> post-herpetic neuralgia,
> migranous neuralgia,
> glossopharangeal neuralgia,
> acoustic neuroma,
> psychogenic facial pain,
> disseminated sclerosis,

The causes of pain in or round the eye may also need to be considered in the differential diagnosis, namely:—

> acute glaucoma,
> herpes zoster,
> frontal sinusitis,
> iritis,
> keratitis,
> retro-bulbar neuritis,

Brachial Neuralgia

A neuralgia involving one or more of the nerves comprising the brachial plexus and usually results from defects in the cervical spine (e.g., cervical spondylosis, prolapsed intervertebral disc). It may also occur as part of the thoracic outlet syndrome or as a result of trauma to the brachial plexus. Females are affected more often than males and are usually at or beyond middle age. Paraesthesiae may occur in the hand or arm and muscle wasting may be seen.

Migrainous Neuralgia

Migrainous neuralgia may occur in bouts lasting several weeks. Patients are usually middle-aged. Migraine is more fully discussed on page 252.

Psychogenic Facial Pain

This condition is not uncommon but may cause great distress. It is important to exclude a structural lesion. There will usually be a history of depression or anxiety.

Glossopharangeal Neuralgia

A condition which resembles trigeminal neuralgia in that the pain is of lancinating character and of episodic occurrence but it is much less common. The pain is triggered by swallowing and is confined to the back of the tongue and pharynx but may radiate to the ear. It may occur confined to the external auditory meatus. The pain arises from isolated lesions of the 9th cranial nerve resulting from its involvement in a fracture of the base of the skull or an invasive tumour. Treatment is with carbamezapine 200 mg t.d.s. which may also be combined with phenytoin 100 mg t.d.s. Occasionally, intractable cases may require section of the 9th cranial nerve.

Post-Herpetic Neuralgia

Post-herpetic neuralgia may occur at any site affected by herpes zoster. There is a persistent burning pain in the area where the eruption occurred, which is sometimes intractable.

Burning Feet Syndrome

May occur in any polyneuropathy (e.g., nutritional, uraemic). The discomfort is aggravated by the touch of bed coverings and by putting the foot to the ground.

Neoplasia

Tumours arising in the cerebello-pontine angle, middle cranial fossa or nasopharynx and spinal cord, may give rise to pain of neuralgic type due to involvement of neighbouring cranial nerves.

Causalgia

A neuralgic-type pain resulting from trauma to a peripheral nerve, or local pressure upon the nerve or its roots. The skin over the affected area may be atrophic and hairless. Sciatic neuralgia (sciatica), an example of this condition, results from irritation of the sciatic nerve or its roots (L4-S3) and is caused by disease of the lumbar spine or a lumbar disc protrusion.

Management

The treatment of trigeminal neuralgia has been discussed above. Specific treatment for other neuralgias is related to the underlying cause. The persistent burning pain often causes considerable distress. Relief may be achieved by analgesic drugs. Simple analgesics should be tried first; pethidine or opiates should never be prescribed. Where neuralgia is due to trauma or root pressure it will be helpful to rest the part concerned, e.g., by a Thomas' collar in cervical spondylosis, a sling in brachial neuralgia and bed rest in sciatic neuralgia. Local heat by radiation or short wave diathermy is also sometimes beneficial. Carbamezapine should always be tried in any persistent neuralgia where the precipitating cause is unknown or uncorrectable, e.g., neoplasia. The effect is sometimes dramatic.

NEUROPATHY

Neuropathy implies a disorder of a single peripheral nerve (mononeuropathy) or more than one (polyneuropathy). Apart from the carpal-tunnel syndrome and meralgia paraesthetica, neuropathy is uncommon in family practice.

The fibres of peripheral nerves may arise from cells situated in the brain stem nuclei, the sympathetic ganglia or the ventral horns of the spinal cord. A disorder resulting in a neuropathy may originate at any of these points. Neuropathy may also be caused by demyelination or compression of axonal processes.

Polyneuropathy

Polyneuropathy is a symmetrical lesion affecting more than one nerve. Symptoms begin distally, usually in the feet, and spread proximally. Both the sensory and the motor components are commonly involved, although the degree of involvement may be unequal. Pure motor or pure sensory disturbance can occur. Sensory disturbances, numbness and paraesthesiae, are initially of glove-and-stocking distribution. Motor disturbances may include foot drop, wrist drop, impairment of hand movements, loss of power and muscle wasting. Muscle pain and tenderness may also be present. The tendon reflexes will be depressed or absent. The plantar responses are flexor.

Mononeuropathy

The symptoms of mononeuropathy are the same as in polyneuropathy but only one nerve is involved, and are therefore confined to the distribution of the affected nerve.

Aetiology

The causes of neuropathy include metabolic disorders, deficiency diseases, infections, allergic reactions, vascular disorders, nerve compression, toxic agents, genetic disorders and malignant neoplasms.

Metabolic Disorders

Diabetes Mellitus   Diabetic neuropathy is most often found in middle-aged or elderly diabetics of long standing and is more common if the diabetes has been poorly controlled.

Symptoms may be minimal. Pain and paraesthesiae may occur and are usually confined to the leg or foot. Involvement of the autonomic system may lead to diarrhoea, overflow urinary incontinence, skin temperature disturbance and postural hypotension. Physical signs include peripheral hyperaesthia, loss of vibration sense, trophic ulceration of the feet and painless arthropathy. Polyneuropathy or mononeuropathy may occur, the latter usually due to ischaemia following atheromatous occlusion of the vasa vasorum.

Other Metabolic Disorders   Neuropathy may occur in porphyria, primary amylodiosis and chronic liver or renal failure.

Deficiency Diseases

Neuropathy may accompany subacute combined degeneration of the cord, chronic alcoholism, sprue, beri beri and pellegra.

Infections

Neuropathy may occur in diphtheria within 3 weeks of the initial infection and involve paralysis of the muscles of accommodation in the eye, the palatal or the pharangeal muscles and may be accompanied by a generalised sensimotor polyneuropathy. Recovery is usually complete. Neuropathy may also occur in association with infectious mononucleosis, sarcoidosis and leprosy.

Post-infective Polyneuropathy (Guillain-Barré Syndrome)

This condition may follow an upper respiratory or gastro-intestinal infection or a surgical procedure. The pathogenesis is uncertain but it possibly results from an autoimmune reaction which causes demyelination of the axon.

Other Disorders

Neuropathy may accompany rheumatoid arthritis, polyarteritis nodosa, systemic lupus erythematosuss, and thromboangiitis obliterans. The mechanism is uncertain but the most likely cause is either occlusion of the small vessels of the vasa vasorum, or an autoimmune reaction.

Nerve Compression

Carpal-Tunnel Syndrome   Neuropathy may result from pressure upon the median nerve as it passes beneath the flexor retinaculum. Most cases are idiopathic but the condition may occur during the second half of pregnancy (usually associated with fluid retention), in myxoedema, obesity or rheumatoid arthritis. The patient complains of pain in the hand which may spread up the arm and which is usually worse at night. There may be complaints of swelling or heaviness of the hand, most noticeable in the mornings. Paraesthesiae or numbness may occur in the area supplied by the median nerve. The symptoms are aggravated by manual work. Weakness or wasting of the muscles of the thenar eminence may also be found.

The carpal-tunnel syndrome is a common cause of pain in the arm, especially in women, and it is important not to overlook the possibility that myxoedema or rheumatoid arthritis may be present. The diagnosis is based mainly on the history.

Meralgia Paraesthetica   This is not uncommon in family practice and results from compression of the lateral cutaneous nerve of the thigh as it passes beneath the inguinal ligament. The patient complains of numbness or paraesthesiae over the lateral aspect of the thigh which is aggravated by walking or standing and is relieved by sitting or lying. Sometimes pain occurs at the same site. It is frequently associated with obesity or pregnancy.

Compression of the Ulnar Nerve   Ulnar nerve compression usually results from fractures or dislocations at the elbow and leads to weakness of the flexor muscles of the wrist, the middle and ring fingers and sometimes of the interossei. Loss of cutaneous sensation may be found over the hypothenar eminence, the little finger and the ulnar half of the ring finger.

Toxic Agents

The absorption of toxic amounts of lead, arsenic or organophosphorus compounds may result in neuropathy. Drugs, including isoniazid, sulphonamides, nitrofurantoin, phenytoin, phenobarbitone and chloral hydrate, may be occasional culprits.

Genetic Disorders

Genetic disorders are a rare cause of neuropathy but include peroneal muscular atrophy (Charcot-Marie-Tooth syndrome) and hypertrophic interstitial neuropathy (Dejernine-Sottas syndrome).

Malignant Neoplasm

Neuropathy may occasionally occur in the presence of malignant neoplasia. Often the cause cannot be determined precisely but it may result from compression of a peripheral nerve by an invasive tumour.

Diagnosis

The diagnosis of neuropathy depends upon a careful history and neurological examination. It is important to consider possible underlying causes. It is usually advisable for the patient to be referred to a consultant neurologist for confirmation of the diagnosis.

Management

Most forms of neuropathy are amenable to treatment which is generally that of the underlying cause. Diabetic neuropathy and neuropathy due to a vascular cause or malignant neoplasia may be difficult to relieve. General measures include splinting of the wrists or foot where they are affected.

Follow-Up and Continuing Care

The continuing care of a patient with neuropathy includes surveillance of the underlying cause. Continuing care should be arranged in association with the appropriate consultant specialist.

TUMOURS OF THE NERVOUS SYSTEM

A tumour of the nervous system may be intra-cerebral or extra-cerebral or involve the spinal cord or peripheral nerves.

General Considerations

Approximately 50 per cent of neoplasms of the central nervous system arise from metastatic deposits, 25 per cent are gliomas and 25 per cent are benign. Primary tumours may occur at any age but appear most frequently in the 40—50 age group. In children primary tumours are usually gliomas and tend to be situated below the tentorium. Primary tumours occurring later in life are usually supratenorial. Meningiomas occur most commonly in middle life.

Intra-cerebral Tumours
Intra-cerebral tumours are the most important group and are always life-threatening. Their incidence is about 12 per 100 000 of the population and their prevalence about 50 per 100 000 of the population.

Tumours of the Peripheral Nerves
Primary malignant tumours of the peripheral nerves are rare. Benign tumours which are usually neuromas or neurofibromas are also uncommon. The

commonest neuroma is an acoustic neuroma which arises from the 8th cranial nerve, usually in or near the internal auditory meatus.

Neurofibromatosis is a familial condition inherited as an autosomal dominant. It involves principally the cutaneous nerves which exhibit tumours of variable size; malignant change may occur.

Tumours of the Spinal Cord

Tumours of the spinal cord are rare. The majority are extradural and are usually the result of metastatic spread. Intradural tumours include meningiomata and neurofibromas.

Clinical Features

Intra-cerebral Tumours

The symptoms and signs produced by an intra-cerebral tumour depend upon its size and site. A tumour situated in a 'silent' area of the brain, e.g., the frontal lobe, may grow to a large size before producing any effect. On the other hand a tumour developing in the motor cortex may produce significant symptoms and focal signs at an early stage. Both symptoms and signs tend to develop progressively as the tumour enlarges.

A tumour in the frontal lobe produces few physical signs. Early symptoms are usually related to minor degrees of mental disturbance such as memory loss, depression and intellectual impairment. Anosmia may result from pressure on the olfactory nerve and usually means an olfactory groove meningioma.

Tumours situated in the motor cortex may produce Jacksonian fits (p. 260), with or without monoplegia.

A parietal lobe tumour may produce various sensory disturbances including apraxia, agnosia, receptive dysphasia and spatial disorientation.

Occipital lobe tumours often cause visual hallucinations and may produce homonymous hemianopia.

Temporal lobe tumours may produce symptoms of temporal lobe epilepsy and auditory, gustatory, olfactory or visual hallucinations.

The space within the rigid skull occupied by an enlarging tumour will eventually lead to an increase in intra-cranial pressure. Raised intra-cranial pressure causes headache, vomiting and papilloedema. Initially the headache may be localised to the same side as the lesion but later it becomes generalised. Characteristically the headache is present in the morning and tends to wear off as the day proceeds. It is eased by standing and aggravated by exertion or by any activity which normally leads to an increase in intra-cranial pressure, e.g., coughing or straining at stool. Only rarely does the headache conform to the classical description of being 'like a band round the head'. Vomiting occurs as the headache becomes more severe.

It is important to remember that a patient with an intracerebral tumour may present with symptoms of raised intra-cranial pressure.

Acoustic Neuroma

An acoustic neuroma is usually unilateral but may be bilateral in neurofibromatosis. It is slow growing, and tends to occur most commonly between the ages of 20 and 40. Symptoms relate to auditory and vestibular dysfunction. The first symptom is usually tinnitus, followed by progressive deafness and evidence of vestibular disturbance. Sometimes vestibular symptoms may precede auditory symptoms. As growth advances the 5th and 7th cranial nerves may become involved.

Neurofibromatosis (Van Recklinghausen's Disease)

Neurofibromatosis is a disease of congenital origin characterised by the presence of single or multiple swellings of cutaneous nerves and irregular brown pigmented spots or patches on the skin (café-au-lait spots). Rarely tumours may also occur in other tissues, e.g., meningioma or glioma. The cutaneous nodules also vary in size and shape.

Diagnosis

The possibility of an intra-cerebral tumour should be considered whenever a patient shows evidence of a focal cerebral abnormality. Epilepsy developing for the first time, or evidence of change in behaviour or intellect occurring at any time, is suggestive of the diagnosis. The history should include enquiry about all systems, since malignant neoplasms of the bowel, breast and lung commonly metastisize to the brain.

The physical examination of the central nervous system should be thorough and unhurried. An important factor which should alert the physician to the possibility of an intra-cerebral tumour is the progressive development of physical signs, which will usually follow a logical pattern dependent upon the site and structures involved. The physical examination should therefore be repeated at intervals. A chest X-ray should always be arranged to exclude a primary neoplasm in the lung.

If a tumour of the nervous system is suspected the patient should be referred to a consultant neurologist for investigation.

Management

There is no treatment for neurofibromatosis except to remove fibromas which are unsightly or causing pressure symptoms.

The subsequent management of other patients will depend upon the degree of residual neurological deficit.

CARE OF THE PARAPLEGIC PATIENT

Paraplegia results from disease or injury of the spinal cord. There is complete or partial loss of motor, sensory and autonomic function below the level of the lesion. Successful domiciliary management depends upon strict attention to detail and the active co-operation of relatives, friends and members of the primary care health team. The key to success is good nursing and paying particular attention to the care of the skin, bladder, bowels and joints.

The Skin

The skin of a patient who remains immobile for long periods whether lying in bed or sitting in a chair, will be subject to sustained pressure over the weight-bearing points, particularly bony protuberances such as the scapulae, spinal processes, sacrum, heels, elbows, and posterior iliac crests when in the supine position; the anterior iliac spines and patellae when in the prone position; and the malleolus, femoral condyle, trochanter and iliac crest when in the lateral position. Long continued pressure leads to tissue necrosis due to ischaemia following compression of cutaneous blood vessels.

The early signs of pressure necrosis is reddening of the skin surface. Any such areas should not again be subject to pressure until the skin has returned to normal. Weight bearing should be avoided for any areas where the skin surface becomes broken.

In order to avoid the effects of prolonged pressure it is essential that tne patient's position should be changed frequently, at least every 2 hours, day and night. Whenever the patient is turned, the areas of skin that have been subject to pressure should be massaged gently to stimulate local blood flow. A bland cream may be used as a lubricant. It is important to avoid vigorous massage which may precipitate skin damage. Bony protuberances may be protected to some extent by the careful placing of pillows. The use of a ripple mattress or water mattress will help to distribute the weight of the patient more evenly and help to avoid concentration of pressure on the prominent bony points.

Hard objects should not be allowed to come into contact with the skin, especially hot water bottles which are a particular hazard since they may also cause a burn. If used at all, hot water bottles should be placed at least one blanket thickness away from the patient's body and never beneath the patient.

With the passage of time the patient's skin will become more resistant to the effect of pressure; after 9—12 months he may be allowed to remain up to 8 hours in one position.

If the skin is exposed to moisture for long periods it becomes water-logged and more susceptible to pressure injury. As most paraplegic patients are incontinent, precautions need to be taken against allowing the patient to lie in a wet bed. A silicone barrier cream will help to protect the skin against the effects of moisture.

Urinary Tract

During the first few weeks following the acute onset of paraplegia the bladder is atonic and readily distensible so that retention of urine with overflow incontinence may result. Retained urine is a potential source of infection and steps should be taken to ensure that the atonic bladder is kept empty. This is best done by means of an indwelling urethral catheter. The potential risk of infection from the presence of the catheter is less than if a full atonic bladder is allowed to remain. While the catheter is *in situ* samples of urine should be examined every second day for evidence of infection and appropriate treatment prescribed if necessary. Later some tone returns to the bladder musculature and function becomes automatic, urine being evacuated involuntarily in response to bladder distention, and the catheter can be removed. However the bladder is rarely emptied completely and the potential risk of infection remains. Evacuation of the bladder can be assisted by manual compression over the hypogastrium.

The presence of residual urine in the bladder is a potential source for the formation of bladder calculi as well as infection, especially if the patient is allowed to remain immobile for long periods. Calculi may also form in the renal pelvis. Therefore frequent turning of the patient is as important for care of the renal tract as it is for care of the skin. Calculus formation is more likely if the urine is allowed to become highly concentrated due to deficient fluid intake, and it should be remembered that an immobile patient lying in bed may lose a significant amount of fluid from sweating.

The management of the patient with urinary incontinence is directed primarily towards preventing the patient from lying in a wet bed and so making skin damage more likely. In the male patient a penile clamp may be used and removed at intervals.

Incontinence pads, cellulose wadding, or other absorbent material, may be placed under the patient but must be changed at frequent intervals. In the female patient the use of absorbent material may be the only practical solution.

Bowels

Constipation may result from a combination of inactivity and reduced fluid intake and may lead to faecal impaction with extra discomfort for the patient. It is best prevented by attention to the diet, and if necessary, a twice weekly enema. Commonly a paraplegic patient nursed at home is given an 'invalid' diet which is low in roughage. The relatives should be given specific instructions to include an adequate amount of roughage and fluid in the diet. In the paraplegic patient the bowel will usually function reflexly in response to bowel distention and this may lead to faecal incontinence. The skin and bed-clothes should be protected in the manner described for the management of urinary incontinence.

Limbs

The immobile patient, whether lying in bed or sitting in a chair, may quickly develop contractures and deformities of the joints. From the earliest stage of the illness the legs should be moved passively through their whole range of movement three or four times a day, not only to maintain joint movement and exercise the muscles but also to stimulate the venous return and thus help to prevent phlebothrombosis.

During the early stages of the illness the muscles will by hypotonic, but some tone will later return. The skilled physiotherapist can take advantage of any surviving postural reflexes to enable the patient to stand. Every effort should be made to encourge the patient to remain independently mobile; various forms of support may be used, including calipers. If a wheelchair is necessary the patient should be encouraged to adopt an active wheelchair life.

The Health Team

All members of the health team, including the district nurse, health visitor and social worker, may be involved at one time or another in the care of the paraplegic patient or in giving support to the patient's family. The district nurse will be the person most concerned with day-to-day care and will play an important part in instructing the relatives in home nursing techniques. The health visitor or social worker may become involved as specific needs arise, and will assist with the mobilisation of community services, including voluntary agencies, for the patient's benefit.

Voluntary organisations may be found who will be prepared to assist with shopping, or taking a patient out in a wheelchair. Some agencies are prepared to provide sitters-in to relieve relatives, and to help with home decorating and repairs. The extent to which voluntary agencies are available and their capacity to help will vary from one locality to another. The provision of home helps, laundry services and meals-on-wheels may be obtained through the local Social Services Department who may also be able to provide information about voluntary organisations.

References

1. Gower, W. R. (1893). *A Manual of Diseases of the Nervous System*, 2nd Ed., vol. 2, (Edinburgh and London: Churchill Livingstone).
2. Russell, R. W. R. (1963). *Brain* **86**, 425.
3. Charcot, J. M. and Bouchard, C. (1868). *Arch. Physiol. norm. Path.* **1**, 10.
4. Acheson, J. and Hutchinson, E. C. (1971). *Quart. J. Med.* **40**, 15.
5. Cole, F. M. and Yates, P. O. (1968). *Neurol. Minneap.* **18**, 255.
6. Acheson, J. Acheson, H. W. K. and Tellwright, J. M. (1968). *J. roy. Coll. gen. Pract.* **16**, 428.
7. Acheson, J. and Hutchinson, E. C. (1964). *Lancet* ii, 871.

15

Gynaecology

G. Lloyd

INTRODUCTION

Most illness associated with the female genital tract occurs after the age of 15 years. Infective conditions and disorders of menstruation are most common between the ages of 15 and 45. Degenerative and malignant disease occur most frequently in women over the age of 45.

Table 15.1 shows the comparative consultation rate for gynaecological and other diseases and Table 15.2 shows the annual number of episodes and the consultation rate for the various types of gynaecological disorders. Clearly gynaecology forms a substantial portion of the family practitioner's workload. Preventive procedures, such as contraceptive advice and cervical cytology, take up a significant proportion of the family practitioner's time. Almost a quarter of two million smears taken in England and Wales each year are taken by family practitioners.

The identification and management of gynaecological problems depend

Table 15.1 Comparative table of various morbidity groups (from Morbidity Statistics from General Practice (1974), HMSO) consultation rates per 1000 female patient per annum.

Diseases of the respiratory system	535.2
Mental disorders	400.5
Gynaecology, including advice on contraception and sterilisation	<u>332.6</u>
Complications of pregnancy and normal pre-natal and post-natal care	299.1
Diseases of the circulatory system	273.3
Diseases of the musculoskeletal system and connective tissue	220.1
Diseases of the nervous system and sense organs	210.0
Diseases of the skin and subcutaneous tissue	202.0
Accidents, poisoning and violence	126.2
Diseases of the digestive system	115.2
Infective and parasitic	109.8
Endocrine, nutritional and metabolic disease	91.0
Neoplasms other than genital	38.7

Table 15.2   Gynaecological consultations in general practice (from Morbidity Statistics from General Practice (1974), HMSO).

	Episodes per annum (per 1000 patients at risk)		Consultations per annum (per 1000 patients at risk)	
	Number	Per cent	Number	Per cent
Contraceptive advice	66.8	35.3	156.7	47.5
Vaginal discharge	23.9	12.6	33.8	10.2
Cervical smear	22.1	11.7	23.2	7.0
Amenorrhoea and hypomenorrhoea (excluding pregnancy)	15.3	8.1	21.5	6.5
Menorrhagia	12.1	6.4	20.4	6.2
Irregular menstruation	11.1	5.9	16.3	4.9
Menopausal symptoms	11.0	5.8	16.0	4.8
Dysmenorrhoea	8.4	4.5	12.0	3.6
Intermenstrual and postmenopausal bleeding	5.8	3.1	8.5	2.6
Utero-vaginal prolapse	4.0	2.1	6.8	2.1
Cervical erosion	2.8	1.5	4.0	1.2
Benign neoplasms of uterus and other female genital organs	1.6	0.8	3.4	1.0
Salpingitis and oophoritis	1.1	0.6	2.5	0.8
Malignant disease of cervix uteri	0.6	0.3	1.8	0.6
Sterilisation	1.2	0.6	1.5	0.4
Ovulation pain	0.5	0.3	0.7	0.2
Disorders of menarche	0.5	0.3	0.6	0.2
Malignant disease of corpus uteri	0.2	0.1	0.6	0.2
Total	189.0		330.3	

upon securing a good history and undertaking an adequate pelvic examination. Yet, despite the commonality of gynaecological disorders, many family practitioners take an inadequate history and some are reluctant to carry out a pelvic examination of any kind.

The emphasis, in this chapter, will therefore be on procedure and management which can be undertaken in family practice. Referral for specialist advice is indicated where appropriate.

History

The component parts of the gynaecological history are shown in Table 15.3. It is prudent to obtain all this history whenever patients present with gynaecological complaints. If necessary, a duplicated pro-forma can be used and included in the medical record.

Table 15.3   Gynaecological history

Age of patient
Single, married or widowed
Duration of marriage
Occupation of husband
Age of menarche
Menstrual cycle — duration of menses
*   — intermenstrual interval*
Menstrual pain
Amount of menstrual loss (pads or tampons per day)
Date of L.M.P.
Has sexual intercourse taken place
Number of pregnancies
Complications of pregnancies
Number of abortions (including termination)
Vaginal discharge
Abdominal pain or discomfort
Backache
Urinary frequency
Urinary pain
Haematuria
Incontinence — stress
*   — urgency*
*   — other*
Contraceptive method used
Timing of last bath or douche
Time bladder last emptied.

To the family practitioner, some of the history may already be known and the full history need only be repeated when a change in the clinical condition presented by the patient is apparent.

Some parts of the history suggested require emphasis or explanation.

The occupation of the husband is a good indicator of social class. Carcinoma of the cervix is more common in the lower social groups.

Knowing if sexual intercourse has taken place helps the doctor to be more aware of the possibility of pregnancy and also gives an indication of the likely ease of pelvic examination.

Urinary symptoms are commonly associated with ovarian tumours and salpingitis as well as utero-vaginal prolapse.

Recent bathing or douching will modify the clinical appearance of the vagina and cervix and minimise supporting evidence of vaginal discharge.

Knowing if the bladder is supposedly full or empty before embarking on clinical examination is often useful. The body of the uterus and the appendages can be difficult to palpate and uncomfortable for the patient, if the bladder is full. An empty bladder does not permit clinical demonstration of stress incontinence. Interrupting clinical examination to allow the patient to empty or fill the bladder can be avoided if the state is established before proceeding to examination.

Pelvic Examination

Examination of the female genital tract has two components. Firstly there is a visual part of the examination and secondly a bimanual palpation of the organs. This is the correct order of the examination so that lubricant used or bleeding which might occur during digital examination, does not obscure visual findings. Such examination should be conducted in the consulting rooms. The circumstances need to be very unusual for a family practitioner to undertake pelvic examination for gynaecological reasons in the patient's home.

The preferred position for the patient is that position with which the examiner is most confident and experienced. However, on the type of couch usually used by the family practitioner, the left lateral or Sim's position, permits easier manipulation of a speculum as well as allowing the patient a better degree of modesty.

The equipment required to undertake an adequate pelvic examination is indicated in Table 15.4. As far as possible, disposable equipment should be used by family practitioners unless there is access to a central sterilisation unit. Perfunctory boiling does not prevent cross infection by trichomonas or monilia. Disposable gloves, which are cheap, should always be used. There are a few varieties of disposable speculum. The best is the clear plastic bivalve variety.

The volsellum should be of the single toothed variety as this causes less pain on application as well as less bleeding. In use the volsellum should grasp the portio vaginalis of the anterior cervix rather than the lip of the cervix where it

Table 15.4   Equipment for pelvic examination.

Examination couch
Source of illumination, which is preferably of the shadow reduced type and which can be readily manipulated into an appropriate position.
Disposable polythene gloves
Speculum, preferably simple, disposable, bivalve
Single-toothed volsellum
Sponge holder
Uterine sound
Ayre spatulas
Lubricant
Glass slides for Ayre smear
Fixative for Ayre smear, liquid or aerosol.

---

obstructs the rotation of an Ayre spatula. The function of the volsellum is to mobilise the cervix into the best visual position.

Pelvic examination begins with visual inspection of the vulva, urethra and introitus. A lightly lubricated speculum is then inserted into the vagina and the cervix identified. Following inspection of the cervix a smear can be taken or a swab or aspirate taken from the posterior fornix of the vagina. The vagina itself is inspected during withdrawal of the speculum.

Bimanual examination follows, palpation of the uterine body and of the appendages taking place in that order. An empty bladder is desirable. The right appendage is usually more easily palpated than the left. Particular attention should be paid to the position and size of the organs palpated and to any tenderness elicited. In the very young, the virgin or the very old, vaginal examination may not be possible in the environment of family practice. Though some clinical information can be obtained by rectal examination, it is preferable to refer such patients to a consulting gynaecologist who can undertake a more adequate examination under anaesthesia.

VAGINAL DISCHARGE

The normal vaginal epithelium produces an acid secretion (PH about 4.5) which contains desquamated epithelial cells and bacteria. The endocervical epithelium contributes an alkaline secretion which contains desquamated cells. The epithelium of the vagina is rich in glycogen which is converted by Döderlein's bacillus into lactic acid. Normal vaginal discharge is called leucorrhoea and needs no treatment. Infection of the vagina occurs more readily when the acidity of the secretion is lowered, in particular before puberty, during menstruation, during the puerperium and after the menopause.

Apart from venereal infections two common vaginal infections are encountered in family practice: *Trichomonas vaginalis* vaginitis and Monilia vaginitis.

Trichomoniasis

The causal organism is a motile flagellated protozoon. In many women, trichomonas does not cause symptomatic infection. In others there is a profuse greenish yellow fluid discharge which only occasionally has a frothy appearance. There is usually an associated cervicitis and a distressing vulvitis characterised by intense irritation rather than itching. Infection is usually transmitted during intercourse. Infection with trichomonas which causes symptoms can be recognised on visual inspection of the vagina. The only satisfactory and reliable supportive diagnostic aid in family practice is a cervical smear. Most cases of trichomonal infection respond to treatment with 200 mg metronidazole thrice daily for one or two weeks. Because the infection is sexually transmitted the sexual partner should receive treatment at the same time. Intercourse should be avoided during treatment.

Monilia Vaginitis

The causal organism is the mycelium *Candida albicans*. The infection is more likely to be encountered during pregnancy, following wide spectrum antibiotic therapy or with glycosuria. Apart from the discharge the usual symptom is vulval itching resulting from associated vulvitis. The appearance of the infection on visual examination of the vagina is quite different from trichomonas infection. The discharge is more solid and white patches are seen on the vaginal wall. The cervix is commonly infected.

Diagnosis is most readily achieved by visual examination. A cervical smear or vaginal aspirate may reveal mycelium but not as reliably as trichomonas. Treatment is by vaginal pessary, nystatin pessaries (100 000 units) inserted twice daily for ten days, being preferred. The sexual partner may harbour mycelium in the urethra or bladder and can be treated with orally administered nystatin.

Other Vaginal Infections

Vulvo-vaginitis in Pre-pubertal Children

Vulvo-vaginitis in children may be caused by a variety of organisms, including coliforms, various cocci, monilia or trichomonads. Discharge is usually purulent. Foreign bodies are rarely a cause. The vulva can be inspected readily in children and evidence of monilial infection detected. Inspection of the vagina is very difficult in children and if required, is better carried out under anaesthesia.

Gentle, one-finger digital examination, in the presence of a parent or guardian, is permissible and a foreign body may be detectable. By gentle rectal examination, vaginal discharge may be milked from the vagina in children and a smear or aspirate taken. When doubt persists or the child is under ten years old, the assistance of a gynaecologist should be sought. Treatment of vaginal discharge in children consists of treatment appropriate to the identified organism together with oral oestrogens (stilbestrol, 0.5 mg daily for 14 days).

Senile Vaginitis

Senile vaginitis may be caused by a variety of organisms and the loss of vaginal acidity encourages coliform or coccal infections. Visual inspection of the vagina usually reveals a thin watery discharge which is commonly blood stained. The walls of the vagina are usually smooth and glossy in appearance in the elderly.

Monilia infection is commoner in diabetic patients. Treatment is the same as for vaginitis in children.

Malignant Disease

Malignant disease as a cause of vaginal discharge should always be suspected, particularly in the post-menopausal, prurulent vaginal discharge being a common presenting symptom of cancer of the endometrium.

ABNORMAL VAGINAL BLEEDING

Normal vaginal bleeding occurs under two circumstances; during menstruation and the third stage of labour. Abnormal bleeding in pregnancy is discussed in Chapter 16. Abnormal bleeding other than during pregnancy can be considered in two main groups. Firstly, abnormalities of menstruation and secondly, bleeding unassociated with menstruation.

Abnormal Menstrual Bleeding

Menstruation is insufficient if the loss occurs at intervals of 42 days or longer or the duration of loss is one day or less, or if both of these occur.

Menstruation is excessive if bleeding occurs at intervals of less than 21 days, or if the duration of loss is longer than seven days or if more than twelve well-soaked pads or tampons are used during a single day or if any combination of these occur.

Having defined the limits of normality, it does not follow that all abnormal menstruation calls for treatment.

Insufficient Menstruation

Five associated circumstances require attention to insufficient menstruation:

1. Oral contraceptives should be prescribed with great caution, if menstruation is insufficient. An already inadequate hypothalamic-pituitary-ovarian function can be further suppressed leading to infertility.
2. Insufficient menstruation may indicate anovular cycles which can be confirmed by means of basal temperature records. Infertility resulting from anovular menstruation can be corrected by suitable hormone therapy, though in the UK the appropriate preparations are not available to family practitioners. Reference to a specialist is indicated.
3. Insufficient menstruation may be caused by anaemia.
4. More rarely, endometrial tuberculosis can cause insufficient menstruation.

5. Anxiety may induce menstrual suppression through a process of cortical stimulation of the hypothalamic-pituitary ovarian axis.

These five circumstances excepted, insufficient menstruation does not require investigation or treatment.

Total amenorrhoea can result from a variety of hormonal or genetic causes, such as dwarfism, Cushing's syndrome, Simmond's disease, Turner's syndrome or Klinefelter's syndrome. All these are rare occurrences and if in any way suspected, indicate referral to a gynaecologist for intensive investigation.

Excessive Menstruation

Excessive menstruation is considerably more common and is a symptom of a wide variety of conditions. It is important to establish as clearly as possible the periodicity and amount of menstrual loss. Excessive menstruation may have been present for many months before the patient consults a doctor, and securing an adequate retrospective pattern of menstruation may be difficult. Prospective recording of menstruation can be undertaken by most women using an ordinary diary. A symbol such as an 'X' can be entered for each pad or tampon used on each day of bleeding. Whilst bearing in mind the need to avoid delay in the search for cancer and anaemia, prospective menstrual records can be of great help to the family practitioner in understanding the nature of excessive menstruation.

At puberty and the menopause, menstruation can result from the action of oestrogens alone, unopposed by progesterones. Under this condition, menstural periods tend to be heavier and longer than normal. In most instances the condition is self-limiting. At puberty, prolonged excessive bleeding of this type can be corrected by means of cyclical progesterone therapy such as norethisterone (10 mg) given orally daily from the 15th to the 25th day of the cycle.

At the menopause it is important to exclude endometrial carcinoma and referral to a specialist is indicated. Presistent heavy bleeding can usually be abruptly arrested by large doses of progesterones, for example Primolut N (norethisterone 10 mg) thrice daily or intramuscular progesterone. Associated anaemia should be discovered and adequately treated.

The cause of most instances of excessive menstruation during the reproductive period is not understood. In some women the ovarian follicles fail to proceed to form corpora lutea so that only oestrogens are produced. These anovular cycles tend to be associated with heavy, prolonged and irregular menstruation. On pelvic examination the ovaries are usually readily palpable, may be enlarged and are frequently tender. Short term relief can be obtained with cyclical hormone therapy.

Excessive menstrual bleeding which remains unresolved after four menstrual cycles is an indication for specialist assistance.

Significant interference with the life-style of the patient or the development of anaemia are good reasons for aggressive treatment which might include hysterectomy.

Bleeding not Associated with Menstruation

The commonest cause, today, of vaginal bleeding, unassociated with menstruation, is the 'break-through' bleeding in women taking the oral contraceptive pill. The usual cause is a hormone imbalance which can be corrected by increasing the dose of progesterone.

Oral contraceptives encourage cervical erosion and monilia vaginitis, both of which may exhibit slight vaginal bleeding, particularly during or after intercourse.

Cancer of the vulva, vagina or more frequently of the cervix, cause fresh bright red vaginal bleeding. Cancer of the body of the uterus is more likely to cause a blood stained discharge or bleeding which resembles menstrual loss.

Other less common causes of vaginal bleeding are vaginitis, urethral caruncle, cervicitis, cervical polyp and endometrial polyp.

Both post-coital bleeding and post-menopausal bleeding demand rigorous examination and investigation to exclude an organic, possibly malignant, cause.

THE MENOPAUSE

At the menopause, the reproductive period of life and menstruation cease. Most women pass through the menopause between the ages of 45 and 50. Early menopause, between 35 and 45, is usually associated with a more severe reaction but also with a sevenfold lowering in the incidence of coronary thrombosis. Over 80 per cent of women experience a menopause without significant adverse reaction.

For those women who suffer at the menopause there is a need for both explanation and effective treatment. Vera Liff has described her menopause as follows:

> 'In the hinterland of feeling,
> hormones with a rock and roll,
> sudden madcap dance concealing
> agonies of human soul'

The clinical pattern of the menopause reflects physiological changes. The ovarian response to pituitary stimulation first fails so that progesterone is no longer produced. This leads to anovular menstrual cycles and, in some women, to excessive menstrual loss due to the unopposed action of oestrogens.

The release of oestrogens eventually ceases and it is this which probably causes most of the symptoms of the menopause which are commonly of two kinds, physical and psychological. The physical effects, which are mainly vasomotor reactions, include amenorrhoea, hot flushes, headache, dyspepsia, vaginal atrophy with narrowing and breast atrophy. Narrowing of the vagina can lead to dyspareunia. The psychological effects are loss of libido and an awareness of loss of fertility. These two can be independent and it should not be assumed that recognising an awareness of loss of fertility will correct a loss of libido. Depression associated with the menopause has not been satisfactorily explained and is usually enountered only in women who have a previous history of depressive illness.

Symptoms of the menopause which the patient expresses to be unacceptable, should be treated. Effective treatment is almost invariably by means of hormones. Excessive vaginal bleeding due to progesterone withdrawal can be relieved by cyclical progesterone treatment. Symptoms attributable to oestrogen withdrawal should be appropriately treated. Ethinyl oestradiol is better tolerated than stilbestrol. A regime of 0.05 mg three times daily for two weeks, followed by a twice daily dose for two weeks, followed by a once daily dose for two weeks, is usually effective and can be repeated at necessary intervals. The small risk of venous thrombosis resulting from oestrogen therapy is acceptable in the presence of disabling symptoms.

UNUSUAL SEXUAL BEHAVIOUR

An appreciation of sexual behaviour can vary between sexual partners and may manifest during gynaecological enquiry. The only abnormal sexual behaviour is that which is unacceptable to one of the sexual partners and in any event, only the unacceptable will be presented as a symptom. The family practitioner should have no fear to seek, understand and counsel on abnormal sexual behaviour. One condition helps both understanding and counsel and that is that both partners should be consulted, independently and together. Should one of the sexual partners be registered with another practitioner, his consent to interview is desirable.

FERTILITY AND INFERTILITY

The ability of man and wife to procreate is a product of the sum of their respective fertility. The one may summate with the other to a degree which requires advice on the avoidance of pregnancy. Otherwise the one may be inadequate for the other, so that the family practitioner needs to advise on appropriate treatment including alternative ways of securing a family. Both these roles are supremely relevant to family practice. It cannot too strongly be emphasised that the managment of fertility, either excessive or insufficient, should not devolve to the gynaecologist, urologist or surgeon. Their advice can and should be sought but only in the strictest terms, as specialist consultation.

The role of the family practitioner begins with recognising the problem. This may occur when, almost invariably, the woman presents with infertility or when the family practitioner, perceptive of the patient's circumstances, can legitimately enquire about the avoidance of an increase in the size of the family.

Excessive fertility, being the commoner, is first considered. The only truly satisfactory method of limiting pregnancy is sterilisation. When both husband and wife request this procedure the family practitioner has a duty to secure suitable arrangements. Gynaecologists and urologists, since the 1968 Abortion Act, will generally accede to sterilisation of one or the other of any couple aged over 25 years who have two living children. It is a matter of marital choice whether the husband or the wife is sterilised. Female sterilisation is instantaneous whilst male sterilisation is delayed.

Some women desire to retain their fertility and are prepared to accept the risks associated with other methods of avoiding pregnancy. The oral contraceptive pill is both effective and popular but may be associated with unacceptable ill-effects, such as excessive weight gain, depression or headache. Venous and arterial thrombosis have exaggerated claims of incidence.

Intra-uterine contraceptive devices have a 10 per cent frequency of unacceptable effects. including excessive menstrual loss, dysmenorrhoea, salpingitis, rejection, as well as an incidence of pregnancy in excess of 5 per cent.

Other methods, such as sheaths, caps, 'C-film' or spermicidal foam, have the very important limitation of allowing intercourse only when the facilitity is available.

Infertility or sub-fertility presents as a primary condition in about 5 per cent of marriages. The problem is one to be shared jointly between the partners as regards to cause, investigation, emotional reaction and management. It is usual to allow twelve montus of regular intercourse to elapse before accepting a state of primary infertility. The family practitioner may be able to identify causes such as infrequent or inadequate intercourse and about which proper advice can be given. Should further investigation be needed, it is advisable to secure this from a single source for both partners, usually by referral to a gynaecologist.

There are practical and emotional advantages to be gained by insisting at the investigative stage, that the problem is normally shared by the married couple. The primary objectives of investigation are to establish the quality and volume of sperm produced by the man and the quality of ovulation and potency of the fallopian tubes in the female. If either or both situations prevail, the assistance of a specialist is required.

Recent progress in the correction of failure of the pituitary to stimulate the female gonads has led to a reduction in overall infertility. Though attention is drawn by the news media to multiple pregnancy associated with pituitary hormone replacement, the accumulated evidence now shows that some 90 per cent of pregnancies so secured are single pregnancies.

In the absence of an adequate physical explanation for infertility, the emotional interaction between partners should be explored and if necessary, the support of a psychiatrist or psychologist, experienced in the management of psychosexual problems, sought.

During any or all of these procedures the family practitioner should maintain a close relationship with the family in order to secure adequate investigation and management. For some couples, adoption may be an acceptable solution.

Secondary infertility calls for a similar pattern of investigation and management as primary infertility. On the other hand, infertility imposed by knowledge of significant genetic inheritance requires separate specialist guidance.

UTERO-VAGINAL PROLAPSE

The aetiology, anatomy and classification of utero vaginal prolapse is irrelevant to the family practitioner. Women do not complain of a first or second degree prolapse but rather of one or more of the following symptoms: a bearing down sensation, frequency of micturation, stress incontinence or feeling a tumour at the vulva. Cystocoele, rectocoele or uterine prolapse can be detected on clinical examination if the patient is asked to strain downward before a speculum is inserted.

Referral to a gynaecologist for surgical intervention is indicated if symptoms are present or if delay would be associated with increased anaesthetic or post-operative complications. The woman who has chronic bronchitis or hypertensive heart disease cannot afford a delay in treatment which awaits the onset of symptomatic prolapse. Supportive pessaries are no longer a satisfactory means of treating prolapse.

STRESS INCONTINENCE

Incontinence of urine occurring on coughing or straining is termed stress incontinence. The incontinence in turn causes emotional stress. The cause of the symptoms is usually damage to the neck of the bladder at the time of delivery. Women of the post-menopausal age are most commonly affected. Some women suffer transient stress incontinence shortly after delivery and recovery is encouraged by pelvic floor exercises. Stress incontinence and prolapse may be associated, though they result from separate injuries to the genital tract.

Many women conceal their stress incontinence for long periods and will rearrange their daily schedule to allow frequent emptying of the bladder. Emotional anxiety and, in particular, a fear of a public demonstration of incontinence, exacerbates the symptoms. Common restrictions which women with stress incontinence place on themselves are — disassociation from public gatherings and inhibition of travel by means of public transport. Gynaecological pads and a variety of proprietary protective garments may be worn to increase personal security and conceal from others the effects of stress incontinence.

Stress incontinence may be seen during pelvic examination if the patient is encouraged to cough lustily and so long as the bladder contains sufficient urine.

Investigations such as a radiological stress cystogram do not help make the diagnosis but can be useful to the gynaecologist to determine the preferred method of treatment.

Stress incontinence which fails to respond to pelvic floor exercises or faradism, can be treated surgically, treatment taking place in hospital. The gynaecologist can be helped to determine the method and urgency of treatment if the family practitioner can indicate the degree of personal anxiety and behavioural change which stress incontinence has caused to the patient.

GYNAECOLOGICAL BENIGN TUMOURS

Vulva

The commonest benign tumour seen at the vulva is a cyst or abscess of Bartholin's gland. The condition is seen during the woman's active sexual life.

Infection can be caused by almost any organism. The treatment of cyst or abscess is surgical, marsupialisation being the easiest and most effective treatment.

Condylomata acuminata, of viral origin, are not uncommon and many respond to the application of podophyllin ointment. Cautery or excision is indicated in resistant cases.

Sebaceous cysts and haematomas of the vulva are occasionally seen. Much rarer are fibromas, lipomas and hidradenoma.

Vagina

Cysts of the vagina are not uncommon and are usually seen in the lower third of the vagina.

The cyst may arise from the vaginal epithelium or from remains of Gartner's duct. They rarely cause symptoms other than dyspareunia and treatment is by surgical excision.

Cervix

The only benign tumour of the cervix is a polyp. There is usually an associated cervicitis and either the polyp or the cervicitis may cause vaginal discharge or post-coital bleeding. Treatment is by surgical evulsion or diathermy.

Body of the Uterus

Three benign tumours occur in the body of the uterus. Fibroids are the most common and are present in 20 per cent of women over the age of 35 years. Fibroids which increase the endometrial surface can cause excessive menstrual bleeding and sometimes infertility. By and large, fibroids are otherwise symptomless. On clinical examination, fibroids are detected more by an irregularity of the uterine outline than by an increase in the size of the uterus. There is an association between fibroids and cancer of the endometrium and some fibroids may undergo sarcomatous degenerative change. Symptomless small fibroids can be ignored. Patients who have symptomatic or large fibroids should be referred for specialist opinion.

Small mucosal polypi of the endometrium can give rise to vaginal discharge or to intermenstrual bleeding. If suspected, curettage of the uterus is indicated.

Ectopic deposits of endometrium in the uterine wall cause tumour formation, adenomyosis. The condition may be localised forming a tumour resembling a fibroid on palpation. More commonly, the condition is diffuse, causing a general enlargement of the uterus. Chocolate cysts are rare in the myometrium, because any bleeding is discharged into the uterine cavity, often causing excessive menstrual bleeding. The only satisfactory treatment is hysterectomy.

Ovary

Benign ovarian tumours can be found at any age and are most common between the ages of 25 and 45.

The commonest symptoms of benign ovarian tumours are frequency of micturation and dysuria. Very large tumours, usually cystadenoma, cause abdominal swelling and discomfort due to pressure. Torsion of the pedicle of an ovarian cyst presents as an acute abdominal emergency.

The clinical diagnosis of ovarian tumour is made on pelvic examination. It is not usually possible to determine the exact nature of the tumour or to exclude malignancy, except at laparotomy. All patients believed to have an ovarian tumour should be referred for specialist opinion.

Fallopian Tubes

Benign tumours of the fallopian tubes are almost invariably infective, being the end result of long-standing and untreated salpingitis. The patient regularly has lower abdominal pain and menstruation is usually excessive. Bimanual examination reveals tumours which are tender, compared with benign ovarian cysts, which are not. The condition is frequently first encountered in a woman complaining of infertility, which may be primary or secondary. Associated urinary symptoms are common.

MALIGNANT TUMOURS

Of all deaths due to malignant disease of women, malignant diseases of the female genital tract account for 20 per cent. For women below age 50, cancer of the cervix alone is responsible for a quarter of deaths due to cancer.

Morbidity surveys in family practice show that cancer of the cervix has a threefold incidence of both episodes and consultation over malignant disease of the body of the uterus.

The Vulva and Vagina

Primary malignant lesions of the vulva and vagina are rare. In the former location there is usually a preceding history of pruritus or leukoplakia, and the cancer presents as an ulcerated nodule.

Primary or secondary cancer of the vagina occurs in the elderly and presents with vaginal bleeding of bright red blood. Secondary vaginal cancer is almost invariably spread from the cervix. On clinical examination both primary and secondary cancer of the vagina are seen to be friable growths which bleed easily on touching.

Treatment of cancer of both vulva and vagina may be by surgery or radiotherapy, usually following consultation between gynaecologist and radiotherapist. Suspicion of cancer in either location calls for urgent consultant opinion.

Cervix

Cancer of the cervix is both the most common and most successfully remedial cancer of the genital tract. The action of the family practitioner is critical to successful management because early detection is well within the limits of possibility in family practice. Screening procedures by means of exfoliative cytology of identifiable at-risk groups of women has been shown to be both practical and valuable. Close collaboration with nursing colleagues improve the practical aspects of screening programmes. A crucial precursor of success is an accurate knowledge of the identity of women within the age groups 25–65. A practice age-sex register provides this information. In the light of current knowledge, it can no longer be regarded as reasonable for the family practitioner to await the presentation of symptomatic cancer of the cervix by his patients or to anticipate that others will undertake pre-symptomatic screening. Every family practitioner has to consider seriously if he can afford to sacrifice opportunities which permit very high curative and survival rates of cancer of the cervix for his patients. It must be a matter of concern to all trainees in family practice to learn the techniques of cervical cytology. Non-invasive (Stage 0) cancer of the cervix, as well as pre-symptomatic invasive cancer, can be detected with an accuracy of about 90 per cent by means of a cervical smear (cervical cytotest).

Some aspects of the cervical cytotest are worth emphasis. A positive test does not diagnose cancer but selects patients who require further investigation. A negative cytotest does not exclude cancer. Cancer is not determined by the appearance of a cell. All smears which are reported to contain suspicious cells (including dyskaryotic or dysplasic cells) demand referral of the patient for cervical biopsy. Infected material obscures the cervical smear and all such reported smears should always be repeated after appropriate treatment of the infection.

The essential requirements for cervical cytology in the surgery are a suitable couch, adequate illumination, a sterile speculum, an Ayre spatula or a cytopipette, a clean glass slide, fixative and a suitable container for the slide.

Specimens obtained by aspirate or scrape should be transferred quickly to the slide and spread thinly. The fixative, either liquid or spray, should be applied while the smear is still wet. The name of the patient should be written on the frosted end of the slide.

Any irregularity of the contour or appearance of the cervix or any bleeding which occurs following digital examination, may indicate more advanced cancer and calls for gynaecological specialist opinion.

The grading and initial treatment of cancer of the cervix takes place in hospital. Non remedial cancer of the cervix often results in protracted and painful illness. Spread of growth, via the parametrium, to the spine, causes debilitating low back pain. Spread of growth into the vagina causes substantial bleeding and anaemia. The family practitioner has the responsibility to secure, for his patients, as high a degree of comfort as is attainable by analgesia and spinal anaesthesia. The assistance of nursing colleagues and of relatives are invaluable in the terminal care of cancer of the cervix.

Body of the Uterus

Two malignant tumours of the body of the uterus are described.

Carcinoma of the uterus arises from the endometrium and is almost invariably a columner celled carcinoma. This is by far the most common malignant tumour of the body of the uterus.

Sarcoma of the uterus is much more rare and may arise in 0.2 per cent of fibroids of the uterus especially in large fibroids at the time of the menopause.

Whilst with treatment, the five-year survival rate for cancer of the endometrium is 60 per cent, survival consequent to sarcoma is very poor because of the rapid growth and spread of sarcomatous tumour.

In both carcinoma and sarcoma, abnormal vaginal bleeding or discharge is the presenting symptom. The cervical scrape or vaginal aspirate will usually only detect less than half of malignant tumours of the uterine body and is not a reliable early diagnostic aid.

Any unusual bleeding or blood stained vaginal discharge particularly at the time of the menopause or consequently, calls for more intensive investigation. Satisfactory diagnosis and treatment of malignant conditions of the body of the uterus take place in hospital.

Ovary

Malignant conditions of the ovary are very rarely identified with certainty in family practice. Pain and rapid growth of a tumour are very highly suggestive of a malignancy.

Any cause for suspicion of an ovarian enlargement or cyst, requires investigation and initial treatment in hospital. Ovarian carcinoma, which is irremedial, leads frequently to ascites. Relieving an ascites by abdominal tap is feasible in the surgery or the patient's home. Nursing colleagues are trained to support the family practitioner in this treatment.

16

Obstetrics

G. Lloyd

INTRODUCTION

During the past decade there has been a considerable change in the obstetric role of the family practitioner.

The rate of delivery in hospital obstetric units has increased dramatically and in some areas of the world, such as parts of Scotland, the hospital delivery rate is already 100 per cent.

This has come about as a result of a reduction in the birth rate, a more general recognition of safety requirements during labour, a sustained level of available maternity beds and a shortening of the duration of stay in hospital after delivery. There can no longer be justification for delivery, any more than appendectomy, to take place in the patient's home, or in a family practitioner obstetric unit which is not an integral part of a hospital unit.

Manipulative and interventive obstetrics is better conducted by skilled teams working in hospital units, fully equipped to deal with any emergency which might occur to the mother in labour or to the new-born. For the future, the role of the family practitioner in intra-natal care will be restricted to the very few who have prolonged and continuing special experience.

The movement towards practice in Health Centres and the development of community based obstetric teams of doctors and midwives, will allow better opportunity for organised ante-natal and post-natal care outside hospital. There is also an increasing awareness, as a result of both objective and subjective observation, of the importance of mental health in pregnancy.

This chapter will therefore be concerned with three aspects of obstetrics: ante-natal care, post-natal care, and mental health, in the context of family practice.

ANTE-NATAL CARE

Optimal ante-natal care may be defined as the accomplishment of those measures which are necessary to achieve a state of physical, mental and social well-being and the maintenance of this state prior to planned confinement. Such optimal care will include the following:

1. Early diagnosis of pregnancy.
2. Evaluation of the physical and mental health of the mother with application of preventive and corrective measures, including selection of the correct place for delivery.
3. Evaluation of the social circumstances of the family and the provision of adequate support.
4. Control of hazards to the foetus.
5. Avoidance of teratogenic influences.
6. Monitoring of maternal health and foetal development and the selection of the optimum time for delivery.
7. Nutritional supplementation and instruction.
8. Consultation with all necessary specialist services.
9. Provision of appropriate emotional support and childbirth education with opportunity for sympathetic and intelligent counselling on matters of parental concern.
10. An active programme of preparation for labour.

Such ante-natal care is achieved by means of organised ante-natal clinics. It is customary for patients to attend ante-natal clinics each month up to the 28th week of pregnancy; each fortnight from the 28th to the 36th week; and each week thereafter until confinement. In certain circumstances, the frequency of attendance may be increased.

The family practitioner who has special facilities and maintains an interest, is well able to undertake optimal ante-natal care and should seek to do so in association with a registered midwife.

The main objectives of regular attendance at ante-natal clinics is the provision of procedures which permit the determination of the management of the pregnant woman and allow for the detection of pre-symptomatic abnormalities of pregnancy.

These objectives are achieved by means of:—

a) The patient's physical, mental and social health history.
b) Clinical examination.
c) Investigative procedures.

The manner or method of ante-natal care may vary according to the family practice situation. In a large Health Centre, organised joint clinics may be shared between groups of doctors. In a rural community, the practitioner may more easily attain the objectives of ante-natal care during ordinary surgery. In so far as it is possible, separate clinics should be arranged at which the family practitioner, the midwife and the receptionist can share in both routine procedures and management of the abnormal.

The First Ante-Natal Attendance

The first ante-natal attendance of the pregnant woman should contain sufficient enquiry to establish the existing state of her health, to make recommendations as to special observations or treatment and to predict the manner of delivery. Clearly, such enquiry has to be extensive and will include at least the information in Table 16.1.

Table 16.1 Information obtained at the first ante-natal attendance.

Patient's past medical history	
	Physical
	Psychological
	Social
Patient's present medical history	
	Physical
	Psychological
	Social
Family history	
Previous gynaecological history	
Previous obstetric history	
Physical examination	
Height	Spine
Weight	Abdomen
Blood pressure	Legs for varicose veins
Heart	Pelvic examination
Chest	
Investigative procedure	
Hb or full blood count	Specific tests for syphilis
Blood group	and gonorrhoea
Rh factor	Midstream urine specimen
Rubella antibody titre	Vaginal aspirate or cervical smear

Whilst the evidence gathered at the first ante-natal examination is very extensive, it is obtained for logical reasons. Two examples are suggested in Tables 16.2 and 16.3.

Table 16.2 Factors which could affect the normality or health of a newborn Infant.

a) Tuberculosis in mother or close relative
b) Previous Rh isoimmunisation
c) Congenital abnormality
d) Inherited metabolic disorder
e) Previous immature baby (small-for-dates baby)
f) Primigravida age over 35 − mongolism
g) Excessive maternal cigarette smoking

During the ante-natal period, special enquiry or advice may be needed by women recognised as having any of the risks listed in Table 16.2.

Table 16.3   Obstetric abnormalities which could recur during the Ante-natal period.

---

a) Toxaemia
b) Premature labour
c) Rh negative with antibodies
d) Breech presentation
e) Twins

Any woman with a history of any of the events listed in Table 16.3 clearly requires special ante-natal surveillance.

It is not an unrewarding exercise to attribute significance to each component of history, examination and investigation, as a basis of rational ante-natal procedure.

Subsequent Ante-Natal Attendances

At each ante-natal attendance, the following information should be obtained for all women and the results recorded:—

1. The general well-being of the mother
2. Any amount of vaginal bleeding or discharge
3. Emotional and social difficulties
4. The weight of the mother
5. The blood pressure
6. The urine for sugar and protein
7. The ankles for oedema
8. The legs for varicose veins
9. The abdomen for the height of the fundus of the uterus.

From the 15th week, foetal parts may be balloted. From the 26th week, the foetal heart may be heard. From the 28th week, the presenting part should be discernible and from the 32nd week, the presenting part should be stable.

The procedure at the ante-natal clinic should include these clinical evaluations from the respective duration of pregnancy indicated. The results should be recorded in each instance. An awareness of common abnormalities helps to make their early and more frequent detection possible. A list of common ante-natal abnormalities is shown in Table 16.4.

The whole of ante-natal care cannot be described in a single chapter of a textbook. However, a number of special circumstances encountered during pregnancy attract special needs. Three examples are offered for consideration:—

Anaemia During the Ante-natal Period

It is generally agreed that a haemoglobin value of less than 10.2 g/100 ml is unacceptable, even allowing for possible physiological phenomena.

Table 16.4   Common ante-natal abnormalities.

9th to 11th weeks

Threatened abortion

9th to 14th weeks

Hyperemesis. Disparity
between dates and size of uterus

14th to 24th weeks

Hydatidiform mole-toxaemia.   Torsion of ovarian tumours
Abortion due to incompetent   Hydramnios − multiple pregnancy.
cervical os.

24th to 32nd weeks

Anaemia   Excessive weight gain
Pyelitis   Oedema of ankles
Hydramnios − multiple pregnancy or First 'bleed' of placenta praevia
foetal abnormality
Rhesus antibodies appear

From 32nd week

Anaemia   Unstable lie of foetus
Pyelitis   Multiple pregnancy
Toxaemia   Hydramnios − foetal abnormality
Pre-diabetes   Premature labour
Ante-partum haemorrhage   Failure of descent of presenting part
Breech presentation

It should be the aim during the ante-natal period, to ensure that anaemia is detected and adequately treated, so that at the time of delivery, the highest possible haemoglobin level is attained. The maximum quantity of iron normally available from food is 2.4 mg per day. Iron deficiency anaemia is not an uncommon event in pregnancy and the risk is increased by inadequate diet or failure to take prophylactic medicinal iron.

Megaloblastic anaemia due to a deficiency of folic acid can be prevented by daily oral intake of medicinal iron of the order of 100 mg per day and of folic acid of the order of 300 mg per day. The significant role of ascorbic acid in the metabolism of folic acid needs to be recognised. Addisonian pernicious anaemia is extremely rare.

Possession of the sickle-cell trait Hb AS by the African mother has been shown to be associated with a significant increase in perinatal mortality when there is anoxic stress. An increase in the African immigrant population of the UK creates a need for special enquiry to detect sickle-cell trait.

The procedure for detection and treatment of anaemia in pregnancy is as follows:−

1. Determine as closely as possible, the dietary habits of all pregnant women.

2. Estimate the haemoglobin value of all pregnant women at the first attendance, and at least twice again between the 28th week of pregnancy and confinement.

3. Estimate the sickle-cell trait of all African women at the first ante-natal attendance.

4. Investigate more fully all women who have a haemoglobin value of 10.2 g/100 ml or less.

5. Ensure increased frequency of haemoglobin estimations of all women with anaemia in pregnancy, particularly following treatment. Additional screening should continue until an acceptable level of haemoglobin is achieved.

Rhesus Incompatibility

'It is a rarity in clinical medicine that, in a single generation, a disease process is discovered, successfully treated, and finally prevented' (Commentary, Clinical Paediatrics, 1968).

Erythroblastosis foetalis was first related to isoimmunisation to the Rh antigen in 1941. This illness of the new-born can be anticipated by screening all pregnant women for the Rh factor. Fifteen per cent of all women are Rh negative and are at risk of reacting with an Rh positive foetus, to the point of producing an adverse isoimmunisation of the foetus.

The mother is rarely sensitised to the Rh antigen in her first pregnancy. In most instances the sensitising transplacental haemorrhages occur during, or shortly after, labour.

An Rh incompatible blood transfusion of a woman produces a severe sensitisation and is much more likely to be associated with erythroblastosis foetalis than sensitisation by an Rh positive foetus. Sensitisation can also occur as a result of abortion.

Procedure for rhesus incompatibility:—

1. Enquire of all pregnant women about blood transfusions prior to pregnancy.

2. Obtain all relevant previous obstetric history.

3. Test the blood of all pregnant women for Rh grouping at the first ante-natal attendance. Previous Rh tests should not be accepted as absolute evidence.

4. Test the blood of all pregnant women for Rh antibodies at the first ante-natal attendance. This permits the early anticipation of isoimmunisation in Rh negative women who may have had a previous incompatible blood transfusion, or who may be concealing information about a previous pregnancy.

5. Test the blood of all Rh negative women for Rh antibodies at the 30th week.

Special attention will need to be given to women who have a history of previous rhesus isoimmunisation and the frequency of tests for antibodies will depend on individual circumstances. Whilst erythroblastosis foetalis is now largely preventable by anti-immunisation, the screening procedure needs to be carefully observed if the occasional stillbirth or neonatal tragedy is to be avoided.

Foetal Maturity

Foetal maturity is traditionally predicted by calculation of the expected date of confinement (EDC) using Naegele's rule, from the date of the last menstrual period (LMP). It has been shown that in about 22 per cent of pregnant women, calculation of the EDC by this method is unreliable and that for the infants of these women, the perinatal mortality is higher.

Measurement of the fundal height has been shown to be an unreliable measure of maturity. Though this measurement continues to be a part of the procedure at each ante-natal attendance, it provides only a crude estimate and at best, can be justified as an indicator for further investigation.

More accurate estimation of maturity can be made by means of ultrasound cephalometry. This technique has been developed to a stage where sophisticated ultrasound equipment is available for the measurement of the biparietal diameter of the foetal skull in utero.

The measurement is accurate between the 20th and 30th week of pregnancy. This facility is not yet universally available. The method is considered to be safe and does not have the genetic hazard of radiography. Serial ultrasound cephalometry allows the separation of those patients 'at risk' with a small-for-dates foetus from those with uncertain maturity.

Procedure for ultrasound cephalometry:—

1. Screen all women between the 20th and 30th week of pregnancy, who have an unpredictable EDC as calculated by Naegele's formula.
2. Screen all women between the 20th and 30th week if the EDC is predictable by Naegele's formula and if they appear clinically to have a smaller-for-dates pregnancy.
3. Screen all women at intervals of one or two weeks, after the 20th week, if there is suspicion that the foetal growth is retarded, or if the mother fails to gain weight, or loses weight.

POST-NATAL CARE

Forty years ago, Blair Bell estimated that 10 per cent of mothers were more or less crippled by childbirth. Haemorrhage with consequent anaemia, renal failure, prolapse, stress incontinence, thrombosis and carcinoma of the cervix were all sequelae of childbirth. Many of these complications are avoidable and measures are now available to correct haemorrhage, to avoid damage to the genital tract and to prevent deep vein thrombosis in the leg.

Genital tract infection following childbirth has been very considerably reduced, though salpingitis remains as a significant sequelae of pregnancy.

The concept of early discharge from hospital, being the outcome of expediency in the early 1960s, has come to be adopted as a normal event, with clear advantage to many patients. A hospital can never be a home.

The changes which have occurred in post-natal care have increased the involvement and responsibility of the family practitioner. There are two special areas of care during the post-natal period, these being — the immediate care after delivery, and the post-natal examination.

Immediate Post-natal Care

By and large, physical complications of the puerperium are uncommon. Venous thrombosis, stress incontinence and anaemia persist, though with diminishing frequency. The family practitioner needs to have an expectant awareness of these problems and secure adequate treatment for his patients.

A much more common problem immediately following delivery is that of breast feeding.

Some women wish to breast feed and usually succeed. Others choose adamantly to avoid breast feeding and should not be encouraged to do otherwise. So long as breast feeding is at no time attempted, suppression of lactation presents few problems and medical intervention is unnecessary. The family practitioner has the responsibility to identify these women during the ante-natal period and to ensure that their convictions are medically supported.

The problem patients are those who are unable to express their misgivings about breast feeding and choose to try to conform with convention and the belief that breast feeding offers advantages to the baby. There is some evidence that the bottle fed infant is less resistant to gastrointestinal infection.

Mothers with confused concepts about breast feeding will usually make the attempt and encounter failure for a variety of reasons at the 4th or 5th day after delivery. The breasts have, by now, been stimulated and suppression of lactation becomes more difficult. The family practitioner may frequently find that he has to assist suppression of lactation under the most difficult circumstances. A balance between successful suppression and comfort to the mother needs to be achieved. Significant discomfort to the mother is intolerable and simple measures of suppression of lactation may be inadequate. The most useful medicinal treatment is 'Estrovis'. The amount required is small and the formulation of the oestrogen has reduced hepatotoxic effects with consequent limitations of the risk of thrombosis. The family practitioner and the midwife should co-operate to ensure a comfortable passage for the mother through the process of suppression of lactation.

Secondary post-partum haemorrhage is a complication of the puerperium confronting the family practitioner. Admission to hospital for curettage of the uterus is the best treatment, though some patients may respond to a three day course of ergometrine, by mouth.

The Post-natal Examination

The post-natal examination has the principle objective of ensuring that the genital tract has returned to normal. Vaginal prolapse and tubal tenderness should particularly be anticipated.

The breasts should be examined to ensure their normality.

The blood pressure and urine should be normal and if found to be abnormal, suitably investigated.

The emotional state of the mother should be established and the health of the baby determined. Problems of interrelationships between the mother, the family and the new baby can be explored at the post-natal examination and necessary intervention initiated.

The post-natal examination is an appropriate opportunity to take a cervical smear, not merely to exclude cancer but more to identify trichomonas infection or monilia vaginitis. The haemoglobin should be estimated and any recognised anaemia corrected.

Relationships between the family practitioner and the midwife are especially important during the puerperium. The day-to-day care of the patient is the responsibility of the midwife, though the family practitioner should promptly respond to any request for assistance.

MENTAL HEALTH IN PREGNANCY

The psychological aspects of pregnancy are perhaps the least well understood. In terms of psychosis, the pregnant woman contributes less than the non-pregnant woman. Schizophrenia, paranoid states, alcoholism, drug dependence, are illnesses usually associated with a lowering of fertility, although the evidence in connection with schizophrenia is a little conflicting. Fourteen per cent of known schizophrenic women who fall pregnant, relapse during pregnancy.

Obsessional neurosis is also less commonly encountered in pregnancy. Obsessional males tend to have a high celibacy rate and both obsessional males and females have a reduced fertility rate.

On the other hand, depressive women are not sub-fertile and it has been shown that 25 per cent of women with a history of depression experience a breakdown associated with pregnancy or childbirth and 80 per cent of these occur after delivery.

It is becoming increasingly evident that physical obstetric complications such as caesarean section, post-partum haemorrhage, instrumental delivery and toxaemia, are not associated with mental illness during pregnancy.

Many emotional reactions in pregnancy are sufficiently common to be regarded as normal. In the first three months, women tend to be anxious and some symptoms may be exaggerated to test the husband's or doctor's concern. In the second three months, there are reactions such as a tendency towards increased confidence and stability in the patient's behaviour. During the final three months there are more significant reactions like emotional lethargy, an increase in under-current anxiety, particularly about confinement and delivery. Towards term, there may be mental and physical restlessness giving rise to insomnia. In labour, women are usually detached and tend to concentrate their attentions on their physical sensations, although women in labour can react very strongly and fanatically to a casual remark which may cause offence or pleasure.

During the post-natal period, women are more emotionally labile, and tend to be more readily influenced by events around them. They show exaggerated responses to quite small events in their lives. The importance of the immediate post-natal period in the development of the mother—child bond and the influence of the trend towards delivery in hospital obstetric units is discussed in Chapter 23, page 529.

Babies who die arouse the usual grief syndrome and this must not be forgotten when babies are still-born. Towards abnormal babies, following an initial shock, most mothers develop a much stronger than normal maternal attachment.

Sleeping Patterns in Pregnancy

Another measurement of mental disturbance during pregnancy is the measurement of sleeplessness.

By means of the EEG we can measure objectively detectable changes in sleep patterns. There is more total sleep time in early pregnancy when women tend to sleep better than average. In late pregnancy, total sleep is slightly less than non-pregnant women. In the last month, the characteristic feature of pregnancy is a complete loss of the deep, stage four sleep and this phenomenon is sometimes associated with significant psychiatric illness and hormone disturbance. There is beginning to emerge a correlation between loss of deep sleep and hormone imbalance. Another characteristic is the sudden and quite dramatic recovery of stage four sleep during the first few days following confinement.

On the subjective level, women can be asked by self-administered questionnaires, about their sleep patterns. When this is done, it is found that 68 per cent admit to some disturbance of sleep — 13 per cent in the first three months, 19 per cent in the second and 66 per cent in the final three months. A high proportion (12 per cent) have a sufficient problem with sleeping to take some kind of sleeping tablet.

Fear during the Ante-natal Period

From personal experience, the following examples of fear are presented: —

1. A young girl, whose expectation was that labour was a very frightening experience, which was painful, discussed her problem with her mother, who told her that it was a waste of time trying to explain it — 'You have to experience it yourself!' This young girl continued through her ante-natal period carrying this fear which her parents had not been able to resolve and her expectation was that she would have a painful, frightening experience.

2. A multiparous patient complained of a fear of the unawareness of the onset of labour. Her first and second labours were artificially induced. We, as doctors, had taken away from her a normal, natural experience. Her anxiety, which is normal in a primigravida, now extended to subsequent pregnancy. Unless we are aware of this problem, we may fail to recognise that a woman has a right to be afraid in her third pregnancy just as much as in her first.

3. One patient had a fear of pain to such a degree as to cause recurrent asthmatic attacks, but it wasn't labour that bothered her, as she had a previous normal delivery which was painless. In the interim period, she also had salpingitis and her fantasy now was that the baby's head would press on her fallopian tubes during labour, giving rise to the same kind of pain as she had experienced with salpingitis. It was not too difficult to reassure her by giving her a simple anatomical understanding of herself.

There are also many ill-defined fears, such as fear of a caesarian section.

Pressures and stresses such as these, which occur during the ante-natal period, have not been adequately explored or investigated. The emphasis that we have given to pain in labour and post-natal depression has distracted our attention away from the psychological and emotional needs of women during the ante-natal period.

Maternity Blues

The abnormal emotional state in pregnancy can be an exaggeration of normal reactions. The most common exaggeration of emotion occurs between the second and the eleventh day after delivery — this is the 'baby blues' or 'maternity blues'. The symptoms are tearfulness, depression, anxiety and confusion. It is interesting that hypochondriasis, headache, insomnia and fatigue are not characteristics of 'maternity blues'. This syndrome is found in some degree in 50 per cent of women. There appears to be no relationship with physical obstetric abnormalities and the only other activity which seems to be disturbed is breast-feeding, which is established with greater difficulty in about 5 per cent of women who have 'baby blues'. It has been suggested that women confined in hospital have this phenomenon more frequently than those confined at home, though the evidence is not entirely convincing.

The syndrome may be organically determined as there is a correlation between its development and the very rapid fall in blood oestrogen and progesterone levels which occur immediately following delivery.

'Maternity blues' is regarded, and tends to be accepted, as a relatively trivial, fleeting phenomenon which needs to be distinguished from the more serious and protracted puerperal depression.

Puerperal Depression

This is the most commonly attributed mental illness in pregnancy. It occurs most frequently in women who have a previous history of mental illness, particularly of the depressive type. It has the same characteristics as depression found in the non-pregnant, though additional associations of guilt, anxieties about motherhood and the burdens of infant rearing are contributory factors. Detecting and defining the problem and its treatment follow the usual patterns, although special attention needs to be given to the possibility of suicide, infanticide and the possible development of a battered baby syndrome (see Chapter 23, page 527).

Mental Health During the Ante-natal Period

The emphasis on 'maternity blues' and puerperal depression has tended to distract our attention from psychological and emotional abnormalities of the ante-natal period. Grantly Dick-Reed evolved the hypothesis that pain in labour resulted from tension and anxiety during the ante-natal period, perhaps arising from fear. Some areas of concern by mothers during the ante-natal period are beginning to be defined. Some of these are — concern about themselves, about the baby, childbirth, subsequent pregnancies, their own appearance, good medical care, money, other members of the family, their doctor, medication and birth defects.

There are certain differences between primigravida and multigravida. The multigravida tend to have a high concern for being able to care for a family and also a concern about the type of contraceptive which they are likely to use after confinement. These concerns are there during the ante-natal period. Concern about a healthy normal baby and concern about the baby's condition at birth have a high frequency. Concern about subsequent pregnancies and of self in terms of attractiveness happen to half of women. Much less than half are concerned that the baby might have a defect at birth.

During pregnancy, women have a significant emotional experience and are able to absorb a large number of favourable and unfavourable stimuli. We doctors feed them unfavourable stimuli such as the casual remark about blood pressure or rhesus group, which can be very significant to a woman who wants to be well.

Childbirth or labour is the culminating point of pregnancy, yet for some women, it is a crisis. The ante-natal period is the period of the gathering storm before the thunderclaps of the crisis. If we are to recognise the components and significance of this gathering storm, we need to modify our attitude to ante-natal care. Whilst accepting the physical and social aspects to be important, we cannot be effective in terms of the whole diagnosis or of whole patient care until we attribute significance to the emotional and psychological elements of routine detection and management during the ante-natal period.

17

The Kidney and Urogenital Tract

D. Brooks

INTRODUCTION

Diseases of the kidney and urogenital tract can be of such complexity that the specialities of urology, nephrology, and more recently transplant surgery have evolved to meet the increasing need for particular skills. Indeed, some disorders requiring intricate diagnostic and treatment facilities, must involve these specialities to a considerable extent. Other disorders, however, often those that are commonly encountered, are best diagnosed and managed largely or entirely by the family practitioner himself given certain facilities for patient investigation. This account concentrates on these common disorders and at the same time, because the family practitioner has the ultimate responsibility for a patient rather than a disease, attempts to describe the contribution that might be made in some of the others.

DIAGNOSIS IN UROGENITAL DISEASE

Certain symptoms such as dysuria and loin pain may be quite characteristic of urogenital disease. Other symptoms however may not bear such an obvious relationship as they reflect abnormalities in body fluid composition or hypertension. These include nausea and vomiting, muscle weakness, pleuritic pain, cardiac pain and blurring of vision. These facts emphasise the importance of a careful history and routine urine examination in family practice. It would be inappropriate to detail here basic history taking and physical examination techniques as these can be found in textbooks of clinical methods but certain features are worth emphasising.

Examination Techniques

It should be remembered that congenital renal abnormalities are often found in association with malformed ears particularly if asymmetrical. Indeed the ear deformity is often on the same side as the renal abnormality. Family practitioners who conduct their own deliveries should be aware that as many as one third of infants who have a single umbilical artery also have a congenital renal anomaly. All infants with these abnormalities should have an intra-venous pyelogram as soon as possible as many of the renal anomalies discovered are surgically correctable. The bladder in infants is an abdominal organ and routine examination of the newborn should include palpation of the bladder, as many of the congenital abnormalities of the urogenital system lead to obstruction of urine flow, which may well manifest as a bladder that does not empty satisfactorily if the obstruction should be distal to it. One of the commoner urethral abnormalities is the presence of valves in the posterior urethra which occurs almost exclusively in the male. These infants may well present with a persistantly palpable bladder which if detected will result in treatment by surgical excision of the valves.

A common failure in family practice is to omit blood pressure examination in children and this should be included in children over the age of two years. A smaller cuff can be fitted to standard sphygmomanometers but the largest cuff that will fit is the better choice as too small a cuff results in an over estimation of the true blood pressure. Londe[1], gives standards for children determined under out-patient conditions.

Finally, it should be emphasised that examination of the genitourinary tract is not complete without a rectal examination and examination of the scrotum in the male, and a vaginal examination in the female, bearing in mind that in the latter the urethra can be directly palpated below the symphysis pubis.

Polyuria

Polyuria and oliguria represent altered renal function and the former needs to be differentiated from frequency which represents altered bladder function. Polyuria can be defined as a persistant increase in urinary output over 2500 ml in 24 hours and it can be caused by conditions in which an osmotic diuresis occurs such as diabetes mellitus and uraemia. It may also be caused by lack of production of anti-diuretic hormone ADH in pituitary disease or lack of response to ADH due to potassium depletion, some forms of chronic renal failure, or hyperparathyroidism. It may be due to psychological polydipsia in which ADH production is inhibited. Most frequently however polyuria is seen in the recovery phase of congestive heart failure.

Oliguria

Oliguria may be defined as the production of insufficient urine to enable the various solutes to be excreted in adequate amounts. A urine volume below 800 ml per 24 hours in our climate should be regarded with suspicion. Oliguria develops when renal blood flow and glomerular filtration rate are reduced, for example, in hypotension, cardiac failure, and diseases giving rise to water and salt depletion. It may sometimes occur in acute glomerulo-nephritis and other parenchymal diseases of the kidney. In conditions in which the ability to produce a concentrated urine is impaired, or alternatively when the solute load is increased such as in infection there may be a relative oliguria when 2 or 3 litres of urine may be insufficient to excrete the solute load. This emphasises the need for extra fluids in severe infections.

Urinary Frequency

Urinary frequency is essentially a subjective phenomenon but it can be said to exist when the amount of urine passed is consistently less than the capacity of a normal bladder which is about 300 ml. Micturition normally occurs every three or four hours during the day and perhaps once at night but frequency may occur in bladder and urethral irritation. It may result from external pressure on the bladder due to fibroids or a pregnant uterus and in contracture of the bladder due to malignancies and fibrosis. It may occur in bladder neck obstruction and neurological disease and may of course result from psychological factors.

Haematuria

Haematuria may be a symptom or a sign and as it is a common and alarming indication of urogenital disease both for the patient and the family doctor it is helpful to consider it from a problem-orientated viewpoint. The patient may rapidly present at the surgery or alternatively (and not infrequently) may request a domiciliary visit out of hours. The practitioner must regard the condition as indicating a malignancy until proved otherwise and yet at the same time manage to temper an appropriate sense of urgency with that quiet confidence which is necessary to calm and reassure his patient.

Although any diagnosis must be speculative until thorough investigation has been carried out a careful history cannot be neglected. It is necessary to enquire into the duration of the haematuria and to ask whether it has occurred previously. It is helpful to know whether blood is seen only at the commencement of micturition which may occur in urethral conditions or whether blood is spread uniformly throughout the specimen. The presence of associated symptoms and signs is of particular importance as 'silent' haematuria is an especially ominous symptom. Pyrexia, headache, sore throat, abdominal pain, dysuria and frequency, and the discovery of anaemia, oedema and hypertension may point to the origin of the bleeding. A specimen should be examined with the naked eye and also microscopically as pus cells indicating possible infection may be seen in association with haematuria, and the diagnosis can be confirmed by culture. Microscopy may also be helpful in differentiating haematuria from haemoglobinuria when the smoky naked eye appearance of the former is not obvious. Chemical tests for blood using 'haemotest' tablets will differentiate a red appearance due to haemoglobin from that due to substances such as eosin or porphyrins. Failure to find evidence of haematuria must not be allowed to lull the family doctor into a false sense of security as haematuria can be, and often is, intermittent and any patient complaining of haematuria, with the possible exception of minimal haematuria associated with acute dysuria and frequency in women, should be referred for a full urological examination. Details of the history and findings should be mentioned in the referral letter as information recorded at the time of the acute episode may be particularly helpful to the urologist, who may see the patient during a quiescent period.

It is worth mentioning that a common error is to neglect to ask a woman complaining of haematuria whether she is menstruating!

Synopses of possible causes of haematuria can be found in any surgical textbook and it is sufficient to emphasise that the age of the patient will have some bearing on the most likely cause. In male infants meatal ulceration and stenosis of the urethral orifice may be found. In young children urinary infection and acute glomerulonephritis may be responsible. In the adult patient infection, calculi, and neoplasms of the kidney or bladder may be found; the elderly may of course suffer chronic blood loss from the urogenital system resulting in chronic anaemia and heart failure.

INVESTIGATION IN UROGENITAL DISEASE

The family practitioner will primarily be concerned with that group of investigations that can be carried out either in or from his practice. This includes simple biochemical tests on blood and urine, urine inspection and microscopy, urine bacteriology, and simple radiological investigaton with plain abdominal films and excretion pyelography. He is less likely to be concerned with the group of investigations that requires a hospital setting such as tests of glomerular and tubular function, retrograde pyelography, cystourethroscopy, renal angiography, isotope renography and renal biopsy.

Inspection and Microscopy

Simple inspection is often neglected and yet further investigation for haematuria may be avoided if it is remembered that certain drugs and other substances such as beetroot, senna and cascara may redden the urine. Self medication for urinary symptoms is not uncommon and phenolpthalein is a popular constituent of many 'backache and kidney' pills. If the urine is alkaline it may turn pink in the presence of phenolpthalein, a colour that disappears on the addition of a few drops of acid. A sediment in the urine may be due to phosphates or pus the former being dispelled by a few drops of acetic acid.

Many family practitioners have a microscope and the skill involved in recognising the cellular constituents of an unstained urinary deposit is worth acquiring because much can be learned about renal disease. If the urine is cloudy or smoky or bloody on naked eye inspection a drop of the specimen is removed with a pipette, placed on a clean slide, and covered with a slip. In a blood stained specimen red cells appear as pale yellowish rings which swell and eventually rupture in a dilute urine. White blood cells are larger and have a granular appearance. Large vaginal squamous cells can be seen in specimens from female patients. Dense amorphous phosphate deposits can be removed with acetic acid. Casts are formed in the renal tubules by the coagulation of protein, and erythrocytes, leucocytes, and epithelial cells may be compressed onto them. Granular casts are described when these cells degenerate. Blood and epithelial casts are found in the early stages of acute glomerulonephritis, epithelial and granular casts indicate tubular degeneration, and hyaline casts (without any cellular impression) are found in chronic glomerulonephritis and occasionally in small numbers in normal urine.

Some family practitioners have a hand centrifuge and 10 ml of the specimen should be centrifuged as slowly as possible at about 1000 revolutions per minute for 5 minutes. The sediment is first examined with the naked eye. A red deposit indicates red blood cells; pus cells and amorphous phosphates appear white or creamy and urates give a brick coloured appearance. The supernatent fluid is then decanted and a little of the remaining fluid is removed with a pipette and re-examined under the microscope. A rough guide to the presence of significant pyuria may be obtained in the presence of more than five pus cells per high power field. Ideally, however, urine should not be centrifuged if pus cells are to be counted and the number of cells per cu mm of uncentrifuged urine should be estimated with a counting chamber in the pathology laboratory. This gives an estimate of the white cell excretion rate, the normal upper limit being 10 per cu mm (400 000 per hour). If infection is suspected, however, the urine must be cultured. Persistant pyuria in the absence of bacteriuria is suggestive of tuberculosis. Many fields must be scanned in normal urine before red cells and especially casts are seen.

Biochemical Examination of the Urine

Biochemical examination of the urine in the consulting room is a straightforward and simple task. Protein and glucose can be estimated routinely with Uristix, and Labstix can be used more selectively to provide information about urinary pH, protein, glucose, ketones, and blood.

Glycosuria

Dip stick tests are specific for glucose in the urine but the presence of glycosuria does not necessarily indicate diabetes mellitus. Renal glycosuria is more common than diabetes in the twenty to thirty age group which frequently undergoes routine medical examination and of course renal glycosuria is common in pregnancy. The discovery of glycosuria, however, should always be followed by a glucose tolerance test.

Proteinuria

Normal urine does not contain more than 50—300 mg of protein in twenty four hours (less than 5 mg per 100 ml). One fraction consists of incompletely reabsorbed glomerular filtrate protein and the remainder is a mucoprotein (Tamm Horsfall protein) secreted by the distal tubules and collecting ducts, which is considered to form the matrix of hyaline casts.

The dipstick (Albustix, Uristix) is capable of detecting proteinuria at about a level of 10 mg per 100 ml and simplicity in use has made it a popular diagnostic tool in family practice. There are a few snags however, that are not commonly appreciated. A high incidence of false positive results with the dipstick, when compared with the traditional sulpho salicylic acid test, may be found in association with febrile illnesses. The urine must be fresh as alkalinity, which may result on standing when urine contains urea splitting organisms such as *Proteus spp.*, can give a false positive result. Conversely an acidified specimen may lead to a false negative result. False positive results may also follow if the dip stick is not absolutely dry (it must be stored in its original container) and if the urine container is contaminated by detergent or soap. Unfortunately the Bence Jones proteinuria of multiple myeloma may be missed if dip sticks are used and if suspected it is necessary to employ the more time consuming boiling test in which the urine is boiled and allowed to cool. The Bence Jones protein precipitates out as the urine cools to about 50 °C. If the urine is cloudy it should be filtered prior to boiling and the pH adjusted with acetic acid to just give an acid reaction, as phosphates may be precipitated in an alkaline urine and the protein may remain in solution if the urine is strongly acid or alkaline.

Causes of Proteinuria Proteinuria may result from four basic causes — increased plasma concentration, impaired glomerular filtration, renal tubular disorders, and the addition of protein to the urine during its passage down the urinary tract in association with infection, calculi and neoplasms. Increased plasma concentration of low molecular weight protein, which then escapes through the glomerular filter, occurs in myelomatosis and in tissue destruction of any kind e.g., burns, surgery and neoplastic processes. Proteinuria most commonly results from impaired glomerular function however, and it may be transient or persistent. Transient proteinuria may occur in fevers, sensitivity reactions, anaemia and purpura. It is found in toxaemia of pregnancy, cardiac failure and certain endocrine disorders, e.g., thyrotoxicosis. Certain drugs or poisons such as gold and mercury may also result in transient proteinuria and it can occur in healthy individuals after exposure to severe cold and after violent physical exercise. It is for this latter reason that proteinuria may occur after a fit. Persistent proteinuria occurs when there is considerable damage to the nephron as in nephritis, malignant hypertension with nephrosclerosis, diabetic nephropathy, gout nephropathy and other kidney disorders.

Proteinuria due to impaired tubular reabsorption is not common but is found in certain inborn errors of metabolism (e.g., renal tubular acidosis; Fanconi syndrome) and it may occur after acute renal failure.

Classification   Proteinuria can accompany many diseases of the urogenital tract but a common problem in family practice is the discovery of isolated proteinuria in an individual who is otherwise perfectly well, perhaps during the course of an insurance medical examination. It is useful prognostically to classify 'idiopathic' proteinuria into four sub-groups: persistent, when isolated proteinuria is noted in all random specimens; intermittent, when proteinuria is found in many but not all random specimens; fixed orthostatic, when proteinuria is consistently found in specimens collected with the patient in the upright posture; transient orthostatic, when protein is present only occasionally in such specimens.

Persistent proteinuria is not common in the apparently healthy but community studies in the United States have revealed that transient proteinuria might be expected in 6 per cent of healthy pre-adolescents and 15 per cent of healthy adolescents. This 'idiopathic' proteinuria may well have certain important social implications as it may affect employment prospects, insurance premiums, emigration plans and in women, future obstetric management; there fore it deserves careful assessment. A full history and physical examination (including blood pressure assessment) must be carried out as if proteinuria is present in association with oedema detailed hospital investigation including renal biopsy may well be necessary.

It is clearly the duty of the family practitioner to define precisely the category into which his patient falls and this may be done by testing a number of specimens over a period of a week or so. The patient can be given 'Albustix' and taught how to use them. Orthostatic proteinuria can be recognised by the following procedure. The patient is asked to empty his bladder immediately before going to bed and again as he gets up the following morning. If the first specimen contains protein and the second specimen is clear a diagnosis of orthostatic proteinuria can be made.

The discovery of proteinuria in family practice should be followed by microscopy and culture of a urine specimen either at a hospital laboratory or in the consulting room as more involved hospital diagnostic procedures may be avoided at a later date if relevant information can be collected at the time of the acute episode. The presence of haematuria and white blood cells and the absence of casts may suggest infection, calculi or malignancy, whereas proteinuria accompanied by cast formation may point to glomerular disease.

Proteinuria will usually require even further investigation particularly if it persists day and night and the albustix readings are ++ or more. Accurate quantitative tests should follow. A full 24 hour specimen can be obtained. The presence of more than 500 mg of protein in such a specimen is abnormal and is an indication for specialist referral even if an orthostatic element is suspected. Blood urea and serum creatini .. estimations may be obtained and an intravenous pyelogram may be ordered while awaiting an out patient appointment at an appropriate specialist clinic. Specialist investigation may include assessment of the glomerular filtration rate, serum complement estimation and even renal biopsy.

Prognosis It is commonly stated that orthostatic proteinuria carries an excellent prognosis and indeed this is true as many long term follow up studies have demonstrated. Ultimately, however, prognosis depends on the histological appearances and it should be remembered that fixed orthostatic proteinuria is associated with renal morphological changes in 8 to 25 per cent of cases. Persistent or intermittent idiopathic proteinuria has been associated with definite renal changes in 60 to 80 per cent of cases. The morphological changes include proliferative and membranous glomerulonephritis but their significance, especially if minor, in terms of future impairment of renal function is uncertain. Clearly the attitude of the family practitioner should be one of cautious optimism.

Blood Biochemistry Proteinuria appears relatively early in the natural history of renal disease but as renal function progressively deteriorates the composition of body fluids becomes more abnormal and these abnormalities may be detected by blood analysis. In particular, metabolites, which are normally filtered at the glomerulus, are retained in the blood as the number of functioning glomeruli diminishes and the glomerular filtration rate drops from 125 ml per minute to about 25 ml per minute. Thus the plasma concentration of urea and creatinine and anions such as phosphate rises, and given a constant rate of production (more likely with creatinine than urea) the level in the plasma becomes a measure of the glomerular filtration rate. As the kidney's efficiency in excreting hydrogen ions deteriorates blood bicarbonate is used up and plasma bicarbonate levels may be a useful guide to renal function as may plasma electrolyte levels.

Urine Bacteriology

An important innovation has been the introduction of a dip slide to be used in the diagnosis of urinary infection; it has been marketed under the trade names 'Uricult' and 'Oxoid'. The Uricult dip slide consists of a glass slide coated on one side with MacConkey agar and on the reverse side with Cystine-lactose-electrolyte-deficient agar. The slide fits neatly into it's sterile plastic container and the unit has gradually established itself as an essential diagnostic aid in family practice.

Urinary infection has been defined as a condition in which bacteria are multiplying in bladder urine. The organisms which cause urinary infection however originate in the bowel flora and consequently may be present in the distal urethra and on the perineum from where they may enter the urine during micturition, though the bladder urine itself may be sterile. It follows that pathological reports using vague terms such as 'slight growth', 'heavy growth' or 'contaminants only' are unsatisfactory because of their inherent lack of objectivity.

In 1956, Professor Kass of the Department of Bacteriology and Immunology at Harvard Medical School was hoping to study the possibility of a relationship between urinary infection and chronic pyelonephritis and he planned to concentrate his attention upon patients with asymptomatic infection, as previous studies of patients with symptomatic infection had proved unrewarding. In this situation objective criteria for the diagnosis of urinary infection were clearly desirable but did not exist. Kass's in vitro experiments[2] demonstrated that if bacteria were introduced into pooled sterile urine specimens they multiplied rapidly within one hour or so to levels of about 10^8 organisms per ml. It seemed likely that a similar phenomenon occurred in vivo and indeed Kass's experimental studies on large numbers of asymptomatic and symptomatic patients demonstrated that if bacteria were multiplying in the urine (i.e., a urinary infection was present) the organism count in that urine would usually be 10^5 per ml or more; conversely if the count was 10^4 per ml or less it was nearly always the result of contamination as bacterial multiplication could not have occurred in urine. On the rare occasions that counts between 10^4 and 10^5 per ml were obtained the result was equivocal and the investigation needed to be repeated. These results have been widely accepted but Kass himself emphasised that anything interfering with bacterial multiplication in the bladder urine, such as the presence of antibiotics in the urine, and marked frequency, could result in lower counts assuming significance, and indeed, as others have pointed out, so could the presence of infection distal to the bladder (see urethral syndrome, (page 332). Kass also emphasised that urine at room temperature needed to be examined within one hour and refrigerated urine within 48 hours if significant multiplication of contaminants was to be avoided. This latter requirement proved almost insurmountable in the context of active family practice until the introduction of the dip slide. This both overcame the transport problem due to the necessity of immediate inoculation of the MacConkey agar, and provided a simple yet accurate semi-quantitative approach, as the colonies on the slide could be counted after incubation. Indeed specimens from family practice have been shown to give reliable results, even when posted to the laboratory, in comparison studies with the time consuming full count techniques upon which Kass himself based his work.

Preparation of the adult patient does not appear to be necessary in the author's experience though some recommend swabbing the perineum with tap water. If the specimen is obtained from an infant or young child however swabbing is advisable as the incidence of contaminated specimens is much higher, due I suspect to the absence of bladder control. The author's experience with infant collecting bags is that the incidence of high count specimens is very high at around 60 per cent and that it is preferable to obtain a clean catch specimen. This can be obtained with much less difficulty than one might imagine as most infants micturate every 20 minutes or so and if the mother sits in a side room holding her infant over a waxed hospital container, her efforts will be rewarded surprisingly quickly. It should be remembered that the technique of suprapubic aspiration (SPA) can be practised in the consulting room without anaesthesia and if one is faced with an ill and fractious child with vague clinical signs the method could be adopted with advantage. The technique may at first sight appear alarming but many thousands of aspirations have now been carried out without mishap and even on the rare occasions when bowel contents have been aspirated the patient has been none the worse for the experience! The urine is obtained with a 10 ml syringe and an intravenous needle, entry being made after preliminary swabbing with ether about 1 inch above the symphysis in the mid line. The author's experience of the technique has been obtained solely in infants and an overall success rate of about 50 per cent is claimed. If the napkin is dry and the bladder palpable the success rate is much higher.

Once the urine has been obtained the dip slide should be inoculated promptly but after inoculation further delay is of no consequence and the slide can be taken or posted to the laboratory. The author has no doubt however that an incubator in the surgery is of inestimable value given the high incidence of urinary tract infection in the community and there is clearly a need for the introduction of reasonably priced equipment so that delay and communication problems with the laboratory may be avoided.* Instructions for interpreting the results are given with the dip slides which can sometimes be obtained from a

---

* Tillotts Laboratories, 44 Lupus Street, London, S.W.1., have introduced incubator for distribution to interested practitioners. They will aslo provide a free dip slide service on request.

local pathology laboratory if they are used in the hospital itself. It is usually assumed that urine obtained by SPA should be sterile in health as local defences should not allow urinary pathogens to enter the bladder urine. There is room for further discussion and research in this area however.

INFECTIONS OF THE URINE AND URINARY TRACT

Infection of the urine exists when bacteria are multiplying in bladder urine and infection of the urinary tract exists when tissue involvement has occurred somewhere along its length. These conditions may occur together or separately, with or without symptoms and they are encountered very frequently in family practice where they have received much attention over the last fifteen years, both from hospital based research workers and family practitioners themselves. This work has done much to improve our knowledge and in particular has emphasised the very real difference between disease as encountered in hospital and in family practice.

Textbooks of hospital medicine have traditionally divided these infections into primary (or simple) and secondary (or complicated) according to whether anatomical abnormalities are found on further investigation. Although useful perhaps in a hospital setting such a classification is less helpful in family practice than one based on the four types of patient who are likely to present with symptoms, since aetiology, prognosis and management may vary accordingly. The largest group consists of women with acute dysuria and frequency of micturition. A second group consists of men with similar symptoms not infrequently accompanied by a mild rigor, a condition often described as prostatitis. Pregnant women in whom renal infection is commoner constitute a third group. A final group consists of children with infection; characteristic symptoms might be less prominent in this group and a significant underlying pathology might be found.

The Syndrome of Dysuria and Frequency in Women

Epidemiology

Acute symptoms referrable to the lower urinary tract have been described as *cystitis*, which in most cases is probably anatomically incorrect, and as the *urethral syndrome*, which may be confusing. Many studies have revealed that only about half of the women presenting to the family practitioner with symptoms have bacteria multiplying in their bladder urines on subsequent investigation. The term urethral syndrome has tended to be used to describe the symptomatology of the women who do not appear to have a urinary infection, although their symptoms do not differ in any way from those present in women who do. This restrictive use of the term is not particularly helpful however, as quite apart from being etymologically incorrect (a syndrome is a collection of symptoms), it could mislead in other ways, as it has been suggested that the two conditions, 'urethral syndrome' and 'urinary infection', represent different stages in the pathogenesis of the same disease process.

This syndrome of dysuria and frequency is common in family practice with an incidence of about 48 per 1000 women at risk per year in the age range 15—75. The incidence of urinary infection in these women is about 25 per 1000 women at risk per year. This means that a practitioner with 2500 patients and an average age — sex distribution can expect to see nearly 50 different women with symptoms each year, although a proportion will attend on more than one occasion. Family practice studies, however, give a misleading impression of the prevalence of the condition in the community as symptoms do not always lead to a consultation with the family doctor. In one recent community survey 3000 women between 20 and 64 years of age were questioned. Twenty per cent had experienced dysuria (defined as burning pain on micturition) within the previous year. In half of these the dysuria had lasted two weeks or more during the year and only ten per cent of the total had consulted a family practitioner. Nearly half the 3000 women questioned had experienced dysuria at some time in their lives.

When the relationship between age in decades and family practitioner consultations is studied attacks of dysuria and frequency occur most commonly in the 25 to 34 age group but are reasonably common throughout life. About one third of women presenting during a twelve month period will be experiencing their first attack of symptoms. First attacks are three to four times more common in the 15—24 age group but do occur throughout life, even in the elderly. This suggests, at least in the young, that a relationship could exist between symptoms and first sexual experience. Although overall half the women with symptoms have a urinary infection there is evidence that up to the age of 45 the younger the patient the more likely that she will have an infected urine. After the age of 45 the likelihood of an infected urine, instead of continuing to decline, starts to rise again with increasing age. These facts could reflect altered urethral defences against ascending infection as a result of sexual intercourse in the younger women and oestrogen deficiency in the older woman. Impaired bladder emptying with resulting residual urine may also play a part in the escalation of bacteriuria in women approaching the age of 65.

Aetiology and Pathogenesis
When a specimen of urine is taken from a woman with the syndrome of dysuria and frequency and used to inoculate a dip slide, Kass's criterion[2] should be used to determine the presence of a urinary infection (see p. 330) which will be

present in about half the women with symptoms. Many studies in family practice have demonstrated that as many as 90 per cent of the organisms isolated from these infections are *Escherichia coli* and the remaining ten per cent are composed of *Proteus spp.*, *Staphylococcus albus*, *Streptococcus faecalis* and *Pseudomonas pyocyaneus.* In hospital acquired infections the relative per centage of *Escherichia coli* is much lower.

The aetiology of symptoms in the remaining 50 per cent who do not have a urinary infection has intrigued clinicians for many years and a study of the literature will reveal that explanations have been many and varied. At the end of the last century authors wrote of conditions mimicking cystitis such as hyperacidity, neurosis, calculus disease and gynaecological disease, and collectively referred to these as the irritable bladder syndrome. It was felt that these conditions predisposed to 'cystitis'. Recent work has suggested a number of factors and explanations including vitamin deficiency, hysteria, anxiety neurosis, diverticulitis, urinary obstruction, bad micturition habits, oestrogen deficiency, allergy, gynaecological disorders and the adequacy of bacteriological techniques and previous antibiotic treatment by the family practitioner. It has also been suggested that a dry vagina following hysterectomy or amputation of the cervix, mini skirts and even bubble baths might be involved. Attempts to incriminate non-bacterial pathogens such as viruses, fungi and protozoa have by and large been unsuccessful.

Although these women do not have a urinary infection (i.e., an organism count in the urine of 10^5 per ml) bacterial counts below 10^5 per ml may well be isolated. In the past these organisms have often been regarded as contaminants but recent research has thrown doubt on this as over 80 per cent of women with acute dysuria and frequency have some bacteria in their urine compared with less than 10 per cent of women who have never had such symptoms; in addition many women with symptoms and insignificant bacteriuria eventually develop significant bacteriuria on follow-up. Kass[2] emphasised that his criterion only applied in a situation where bacteria had the opportunity to multiply in bladder urine. It is possible that a lesion in the dysuria and frequency syndrome is, initially at least, in the urethra when such an opportunity might not occur. For this reason as well as the possible effect of urinary frequency Kass's criterion needs to be applied with caution in the bacterial assessment of urine from women with the dysuria and frequency syndrome. It seems reasonable to conclude that on using Kass's criterion half the women with the dysuria and frequency syndrome will have bacteria multiplying in their bladder urines i.e., a urinary infection and that the majority of the remainder may have the same organisms involved as pathogens in a urethral lesion or urinary tract infection, which may or may not eventually escallate into the former condition.

In order to explain the observation that not all women have urinary tract infection the existence of defence mechanisms and precipitating factors have been postulated. Defence mechanisms which prevent urinary pathogens in the rectal flora entering the bladder include a residual urethral flora, a normal urethral flow and adequate bladder emptying. Precipitating factors interfere with the normal functioning of these mechanisms and include sexual intercourse, allergy, catheterisation, menstruation, and bouts of diarrhoea. Perhaps in some women acute dysuria and frequency is produced by precipitating factors alone which may cause a local urethritis. In others urinary pathogens may become involved in this lesion which may progress and bacteria may then multiply in bladder urine to levels satisfying Kass's criterion. These ideas are being researched but as yet there is no firm evidence of the existence of a urethral lesion in women with the dysuria and frequency syndrome.

Clinical Features
Many women do not regard the syndrome of dysuria and frequency as an indication for a consultation with a doctor and will try some form of home remedy first of all, commonly barley water. The pharmacist is often consulted and he will sell the patient a variety of proprietary preparations which are usually of the 'shotgun' variety containing substances such as buchu, hexamine, senna leaf and phenolpthalein and the latter may result in a urine of unusual hue. As a result of this home treatment and the belief that the problem will go away the patient will often attend the surgery after the first 48 hours of symptoms.

The symptoms and signs which are associated with the dysuria and frequency syndrome are listed in Table 17.1. Although dysuria and frequency are the commonest complaints other symptoms can be obtained. The patient often notices that her urine has an offensive smell even when subsequent bacterial investigation fails to demonstrate a urinary infection and loin pain and haematuria might be noticed. It has been suggested that loin pain might be referred from the urethra. The most striking observation however, is the similar symptomatology in all women with the syndrome whether or not their urine is infected. Clearly one cannot forecast the result of a urine culture from a consideration of symptoms and signs although as judged by requests for a domiciliary visit and blood tests there is some evidence that the presence of significant bacteriuria is associated with a more upsetting illness.

A relatively small group of women suffer from frequent attacks of distressing symptoms but on a national scale their numbers are considerable. These women may have attacks of symptoms every month or two and the inadequacy of traditional courses of antibiotics has been emphasised by the existence of U and I clubs whose writings have little praise for traditional medical attitudes towards this common problem.

Table 17.1   Individual symptoms and signs in 71 infected and 68 non-infected females (from Brooks, 1973[3]).

Symptoms	Frequency of Occurrence (Percentages)	
	Infected	Non-infected
Frequency	86	95
Dysuria	80	85
Loin pain	37	29
Loin tenderness	18	7
Suprapubic pain*	17	19
Suprapubic tenderness	25	14
Haematuria	31	20
Fever	18	10
Smelly urine	49	30
Backache*	17	27
'Flu-like' symptoms*	15	19
Perineal irritation	—	12

* These symptoms were not directly enquired about but were volunteered in response to a request for any other symptoms.

Diagnosis
The family practitioner needs to decide not only whether his patient has a urinary infection but also why she has got it at that particular time and what its relevance is in terms of continuing morbidity and underlying genito-urinary tract disease. History, examination and investigation are directed to these ends.

History   The family doctor should not only explore the presenting symptoms but in addition should help the patient to find precipitating factors along the lines previously described. An attempt should be made to define a patient profile revealing why she suffers from the dysuria and frequency syndrome. Asking the patient to cast her mind back to her very first attack is often helpful in this context. It is important to know if attacks occurred during childhood or during pregnancy. The possibility of an early pregnancy should be kept in mind and a menstrual history taken.

Examination   During the examination a particular attempt should be made to exclude acute pyelonephritis by palpation and percussion of the loin area. Inspection of the external genitalia may reveal evidence of senile vaginitis in older women due to hormonal deficiency. A pelvic examination does not often reveal useful information in the context of the dysuria and frequency syndrome. A recent study did not demonstrate any association between the syndrome and cervicitis, cervical erosion, vaginal discharge or uterine prolapse. Recent blood pressure levels should of course be recorded in every patients' notes but it is not especially raised in the context of the dysuria and frequency syndrome.

Investigations

Bacterial examination of a urine specimen is required for adequate management, not only because it is essential if a diagnosis of urinary infection is to be made with certainty, but also to identify the organisms for the sensitivity studies that are sometimes necessary when there is a poor response to therapy. The technique has been outlined previously (p. 330).

Since pyuria reflects the presence of inflammation in the urinary tract, which may or may not be due to infection, the white cell content of a urine specimen is not an adequate diagnostic criterion. Although the presence of significant pyuria is helpful false positive and false negative values may be obtained. In a recent study in family practice 80 per cent of women with symptoms and significant bacteriuria had more than 5 white cells per high power field compared with 29 per cent of women with equivocal organism counts and 18 per cent of women with counts below 10^4 per ml.

An IVP is not indicated in the syndrome of dysuria and frequency in women unless attacks are particularly frequent when it may be helpful as part of a more intensive investigation of the lower urinary tract. If, however, a diagnosis of pyelonephritis has been made or childhood attacks are recalled an IVP should be carried out as a higher incidence of renal abnormalities might be expected.

Management

The isolation of significant bacteriuria is generally regarded at present as an indication for the administration of an appropriate antibacterial agent and when taken symptoms can be expected to disappear within four days in nearly 80 per cent of cases. The choice of agent from the wide range available will be based on a number of factors including cost, side effects, and the *in vitro* resistance patterns of the organisms isolated. Ideally the choice should be made after *in vitro* sensitivity tests but this usually requires hospital laboratory facilities and unavoidable delay. Since their introduction in 1935 the first choice has been a sulphonamide but recent claims of increasing resistance in *Escherichia coli* require that this policy should be critically examined. The incidence of sulphonamide resistance in family practice is a matter of some dispute. There is certainly geographical variation but whether this reflects real differences in the organisms themselves which could result from different prescribing habits, or whether it merely reflects the difficulties inherent in sulphonamide sensitivity testing is difficult to resolve. Ideally each practice should determine its own prescribing policies based upon effectiveness, safety and cost. The effectiveness of antibacterial therapy may be modified not only by the type of organism isolated and its likely *in vitro* resistance pattern[4] (which should be discussed with a local consultant bacteriologist) but also by the type of patient and the site of the infection. One approach to therapy is suggested below.

Sulphadimidine 0.5 g in a dose of four stat and two six hourly for seven days is still the drug of first choice in the majority of women with the dysuria and frequency syndrome as it is effective, cheap and relatively free from side effects. In the author's experience 75 per cent of women experiencing a first infection will have organisms in their urine exhibiting *in vitro* sensitivity. *In vitro* resistance to sulphonamides may be increased however in women who have had sulphonamides frequently in the past because of recurrent infection. When attacks are frequent sensitivity studies are particularly desirable and an alternative first choice might be preferred such as ampicillin or co-trimoxazole.

When smaller numbers of organisms are isolated the decision whether or not to administer antibacterial agents is more difficult. Some guide lines can be given however. We might wish to give these drugs either to relieve symptoms or to prevent the later development of significant bacteriuria or both. It is possible to measure the effectiveness of antibacterial therapy against these criteria and consider the result in the light of the known hazards of such therapy.

When placebo therapy was compared in a double blind trial with co-trimoxazole in women with dysuria and frequency and insignificant bacteriuria 40 per cent recovered from their symptoms in 48 hours on the placebo alone and this figure rose to 60 per cent within four days[4]. On co-trimoxazole therapy 76 per cent of women recovered in four days. When women with the dysuria and frequency syndrome and insignificant bacteriuria were followed up in double blind fashion after treatment with co-trimoxazole and a placebo 25 per cent of those previously given co-trimoxazole developed significant bacteriuria within three months compared with 35 per cent given the placebo.

On the other hand antibacterial agents are not inocuous. Certain side effects are well known but it is perhaps not so commonly realised that organisms isolated from the inevitable recurrent infection can be modified by the drugs previously administered. In this same study[4] 38 per cent pf organisms isolated from urinary infections were resistant to sulphonamides. This figure fell to 25 per cent in women experiencing their first attack of symptoms and increased to 46 per cent in those with a previous history. When organisms were examined from follow up infections within three months of a course of co-trimoxazole or a sulphonamide 66 per cent had developed resistance to sulphonamides. In addition however, when the number of drugs to which each organism had resistance was studied, resistance to two or more drugs increased threefold from 24 per cent before therapy to 73 per cent after therapy.

The conclusion must be that a decision about antibiotic therapy should not be taken lightly. When symptoms are trivial and significant bacteriuria is not discovered, the elimination of any organisms isolated is probably best left to the patient's own natural defence mechanisms, as it is possible that an antibacterial agent may induce resistance in rectal flora which may subsequently infect the urine. If a prescription is felt to be necessary Mistura Potassium Citrate or flavoxate hydrochloride 100 mg in a dose of two tablets three times daily for five days might be tried. The patient should be told that if symptoms do not improve after this time an antibiotic will be given because it is unreasonable to allow symptoms to continue for too long, and in any case the persistence of symptoms may indicate a progression of the disease process to produce urinary infection.

The women who suffer frequent attacks require a different approach, not least in importance is sympathy and interest and an active desire to help as with a little care much can be done. The patient can be given a supply of dip slides, taught how to use them, and told to deliver them as soon as symptoms start. At the same time she can make an appointment to see the doctor the following day when the result of the dip slide culture should be available. Perhaps the most important measure is to prepare a patient profile along the lines previously indicated, after which management is self evident as the aim is to eliminate the precipitating factors. If sexual intercourse is incriminated scrupulous cleanliness in both partners before intercourse is desirable, and the use of KY Jelly as a lubricant and the adoption of alternative positions during intercourse might help to reduce the trauma. Immediately after intercourse double micturition should be practised. If these measures fail, nitrofurantoin 50 mg at night for two or three days at the time of intercourse may be successful. If the onset of the syndrome coincides with the menopause the use of dienoestrol pessaries or cream may be helpful. Obstinate cases may benefit from quinestradol which has a selective action on the mucosa of the urethra rather than the uterus. The dose is two tablets twice daily for two to three weeks at a time depending on the severity of symptoms. A careful history may reveal an allergen such as eggs or citrous fruits. If menstruation is incriminated the use of a simple diuretic for a few days before menstruation should help as should scrupulous hygiene and a trial of pads instead of tampons and vice-versa. All intractable cases should have a high fluid intake whatever the precipitating factors and should avoid delaying micturition for social reasons.

In the event of these measures failing referral to a specialist unit should be considered as although significant underlying renal abnormalities are unlikely to be found the patient may be worried about this. In any case urethroscopy, cystoscopy and cystometry including studies of the urine flow properties should be undertaken in an attempt to elucidate local causes. When all else fails nitrofurantoin in a dose of 50 mg nightly for three to six months may be of real benefit.

Follow up and Continuing Care

Despite adequate therapy and a bacteriological cure as judged by a post treatment urine culture one third of those treated will develop significant bacteriuria over a 3 month follow up period and this raises the question of routine follow up. In the authors opinion demands on the family practitioners time are such that post-treatment urine examination and routine follow-up should be limited to pregnant women, those with known renal involvement or urogenital tract abnormalities and those with frequent attacks. Until there is evidence that routine follow-up can be of benefit to any other group, or firm evidence that urinary infection can be linked aetiologically with chronic pyelonephritis, therapeutic enthusiasm must be tempered by prudence.

It is now generally accepted that with rare exceptions scarring occurs only in the growing kidneys of infants and young children and that in the absence of obstruction and pregnancy, urinary infection, even with renal parecnchymal involvement, usually follows a benign course. In terms of declining renal function phenacetin ingestion may prove to be more of a threat than acute pyelonephritis and recurrent urinary infection (see chronic pyelonephritis p. 350).

Conclusion and Future Development

It is probably true to say that definitive studies into the aetiology and pathogenesis of the dysuria and frequency syndrome are just as likely to emerge from the family practitioners surgery as they are from the research laboratories of our major hospitals. The discovery of a new precipitating factor for example is well worth a letter to a medical journal. Perhaps the most important advance of recent years has been the realisation that these attacks do not carry a serious prognosis and that successful management does not depend solely on a bottle of antibiotic tablets.

Urinary Tract Infection in the Adult Male

Epidemiology

Symptoms referrable to the lower urinary tract in women are not always accompanied by significant bacteriuria and this is also a noticeable feature of similar symptoms presented by the male. The incidence of urinary infection in men between the ages of 15 and 75 has been reported to be 5 per thousand men at risk per year i.e., one fifth of the incidence in women of comparable age. This means that a practitioner with a list of 2500 patients can expect to see about ten men with symptoms during the course of the year and four of these should have significant bacteriuria.

Aetiology and Pathogenesis

When urinary infection is present the causative organisms are similar to those isolated in women with the syndrome of dysuria and frequency, with

Escherichia coli predominating. The site of the pathology in the lower urinary tract is often difficult to determine in any individual patient as it may be in the prostate gland, the posterior urethra, the bladder wall, or sometimes all these. On occasions infection may spread to involve the epididymis and testes and if tissue oedema provokes obstruction acute retention may occur. This is usually a complication of benign prostatic hypertrophy.

Failure to isolate organisms may be due to bacterial multiplication in prostatic fluid rather than urine and their existence in such small numbers that they can only be demonstrated by special techniques. It has been demonstrated that prostatic fluid contains a substance with bactericidal properties which might explain a low organism count and might be a major reason why urinary infection is more common in women.

If the prostate gland becomes chronically inflamed as a result of acute prostatitis or for other obscure reasons the condition may remain symptomatically silent for long periods and the existence of white blood cells in the prostatic fluid may be the only indication of its existence. Chronic prostatitis however, is believed to be a major source of relapsing urinary infection in the male. It has been emphasised that in some men with symptoms resembling chronic bacterial prostatitis organisms are never found (a condition that has been described as 'prostatosis') but it is generally believed that chronic prostatitis is primarily caused by gram negative bacteria. The route of infection is unknown but it is suspected that the urethra might become colonised by pathogenic vaginal bacterial during sexual intercourse and indeed evidence that this might occur has recently emerged from the authors own practice. On two occasions during a 12 month study a husband and wife presented together both complaining of the onset of dysuria and frequency within 48 hours of sexual intercourse. In the first couple the husband had significant bacteriuria and the wife had an equivocal organism count. In the second couple, husband and wife had significant bacteriuria. When swabs were taken from the rectum and vagina in the wife and the rectum in the husband, *Escherichia coli* serogroup O6 was found in all swabs. The urinary organisms were also group O6. As identical organisms were found on all swabs the route was not proven but the case demonstrated the likelihood of the husband receiving a sexually transmitted inoculum from his wife's vagina rather than from his own bowel flora.

Little is known about other precipitating factors but obstruction to urine flow is frequently associated with urinary infection in males and most commonly this results from benign prostatic hypertrophy.

Clinical Features
Three fundamental types of presentation are seen in family practice although some overlap might occur. The older man may present primarily with mild obstructive symptoms such as hesitancy, urgency and an altered urine stream,

when the urine is cultured infection may accompany these symptoms. Other men present primarily with symptoms suggesting acute infection such as dysuria and frequency, haematuria, offensive urine, mild rigors and loin pain; culture of the urine may or may not reveal significant bacteriuria. Yet another group however present with vaguer symptoms such as varying degrees of low back and perineal discomfort and vague micturition dysfunction. Urinary infection is uncommon in this group but evidence of infection may exist in the prostatic secretions. Occasionally flu-like symptoms are the major presenting feature and lower urinary tract symptoms are only mild and can only be elicited on direct questioning.

As with women there is evidence that when symptoms are associated with infection of the urine the patient tends to be more ill as judged by a request for a domiciliary as opposed to a surgery consultation and by blood investigations. There is also some evidence that urinary infection evokes a more marked tissue response in men than it does in women.

Diagnosis

Many features of diagnosis in males differ in no way from those in females but some are worth emphasising. It is particularly important to establish the earliest date of onset of symptoms referrable to the lower urinary tract as this may establish a background of prostatism upon which infection has become superimposed. Examination should include palpation of the testicles and epididymis for evidence of local spread of infection. A rectal examination may demonstrate prostate tenderness although this is uncommon and possibly hypertrophy may be clinically apparent. Culture of the urine is of course necessary if urinary infection is to be confirmed but unlike the situation in women, intravenous pyelography is required routinely as there is a high incidence of underlying abnormality, usually prostatic hypertrophy.

Management

The first priority in management is to eradicate urinary infection. The concentration of most agents active against gram negative organisms is considerably less in the prostate than in the plasma and because of this co-trimoxazole may be preferred in the male with urinary infection. Two co-trimoxazole tablets twice daily for seven days have given good results. There is evidence in the dog that trimethoprim achieves peak concentrations in the prostatic fluid two to three times higher than in the blood whereas sulpha-methoxazole has a lower concentration in the prostate than in the blood. It should be remembered that significant bacteriuria is not necessarily isolated in bacterial prostatitis and that smaller numbers of organisms may be clinically significant. When symptoms are minimal and no organisms are isolated the clinician may well decide not to employ antibacterial agents in expectation of a spontaneous resolution.

Referral to a urological surgeon is advisable in all cases and as an IVP examination is mandatory in all cases, with the possible exception of young men who usually have no underlying lesion, this can be requested by the family practitioner so that it is available at the time of the specialist appointment. In a recent study of men with symptoms suggesting lower urinary tract infection in the author's practice 40 per cent of the intravenous pyelograms were in some way abnormal. Although the abnormality usually consisted of a prostate filling defect in the bladder associated with a residual urine, half of the abnormalities involved the upper urinary tract and consisted of radiological evidence of renal infection and hydronephrosis. Of 26 men referred to a consultant urologist 5 required prostatectomy and a further 2 had laparotomies because of their upper tract lesions.

Urinary Tract Infection in Childhood

Epidemiology

Urinary tract infection in children in family practice is often neglected in the sense that the diagnosis is easily missed and even when it isn't missed it is often taken lightly. Very few incidence studies have been reported. One study reported an incidence of 17 per 1000 girls at risk per year and 4 per 1000 boys at risk per year, in children under the age of 15. No cases were seen between the ages of 10 and 15. Another study gave figures of 21 per 1000 girls at risk per year and 7 per 1000 boys at risk per year in the age range 0 to 10. These figures imply that a practitioner in the UK with a list of 2500 patients and an average age-sex distribution could expect to see between 3 and 5 girls and 1 or 2 boys with infection each year.

Aetiology and Pathogenosis

Organisms isolated from childhood urinary infections are the same as those isolated from adult infections and ascending infection is believed to be the prominent mode of infection but it is possible that in neonates descending infection may occur. Factors influencing and encouraging infection in children are as yet incompletely explored but screening studies are suggesting that they seem to be associated to some extent with poor housing and poor home care. The relevance of this to acute symptomatic episodes as seen in the surgery is uncertain. It is believed that the majority of these infections begin in the first three years of life and perhaps 20 to 30 per cent of relapses may be associated with an upper respiratory infection. Occasionally a family history is found.

It is generally accepted that there is a close relationship between recurrent urinary infection in childhood, vesico-ureteric reflux and radiological evidence of chronic pyelonephritic scarring. The development of this radiological lesion has only been observed in children and moreover in the absence of reflux recurrent urinary infection is much less likely to have serious consequences. Work at University College Hospital has demonstrated that a radiological abnormality can frequently be demonstrated in children with urinary tract infection, being present in 35 per cent of children with a history of one infection and 65 per cent of children with recurrent infection. Micturating cystograms reveal that vesico-ureteric reflux can be demonstrated in between 30 and 40 per cent of all children with infection and up to half of the children with recurrent infection. Reflux not only aids the ascent of bacteria towards the renal parenchyma but also helps to maintain an infected residual bladder urine as after the act of micturition refluxing urine descends into the bladder again. Reflux is often associated with chronic pyelonephritic scarring and intravenous pyelography reveals that the lesion can be found in 26 per cent of children with recurrent infection and 13 per cent of all children with infection. As well as information about the possible effects of infection radiography also gives information about congenital abnormalities possibly predisposing to infection which may be amenable to surgery. Overall 35 per cent of IVPs revealed some abnormality (including 13 per cent with renal scarring) and 46 per cent of micturating cystograms revealed some abnormality (including 34 per cent with reflux).

It is of course tempting to translate these alarming figures into the context of family practice but this can only be done with reservation as hospital studies are highly selective. Studies of the presenting features and the outcome of symptomatic urinary infection in childhood have yet to appear from family practice.

Reflux clearly plays an important part in the pathogenesis of infection and it is believed that reflux *per se*, without infection, may result in hydronephritic renal damage and even chronic pyelonephritis. However, spontaneous resolution of reflux may occur in as many as 80 per cent of children by the time adolescence is reached. Attempts to identify the 20 per cent or so that do not so resolve have not yet been successful, making decisions about the surgical management of reflux somewhat controversial.

Clinical Features

The clinical features of childhood urinary tract infection vary according to age. In the neonate infection may be present as a severe systemic illness with septicaemia and secondary renal parenchymal involvement and possibly jaundice. It may be associated with serious congenital abnormalities of the urinary tract with clinical evidence of pyelonephritis; the mortality in these cases may be high. Other infants may have vague symptoms and signs such as anorexia, vomiting and loose stools, fever and general lethargy. Yet another group may be entirely asymptomatic. In a recent hospital review of 66 cases in the first month of life with clinical illness attributed to urinary tract infection 30 per cent had a positive blood culture, half had a blood urea above 50 mg per cent and the overall mortality was 11 per cent. Forty five per cent of the mothers of infected infants were known to have some type of infection during labour or the puerperium. In contrast with infection later in childhood boys are more frequently infected than girls.

Between the age of one month and two years poor weight gain is a major sign as is the presence of fever and vomiting attacks. Disturbances of micturition are unusual. Sometimes the fishy odour of a urine infection may be noticed by the mother or the doctor and, although this can be confused with the odour of stale urine, it can be a pointer to the diagnosis and is usually an indication for culturing the urine. Gastroenteritis, pyloric stenosis and maternal inadequacy are commonly diagnosed.

Between 2 and 5 years fever remains an important sign but abdominal pain may be complained of and mother may emphasise enuresis of recent onset. Infections of the upper respiratory tract are often diagnosed and indeed such infections may often co-exist.

After the age of 5 conventional urinary tract symptoms are more prominent such as frequency, dysuria, abdominal or loin pain and possibly enuresis. Enuresis is an interesting symptom. There is not a particularly high incidence of urinary infection in children presenting with enuresis and nothing else: studies have claimed that 5 per cent of enuretic girls and 1.2 per cent of enuretic boys have urinary infection. On the other hand enuresis may be associated with, although often obscured by, other symptoms of infection and mothers may admit to this on direct questioning. It has been claimed that 45 per cent of bacteriuric girls are currently bedwetting compared with 17 per cent of normal girls up to the age of 15. (Enuresis is discussed in Chapter 23).

Diagnosis
From what has been said it is clear that, in young children at least, symptoms and signs may not necessarily point to the possibility of urinary infection and bacteriological examination of a urinary specimen is necessary in view of the vague clinical syndrome in infancy and childhood. Techniques of urine collection have been discussed previously (p. 330).

Any child with a urinary infection should be referred to a paediatric nephrologist or urologist for further assessment which will include intravenous pyelography and possibly micturating cystography. Cystourethroscopy and retrograde pyelography may be required in some cases.

Management
The demonstration of significant bacteriuria should be followed by identification of the pathogen at the local pathology laboratory and an antibiogram indicating drug sensitivities. While awaiting sensitivity studies co-trimoxazole can

be administered in appropriate dosage for a period of 15 days. A post-treatment urine examination is advisable to ensure that the organisms have been eliminated. The medical records should be studied as previous illnesses may have occurred which, with the benefit of hindsight, could have been caused by urinary infection. This information should be included in the referral letter with a description of the clinical symptoms and signs. Care should be taken to ensure that the parents understand just why the child is being referred to a specialist. Anxiety is often allayed when it is pointed out that this is routine in all children who develop infection, not only to ensure that no serious abnormality underlies the condition but also to ensure that adequate care can be given in the future to prevent any recurrence.

Thorough investigation will result in four categories of patient. Children with no obvious abnormality, children with reflux but no scarring of the kidneys, children with renal scarring and children with congenital abnormalities other than reflux, some of which e.g., urethral valves and ureterocoeles, may be surgically correctable. All of these children will need careful follow up until adolescence is reached when further renal damage as a result of infection is unlikely. Ideally monthly urine examinations should be arranged at the surgery until it has been demonstrated that recurrences are infrequent when three monthly examinations can be allowed.

More controversial aspects of management arise when the surgical correction of reflux and long term chemotherapy are considered. Factors influencing a decision to operate on reflux include the degree of dilatation of the ureter, the appearance of the ureteric orifice at cystoscopy, the cause of the reflux, the frequency of recurrent infection, the amount of reflux and the presence of renal scarring. Some experts have emphasised their uneasiness about the lack of consistent standards among surgeons about the criteria for operation as a childs fate often depends more on which surgeon happens to be consulted than it does on the pathological processes in the renal tract, which places a considerable responsibility on the family doctor. Experienced surgeons can abolish reflux in about 90 per cent of the ureters they reimplant but infection may persist after successful surgery in 20 to 30 per cent of cases.

When recurrent infections are frequent prolonged antibiotic therapy with double or triple micturition is often tried before surgery of reflux is considered; frequent urine assessments are required as reinfection with resistant bacteria is common.

The Future

Future studies need to concentrate on the relevance of urinary infection in childhood from the point of view of the family practitioner. Continuing studies in the authors practice, as yet unpublished, are beginning to suggest that although urinary infection is common, abnormalities are not found as frequently as they are in hospital studies. Even when renal scarring is discovered it should be remembered that a recent study of the function of the kidneys which appeared to show scarring on radiological examination concluded that the radiologically estimated size of the kidney bore no relation to its function. Indeed it was suggested that the function of such kidneys might be far better than radiographs would have lead one to suspect. Clearly this work is of considerable significance and before adopting a pessimistic prognosis when children with chronic pyelonephritis are identified in family practice we need to be certain that the radiological diagnosis of chronic pyelonephritis matters. Until these aspects are clarified however, we cannot afford to neglect the continuing care of these children.

Asymptomatic Bacteriuria

Significant bacteriuria may be isolated, not only in association with the clinical syndromes described above, but also in screening programmes in patients who do not complain of any symptoms and do not appear to be ill. In discussing this problem it is important to understand the difference in meaning between the two terms prevalence and incidence as they are often confused. Prevalence is defined as the number of cases existing in a community at any given *point* in time. Incidence is defined as the number of cases arising in a population over a specified *period* of time. Thus in terms of symptomatic infection the incidence of urinary infection in women in family practice may be 25 per 1000 women at risk per year, whereas the prevalence would be the percentage of practice females infected at any one moment of time.

The problem is further complicated by the observation of a number of workers that the term asymptomatic bacteriuria is often a misnomer in that, on direct questioning, a considerable proportion of infected patients, perhaps as many as 70 per cent will often admit to minor symptoms of dysuria, frequency, and enuresis, which had not prompted them to seek medical advice. This situation has been described as covert bacteriuria. The prevalence of bacteriuria on screening has been estimated in various populations at different times. Recent studies in New Zealand have demonstrated a prevalence in the neonate of 1 per cent with a male : female ratio of 3 : 1. The male preponderance commonly found at this age has been attributed to the higher incidence in boys of urinary tract abnormalities such as urethral valves. Recent screening studies in Dundee, Scotland in primary school girls have revealed a prevalence of 1.6 per cent and an annual incidence of 0.9 per cent. This means that, as there is an annual acquisition rate of 0.9 per cent, the incidence of urinary tract infection through childhood could be between 5 per cent and 10 per cent. The prevalence of bacteriuria in schoolboys has been agreed to be about 0.04 per cent i.e., a female : male ratio of over 30 : 1.

The prevalence in adult males is 0.5 per cent and about 4 per cent in adult females, but the annual incidence in females is about 1 per cent which means that the incidence over a lifetime in females is about 10—20 per cent of the female population. The prevalence in pregnant women at 4 per cent is about the same as the prevalence in non pregnant women. Prevalence increases among the elderly of both sexes particularly in the hospitalised in whom it is 20—30 per cent. The significance of these findings is as yet uncertain. In the New Zealand study 14 infants with urinary infection were investigated and all had normal pyelograms but eight had slight or moderate vesico-ureteric reflux. The Dundee study in schoolgirls revealed that 23 per cent of the girls with bacteriuria had radiological evidence of pyelonephritis and 35 per cent had vesico-ureteric reflux. These figures might seem alarming but the authors emphasised that a relationship between bacteriuria and radiological pyelonephritis is not sufficient to justify mass screening programmes as it is necessary to show that covert bacteriuria relates in some way to acute symptomatic disease and that radiological pyelonephritis causes ill health. Certainly it would appear that screening at primary school entrance is too late and that the key years lie between infancy and the pre-school years.

In the adult, studies in Cardiff, Wales have demonstrated that screening for asymptomatic bacteriuria in non-pregnant women is unlikely to be of preventive value as there was no evidence that bacteriuria led to a rise of blood pressure, serum urea concentration, or kidney scarring. Furthermore although symptomatic infection was commoner in the bacteriuric group than the control group there was no evidence that antibacterial agents prevented episodes of symptoms. It is generally accepted that the only screening procedure of value is in the pregnant woman as treatment of asymptomatic bacteriuria in this context prevents the development of symptomatic infection at a later stage of pregnancy or during the puerperium.

Urinary Tract Infection and Pregnancy

Screening for asymptomatic bacteriuria at the ante-natal clinic is well worth the effort as studies have revealed that between 14 per cent and 63 per cent of mothers with bacteriuria will develop acute pyelonephritis during pregnancy. This enhanced susceptibility of pregnant women to renal involvement has been said to be due to a combination of stasis in the urinary tract and a higher urine pH favouring bacterial multiplication. Therapy with ampicillin has been shown to largely prevent this pyelonephritis though not all cases can be predicted on screening. Some studies have suggested increased risks to the mother of hypertension, preeclamptic toxaemia and anaemia when bacteriuria is discovered and increased risk to the foetus of prematurity, neonatal death, stillbirth and abortion but definitive studies are still awaited and there is less ground for thinking that treatment removes these risks.

Various disadvantages have been postulated for most agents used to treat bacteriuria in pregnancy. Tetracyclines should not be given because of teeth staining in the foetus. In one study one week of sulphonamide therapy cured 75 per cent of patients without mishap and ampicillin has been in use for many years, although it is excreted through the foetal kidneys. Nitrofurantoin in normal dosage is only found in very low concentration in milk, amniotic fluid, and cord blood and there should be little danger of foetal toxicity.

If an IVP is carried out in women who have demonstrated pregnancy bacteriuria it must be delayed until 6 months post partum to allow pregnancy changes to resolve. Between 20 per cent and 50 per cent may have renal abnormalities but the significance of these findings in terms of eventual deterioration in renal function is similar to their significance in non pregnant women.

Pyelonephritis

Although many of the features of acute and chronic pyelonephritis have been discussed above certain aspects require emphasis. The term pyelonephritis by definition involves an inflammation of the pelvicalyceal system and interstitium of the kidney in contrast with the primary corpuscular involvement of a glomerulonephritis. In its acute form it is a complication of an ascending urinary infection although in infancy pyelonephritis may complicate a septicaemia. The term chronic pyelonephritis has been used to cover a chronic interstitial nephritis but it is rather difficult to define clearly any disease process to go with it.

Acute Pyelonephritis

Pyelonephritis has a patchy distribution in renal parenchyma tissue characterised by collections of polymorphonuclear leucocytes in the interstitial tissue between the tubules and in the lumina of the tubules themselves. Chronic inflammatory cells such as lymphocytes and plasma cells may also be seen early in the course of the disease. In the more severe cases microabscesses and even necrosis of the papillae may occur. In ascending infection the renal medulla is mainly involved but in blood-borne infection the cortex receives much of the damage.

Diagnosis

When symptoms of dysuria and frequency are accompanied by loin pain, loin tenderness, general malaise, rigors and significant bacteriuria the diagnosis of acute pyelonephritis is relatively straightforward. It may be argued however that acute pyelonephritis can occur in the presence of symptoms referable solely to the lower urinary tract and even in the absence of symptoms, but it would seem reasonable to assume that renal tissue involvement in such circumstances is less extensive. In view of this uncertainty investigations have been introduced to help decide the site of infection. These include the presence of leucocyte casts in the urine, a raised serum antibody titre to the infecting organism, and defects in the maximal urine concentrating ability, but, with the possible exception of the former, these tests have little place in the management of acute urinary infection in family practice. In contrast with the dysuria and frequency syndrome acute pyelonephritis may be associated with underlying renal abnormalities, either congenital or acquired, and a post treatment IVP examination is often worthwhile.

Management

The management of acute pyelonephritis is essentially the management of acute urinary infection but constitutional disturbances may be more pronounced and bed rest in the acute stage is desirable. Patients with renal involvement respond less well to therapy and attention should be paid to the concentration of the drug in the blood and tissues as well as in the urine and because of this ampicillin or co-trimoxazole might be preferred as the drugs of first choice. Ampicillin can be given parenterally.

Course and Outcome

Evidence is accumulating that non-obstructive acute pyelonephritis follows a benign course in adults even when followed by recurrent bacteriuria. Renal scarring is a complication associated with urinary infection in infancy and early childhood when vesico-ureteric reflux is often found.

Chronic Pyelonephritis

In 1933 Longcope and Winkenwerder described nine patients with grossly shrunken kidneys, seven of whom (including five females) had advanced renal failure. The five females had suffered from urinary infection and attention focussed on a possible relationship between urinary infection and this chronic pyelonephritis. It was hoped that adequate treatment for urinary infection would prevent chronic pyelonephritis and consequently many cases of chronic renal failure.

Since this time however a major difficulty has arisen due to the use of the term chronic pyelonephritis in different contexts. Clinicians have emphasised hypertension and renal failure not associated with glomerular disease. Bacteriologists have emphasised recurrent and perhaps asymptomatic bacteriuria. Pathologists have emphasised certain histological features and radiologists have additional criteria which have proved the most helpful from a clinical point of view. Attempts to weld the above features into a recognisable disease process beginning with ascending urinary infection and ending with terminal renal failure have been unsuccessful.

Aetiology and Pathology

The term chronic pyelonephritis is probably best reserved for a description of certain pathological features. On macroscopic inspection the kidneys are scarred and may be of unequal size and shape. On cut section scars may run from cortex to medulla and the calyces may be dilated and deformed. On microscopic examination the essential features include a focal chronic inflammatory reaction primarily involving the interstitial tissue in the medulla but extending into the cortex as well. Fibrosis varies with the duration and extent of the inflammatory process and blood vessels, tubules and glomeruli may be secondarily involved in this.

For many years it was believed that these features were the result of chronic bacterial inflammation but it is now realised that many other non-bacterial processes may produce them including renal arteriosclerosis, analgesic abuse, gout, renal artery stenosis, renal infarction, drug allergy, urinary tract obstruction, irradiation and even chronic glomerulonephritis. These changes are found in 3—15 per cent of all autopsies and it is by no means certain that bacteria play a major aetiological role although chronic pyelonephritis has been associated with ascending urinary infection and vesico-ureteric reflux in childhood. In the absence of obstructing features within the urinary tract, congenital or acquired, which may predispose to infection such as nephro-calcinosis, scarring of the kidneys due to bacterial infection is believed to be rare in adult life.

Clinical Features

These may be so variable as to be non-specific and may range from the demonstration of recurrent asymptomatic bacteriuria with leucocyte casts to overt symptoms and signs of renal failure. The isolation of significant bacteriuria of course does not necessarily imply any aetiological relationship with chronic pyelonephritic changes as infection may be secondary to some other disease process. In some patients the predominant features may be those of the underlying disease process such as urinary lithiasis. Hypertension has been reported to be present in between 22 per cent and 70 per cent of cases especially in association with marked atrophy of one or more kidneys but unlike glomerulonephritis there is no close correlation between the level of the blood pressure and the degree of renal failure. Proteinuria is variable.

Diagnosis

In a disease of uncertain natural history diagnosis must be difficult. Attention should be focussed on vulnerable groups. These will include patients with a history of urinary infection in childhood who may well have developed renal scarring at this time. Patients who are known to have taken large quantities of analgesics, particularly phenacetin, should have their urines examined for bacteria and protein, a blood urea estimation and possibly an IVP. Analgesic abuse may be suspected in the presence of abuse of other drugs including alcohol. Peptic ulceration and anaemia are the presenting features and in these groups withdrawal of analgesics carries a good prognosis. Any patient with a known renal abnormality may develop chronic pyelonephritis and renal abnormalities or chronic pyelonephritis may be found in any patient with acute pyelonephritis clinically. Any male or child with urinary infection may reveal an underlying congenital or acquired lesion which may progress to chronic pyelonephritis.

Clinically the diagnosis is best made from the radiological features. A plain film may demonstrate contraction and scarring of the renal outline and asymmetry between the two kidneys; the major diagnostic features however are revealed by excretion or retrograde pyelography. The earliest changes are minimal blunting of one or more of the calyces in either or both kidneys which progresses to frank clubbing and caliectasis with thinning of the cortex above the dilated calyx.

An early functional change is detectable loss of renal maximal concentrating power but the X-ray changes are the most helpful as the concentration test is not often carried out from family practice.

Management and Prognosis

Although particular care should be made to control any other renal disease and hypertension, and to provide effective treatment and follow up for recurrent urinary infection, the patient should be told that kidneys that may look scarred and distorted on X-ray can nevertheless function very well. There is no convincing evidence that prophylatic long term antibiotics are of value but the family practitioner will want to obtain specialist advice during pregnancy. Other aspects are discussed in the section on chronic renal failure (p. 359).

GLOMERULONEPHRITIS, NEPHRITIC SYNDROME AND NEPHROTIC SYNDROME

Glomerulonephritis is a pathological term implying inflammatory change within a glomerulus and is therefore best avoided when describing clinical situations. The observable histological responses of the glomerulus to injury are limited and a minimal lesion glomerulonephritis, membraneous glomerulonephritis, focal glomerulosclerosis and proliferative glomerulonephritis have been described. The first three lesions are believed to represent histopathological entities whereas the latter is believed to be an heterogenous mixture of changes including different stages of the same disease process and more discrete conditions.

The ways in which glomerular damage can present clinically are also limited and these include an acute nephritic syndrome (acute onset with haematuria), a nephrotic syndrome (oedema, proteinuria, hypoproteinaemia), and a persistent urinary abnormality without symptoms (proteinuria, haematuria); chronic renal failure and acute renal failure are discussed separately at the end of this section. Both the pathological and clinical features may be subdivided still further in that proliferative glomerulonephritis has itself been subdivided into seven distinct entities and several syndromes of an acute nephritic type have been described.

Recent work using electron microscopy of material obtained by percutaneous renal biopsy has revealed that the notion that the basic clinical syndromes of acute haematuric illness, and insidious oedema with proteinuria (Ellis type I and type II nephritis) could be associated with specific histological appearances was mistaken. Each of the two clinical groups is believed to be the outcome of a variety of structural changes most of unknown aetiology, and a further complication is that occasionally nephritic patients have nephrotic changes such as heavy proteinuria or oedema making them difficult to classify. Some patients with systemic vascular disorders such as systemic lupus erythematosus may present with either nephritic or nephrotic features. Clearly when renal biopsy reveals a group of structural changes that can be associated with a certain prognosis there is no implication that they represent a disease in their own right as aetiology may well be multifactorial.

Aetiology

It is now clear that the concept that 'acute nephritis' follows infection with nephritogenic strains of beta haemolytic streptococcus is not entirely true. Although immunological mechanisms are commonly, but not invariably, involved they are not always associated with infection. It has been suggested that vulnerability is enhanced by inherited factors and previous exposure.

The beta haemolytic streptococcus is certainly involved but non haemolytic streptococci, staphylococci and rarely syphilis have been incriminated. Virus infections such as mumps, varicella and influenza may occasionally be involved and recent work has incriminated the Australia antigen of virus B hepatitis. An acute nephritic syndrome and the nephrotic syndrome can occur without any known infective cause as part of a generalised vascular illness such as systemic lupus erythematosis, Goodpastures syndrome and Henoch Schonlein purpura.

Pathogenesis

The immune response is believed to be a major factor in the production of damage which may theoretically occur in two different ways. If an antiserum develops in one species to the glomerular tissue of another then the reinjection of that antiserum into the first species will lead to glomerulonephritis; these antikidney antibodies however, are believed to play only a small part in human glomerulonephritis. A second mechanism involves an antigen that need have no connection with the kidney; the type, dose and time exposed to it however are important factors as is the inherited reaction of the patient and the amount of conditioning that has resulted from previous exposure. Antibody is produced and soluble antigen-antibody complexes fix complement and become deposited in small capillaries in the kidney glomerulus aided by the considerable blood flow to these organs. Most of these antigens have yet to be discovered and it is not even certain that streptococci, although capable of forming soluble complexes, are the major source of antigen.

Glomerular damage however, does not result from the antigen antibody complex but from the secondary reaction to it. This involves complement activation and coagulation. Complement releases inflammatory factors which attract leucocytes, as does the formation of fibrin plugs. Coagulation is normally followed by fibrinolysis and the resolution of the inflammatory process. Why this does not occur in some patients who proceed to chronic glomerulonephritis and chronic renal failure is uncertain but it may be related to the delicate glomerular structure which could readily scar as a result of minimal distortion rendering it functionally useless.

Histological Classification

Electron microscopy of percutaneous renal biopsy material has improved our knowledge of acute glomerulonephritis as various biopsy appearances have been found to correlate to some extent with both the immediate outlook for the patient and the long term prognosis.

Minimal Lesion Glomerulonephritis
The kidney appears normal on light microscopy but on electron microscopy characteristic changes are found involving the foot processes of the epithelial cells of Bowman's capsule. These changes are extensive and involve the disintegration of the foot processes resulting in only a thin smear of protoplasm on the capsular side of the basement membrane.

These histological changes are usually associated with the nephrotic syndrome which commonly presents between the age of one and five years after which the incidence falls. Overall the incidence in the UK is 18 per million children per year under the age of 14 years rising to a peak of 30 per million children per year at the age of three years. The prognosis with treatment may be good and a five year survival rate of up to 90 per cent has been reported.

Membraneous Glomerulonephritis

In membraneous glomerulonephritis there is a marked thickening of the capillary basement membrane with little cellular proliferation. The result is the eventual obliteration of the capillary lumen, and the glomeruli and tubules deprived of their blood supply become replaced by fibrous tissue.

These changes are usually associated with proteinuria but in two thirds of cases it is not severe enough to cause the nephrotic syndrome. It is not found in acute nephritic syndromes but abrupt onset and microscopic haematuria may be present and the latter is occasionally marked. The condition is not common in children with the nephrotic syndrome but when it is found in children the prognosis may be better than in the adult in whom a generally progressive disease usually develops. Survival rates of 70 per cent at 5 years and 40 per cent at ten years have been reported.

Focal Glomerulosclerosis

The essential lesion is a small area of sclerosis, in one or two glomeruli initially, but eventually becoming progressive to involve not only the whole of the glomerulus but also an increasing proportion of glomeruli. Focal tubular atrophy is an inevitable consequence. Frequently described in children associated clinical features include proteinuria, occasionally with oedema and microscopic haematuria. The prognosis is poor, the majority progressing eventually to chronic renal failure.

Proliferative Glomerulonephritis

In proliferative glomerulonephritis the pathological process affects the endothelial cells of the glomerulus which swell and increase in number. The basement membrane of the glomerular capillary wall is damaged by fibrin deposition and protein and red blood cells and white blood cells escape into the tubular space of Bowman's capsule where they form crescent-shaped deposits. Eventually the glomeruli may become obliterated and loss of blood supply results in replacement of glomeruli and tubules by fibrous tissue.

Unlike the three previously described histopathological entities which appear to have a consistent prognosis proliferative glomerulonephritis is more confusing. In the first place, whereas the former three invariably present with a proteinuria or a nephrotic syndrome, proliferative glomerulonephritis may be found in any syndrome of glomerular disease and there may be an acute nephritic syndrome, proteinuria with or without a nephrotic syndrome and occasionally acute renal failure. In the second place several different histological subclassifications of proliferative glomerulonephritis have been described which may represent different entities or different stages of the same entity. Overall there is a steady mortality of about 30 per cent at four years and 40 per cent at 8 years but different subgroups have different prognoses. For example the acute proliferative glomerulonephritis associated with the classical 'acute nephritis' of macroscopic haematuria, mild proteinuria and oliguria consequent to beta haemolytic streptococcal infection carries a good prognosis and it has been said that at least in children chronic disease is never seen in the typical case. This is not necessarily true of other types of proliferative glomerulonephritis some of which may be commoner in adults than children.

Clinical Features

Acute Nephritic Syndrome

This consists of haematuria, oliguria, oedema and hypertension and it may be associated with beta haemolytic streptococcal infection, other bacterial and viral infections, acute glomerulonephritis without known infective cause and certain multisystem diseases. The onset is abrupt and classically occurs 10—14 days after a streptococcal throat or skin infection. Many of these features may be absent; proteinuria is constant but variable in amount usually below 3 g per day. Haematuria may be readily visible or may be detected only on microscopy, and oedema is usually slight and apparent around the eyes. The oedema is a feature of sodium retention and a diminished glomerular filtration rate with consequent circulatory overload. The jugular venous pressure may be raised and blood pressure is elevated in about 70 per cent of cases. Occasionally hypertensive encephalopathy with fits and severe headaches may occur. Hypertension may lead to pulmonary oedema. The oliguria is also a feature of sodium retention and diminished glomerular filtration rate and occasionally acute renal failure with prolonged oliguria or even anuria may intervene.

Typically a diuresis occurs after a few days of oliguria and the clinical features recede leaving microscopic haematuria and slight proteinuria which may remain for many months. Over 90 per cent of children and 50 per cent of adults eventually recover completely. It is said that those who fail to recover and who have persistent hypertension or proteinuria and who progress ultimately to chronic renal failure do not have post streptococcal nephritis.

There is a condition known as primary (recurrent) haematuria in which careful investigation reveals no cause such as stones or tumours. The haematuria may be microscopic or macroscopic and may be related to exertion. Other nephritic features are usually absent and when symptoms are present they consist only of clot colic and dysuria but occasionally episodes of nephritic symptoms may punctuate the course of the illness. The prognosis is said to be excellent.

The Nephrotic Syndrome

This syndrome is characterised by massive proteinuria, oedema, hypopro-teinaemia and a raised blood cholesterol and as any renal disorder that is associated with marked proteinuria can produce it, it can be a feature of many renal diseases. In one study 77 per cent of patients with the nephrotic syndrome had primary glomerulonephritis (membraneous in 30 per cent, proliferative in 22 per cent, minimal lesion in 18 per cent and mixed membraneous and proliferative in 7 per cent). In the other 23 per cent the renal damage was caused by diseases such as systemic lupus erythematosus, renal amyloidosis, diabetic nephropathy and renal vein thrombosis. The presenting complaint is dependant oedema which in children is usually apparent around the face and in the abdomen as ascites. In adults the oedema is usually most obvious in the legs especially in the evenings. It is relatively rare but although it may occur at any age it is commoner in childhood with an incidence of 20 per million children per year. Patients with the nephrotic syndrome are particularly vulnerable to infection.

Diagnosis

Clearly the history is of particular importance and may help to exclude a multisystem disease but particular attention should be paid on examination to the presence of oedema in the face and lower limbs. Pleural effusion and ascites may be present. The blood pressure should be recorded. A number of basic investigations can be initiated in family practice. The urine can be examined not only for protein but also for casts, red blood cells and white blood cells (see p. 326). Bacteriuria needs to be excluded (see p. 330). Swabs of the throat need to be taken as streptococci may be demonstrated. Blood investigation may reveal a high ESR (up to 100 mm per hour), hypoproteinaemia, hypocomplementaemia, an elevated antistreptolysin O titre and a raised blood urea or serum creatinine. Renal biopsy is not usually indicated in the acute nephritic syndrome unless a multisystem disease is suspected or the course is unusually protracted. Persistent hypocomplementaemia and transition to a nephrotic phase are indications for renal biopsy. Renal biopsy is often necessary in the nephrotic syndrome as it is crucial to differentiate between patients having a minimal lesion glomerulonephritis and those having greater structural damage. In general 85 per cent of childhood nephrotic patients between 1 and 5 show a minimal change pattern. After the age of 5 the percentage falls and after 10 years only 20—30 have this lesion. Renal biopsy is therefore usually necessary after the age of 10 but may not be so between the ages of 1 and 5.

Management

Few family practitioners would consider themselves competent to manage nephritic or nephrotic syndromes without specialist advice as accurate diagnosis, correct treatment and a reliable prognosis may well depend on the results of renal biopsy. Patients with the nephritic syndrome may require penicillin in appropriate dosage for 7—10 days if streptococci have been isolated. Bed rest may be of value during the acute stage until a diuresis supervenes and dietary restriction of sodium may be helpful in this period. While oliguria persists a fluid balance chart should be maintained and water intake should be restricted to 500 ml per day plus the equivalent volume of urine passed the previous day in an adult. Frusemide in large doses (up to 1 g for an adult) may be helpful especially in the presence of pulmonary oedema and ascites. Hypertension usually needs no drug therapy but hypotensive therapy should be initiated if the diastolic pressure rises to about 110 mm of mercury. Fits or even restlessness and confusion due to encephalopathy can be controlled by intravenous diazepam 2—10 mg. There is no indication for steroids.

The management of patients with the nephrotic syndrome depends on the lesion identified. Corticosteroids produce a rapid remission in almost all patients with a minimal change lesion within 4 weeks. Bed rest is not especially indicated but diet should be high in protein and low in salt. Diuretics are helpful but care needs to be taken in severe oedema. Prophylactic penicillin may be considered during the oedematous phase. When other histological lesions are identified management is limited to maintaining the patient in an oedema-free condition, treating hypertension and giving palliative treatment for uraemia. There is evidence that corticosteroid therapy may actually be harmful. Bendrofluazide and frusemide (or amiloride in the presence of hypokalaemia) have proved beneficial. Sometimes high doses of frusemide need to be given.

Follow up and Continuing Care

Ninety per cent of patients with an acute nephritic syndrome make a complete recovery. This may, however, take some time and in one study in children slight proteinuria and haematuria continued intermittently in 36 per cent of children for over 2 years, despite the eventual recovery of 95 per cent of the group. These findings therefore need not cause alarm. Of the remaining 10 per cent one quarter die of hypertension or cardiac failure early in the disease and the remainder have persistant proteinuria and hypertension and progress to ultimate renal failure. The family practitioner therefore must ensure that blood pressure levels are estimated and urine examinations performed until the outcome has been clarified.

When a minimal change nephrotic syndrome has been identified it can be anticipated that 50 per cent will remain well indefinitely once a steroid induced remission is complete. Until a remission has occurred daily proteinuria estimations and daily weighings are necessary. The remainder may experience relapses often associated with infections of the upper respiratory tract, but these are rare if one symptom-free year elapses after the initial attack. In the presence of relapses a decision has to be made about treatment with corticosteroids on an *ad hoc* basis, or prophylatic therapy in low dosage. When relapses are frequent alternative therapy with cytotoxic agents such as azathioprine has been tried and found effective. Cyclophosphamide has been found to be particularly effective in this respect but the long term hazards are uncertain.

CHRONIC RENAL FAILURE

Chronic failure implies a gradual deterioration in the various functions of the kidney resulting in an accumulation of metabolic waste products in the blood stream and impaired homeostasis. It has been estimated that about 7000 people die each year from chronic renal failure and although many are elderly nearly half of them are still in their prime. There may be an annual incidence of 40 new patients per million at risk.

Aetiology

Chronic renal failure can be the terminal stage of any chronic bilateral renal disease but in practice glomerulonephritis, chronic pyelonephritis and malignant hypertension account for more than half the cases, with congenital lesions such as polycystic kidneys, or obstructive lesions accounting for a further 20 per cent. Chronic pyelonephritis is the commonest lesion in children and in the elderly whereas chronic glomerulonephritis is commoner in adolescents and young adults.

Pathology

One of the difficulties in deciding the relative importance of different renal diseases in chronic renal failure is that the ultimate stages of many renal diseases and pathological processes may be identical. Indeed any renal lesion may become infected when it may be difficult to decide for example whether the primary lesion was glomerulonephritis or pyelonephritis. For this reason the pathological term 'end stage kidney' has found favour amongst some authors.

Natural History

As 50 to 70 per cent of renal function needs to be lost before any detectable effect on blood chemistry can be observed it is useful to divide the progression of chronic renal failure into two stages of renal impairment and renal failure, that is before and after the development of significant nitrogen retention. In the stage of renal impairment there is at the most minimal nitrogen retention with urea levels up to 100 mg per cent on a normal diet. The patient is as a rule asymptomatic but some nocturia is common as the ability to produce a concentrated urine is impaired. There may be a sudden reduction in renal function associated with the development of electrolyte abnormalities during the course of intercurrent illness, especially when accompanied by diarrhoea and vomiting. Renal failure is associated with considerable nitrogen retention and anaemia and electrolyte disturbances are common; marked symptoms are usually present. The terminal stages are often described as uraemia and the clinical picture is dominated by the mental, neuromuscular, and cardiovascular complications of severe renal failure. These stages inevitably merge into each other and the patient may present at any one of them. The rate of progression in chronic renal failure is determined by the nature of the underlying disease and the success with which hypertension if present, is controlled. Other important factors include renal infection, cardiac failure and therapeutic mismanagement.

Functional Disturbances

The progressive reduction of the nephron population must interfere with the functions of the kidney. Initially each remaining nephron becomes more active than normal in an attempt to maintain homeostasis and each accepts an increased load. Ultimately however, the total amount of solute excreted is reduced and blood urea rises. Since urea is an osmotic diuretic this helps to maintain the urine volume. Inability to concentrate the urine is an early sign of progressive renal disease.

The systemic acidosis of chronic renal failure is produced by reduced bicarbonate reabsorption and reduced ammonia formation in the tubular cells.

Another feature of chronic renal failure is the inability to conserve sodium in response to varying intake and varying body requirements. As plasma sodium and potassium remain fairly constant in chronic renal failure despite a reduced glomerular filtration rate the implication is that the amount of sodium and potassium reabsorption is reduced. Thus a greater percentage of the filtered load is excreted in the urine. Altered sodium intake may affect the kidneys however. Sodium excess is the commonest complication and results in oedema and pulmonary congestion and exacerbation of any existing hypertension. Sodium deficiency however, may occur due to the inability of the failing kidney to reduce sodium excretion. The danger with potassium handling in chronic renal failure is that in the presence of oliguria for any reason, hyperkalaemia may occur as there is a limited capacity to excrete a potassium load. Potassium intake therefore needs to be controlled.

Bone complications in chronic renal failure tend to develop late in the course of the disease except in children who are laying down new bone more rapidly. Serum calcium is low because of poor absorption in uraemia (related to

Vitamin D resistance) and mineralisation of the osteoid framework laid down by the oesteoblasts is retarded. Thus osteomalacia in adults and renal rickets in children may occur. A low serum calcium stimulates the parathyroid glands to secrete parathormone. Increased parathormone levels may mobilise calcium from bone as a result of osteoclastic activity resulting in osteitis fibrosa cystica in some patients. In other patients however parathormome has no effect. It should be remembered that a low serum calcium increases neuromuscular irritability and may lead to tetany but this is not as common as it otherwise might be because of acidosis which tends to counteract the effect.

Anaemia is a common feature in chronic renal failure and there are at least two major causes. One is depression of erythropoisis due to loss of erythropoietin production in the diseased kidney and the other is haemolysis which occurs in the presence of blood urea concentrations above 200 mg per cent. It is typically normochromic and normocytic and resistant to treatment, unless it happens to be due in part to the bleeding tendency manifested particularly in the gastro-intestinal tract, which is sometimes a feature of uraemia.

The most characteristic change in chronic renal failure however is the retention of nitrogenous products. Urea production varies with the protein content of the diet but in renal failure its excretion in the urine is impaired due to the reduced glomerular filtration rate.

Clinical Features

Work at St. Thomas's Hospital, London on patients presenting with chronic renal failure has revealed that less than half developed failure by progression from a previously identified renal disease. Most presented in advanced failure. The commonest complaints were oedema, vomiting, headaches and dyspnoea. On direct questioning 75 per cent admitted to nocturia. Certain patterns of presentation were common. The condition might present as hypertension and its complications. If hypertension is absent failure may progress and anaemia may be the presenting feature. If failure is advanced any infection or gastro-intestinal upset may precipitate severe uraemia and even coma; certain drugs especially tetracycline have been known to do this.

The clinical course of chronic renal failure depends to a large extent on whether hypertension is a complicating factor. Hypertension not only results from renal disease but more commonly produces it and when it is severe chronic renal failure progresses to terminal uraemia relatively quickly. Urea levels are only a rough guide to the severity of renal failure but as a rule it is rare for patients to have uraemia symptoms below 150 mg per cent and rare for them to escape symptoms above 250 mg per cent. Between 100 mg per cent and 150 mg per cent nocturia may be the only complaint. Every tissue and organ in the body may be involved in the uraemic syndrome. Cardiovascular symptoms may include orthopnoea, oedema and chest pain; hypertension, cardiac failure and pericarditis may be found on examination. Gastro-intestinal symptoms are common and include nausea, vomiting, hiccoughs, thirst and diarrhoea. Neuromuscular features include cramps, weakness, fits and tremor; twitching and impaired consciousness may be apparent on examination. Loss of vibration sense may be an early feature of peripheral neuropathy. Ocular complications include retinopathy and retinal detachment, and haematological complications result from a bleeding tendency which with the characteristic normochromic normocytic anaemia tend to produce fatigue and breathlessness. Cutaneous manifestation of pigmentation and pruritus may be apparent, and skeletal complications may result in bone pain and rickety deformities in children.

Diagnosis

In view of the many different manifestations outlined above and the comparative rarity of chronic renal failure in family practice diagnosis must be difficult. Routine investigation for proteinuria may reveal impairment and the condition should be kept in mind when a normocytic normochronic anaemia is discovered. A blood urea or serum creatinine estimation is mandatory in this situation, is easily carried out from practice and is also worthwhile when hypertension is discovered, particularly if treatment is contemplated. It should also be carried out in the presence of oedema.

Having confirmed renal failure (normal values of blood urea are 20—40 mg per cent and of serum creatinine 1.0—1.5 mg per cent) further investigation depends on specialist advice but electrolyte estimations and, if indicated, calcium, phosphate and alkaline phosphatase estimations can be carried out from family practice.

Management

The management of chronic renal failure can be divided into three categories — conservative treatment, regular dialysis and kidney transplantation. These measures are not mutually exclusive and of course the family practitioner will need to follow the advice of a consultant nephrologist.

Conservative Therapy

Conservative therapy includes dietary measures and the control of fluid and electrolyte balance and other complications without operative intervention and the family practitioner may play an important part in this.

The treatment of advanced renal failure with a low protein diet is traditional and indeed uraemic symptoms do improve but it is important to emphasise that renal function does not improve, in fact the rate of glomerular filtration remains unchanged. Blood urea levels will of course fall as less urea is produced but this is of little consequence with regard to prognosis. Possibly many of the unpleasant symptoms of the uraemic state are related to the accumulation of products of protein catabolism which have not been excreted at their optimum rate. It is generally considered that asymptomatic patients in early renal failure are best managed on a diet containing 40 g of protein per day. Symptoms may appear with a blood urea over 100 mg per cent when further reduction of protein intake may be required. A major problem however, is the unpalatability of these diets particularly if the protein is reduced as low as 18 g per day when the skills of the dietician are particularly important. If uraemic symptoms are trivial the patient may consider the diet worse than the disease and indeed Vitamin B supplements may be required. It should be remembered that several calorie boosting foods of low protein content are available such as Caloreen and Hycal and low protein pasta biscuits. Recent research suggests that it might be possible to use adsorbent substances such as activated charcoal, or ion exchange resins to trap urea, ammonia and other uraemic toxins in the gut, and consequently to reduce blood levels.

Salt and water imbalance may be a major problem involving over-hydration on the one hand and dehydration and salt depletion on the other. In both cases variation in weight may be an early sign and an increase or loss of 1 kg or more should be regarded with suspicion. Salt restriction or supplements of sodium chloride (or bicarbonate in the presence of acidosis) require careful biochemical control and specialist advice is needed. Hyperkalaemia may be a dangerous complication in advanced renal failure and so the patient should be advised to avoid foods with a high potassium salt content such as soups, pure fruit juices, dates, bananas or salt substitutes, and of course medicines such as potassium citrate should be avoided.

The bone pain of renal osteodystrophy may be relieved by Vitamin D beginning in low dosage such as dihydrotachysterol 1 gm per day in the adult. The family practitioner may prefer to seek specialist advice however as if plasma phosphate levels are high, a rise in serum calcium consequent to Vitamin D administration may precipitate calcium phosphate in the eyes (causing conjunctivitis and superficial calcification) and the blood vessels. Aluminium hydroxide can be given to reduce serum phosphate levels. If gout should develop due to uric acid accumulation in renal failure allopurinol is best avoided as it may accumulate to give toxic effects but standard analgesic therapy may be used. Calcium gout may produce a similar clinical picture.

As hypertension is an important cause of deterioration in renal function it is well worth keeping it under control in family practice. Indeed it has been demonstrated that if the blood urea is below 60 mg per cent control of hypertension materially prolongs life. In more advanced renal failure therapeutic over enthusiasm may well reduce renal blood flow to such an extent that renal function declines still further. A diastolic pressure of around 100 mg of mercury should be aimed for. Methyldopa is a useful drug but initial doses should be low. In rapidly advancing or malignant hypertension conventional drugs are usually ineffective but the alpha adrenergic blocker phenoxybenzamine has been found effective in a dose of 10 mg daily initially increasing the dose until gastric intolerance develops or the blood pressure falls. In the presence of hypertensive encephalopathy or acute left ventricular failure frusemide 20 mg intravenously produces a dramatic improvement.

Frusemide and ethracrynic acid are useful in managing oedema in chronic renal failure but triamterene or spironolactone can be added in resistant cases. Sodium intake should also be restricted.

The characteristic normochromic normocytic anaemia of chronic renal failure is resistant to all oral therapy other than erythropoetin which is not currently available, and unless there is a haemorrhagic component when iron may be beneficial the only way of raising the haemoglobin is by blood transfusion which should only be given in an emergency in the presence of severe symptoms when dialysis can be carried out at the same time.

Pruritus is of unknown aetiology. It is said to respond for some reason to sauna baths but these are often impracticable. Small doses of chlorpromazine or antihistamines may be beneficial.

Dialysis and Transplantation

The practitioner needs to be constantly aware that a patient managed on conservative therapy may be a candidate for dialysis or even transplantation surgery. The main indications for dialysis are clinical deterioration especially with neurological complications, circulatory failure and oedema, and hyperkalaemia. Criteria for selection are becoming more liberal as a result of improved techniques and favourable experience with older patients but it is still true to say that due to scarcity of resources not all who could benefit are receiving definitive treatment. The only medical contraindication may be the presence of another serious disease process and in the absence of this complication the family practitioner should be prepared to press the interest of his patient as early as possible during the phase of conservative management as it is clearly of considerable benefit to the patient and his family to know that he is not doomed to die from renal failure and that careful watch is being kept on his progress so that dialysis can be commenced before time is lost from work due to uraemic symptoms. Certainly the patient should not be allowed to become bed-ridden or sick and the family practitioner should be alert to the possibility of rapid deterioration during intercurrent illness.

Maintenance haemodialysis has become a relatively simple procedure and indeed in the United Kingdom nearly 60 per cent of the patients receiving maintenance dialysis therapy are at home. The majority of patients require dialysis at least three times weekly for 6 to 12 hours and this is often performed overnight. When not undergoing dialysis the patient leads a normal life and severe dietary protein restriction is not necessary. Complications include hepatitis, anaemia, bone disease, infertility and psychological problems. Sleep may be broken by fail safe audiovisual monitor alarms and there may be anxiety about machine failure. There may be financial problems in adapting a room, and extra light, heating, telephone and transport costs. Holidays may be a problem and may have to be restricted to no more than five days away from the machine. Most patients become oliguric shortly after starting dialysis and fluid restriction may be needed at this time or else oedema may result. Hypertension and anaemia may be difficult to control although hepatitis, a serious complication in hospital is rarely seen in the home. Anticoagulant usage can give rise to problems and prompt antibiotic therapy may be required for minor infections in order to prevent septicaemia. It has been suggested that home peritoneal dialysis is an acceptable alternative to haemodialysis and might even have some advantages.

Transplantation may offer the advantages of the correction of anaemia, greater fertility and possible pregnancy, and greater social mobility but unless a related donor is available survival rates are not as good as with home dialysis and continuous immuno suppressive therapy may pose problems due to infection with resistant organisms.

A major problem of the day is a decision as to whether dialysis or transplantation is better for a given patient at a particular time but guide lines are beginning to emerge. Although haemodialysis is perfectly feasible in children, if a well matched related donor is available, transplantation is preferable as continuing growth and development will be superior. Growth following cadaveric transplantation is less certain due to steroid suppression. Most adolescents make poor adjustment to long term dialysis and cadaveric transplantation is favourable as immuno suppressive therapy can be tolerated if rejection occurs. If there is a matched related donor the indications are even stronger. As age increases however the indications for long term dialysis become stronger particularly having regard to the shortage of suitable donors.

Follow up and Continuing Care

The family practitioner will need to exercise considerable care in the management of intercurrent illness in patients with chronic renal failure, not only because of the possibility of exacerbations but because of the toxic effects of the drugs he might use. Antibiotics should be restricted to penicillin in initial dosage of 1 mega unit per day and 250 000 units per day subsequently, ampicillin in a dose of 500 mg stat and 250 mg 4 times a day, and co-trimoxazole in normal dosage. Tetracycline should be avoided. Nalidyxic acid may be given in unmodified dosage in urinary tract infection but nitrofurantoin should be avoided. Frusemide is the diuretic of choice and it can be given in high dosage up to 2 g daily. Hypotensive drugs need to be given with caution as they may accumulate. Barbiturates are best avoided but if necessary they can be given as phenobarbitone in a maximum dose of 30 mg 3 times a day. Diazepam can be given with caution in a dose of 2 mg 3 times a day. Chlorpromazine in normal dosage of 25 mg 3 times a day may produce profound hypotension and Parkinsonism and the dose should be reduced to 25 mg daily.

Evaluation of Definitive Therapy

The improvement in the quality of life after dialysis or transplantation cannot be denied and about 85 per cent can lead a normal working and social life. Patient survival rates are very encouraging and in the UK in 1972 five year survival rates were reported to be 73 per cent for home dialysis, 72.8 per cent for living donor transplants, 55 per cent for hospital dialysis and 50.6 per cent for cadaver-donor transplants.

ACUTE RENAL FAILURE

Acute renal failure is very rare in family practice and its management is entirely in the hands of the renal physician unless the condition progresses to chronic renal failure when the family practitioner might become involved. It can be defined as a sudden reduction in renal function with retention of waste products and impaired homeostasis, usually associated with oliguria or even anuria; it can occur however in the presence of a normal or even increased urine output.

Aetiology

The family practitioner need only be aware of the conditions in which acute renal failure might occur and in this context the traditional differentiation into pre-renal, renal and post-renal causes is clinically useful. Pre-renal causes are the causes of hypo-volaemia and hypotension such as blood loss, plasma loss as in burns, loss of water and electrolytes, myocardial infarction, massive pulmonary embolism and septicaemia. Renal causes include acute tubular necrosis resulting from ischaemic or toxic injury, renal cortical necrosis, acute glomerulonephritis and malignant hypertensive nephrosclerosis. Post renal failure may result from obstruction due to any cause.

Clinical Features

The clinical features that predominate are those of the cause of the acute renal failure but uraemic symptoms may be superimposed. Patients with acute tubular necrosis will normally recover renal function if they survive the underlying cause, as the initial oliguric phase is replaced after a short period by a diuretic phase but if the much rarer renal cortical necrosis, often associated with obstetric accidents, occurs the outlook is more serious.

Management

This involves correction of pre-renal factors where possible, the administration of an osmotic diuretic such as mannitol and attention to the underlying cause. There is no specific treatment for acute tubular necrosis or cortical necrosis and control of the renal failure may involve conservative measures or dialysis.

Prognosis

If recovery does not occur in 2–6 weeks renal cortical necrosis might be the dominant feature. The overall mortality in acute renal failure is around 50 per cent but it is related to the severity of the underlying illness ranging from about 15 per cent in cases of incompatible blood transfusion to 70 per cent or more in burns and major trauma. The mortality also rises with age being about 20 per cent overall in the twenties rising to 70 per cent in the seventies.

URINARY LITHIASIS

Urinary lithiasis is one of the commoner diseases of the urinary tract. Nearly all urinary calculi in adults are believed to originate in renal papillae from where they subsequently work loose and travel down the ureter producing a series of attacks of ureteric colic until they eventually enter the bladder. Once in the bladder the stones will be voided unless obstruction occurs at the prostate or bladder neck, a complication commoner in older men. The stones may then continue to grow in bladder urine as secondary bladder stones, especially if the urine becomes infected with urea splitting organisms such as *Proteus spp.* which renders the urine more alkaline.

Epidemiology

Not all adults are equally at risk. Lithiasis is twice as common in men as it is in women although in both the average age of onset is in the mid thirties. Studies have demonstrated that the incidence of urinary lithiasis has varied not only at different times throughout history but also in different geographical areas and in different occupations but the reasons for these variations are far from clear. Burkitt, for example, in a description of surgical pathology along the course of the Nile, asked 'Why should stones occur in mountainous cool Rwanda, be almost absent in warm green and hilly Uganda, and appear again in enormous frequency in flat hot desert Sudan?' It has been pointed out that in Northern Europe hospital admissions are commonly for upper tract stones in adults, and the bladder stones that were relatively common in children at the end of the last century seem rare today, yet common in developing countries such as Thailand and India. Countries with an intermediate economic development such as those in the Middle East show a relatively low and variable incidence of stones of both the lower urinary tract in children and the upper urinary tract in adults.

It has been discovered that in Czechoslovakia agricultural workers have the lowest rate of urolithiasis whereas sedentary workers and administrative employees have the highest; railwaymen have more than ten times the average for other occupations. A higher rate of stone formation has been demonstrated particularly in Scottish surgeons and anaesthetists, and also in family practitioners. The hot humid operating theatre environment might be thought to play some part but a review of all cases of upper tract stone occurring in Royal Navy personnel over a ten year period revealed a relatively high incidence in cooks and engineers working in higher environmental temperatures. Yet temperature could only be one of many relevant factors since Royal Marines who had frequently served for long periods in jungle conditions with a low fluid intake had remarkably few stones.

The incidence of urolithiasis in family practice has not been well documented but a Danish study reported an average incidence for men of 3 per 1000 males at risk per year and for women 1 per 1000 females at risk per year. Ureterolithiasis was commoner in men and nephrolithiasis in women.

Overall between 3 per cent and 5 per cent of men suffer from urinary lithiasis at some time in their lives and although the aetiology is not fully understood it is probably correct to say that multiple factors are involved and that broadly speaking in developed countries upper tract stones composed largely of calcium tend to occur in adults whereas in underdeveloped countries lower tract stones composed of acid ammonium urate tend to occur in children.

Aetiology and Pathogenesis

Stones probably form as a result of precipitation from oversaturated urine and it follows that factors that have been identified in aetiology and pathogenesis can be divided into two groups — causes of increased excretion of certain relatively insoluble biochemical components, and mechanisms which trigger off stone precipitation. Important biochemical substances in the first category are calcium, oxalate, cystine, uric acid, xanthine and silicon dioxide. Important factors in the second category are reduced urinary volume, urinary pH, stasis, infection and foreign bodies.

Calcium

Hypercalciuria is found in the majority of stone sufferers and it may occur in four ways: increased dietary calcium, increased absorption from the bowel, increased bone resorption and from renal tubular defects. The term is difficult to define as 24 hour urinary calcium excretion varies so much in different individuals on a normal free diet but total outputs over 300 mg per 24 hours in men and 250 mg per 24 hours in women have been generally accepted as hypercalciuria.

The major calcium containing foods are milk and cheese and marked hypercalciuria can be seen in the adult who drinks four pints of milk or more per day and it has been said to be a hazard for the very thirsty in hard water areas. Increased bowel absorption of calcium occurs in hyperparathyroidism. Seventy-five per cent of hyperparathyroid patients have stones at some stage as primary hyperparathyroidism causes hypercalcaemia and hypercalciuria as well as hyperphosphaturia and hypophosphataemia. It occurs in 2 per cent of male stone formers and 5 per cent of females with stones. Increased bowel absorption of calcium may also occur in Vitamin D intoxication and idiopathic hypercalciuria, the latter condition being common in overweight males; indeed one third of male stone formers have high urinary calcium values in the absence of hypercalcaemia. It is however rare in females. Bone resorption hypercalciuria is maintained even on a low calcium diet and occurs in hyperparathyroidism, hypervitaminosis D, prolonged immobilisation for any reason, and in certain bone diseases such as metastatic carcinoma, myeloma and Paget's disease. Renal tubular hypercalciuria is rare but it may occur in renal failure and renal tubular acidosis. In all stone sufferers idiopathic hypercalciuria is found in about 50 per cent, other causes of hypercalciuria in about 10 per cent and no defect at all other than the stone in about 40 per cent.

Oxalate

The normal excretion of oxalic acid is less than 50 mg in 24 hours. The major source of body oxalate is endogenous but considerable oxalate is found in cabbage, spinach, celery, tomatoes, rhubarb and cocoa. Primary hyperoxaluria is rare but does occur in children and is then often lethal. It is a recessive genetic abnormality in which glyoxalic acid forms oxalate rather than the amino acid glycine.

Uric Acid

Uric acid stones result from one or more of the following factors — low urinary volume, high total uric acid output and low urinary pH as the solubility of urates increases with rising pH. Increased blood uric acid levels and hyperuricosuria occur in gout. Many patients with gout form uric acid calculi but gout is not a necessary prerequisite for the formation of uric acid stones. They may also occur when there is rapid tissue breakdown e.g., in the chemotherapy of leukaemia, polycythaemia and carcinoma. Some Jews and Italians have a persistently low urinary pH which may be caused by a decreased tubular formation of ammonia and these patients may form uric acid stones. Therapy with thiazide diuretics may cause increased serum uric acid levels.

Cystine
Some amino acids may be lost in the urine in excessive amounts in the presence of renal tubular reabsorption defects. Most of these are soluble but cystine is relatively insoluble. Hereditary cystinuria is rare and only a small percentage of these patients form stones, usually in childhood.

Xanthine and Silicone Dioxide
Very rarely xanthine and silicone dioxide may be excreted in the urine in increased quantities, the former as a complication of allopurinol therapy and the latter as a complication of magnesium trisilicate therapy for peptic ulceration.

Precipitating Factors
Given the increased excretion of certain products of metabolism described above other factors are accepted as playing a part in the production of stones by increasing the likelihood of stone precipitation.

The solute concentration in the urine may be increased secondary to a low urinary volume. This may result from a low fluid intake or excess water loss due to sweating which may occur in prolonged fevers, hot climates, or certain occupations. It may also result from diarrhoea and vomiting.

Urinary pH is normally maintained between 7.35 and 7.45 but it is influenced by diet, drugs and proteus urinary infection. Inorganic salts such as calcium and magnesium are less soluble in an alkaline urine and organic substances such as cystine and uric acid are less soluble in an acid urine. Stasis of urine may predispose to urinary stones by encouraging infection and precipitation from a saturated urine according to physico-chemical laws. Infection may encourage stone formation by altering pH towards the alkaline side in the case of proteus species and by producing necrotic material within the urinary tract which may then act as a nidus upon which stone constituents are precipitated. Foreign bodies such as insoluble sutures and those self-introduced into the bladder may also act as a nidus for stone formation as indeed may a permanent indwelling catheter.

More speculative triggering mechanisms may include mucoprotein material in the urine which may act as a nidus in some cases as it forms the matrix of most stones. Randall's calcium plaques are sometimes seen on renal papillae and he postulated in 1940 that ulceration on collecting tubules secondary to infection elsewhere might result in calcification which could act as a nidus for stone formation. Analgesic abuse may cause papillary necrosis with ulceration of the necrotic material and stone formation. It has been suggested that normal urine may contain inhibiting substances which prevent calcification or crystal growth. These may include peptides, pyrophosphate, magnesium, manganese and citrate.

Classification of Urinary Stones

Stones are best classified according to their chemical composition and a knowledge of composition is clearly a necessary prerequisite for specific prophylactic therapy. Most stones contain a significant proportion of mucoprotein which makes up 5—15 per cent of their composition by weight and which acts as a matrix for the other constituents.

Calcium oxalate stones form about 68 per cent of the stones analysed in Britain; they are often small and hard with rough spicules radiating from a centre core. About 15 per cent of stones are calcium phosphate stones; they may be soft or hard in consistency and commonly have a dendritic or staghorn shape. Magnesium ammonium phosphate stones also commonly have a dendritic shape and are often found in association with an alkaline urine; they form about 10 per cent of stones analysed in Britain. Uric acid stones, forming about 5 per cent of the total are usually small, hard and multiple. Cystine stones, xanthine stones and silicate stones are rare and may be associated with the metabolic abnormalities listed above.

Pathology

Urinary tract damage resulting from stone formation is related to the size of the stone and its anatomical position. A small stone lodged in the pelvi-ureteric junction or the ureter may completely obstruct the outflow of the kidney and slowly destroy it, yet a large stone may be in such a position that little renal damage may occur. When stasis occurs secondary to obstruction, infection may result and accelerate renal damage. An enlarging staghorn calculus may cause local ischaemia as a result of pressure which can also damage a kidney. Prolonged ureteric obstruction may result in hydronephrosis and a palpable kidney.

If calcium is precipitated in the tubules themselves or the renal parenchyma or glomeruli the condition is known as nephrocalcinosis and is an indication of more serious renal impairment although the kidneys may appear grossly normal.

As far as symptoms are concerned the severest and most acute pain is usually caused by the smaller stones travelling down the ureter and causing colic by reflex peristalsis. Staghorn calculi may be relatively asymptomatic as may those stones that are adherent to renal papillae. Infection may cause fever and renal tenderness and haematuria is often related to the rougher stones.

Natural History

The formation of a urinary tract stone is not usually an isolated incident in the patient's life but part of a continuous process with a high incidence of recurrent stone formation. Both sides of the urinary tract are commonly involved and there is a strong likelihood of surgical intervention at some time in the patient's life.

A recent study[5] of 538 patients referred to a Leeds Hospital for a minimum period of ten years reported the commonest age at onset to be the third or fourth decade. Twenty per cent of the patients had a history of stone formation going back over 25 years. The 538 patients had 1949 incidents of stone formation and spontaneous passage of a stone accounted for 62 per cent of these, surgical operation for 28 per cent and X-ray diagnosis for 10 per cent. This last group either refused operation or did not require surgery.

It is of interest that stone formation was secondary to some other primary aetiology in only a small number of patients. This was an anatomical abnormality in about 4 per cent, a prolonged history of immobilisation in about 2 per cent and hyperparathyroidism in about 2 per cent. Like other researchers the Leeds workers found a male : female ratio of 2 : 1 but although single stones were equally distributed among the sexes males predominated in the recurrent stone formers. When the type of surgery performed was analysed it was found that nephrolithotomy and pyelolithotomy were commoner in women whereas uretero-lithotomy was predominantly a male operation. Nephrectomy was commoner in women due to the production of large staghorn magnesium ammonium phosphate calculi secondary to urinary infection. It was inferred from this data that males tend to form smaller calculi which can descend into the ureter whereas women form larger calculi on first attendance.

Seven per cent of patients had bilateral calculi on first attendance but this rose to 42 per cent in follow up which was an average of 18.5 years. During this time each patient had an average of 3.6 incidents with 2 incidents having the highest frequency. 394 out of 538 patients had more than one incident, a recurrence rate of 75 per cent half of which occurred in the first five years after hospital attendance.

Urinary infection has been reported in 12 per cent of men and 32 per cent of women with urolithiasis but 69 per cent of staghorn calculi are associated with urinary tract infection.

Clearly the eventual outcome of untreated urinary calculi can be hydronephrosis or pyonephrosis leading to chronic renal failure in some cases but this depends on the degree of obstruction and infection which the individual patient has experienced and these factors are often amenable to therapy given careful follow up.

Clinical Features

The clinical features of urolithiasis follow naturally from an understanding of the aetiology and pathogenesis. The patient is often a man in his thirties or forties and the presenting feature is often abdominal pain. In one hospital study 84 per cent of patients presented with some form of pain although approximately half this number denied that it was of the fluctuating kind we often describe as colic. If a stone obstructs a calyx or the pelvi-ureteric junction there is parenchymal and capsular distension in the kidney and pain is dull in character and situated in the loins. If hyperperistalsis of the calyx or pelvis occurs associated with smooth muscle spasms there will be the characteristic colicky pain associated with urinary lithiasis. If the calculus passes from the renal pelvis into the ureter it is very likely to be passed spontaneously and it has been estimated that this may occur in as many as 80 per cent of cases. This may be associated with haematuria, severe colic radiating to the groin and nausea and vomiting, frequency of micturition and the passage of solid material per urethra. If however the stone becomes impacted in the ureter abdominal distension and paralytic ileus may occur. Chills and fever may result from associated infection. It follows that many of the above symptoms will tend to be acute and the patient will usually request an urgent domiciliary visit as an abrupt onset can be followed by severe colic radiating to the testicle, scrotum or vulva within a matter of minutes. The patient is usually in agony pacing the floor restlessly as nothing he can do will give relief. There may be signs of shock and marked tenderness in the costo vertebral angle. Fever may be a sign of infection and retraction of the ipselateral testicle and hypersensitivity of the scrotal skin and testicle may be found.

Diagnosis in the typical case is usually straightforward but there is a group of patients who may present at the surgery with mild symptoms due to capsular distension which may be rather vague sometimes simulating peptic ulcer or gall bladder disease. If marked hydronephrosis occurs it may be possible to palpate a mass in the loin.

Patients with nephrocalcinosis may have few symptoms and signs other than those associated with the primary disease i.e., hyperparathyroidism or the complications i.e., chronic renal failure unless they should pass gravel or blood per urethra.

Bladder stones are more commonly found in elderly male patients with prostate hypertrophy and proteus infections and they may be associated with anaemia which may of course occur in any patient with chronic lithiasis.

Diagnosis

Diagnosis in urinary lithiasis should be concerned not only with a decision as to whether the patient has a urinary stone but also with the possibility of an underlying cause and the presence of complications. In family practice we cannot afford to neglect social and psychological factors which can have a considerable influence on patient management.

History

A careful history of the presenting features must of course be taken. Questions should be asked about the fluid intake and diet particularly with reference to milk and cheese. Drug therapy should be assessed and the possibility of self medication with analgesics, vitamins and alkalis must not be forgotten. The medical records may reveal previous episodes of urinary lithiasis that the patient, particularly if elderly, may have forgotten about or alternatively episodes of abdominal pain which with the benefit of hindsight could have been due to stone formation. There may have been previous episodes or urinary infection and the family history may be helpful if a near relative suffered from stones or perhaps gout. Immobilisation could possibly be a factor in the chronically ill patient and the patient's work must be enquired into.

A careful social history should be taken. Who lives with the patient? Will he be adequately looked after if he is managed at home? A psychological assessment must be made. Is the patient or his wife intelligent enough to follow instructions and to accept medical advice? Is the patient's pain threshold likely to be low or high as judged by our previous knowledge of him? Is the spouse likely to be able to cope adequately from both a practical and emotional point of view? Will the patient use potent analgesics sensibly? What effect would hospital admission have on the patient and his family? These points are assessed almost subconsciously be the experienced family doctor.

Examination

This is usually straightforward and should be performed along the lines that have been indicated. A rectal examination should not be omitted in the male as a stone might be secondary to urinary stasis resulting from benign prostatic hypertrophy or a prostate carcinoma. A general examination may help to exclude primary diseases and other diseases causing similar symptoms which might confuse such as acute pyelonephritis and renal tuberculosis. Blood pressure readings should be taken at some stage as, if persistently raised, this might indicate renal hypertension and, if normal, provide baselines for future reference.

Investigations

Many investigations can be carried out from family practice and where feasible this is preferable.

The Stone

If solid material is passed per urethra it should be inspected and sent for analysis to the local pathology laboratory. The chemical nature of the stone may provide information useful in prophylaxis against recurrent stones.

The Urine
Urinalysis must be performed, either at the surgery or the local laboratory. Proteinuria due to red blood cells may be present and microscopic haematuria, though not diagnostic, may provide the only objective evidence of stones. Examination of the sediment may reveal crystals and the type may give a clue to the type of stone. If the pH is over 7.6 urea splitting organisms may be present and this suggests magnesium ammonium phosphate stones. If a dip slide culture reveals a urinary infection the slide should be sent to the laboratory so that the organism can be identified and sensitivity studies performed.

The Blood
A specimen of blood should be taken for a full count which may show a white cell response to the presence of infection and confirm the presence of anaemia. A raised serum calcium may point to hyperparathyroidism, a raised alkaline phosphatase may mean bone resorption and a raised serum uric acid may be helpful as it is found in 50 per cent of uric acid stone formers. Impaired renal function may be indicated by raised urea and creatinine levels.

Radiography
A plain film of the abdomen should be obtained (this can be obtained if necessary on a domiciliary basis — though interpretation could prove more difficult) as 90 per cent of stones in this country are radio-opaque and the morphology of the stone may give a clue to its chemical nature. This should be followed at a later date by an IVP which will not only accurately localise radio-opaque stones but also demonstrate urinary obstruction and anatomical abnormalities of the urinary tract.
should be considered on every patient with a suspected stone. Recurrent stone formers require more detailed metabolic investigation which will include the biochemical analysis of 24 hour urine specimens; this will be carried out at a specialist unit.

Management

The most pressing aspect of the management of the patient with urinary lithiasis will be the emergency relief of pain and potent analgesics are usually required. Intramuscular pethidine 100 mg is probably superior to intramuscular morphine 15 mg and both are superior to anticholinergic smooth muscle relaxants. Copious fluids and bed rest are traditional and may be of some value. Pethidine tablets 50 mg may be left with the patient and prescribed in a dose of 100 mg 4 hourly but if necessary the district nurse can repeat an injection during the day and on her evening round.

If the social and psychological circumstances are such that the patient cannot be nursed at home, or pain cannot be controlled or persists longer than 48 hours on the above regime, hospital admission or a domiciliary consultation with a urological surgeon will be needed. This will also be the case if acute retention of urine develops or more rarely renal failure.

Often however, the acute episode will settle after 24 to 48 hours and if the stone is passed it should be sent for analysis. This information together with the results of the blood and urine tests and radiography can be assessed so that infection if present can be treated and prophylaxis can be planned. If the stone is not passed by the time the IVP results are available or if residual stones are still present the advice of a urological surgeon should be obtained. Indications for surgery will include persistent ureteric obstruction, partial ureteric obstruction if the shape of the calculi is such that spontaneous passage is unlikely, persistent or recurrent infection and persistent or recurrent pain. If pain is atypical however and the calculus is of the staghorn variety nephrolithotomy often fails to improve the patient's condition.

Prophylaxis, Follow up and continuing care

Recurrent stones are common and therefore it is mandatory for every family practitioner to ensure that his patients who suffer from urinary lithiasis are adequately investigated and followed up, particularly if recurrent stones have actually occurred when detailed investigation will be required. Occasionally the urological surgeon concentrating on preserving renal function by nephrolithotomy or ureterolithotomy or other techniques may neglect the biochemical aspects and it then falls upon the family doctor to ensure that appropriate investigations have been carried out. The measures indicated for prophylaxis depend on the type of stone isolated. If this is not available its composition may be surmised by X-ray density and morphology, the types of crystals in the urine and abnormalities in blood chemistry. Measures may be general and specific. The former include the maintenance of a high urine volume by a generous fluid intake of around 3 litres per day and regular urine bacteriological examination by means of the dip slide to combat infection, which may be asymptomatic. Recumbency should be avoided and exercise stressed and obstruction should be dealt with by appropriate surgery.

Calcium Phosphate and Magnesium Ammonium Phosphate Stones
If primary hyperparathyroidism is confirmed the parathyroid glands should be explored surgically. The diet is important and dairy products particularly cheese and milk should be avoided. The stones form most readily in a neutral or alkaline urine and the pH of the urine should be kept below 6.0. Diagnostic strips can be used by the patient to check this. Ascorbic acid is a useful

acidifying agent. It has been claimed that thiazide diuretics (e.g., hydrochloro-thiazide 50 mg twice daily) reduce the amount of calcium in the urine by 50 per cent in patients with idiopathic hypercalcaemia by enhancing proximal tubular reabsorption and that calcification is inhibited by substances such as potassium acid phosphate in a dose of 4 to 6 g per day. Recent work suggests the use of calcium binding exchange resins such as cellulose phosphate 15 g per day.

Calcium Oxalate Stones

In the case of calcium oxalate stones calcium intake should be reduced and the above therapy may be described. As most oxalate is endogenous in origin it is questionable whether reduced intake of high oxalate foods such as rhubarb and cabbage is of any value.

Uric Acid and Cystine Stones

In the case of these metabolic stones the urine pH should be kept high at pH 7.0 or above and this can be achieved by mistura potassium citrate 10 ml 4 times a day in addition to a low protein high vegetable and fruit diet. A low purine diet can be prescribed for the uric acid stone former and in addition allopurinol 300 mg twice daily may be taken.

The prognosis for the patient with renal stones is usually good but depends on the success with which recurrent stones are prevented and the prevention of further renal damage from obstruction and infection. The family practitioner is a key figure in long term management. There is no reason why urine specimens should not be cultured regularly, particularly if dip slides are made generally available, and the prompt treatment of infection will clearly be beneficial.

Future Research

Much research is needed, particularly in family practice. We need to establish incidence figures and the results of long term prophylaxis. A number of patients are not referred to specialist clinics and the overall prognosis in family practice needs to be clarified.

BENIGN PROSTATIC HYPERTROPHY

Benign hypertrophy of the prostate gland is common. It has been estimated that a man aged 40 has about a ten per cent chance of requiring prostate surgery if he lives to the age of 80 and that 4 per cent of men over the age of 80 need prostatectomy although 75 per cent have necropsy evidence of hypertrophy. Problems arise, however, not so much from the lesion itself but from progressive obstruction to urine flow resulting in difficulty with the urine stream, increased risk of urinary infection, acute and chronic retention and back pressure effects on the proximal urinary tract.

Aetiology

Aetiology remains obscure but what evidence there is suggests that hormonal changes must play some part. Animal experiments for example reveal that the condition normally occurs in elderly dogs but if the animal has been castrated previously it does not occur. Androgens cannot be the only factor involved however, as levels are decreasing as prostate size is increasing. Dogs with oestrogen tumours of the testis do not develop hypertrophy of the prostate but in man the administration of oestrogen has no effect on the enlarged gland. It is fashionable at present to incriminate androgen/oestrogen imbalance or the relative concentration of testosterone and its metabolites but the possibility of a virus as the initiating factor has not been excluded.

Pathology

The prostate gland is a firm body about the size of a chestnut which has a structure composed partly of fibromuscular tissue, either or both of which may undergo hypertrophy. A large proportion of glands removed surgically show other pathological processes in addition to hypertrophy such as recent or healed infarcts, acute or chronic inflammation or unsuspected carcinoma; the hyperplastic tissue may consist of varying proportions of acinar, vascular, fibrous or muscular tissue and cystic changes are common.

The gland is situated at the bladder neck where it is perforated by the urethra and ejaculatory ducts and it is enclosed by a capsule which is adherent in young men. The hypertrophied gland however, has a surgical capsule composed of capsule proper and compressed extra-urethral prostate and the central obstructing tissue is easily shelled out. The gland itself is divided anatomically into two lateral lobes and one median lobe which in the latter case cannot be felt per rectum.

Progressive obstruction to urine flow, which may result from benign hypertrophy, secondary changes in the bladder, or both, produce the symptoms of prostatism and the pathogenesis of these symptoms has been explained in the following terms.

Like the heart the bladder is a hollow muscular organ receiving fluid which it expels under pressure. Increased work load results in phases of bladder compensation and eventually decompensation. Urination occurs when contraction of the detrusor muscle and trigone opens the bladder neck allowing contraction of the bladder wall musculature to expel the urine under a normal pressure of about 20–40 cm water, a force which in itself further widens the bladder neck. If bladder neck obstruction occurs the vesical musculature compensates by hypertrophy in order to overcome the urethral resistance with the result that the force and size of the urinary stream remain normal. In a normal individual distension of the bladder produces a need to void urine which can be resisted but if the detrusor is hypertrophied the bladder becomes hypersensitive as detrusor spasm may occur producing urgency and frequency.

With increasing obstruction the power to empty the bladder completely is maintained by further hypertrophy of muscle fibres resulting in trabeculation of the bladder wall. In addition to urgency and frequency the patient may notice hesitancy in initiating micturition and there may be some loss in the force and size of the urinary stream. Once urethral resistance exceeds detrusor power the phase of bladder decompensation sets in and residual bladder urine results after micturition. This may occur suddenly after a high fluid intake resulting in an overstretched bladder and marked hesitancy and straining and a poor stream, and painful acute urinary retention may occur. With more gradual decompensation an increasing residual urine volume decreases the effective volume of the bladder with progressive frequency of micturition in addition to obstructive symptoms. As the bladder stretches it may eventually lose its power to contract and relatively painless overflow incontinence may occur.

During the decompensation phase loss of the normal valve action at the ureteric orifice in the bladder may occur with the resulting vesico-ureteric reflux transmitting pressure effects to the kidney which may eventually lead to hydronephrosis. Infection and sometimes stone formation is encouraged not only by stasis due to a residual urine but also by stasis in diverticulae forming in a weakened bladder wall. Progressive renal infection and hydronephrosis may lead eventually to loss of renal concentrating power, diminished glomerular filtration and terminal uraemia.

Clinical Features

As detailed above symptoms are produced by hypertrophy of muscle at the bladder neck, adenomatous prostate hypertrophy or more usually by a combination of both. Significant symptoms rarely occur before the age of 50 and in family practice three types of presentation are seen. One group consists of the men who complain of persistent mild symptoms of obstruction such as urgency and hesitancy, another consists of those who develop symptoms of acute urinary infection as a result of prostate hypertrophy and the third group develop acute or chronic retention. Symptoms and signs will therefore vary according to group, but the second group is probably the most numerous.

In the first group the patient may complain of mild urgency and frequency and if the bladder overfills there may be some hesitation in starting the stream and some loss of force and calibre. Frequency and urgency eventually become more severe and occur both during the day and at night.

If acute infection supervenes it may initiate obstructive symptoms or aggravate them due to oedema of the prostate or bladder neck which increases the degree of obstruction. In addition other symptoms peculiar to infection may develop (see p. 340 to 342). Haematuria may be present as straining may rupture veins at the bladder neck.

Acute retention of urine may occur suddenly in a man who has few symptoms or develop after months or years of prostatism. It not uncommonly develops after a bout of heavy drinking or after the administration of a potent diuretic during the management of pulmonary oedema. Constipation may also precipitate acute retention and the author has seen this occur as a sole cause in an eleven year old boy.

Renal pain as a rule is an indication of infection as hydronephrosis without infection is usually silent but loin pain on micturition has been described in some men with vesico-ureteric reflux due to prostate hypertrophy.

Signs may be minimal depending on the presence of infection and on whether bladder distension has occurred. As far as the family practitioner is concerned symptoms are a better guide to the degree of bladder neck obstruction than the size of the prostate on rectal examination as the former rather than the latter is an indication for further investigation but both are notoriously unreliable as an indication for surgery. Rectal examination however, may reveal smooth and firm enlargement of one or both of the lateral lobes if fibro muscular hyperplasiz has occurred, or soft and boggy hypertrophy if adenomatous hypertrophy has occurred, but its chief value lies in detecting the hard indurated nodules which may indicate carcinoma. If infection is present renal tenderness may be elicited, and bladder distension may be felt as a tender abdominal mass if acute or detected by percussion if chronic. It should not be forgotten that chronic retention may result in uraemia, and prostate obstruction needs to be excluded in confusional states in elderly men.

Diagnosis

Diagnosis can be considered at two levels. First a decision as to whether symptoms result from bladder neck obstruction and secondly an estimation of the degree of prostatic hypertrophy and/or the presence of malignancy so that a decision about surgical management can be taken. The first area is largely the province of the family practitioner and the second is largely the province of the urological surgeon.

History

The symptoms of bladder neck obstruction are characteristic enough to immediately point to their source. The date of onset of the earliest symptoms should be carefully enquired into and the presence or absence of symptoms of infection such as rigors is important. Regrettably too many men ignore minor symptoms with the result that severe back pressure effects may be present on first presentation at the surgery. The history should help to exclude other differential diagnoses such as diabetes. Identical symptoms can be produced by multiple sclerosis although this is rare in this age group and in particular cord compression from an acute disc prolapse or spinal cord tumour. Drug therapy should be enquired into as the anticholinergic group such as atropine and propantheline, the sympathominetic group such as adrenaline, orciprenaline, ephedrine and isoprenaline, and the antidepressives such as imipramine may aggravate or initiate prostatism and even precipitate acute retention. The past medical history is of particular importance as evidence of bronchitis may influence the choice of operation. Severe mental instability is a contraindication to surgery as demented old men do badly after all forms of prostatectomy in that urinary continence is rarely achieved.

A social history is important as urinary incontinence due to hypertrophy may be a considerable embarrassment to an elderly man living with his son or daughter and the extra washing is yet another burden for them to bear. Urinary continence is often an important factor in deciding on accommodation for an elderly man living alone and requiring institutional care. Since it is clearly desirable to preserve as much independence as possible the social history may become a major factor influencing surgery.

Examination
Every man complaining of urinary symptoms should have his abdomen palpated when evidence of bladder enlargement might be found, and a rectal examination when areas of induration may be apparent. Renal tenderness may indicate infection but the examination should also include the heart and lungs with an estimation of the blood pressure. Neurological examination, of the lower limbs in particular, is needed to identify the neurogenic bladder.

Investigations

Many investigations can normally be carried out in family practice, for example it is important to know whether the urine is infected when the patient presents with acute urinary symptoms, whether of prostatism and bladder neck obstruction or whether of urinary infection and pyelonephritis. The IVP is a most helpful investigation as quite apart from information about the kidneys themselves, the presence of residual urine and trabeculation and hypertrophy of the bladder may be demonstrated, as well as complications such as diverticula and stones. A chest X-ray should be a matter of routine and blood can be taken for full blood count, urea and creatinine and acid phosphatase estimations.

Full investigation including cystoscopy is mandatory in the presence of symptoms of bladder neck obstruction as prostate hypertrophy may not be the cause. Phimosis, urethral stricture, vesical calculi and bladder tumours may eventually be held responsible.

Management

The ultimate aim in the management of the patient with benign prostate hypertrophy is the preservation of renal function but the quality of life is of no lesser importance and with this in mind the preservation and attainment of control over micturition is utmost in the mind of the family practitioner. Infection if present must obviously be eradicated but management by and large varies according to the mode of presentation.

Acute retention is normally an indication for emergency hospital admission as in the author's opinion little is gained by initial catheterization in the patient's home unless there is to be delay over admission or unless the patient's general condition is so poor that surgery is contraindicated.

Chronic retention with overflow is best managed after domiciliary consultation with a urological surgeon when a decision will be made about priority admission for surgery in terms of the findings on examination and the social, psychological and physical factors in the history. Catheterization may be required while awaiting surgery or permanently if surgery is contraindicated.

If the patient presents with prostatism or symptoms of urinary infection out patient referral to a urological department is necessary. The referral letter should include the findings on examination, and the results of the various investigations that have been carried out, such as urine microscopy and culture and the blood and X-ray findings. It should also include the relevant history, especially details about chronic chest conditions, important social factors and of course, drug therapy.

Prostatectomy is normally indicated in the presence of acute or chronic retention but ideally the aim of the family practitioner should be to avoid this complication whenever possible by early diagnosis as prostatectomy will usually be advised if compensating changes are seen in the bladder musculature or if a residual urine is present. The most difficult patients to assess are those with minimal residual urine whose symptoms are not severe, as many improve if nothing is done but others return later with a decompensated bladder and upper tract distension. If prostatectomy is deferred careful follow up is necessary. Conservative measures that are emphasised for this group include the avoidance of a large fluid intake and frequent emptying of the bladder so that distension does not occur. The family practitioner needs to be wary of diuretic therapy in the presence of bladder neck obstruction.

The family practitioner has a particular responsibility over the question of specialist referral. Data on all hospital discharges over a period of three years in Scotland when a diagnosis of benign prostate hyperplasia had been made has recently become available. Out of a total 9986 cases there were 376 deaths but the death rate varied according to where the operation was performed being 5 per cent in general surgical units and 2.3 per cent in urological units. The death rate varied between 0 and 20 per cent for different consultants and 0 and 13 per cent for other surgeons but only one urologist had a death rate above 5 per cent compared with 52 out of a total of 110 general surgeons. Clearly urologists should be treating the high risk cases and it is up to the family practitioner to ensure that this occurs. The high risk cases are patients over the age of 80, emergency admissions, those not operated upon and those with an associated diagnosis not involving the urinary tract. There are few absolute contraindications to surgery as if the patient can get about and is not entirely demented the operation is feasible by one route or another.

Follow up and Continuing Care

It is the responsibility of the family practitioner to ensure that adequate follow up is arranged either at the hospital or surgery for the patients who have been referred and are awaiting prostatectomy. At follow up particular attention should be paid to deteriorating symptoms and the development of urinary tract infection as it may be necessary to expedite surgery or to refer the patient back for a further opinion. Post-prostatectomy patients should be encouraged to re-attend the surgery if further symptoms develop as this may indicate the development of a stricture in the posterior urethra.

The Permanent Indwelling Catheter
There will be a small group of patients in whom a decision has been made to insert a permanent indwelling catheter and close liason between the family practitioner and the district nurse is essential if this group is to receive adequate care.

Types of Catheter
There are two types of Foley Self Retaining Catheter. The gum elastic requires to be changed every two weeks. The Silastic is silicone coated and firmer and therefore passes more easily. A particular advantage is that it can be left *in situ* for six months without debris formation and blocking and as changes are made much less frequently the incidence of urethritis is reduced. Unfortunately this catheter is only available at hospital where the patient must attend for insertion.

Catheter Changes at Home
The procedure requires a pre-sterilised dressing pack, a pre-sterilised catheter in a separate pack, a tube of KY jelly for lubrication and a suitable disinfectant such as cetrimide lotion. In addition a kettle of boiled water which has been allowed to cool is required for inflation of

the catheter bulb using a pre-sterilised 10 ml syringe and a $1\frac{1}{2}''$ needle. In hospital all these items are available in one complete sterilised pack which also includes sterilised disposable gloves making an aseptic technique easier to approach than it is in the patient's home but even when such a technique is attempted a catheter change can present further problems.

The insertion of a catheter for the first time may prove difficult due to obstruction in the urethra and the condition of the prostate gland but once *in situ* for a fortnight successive catheter changes should be less traumatic. Occasionally the prepuce may be so tight that it is impossible to cleanse the glans or to find the meatus easily thus increasing the risk of introducing infection. Concretions may sometimes occur forming sharp edges on the deflated bulb which on withdrawal of the catheter may cause pain and damage the urethra.

Catheter Management

As the majority of patients are elderly and may live alone there may be a problem in releasing the spigot to empty the bladder when drainage into a disposable urine bag might be preferrable. The patient will require supervision from the district nurse to ensure an adequate fluid intake, advice on problems, and to ensure that medication is taken. Intermittent courses of urinary antiseptics may be required according to sensitivity studies if infection is symptomatic but long term therapy is unhelpful as drug resistance rapidly develops. An elderly or confused patient may be concerned about 'having a tube in' and may play frequently with the catheter or spigot and stretch the opening of the catheter with the result that the spigot may not fit properly and drop out on movement or on coughing. Occasionally a faulty bulb may deflate allowing the catheter to slip out. Where successfully managed a patient should be comfortable and dry in day clothes as well as in bed. He can be fully ambulant and bathe normally.

Future Research

Further research is needed into the aetiology of benign prostate enlargement as medical treatment, at present unsatisfactory, may eventually emerge. The incidence of referrals from family practice and the outcome needs to be established as does the outcome in that group in whom surgery is deferred, both from the point of view of the eventual need for surgery and the incidence of symptoms and infection in the interim period.

CANCER OF THE PROSTATE

The Registrar General's figures for 1970 reveal that out of 63 236 deaths in males from cancer in England and Wales 3906 were recorded as due to carcinoma of the prostate. This is an average of over ten per day and in fact cancer of the prostate is the fourth commonest cause of cancer death in the male and the commonest cause in the genito-urinary tract. When these figures are related to the population they suggest that one in every 1700 men over the age of 50 die with this condition each year.

Prostate cancers are divided into clinical when symptoms are produced, latent when foci (which are not producing symptoms) are found accidentally in prostate tissue and occult when metastatic symptoms are produced while the primary remains hidden or insignificant in size. Latent carcinoma may be found in 20 per cent of men over the age of 50 and 95 per cent of histologically examined prostates in the eighth decade.

Aetiology

As in the case of benign hypertrophy the causes of carcinoma of the prostate are not known but three aetiological factors appear to play some part although little knowledge exists about any of them. Hormones are considered to play an aetiological role, not so much in the genesis of the tumour but in stimulating and maintaining the prostatic epithelium, as its growth is strikingly influenced by sex hormones. Androgens usually increase the rate of growth whereas oestrogen therapy or orchidectomy slows the growth of these tumours. Secondly age has a bearing on the disease as it is rare before the age of 50 but increases rapidly up to the age of 80 after which the incidence slows. Lastly race may be an aetiological factor as the incidence is high in negroes in Alameda County USA yet low in oriental races. Environment may play some part in this observation as the low incidence in the Japanese is not matched in Japanese residents in the United States, although incidence in the latter does not reach Caucasian levels.

Pathology

As cancer of the prostate is apt to develop in the same age group as benign hypertrophy the two conditions may co-exist. Indeed some workers have reported an increased incidence of clinical cancer of the prostate in patients with benign prostatic hyperplasia. Most tumours originate in the periphery of the prostate in the compressed surgical capsule of the posterior lobe and are therefore easily felt on rectal examination as an indurated area which distorts the normal contours of the gland. The tumour gradually spreads locally to involve the rest of the prostate tissue within the capsule and eventually involves extra capsular structures such as the seminal vesicles, bladder wall and urethral mucosa. Extension around the rectum may occur but direct infiltration is rare.

Metastatic spread occurs through the lymphatic system involving vesical, sacral, external iliac and lumbar lymph nodes and also by way of the venous system to the pelvic bones including the heads of the femurs and the lower lumbar spine. Visceral spread to the lungs and liver is also seen and infiltration of the bone marrow resulting in anaemia is not uncommon. Latent foci are common in the elderly and are usually discovered on histological examination of prostatectomy material or at autopsy. Their biological significance is uncertain. It could be that they are a distinct disease and not destined to develop into clinically active cancer.

Since the primary focus is far removed from the bladder and urethra and 95 per cent of tumours present with obstructive symptoms early symptoms are uncommon and most symptomatic cancers have already extended beyond the scope of radical surgery. A few operable tumours may be discovered on chance rectal examination or as a result of obstructive symptoms from benign hypertrophy. Untreated, it is possible that a tumour may lie dormant for years until some trigger factor operates leading to rapid progressive obstruction due to benign hyperplasia complicated by infection and possibly stone formation. Metastatic complications may occur including oedema of the legs from enlarged iliac nodes obstructing great vessels or spontaneous fractures developing at the site of bony metastases.

Clinical Features

About 95 per cent of patients present with bladder neck obstruction as described in the section on benign prostatic hypertrophy, but 5 per cent present with symptoms due to metastases. In the former group a variable period may elapse before clinical evidence of secondary spread occurs, which is often extended by palliative treatment, but in the latter group death can occur from widespread metastatic disease before the onset of significant obstructive symptoms. It has been suggested that this behaviour could reflect an immunological variation in the tumour-host relationship.

Metastatic spread may result in lumbosacral pain radiating down the lower limbs, or haematuria if the posterior urethra or bladder wall is invaded. If the seminal vesicles are involved haematospermia may occur. General symptoms will include weight loss and anaemia.

Signs on examination can be grouped into those discernible on rectal examination and those resulting from secondary spread. Irregularity and firmness of the prostate gland should raise suspicion. A cancerous nodule is not usually raised above the surface of the gland and there is a sudden change in consistency between it and the surrounding prostate tissue and in fact the advanced lesion may be stony hard and induration of the seminal vesicles may be felt. The median furrow and lateral sulci may be obliterated by capsular extension. Distal signs may include an enlarged nodular liver, pathological fractures, and an enlarged hard left sided supraclavicular gland.

Diagnosis

Although the history as a rule does not differentiate between benign and malignant prostate hypertrophy local examination is often diagnostic. Occasionally benign firm nodules in the prostate may be produced by tuberculosis, chronic granulomatous prostatitis or calculi but tuberculous nodules are often multiple and the nodules of granulomatous prostatitis may be raised above the gland surface. Prostatic calculi may cause crepitations on palpation. Physical examination may also reveal evidence of metastatic spread to the chest or liver or supraclavicular nodes, and the presence of anaemia.

Accurate diagnosis, particularly of the extent of metastatic spread, demands further investigation and some of these investigations can be carried out from family practice while awaiting an out-patient appointment. A full blood count may reveal a profound anaemia due to metastatic infiltration of bone marrow and urea and creatinine estimations may be raised. The serum acid phosphatase level is the only specific laboratory test for prostatic cancer. The normal adult prostate epithelium secretes this enzyme and the function is retained by most carcinomatous cells. The normal serum acid phosphatase in men is 1–5 King Armstrong units and when the cancer extends outside the prostatic capsule and metastases are present 75 per cent of patients will have levels above 10 units. False positive values may occur after vigorous massage of the prostate and a carcinoma limited to the capsule may not produce raised values.

A chest X-ray may show metastases in the hilar nodes, lungs, or ribs and a plain X-ray of the abdomen may reveal osteoblastic metastases in the lumbar spine, pelvis or femoral heads. Hospital investigation will usually include fine needle transrectal aspiration biopsy of suspicious nodules under xylocaine anaesthesia and if conventional radiography is unhelpful isotope scintigraphy may demonstrate latent bone involvement. Occasionally cystoscopy will be employed.

Management

Nearly all patients with suspected carcinoma prostate will require referral to a urological surgeon for confirmation of the diagnosis, determination of the extent of metastatic spread and a decision as to the most appropriate treatment.

Surgical treatment is controversial and ranges from radical surgery through oestrogen therapy to radiotherapy. Controversy is inevitable given our lack of knowledge of the natural history of prostatic cancer. Only about 2–4 per cent of patients present early enough to ensure that a radical cure by prostatectomy or prostatovesiculectomy yet the operation has a 90 per cent ten year survival rate in those patients whose lesions were less than 1 cm in diameter and a 67 per cent ten year survival rate when the lesion was 2 cm in diameter. On the other hand radical surgery carries the penalty of total impotence and the risk of incontinence, and as it is suspected that many latent carcinomas may remain silent for many years, or even indefinitely, it may often be quite unnecessary. Fortunately or unfortunately a decision about radical surgery is not often required, as most patients present when the lesion has undergone considerable local spread, and when metastatic disease is present, and only palliative surgery is possible. Transurethral resection offers considerable temporary relief however for most patients, which is usually of greater value than it sounds, due to the fact that most cases of prostate cancer occur in later life when the impact of the disease is less intense and in fact death is often due to intercurrent illness rather than the carcinoma itself.

Controversy also exists over the case selection for oestrogen therapy and its timing and dosage. Oestrogen therapy was originally given in an attempt to eliminate the main sources of androgen production, prostate cancers being androgen dependent, but it is now believed that oestrogen may also interfere with the metabolism of cancer cells. Unfortunately resistant and relapsing cases occur and in addition patient intolerance often limits the dose that can be given. Fluid retention may be a particular hazard in the presence of heart disease, and hepatic damage and thrombotic and cardiovascular complications have been statistically related to oestrogen therapy for prostate cancer.

There seems to be some agreement however that asymptomatic cancers confined to the primary site are best not treated with oestrogens. In symptomatic cases confined to the primary site alternative treatment by transurethral resection, radiotherapy or castration might be considered. When there is advanced local or metastatic spread oestrogen therapy should not be withheld however although dosage is still disputed. A recommended regime consists of stilboestrol 1 mg 3 times a day. About 85 per cent of prostatic cancers respond and within a few weeks will show definite regression in size. Obstructive symptoms improve and pain due to metastases improves or even disappears.

Follow up and Continuing Care

After hospital discharge the patient should be seen regularly in family practice until he is well established on maintenance oestrogen therapy without undue side effects. If side effects are troublesome they can sometimes be helped by leaving out two or three doses in one week. If side effects are not improved by this method or a trial of other oestrogens such as Honvan 100 mg daily and if bilateral orchidectomy or radiotherapy has not been performed the patient can be referred back for the consideration of these procedures.

If simple methods of endocrine control cease to be effective and increasing pain, progressive anaemia and urinary infection point to relapsing disease, referral back to the consultant urologist is indicated for consideration of further measures. Transnasal irradiation hypophysectomy with yttrium 90 has been recommended, as although requiring a brief anaesthetic the procedure is a relatively minor one and well tolerated by patients even in the penultimate stages of the disease. A dramatic relief of symptoms can be expected in about half the patients treated but it should not be forgotten that substitution therapy with cortisone will be required. If such treatment is not desired a medical adrenalectomy can be accomplished by the administration of cortisone 50 mg per day in divided doses but salt should be restricted and potassium supplements given. When all else fails the administration of testosterone can be tried. In some patients it increases existing pain which will require further analgesia but in some considerable relief may result; the mechanism for this effect is not clear.

It has been said by some hospital based research workers that palliative treatment usually results in death within three years but in the absence of firm knowledge of natural history and means of identifying high risk and low risk patients such statements should be accepted with caution. In the author's experience many patients do well and every practice has its group of elderly men who regularly require repeat prescriptions for oestrogen tablets and who in the end die from intercurrent illness unrelated to their malignancy or its therapy. These patients are often lost to urological follow up and there is clearly a need for family practice studies into the prognosis of carcinoma of the prostate.

CANCER OF THE KIDNEY

Carcinoma of the Kidney

Tumours can develop from any component of the renal parenchyma, the pelvicalyceal system, or the capsule and extracapsular structures but in practice 80 per cent of renal neoplasms are adenocarcinomas.

Aetiology, Pathogenesis and Pathology

Recent histological research suggests that renal adenocarcinomas arise from the cells of the renal tubules. Aetiology is unknown but smoking has been incriminated in some reports. There is usually a well defined capsule of compressed tissue which may have liquified in parts to form cysts. The tumour spreads by direct growth into the perinnephric tissues and adjacent viscera producing distortion of the calyces, renal blood vessels and pelvis. It spreads by the blood stream to any part of the body but particularly to lungs, bone and liver. It may also spread by the lymphatic system to the regional lymph nodes surrounding the aorta. Vascular spread is the commonest however and occasionally the metastasis is solitary when removal of the primary tumour and the metastasis may be curative. Very rarely an adenocarcinoma may produce erythropoiesis causing polycythaemia. Occasionally a renal adenocarcinoma may be secondary to a carcinoma elsewhere especially the lungs.

Clinical Features

The commonest presenting feature is haematuria which is usually silent and may be heavy; it is found in 75 per cent of patients. Pain is usually a late manifestation and may be dull or colicky according to whether it is produced by capsular distension or blood clot or tumour cells in the lumen of the ureter. Symptoms from metastases may be a presenting feature and these include weight loss, anaemia, bone pain and pulmonary symptoms.

Physical examination may reveal a mass in the loin. Metastatic signs include palpable lymph nodes in the left supraclavicular region and oedema of the legs; dilated abdominal veins may be apparent due to venacaval involvement.

Diagnosis

When the history and examination point to the possibility of an adenocarcinoma of the kidney referral to a urological surgeon is indicated for a definitive diagnosis but a blood examination may reveal anaemia or an elevated ESR. A plain X-ray of the abdomen may show an enlarged kidney and excretory pyelograms may show a filling defect due to a space-occupying lesion and dislocation of the pelvicalyceal system. Ureteric catheterisation and retrograde pyelography may be required. A chest X-ray is necessary to exclude pulmonary metastases. These investigations will help to exclude hydronephrosis, polycystic kidney and solitary renal cysts.

Management

Radical nephrectomy is the treatment of choice in the absence of metastases but in the presence of a solitary metastasis surgery may be considered. X-ray therapy is unhelpful but progesterone or testosterone may be tried in patients who have incurable or recurrent tumours.

Follow up and Continuing Care

The five year survival figures after nephrectomy for carcinoma kidney are about 35 per cent. The prognosis is poor if renal vein involvement has occurred and metastases can occur 10–15 years after removal of the primary growth. These figures emphasise the importance of early investigation of haematuria in family practice.

Nephroblastoma

A nephroblastoma is the commonest abdominal tumour in children under six years of age; in ten per cent of cases the tumour is bilateral.

Aetiology, Pathogenesis and Pathology
Nephroblastomas develop from embryonic cells in the kidney before differentiation into renal parenchyma has occurred. It is a highly malignant tumour and it accounts for 20 per cent of childhood malignant tumours particularly in boys in whom it is twice as common as in girls. It grows rapidly to destroy renal parenchyma and metastases occur via the blood stream to the lungs, liver and brain.

Clinical Features
The most common clinical finding is a palpable mass in the loins which may have been noticed by the parents of the child. Any palpable mass in the loin of a child must be regarded as a nephroblastoma until proved otherwise. Hypertension is a common finding and normal levels are restored after nephrectomy. Pain and haematuria may also occur.

Diagnosis
Definitive diagnosis requires referral to a paediatric urological surgeon. Plain X-rays may reveal enlargement and pulmonary metastases and excretion pyelograms will reveal a distorted pelvicalyceal system. Retrograde pyelograms are usually required for greater definition.

Management
Although nephrectomy is the treatment of choice the tumour is radiosensitive and preliminary X-ray therapy may be carried out if the tumour is considered too large.

Follow up and Continuing Care
In the absence of demonstrable metastases up to 90 per cent of children will be cured by a combination of surgery and radiotherapy and the younger the child the better the prognosis. Even in the presence of pulmonary metastases about 50 per cent of children may be cured. Because of the embryological origin of the tumour it may be presumed that a cure has been obtained if the child lives for a period equal to nine months plus its age at the time of surgery.

BLADDER CANCER

Bladder tumours are second only to prostatic tumours as the source of neoplastic disease in the genitourinary tract and about 75 per cent of cases occur in men, usually after the age of 50. In 1969, 3764 deaths due to bladder cancer were recorded in England and Wales.

Aetiology, Pathogenesis and Pathology

Perhaps as many as 20 per cent of bladder cancers are occupational in origin and workers in the chemical dye industry, tailors, textile workers, and some engineering workers are particularly at risk. There is a consistent but probably low risk to cigarette smokers, possibly due to tryptophan metabolites in the urine; it has been estimated that smokers are two to five times more likely to develop bladder cancers than non-smokers.

Eighty per cent of tumours are found at the base of the bladder and although papillary in type most are malignant. They may be single or multiple and usually metastasise to the local lymph nodes although at times the liver, lungs and bone may be involved. They are usually transitional in type and begin as a small focus of cell proliferation upon the transitional epithelium.

Clinical Features

The commonest symptom is painless haematuria which is usually intermittent. If the neoplasm obstructs the urethral orifice bladder neck obstruction may occur and similarly loin pain may be present if a ureter is obstructed. Physical examination is usually unrewarding unless metastatic disease is present.

Diagnosis

The diagnosis is usually made after referral to a urological surgeon when cystoscopy and biopsy can be undertaken.

Management

Management is influenced by two important characteristics of bladder tumours, namely a tendency to recur and a tendency to multiple lesions. Techniques include cystoscopic diathermy, suprapubic diathermy, irradiation, cystectomy and palliative measures.

Cystoscopic diathermy is the method of choice even with large tumours provided there is no demonstrable induration. Suprapubic diathermy is better avoided where possible because of the risk of implantation of malignant cells in the scar. Interstitial irradiation with gold grains implanted into the bladder wall is effective in tumours below 4 cm diameter and external megavoltage irradiation is useful in those patients with highly malignant tumours which may infiltrate to such an extent that surgery is impossible. Partial cystectomy is rarely indicated but total cystectomy is indicated for recurrent tumour after megavoltage irradiation, and multiple tumours too extensive for cystoscopic diathermy.

Course and Outcome

The prognosis is often excellent after cystoscopic diathermy combined with frequent cystoscopies thereafter. There is a five year survival rate of 60 per cent after interstitial irradiation and a three year survival rate of 30 per cent after total cystectomy. The family practitioner may be asked about the management of recurrent tumour presenting with such features as progressive pain, frequency and dysuria and strangury due to the passage of blood clots. Reimplantation of the ureter into the colon may relieve micturition symptoms and bleeding can be controlled by bladder instillations of silver nitrate starting with a 1 : 5000 solution and increasing to 1 : 1000 if necessary; this procedure can be carried out at home by the district nurse. Thiotepa 60–90 mg in normal saline can be used for the same purpose; it is administered on alternate days and should be retained for three hours.

TESTICULAR TUMOURS

With rare exceptions all testicular tumours are malignant and occur mostly between the ages of 20 and 35.

Aetiology

The aetiology of testicular tumours is unknown and all that can be said is that they occur at the age of greatest sexual activity. It has been suggested that the undescended testicle is more likely to undergo malignant change but the evidence is inconclusive.

Fifty one per cent of testicular tumours are seminomas arising from adult cells in the seminiferous tubules and 46 per cent are teratomas derived from all three primary germinal layers of the embryo; the remaining 3 per cent of tumours are composed of chorionepitheliomas, interstitial cell and other tumours.

Metastatic spread may be via the lymphatics or blood stream or both but especially the former to the lumbar and mediastinal nodes. Metastases are commonly found in the lungs and liver.

Clinical Features

A painless lump in the testicle is the usual presenting symptom and any such lump must be regarded as malignant until proved otherwise. On average, patients with a teratoma wait six months and patients with a seminoma wait 12 months before seeking medical advice with the result that about 30 per cent of patients have metastases when first seen.

Diagnosis

The differential diagnosis lies between other painless scrotal swellings such as a hydrocoele which transilluminates but it should be remembered that a hydrocoele can be secondary to a testicular neoplasm. A spermatocoele is a free cystic mass arising above and behind the testis.

A chest X-ray should be requested which may show evidence of metastases and an IVP is mandatory as the ureter or kidney might be displaced by metastases in regional lymph nodes.

Management

If a testicular tumour is palpated exploration is indicated. Orchidectomy is the treatment of choice but seminomas are radiosensitive and therefore radiotherapy is often combined. Pulmonary lobectomy has been successfully performed in a few instances of solitary pulmonary metastases. Chemotherapy with chlorambucil and methotrexate may be tried in relapsing disease.

Follow up and Continuing Care

The presence of demonstrable metastases carries a poor prognosis except in the case of seminomas where radiotherapy is often successful. The type of tumour has considerable prognostic significance. Seminomas carry the best prognosis as there is a 90 per cent five year survival rate compared with 55 per cent in the case of teratomas. Chorionepitheliomas are highly malignant and very few patients with such tumours survive five years.

COMMON DISORDERS OF THE TESTIS AND MALE EXTERNAL GENITALIA

Imperfect testicular descent

The testes are formed in the region of the kidneys and during intrauterine life they migrate, behind the peritoneum, towards the scrotum. In a recent Copenhagen study involving 4500 boys it was found that 17.2 per cent of pre-term infants had undescended testicles at birth, a figure falling to 1.8 per cent in full term babies. At the age of 3 years the figure for full term babies was 0.8 per cent and that for premature babies 2.3 per cent; three quarters of those babies with undescended testicles at birth had normally situated testicles at the age of one year. The prognosis for unilateral maldescent is not good.

An attempt should be made to identify the boys with imperfect testicular descent so that surgery might be considered between the ages of 4 and 5 years in order to avoid the hazards of imperfect descent, the most important of which is impaired spermatogenesis.

During the course of the physical examination the hands must be warm otherwise the cremaster reflex will cause a normal but retractile testis to leave the scrotum and enter the inguinal canal in the suprapubic region; a retractile testis can be pushed back into the scrotum. If a testis can be palpated in the inguinal canal but cannot be pushed into the scrotum, or alternatively, if no testis can be palpated, referral to a paediatric urological surgeon is advisable before the age of 4, as 5 years is believed to be a critical age for testicular growth. If the testes cannot be found in the inguinal canal a laparotomy may be required although this might be considered unjustifiable in the presence of one normal scrotal testicle. Hormone treatment is probably unwise as it is said to be both useless and potentially hazardous.

Torsion of the testicle

Torsion of the testicle is common in adolescents and indeed in this age group is the second most common type of surgical emergency. It can only occur in the presence of a congenital anomaly of the mesorchium allowing the testis and epididymis to twist on a pedicle inside the tunica vaginalis. Precipitating factors include exercise and masturbation possibly accounting for the fact that the condition often occurs during sleep; there may however be no obvious precipitating cause.

Any adolescent with a painful swollen testicle should be considered as having a torsion until proved otherwise as epididymitis and orchitis are rare in this age group; in any case involvement of the testicle in epididymitis is a late complication.

Every patient should be referred immediately to hospital for exploration of the testicle but before doing so an attempt should be made to untwist the testicle by manipulation. A gentle attempt is made to twist the testicle first in one direction and then in the other. In general the right testicle should be 'unscrewed' and the left testicle 'screwed up' to undo the twist. If the pain is made worse the direction of the twist is wrong. The manipulation is continued until pain is relieved bearing in mind that the testicle may have rotated more than once. It should be remembered that spontaneous reduction can occur and nearly half the adolescents admitted to hospital may have had previous warning episodes. If such a history is obtained, of an acute testicular pain which goes away, referral to hospital is indicated as the problem will always recur. Both testicles are usually fixed if one has undergone torsion as the condition is bilateral.

Epididymo-orchitis

Epididymitis may be acute or chronic and when acute it is usually associated with a lower urinary tract infection and will have a similar aetiology and management (p. 340). When chronic it may be tuberculous and secondary to such infection elsewhere.

Orchitis may be the result of mumps or syphilis. Mumps orchitis occurs in one out of every four males who contract mumps after puberty developing about one week after the onset of the disease. It is usually unilateral but may be bilateral and has an acute onset with pain, which may be severe, and swelling of a testicle, which may be very tender. It may be difficult to differentiate the condition from torsion and it is right and proper that the correct management might frequently involve surgical exploration, particularly in the young, but failing this bed rest, local heat, a scrotal support, and analgesics are indicated. The infiltration of 20 ml of 1 per cent procaine into the spermatic cord just above the involved testis sometimes causes rapid resolution and pain relief.

As perhaps half the infected testicles atrophy and become infertile, prophylactic measures might be considered. The incidence of mumps orchitis might be lessened by the administration of mumps convalescent gamma globulin during the incubation period or early in the disease.

Hydrocoele

A hydrocoele is a collection of excess fluid between the visceral and parietal layers of the tunica vaginalis surrounding the testis. It may be unilateral or bilateral, unilocular or multilocular, acute or chronic, and is the commonest cause of a swelling in the scrotum. It may occur at any age but the incidence increases with age although in most instances the cause is unknown. It occasionally follows repair of an inguinal hernia or varicocoele and may be secondary to a testicular neoplasm.

Diagnosis is usually confirmed by transillumination and unlike a scrotal hernia it is possible to get above the swelling.

When a hydrocoele occurs in an infant or young child it should be left alone as in most instances it will disappear. In an older patient treatment will consist of aspiration, with or without the injection of a sclerosing agent, or in some cases operation particularly if any doubt exists about primary testicular disease.

Aspiration can be carried out quite simply in family practice with a trocar and cannula or a 20 syringe and a $1\frac{1}{2}''$ needle. A small area of scrotal skin is infiltrated with a local anaesthetic and the needle is inserted about two centimetres into the hydrocele so that the clear straw coloured fluid can be drained off. Although the procedure is rarely curative it may be entirely satisfactory in the elderly. A better procedure is to inject 2 to 4 ml of urethane and quinine hydrochloride as the sac is emptied which results in the formation of a fibrinous inflammatory reaction in the tunica vaginalis which obliterates the space between the visceral and patietal layers. If after three weeks additional fluid has formed the procedure can be repeated. In a younger man however, referral to a surgeon may be preferred. The testes should always be palpated thoroughly after the hydrocoele has been drained.

Balanitis, Phimosis and Paraphimosis

The incidence of balanitis has been reported as 3 per 1000 patients at risk per year in family practice and the diagnosis is readily made from the red excoriated appearance of the foreskin and an associated discharge. It is commonly seen in young boys. when poor hygiene or an associated napkin rash may be a contributory factor. Its presence in older males may be a sign of diabetes mellitus or carcinoma penis. The condition readily responds to bland cleansing creams and, in resistant cases, nystatin cream applied locally. Failure to respond to treatment should raise the possibility of an underlying cause.

Phimosis is sometimes an aetiological factor in balanitis. It is best left untreated other than by simple measures necessary to maintain cleanliness as over enthusiastic stretching of the foreskin is the commonest cause of a paraphimosis. It should be remembered that the prepuce is still undergoing development at birth and as the child grows older the preputial orifice will widen; only 4 per cent of newborn boys have a fully retractable prepuce and in nearly half the foreskin cannot be retracted sufficiently to reveal the external urethral meatus.

When circumcision is suggested by a parent it should be remembered that in the UK the Registrar General's figures still show that 16 children die each year from circumcision and that the operation has a considerable morbidity ranging from the removal of too much skin to urethral fistula and partial amputation of the glans. Genuine medical indications for circumcision must be uncommon when one considers that significant obstruction to urine flow practically never occurs (ballooning is normal). In addition doubt has been expressed about the statement that cancer of the penis does not occur in circumcised men and that cervical cancer is commoner in the wives of uncircumcised men.

Paraphimosis is an emergency that can usually be dealt with in family practice by taking the penis in one hand and squeezing and elongating the glans with the other in order to compress it under the constriction ring. If this fails an ampoule of hyaluronidase (1 : 500) can be dissolved in 4 ml of 1 per cent plain xylocaine and used to inject at four equidistant sites around the constriction ring. If the penis is then wrapped in lint soaked in ice cold water the swelling will quickly reduce.

References

1. Londe, S. (1968) *Clin. Pediat.* (*Phila.*) 7, 400.
2. Kass, E. H. (1956) *Trans. Ass. Amer. Phys.* 69, 56.
3. Brooks, D. (1973) *Update* 7, 1129.
4. Brooks, D., Garrett, G. and Holihead, R. (1972) *J. roy. Col. gen. Pract.* 22, 695.
5. Williams, R. E. (1969). The natural history of renal lithiasis. In A. Hodgkinson and B. E. C. Nordin (eds.) *Renal Stone Research Symposium* (London: J. A. Churchill).

18

The Skin: Its Care and Abuse

G. B. Walker

THE SKIN IN FAMILY PRACTICE

Gulliver faced many difficulties in his journey to the land of Lilliput and then to the land of Brobdingnag; not least was the effort required in adjusting himself to different scales of value. If these seemed great to him, they are no greater than those which appear to the physician about to enter family practice from hospital. That which appeared rare in hospital becomes common practice, and that which appeared common place becomes rare. From a subject which attracted only a small proportion of his time, he is confronted with the fact that dermatology will occupy a major part of his time, and although a minor speciality in teaching hospital practice it is a major one in family practice. In the UK skin disorders are the third most common disorder in family practice. Of the total work load of a family practitioner approximately one tenth is devoted to dermatological work and over 75 per cent of the family practitioner's work in dermatology is devoted to infections and eczemas.

It has been said that patients with skin affections are more disturbed by their complaints, than patients with other medical disorders. At least 40 per cent of skin conditions have an emotional component, which if not treated will lead to the skin condition becoming chronic. Although often mild in nature the psychological changes may be profound; depression and anxiety may be so manifest as to render the patient unable or unwilling to carry out treatment. On these occasions full co-operation from nurse and health visitor may be necessary to ensure treatment. In considering the skin, do not attempt to separate the skin from the person beneath it; the skin is now realised to be intimately related to psychological and pathological changes in the body.

The changes that are seen on the surface of the skin often merely reflect those deeper within the body. It should not be forgotten that both skin and brain are derived from the neural crest.

Care of the dermatological patient is therefore care of the whole person and to see dermatology as merely a number of spots upon a surface is to see the sea as a mere succession of waves, without being aware of the tides and the winds which produce them. Failure to take account of this has wrecked many a sailor and many a dermatologist has floundered because he has seen only the skin and not the person.

THE SKIN AND ITS CARE

The epidermis is the tissue of the body which often receives the least care and greatest abuse. In a sense, nature has designed it so because the integument in man is the barrier between the organism and his environment. Its functions are several: it provides a thermo regulatory mechanism; it acts as a semi-permeable membrane to foreign materials and radiation; it mediates sensation. Its function is dependent upon the integrity of the epidermal layers, the epidermis absorbing most of the ultra violet radiation and the stratum corneum being the main barrier affecting percutaneous absorption and hydration. Diseases of the skin are factors which increase percutaneous absorption and decrease the efficiency of the barrier; some absorption can also take place by glandular orifices. Care of the skin therefore lies in the prevention of the skin being placed in an environment in which it cannot maintain a normal physiological function and equilibrium. Clothing therefore should be light and loose in texture and allow sufficient ventilation but provide insulation. Close textured fabrics and plastic clothing, especially those which are used in babies should be avoided especially where there is the presence of a skin disorder. Dressings in dermatology should also be light in texture and allow ventilation. Absorbent gauze tends to be too adherent especially in moist lesions and strips of linen or Regal gauze squares (Johnsons and Johnsons) are preferable. Lint and cotton wool should be avoided.

Stockingette, neat-a-last or old nylon stocking are useful to hold dressings in place. Ointments when applied should be applied generously but not lavishly, the aim should be to cover the lesion but not with too thick a layer of ointment. In the case of steroid topical preparations the ointment should be applied sparingly. An important factor in the use of ointments is the quantity dispensed. In small areas too much is often dispensed but the converse applies with more extensive lesions. Between 12 and 26 g applied sparingly are required to cover a total body by a trained operator, higher figures being required by an untrained operator, or when pastes are used. It can be seen that to cover only half the body daily with an ointment will require at least 100 g per week, and if the skin is roughened or a paste is used, up to 500 g per week may be needed.

Contrary to what has been thought washing has little effect on the bacterial content of the skin. Acute and weeping eczemas do not tolerate washing well and ointment is best removed by liquid paraffin or vegetable oils. In most cases all that is required is to repeat the application of ointment and merely change the dressing; the skin need only be cleaned if the ointment or paste begins to 'cake'.

THE SKIN AND ITS ABUSE

It is probably fair to say that the difference between dermatology in family practice and in hospital practice is that the first has to recognise untreated lesions and the second has to be able to recognise them after treatment with steroid ointments. The increasing amount of persistent skin damage being seen by dermatologists, following the long continuing use of potent topical corticosteroid preparations in the treatment of chronic skin disorder is causing alarm[1]. In 1967 10 million prescriptions for topical steroids were issued by practitioners in England and the figures are probably higher today. It is necessary to be aware of the damages and clinical presentation of steroid iatrogenic disease. The dangers can be divided into two groups:

1. *General Effects* Steroids applied to the skin are absorbed and can produce adrenal suppression[2,3]. This most easily occurs with use of fluorinated steroids, but is rare with the use of the hydrocortisones. The effects of absorption are often increased by the use of occlusive polythene or plastic film[4]. It commonly occurs in those conditions which have been allowed to become chronic.

2. *Local Effects* Steroids applied topically have an anti inflammatory reaction which reduces itching and inflammation, there is also a vasoconstrictor effect which produces pallor. Prolonged use of steroids produces premature ageing of the skin in the form of striae, atrophy and telangectasia, especially on the face, thighs and intertriginous areas.

There is a decreased resistance to fungal, viral and bacterial infections. Occasionally a rosacea like appearance may develop. Exacerbations may follow the withdrawal of steroids (rebound phenomena).

From the above facts we can formulate several basic rules for the use of topical steroids in family practice:—

1. use the potent steriods to bring lesions quickly under control, and then change to the hydrocortisone preparations, if prolonged use is required.
2. try to avoid using them in chronic conditions where alternative preparations are effective.
3. on the face use only hydrocortisone preparations.

ECZEMA

Aetiology

Eczema can be defined as a papulo-vesicular reaction of the skin which is inflammatory in nature. It is an important and common condition for the family practitioner who will see several cases each week. It can result in industrial disability and if incorrectly managed in chronicity.

There is a variety of types of eczema which can be separated into two basic groups: those which arise from internal causes and those which arise from external causes. There is however some overlapping between the groups. From long usage the word *dermatitis* is sometimes used where the eczema is externally produced.

Pathology

There is epidermal oedema (spongiosis) which eventually results in the formation of primordial vesicles, there is also an increase in the malpighian layer (acanthosis) and in the horny layer cells retain their nuclei (parakeratosis).

Contact eczema has an allergic basis and is a cell mediated response; chemicals applied to the skin are absorbed through the skin and passed to the lymphatic system. The T-lymphoctyes are the lymphocytes which are mainly affected and only a small proportion are carriers of the sensitivity. In atopic eczema there is probably endogenous (non antigenic) stimulation of cells with release of lymphocyte substances which produce eczema; stimulation is due to a defect of the self regulatory mechanism between T and B lymphocytes.

Clinical Features

Eczema presents as an itching rash of small (1—2 mm) papules which become vesicular. Although this is the basic lesion the presentation may differ according to the stage and site of the pathological process.

Stages of the Pathological Process

1. Spongiosis produces papules which lead to vesicles; itching is marked.
2. Rupture of vesicles: the surface becomes 'raw', moist, erythematous and exudative.
3. Parakeratosis: the surface becomes intact, erythematous and crusted. Fine scaling may occur.
4. Lichenification: thickening and heaping up of epidermal layers occurs with keratinization.
5. Recovery: the process from 1—5 may be rapid, stop at any stage or may be prolonged.

The Site of the Pathological Process

1. *Hands and Feet*   Clinically the lesions look like translucent areas under the skin which are indurated (pompholyx). The lesions are described as looking like sago grains. If the process is acute the epidermal layers may be shed in large sheets. A hyperkeratotic form can occur with thickening of the keratin layer and minimal scaling.
2. *Nails*   Here the eczema presents as irregular transverse ridges. Slight discolouration of the nail occurs. Superficial pitting may be present.
3. *Axilla and Gluteal Region*   Due to perspiration the lesions are moist and erythematous. Large plaques are formed, and the edge is often clearly defined with outlying papules.

Atopic Eczema

The word 'atopic' means out of place and was chosen by Coca to describe a group of people who had a tendency to inherit either eczema, hay fever or asthma. A family history is present in about 2/3; in over 50 per cent of cases there is a tendency to have associated hay fever, asthma, urticaria, migraine headaches, or allergic rhinitis. The condition usually starts between 6 months and 2 years of age. The face may be first involved and later the flexures of the knee and elbow. In these areas it rapidly passes into the chronic phase presenting as large lichenified plaques with associated itching papules. Localised patches of vesicular eczema may occur elsewhere. Impetiginization is not uncommon. Congenital dryness of the skin (xeroderma) is often associated. Fortunately in most cases the affection has disappeared by about the age of 10 although in a few it may continue into adult life. Infection by the herpes simplex or vaccinia virus may produce generalized spread in the atopic patient, he should therefore not be vaccinated and be kept away from relatives or persons who have been vaccinated or who are suffering from a herpes simplex infection.

General Management

In most there is an element of xerodema and washing should be restricted. In acute cases corn or nut oil can be used for cleaning instead of water. The use of Ung-Emulsificans in the bath or used as a soap is helpful and Boots E45 can be applied after bathing and as required.

Seborrhoeic Eczema

This occurs in a group of people who are characterised by the presence of a greasy yellow skin, dilated skin follicles and pallor. The condition is probably genetically determined and is related to the activity of the seborrhoeic glands, which are found in greatest numbers on the face, interscapular areas, external auditory meatus, and intergluteal areas. It appears to be related to the secretion of androgens and oestrogens. Bacterial infection is common in the seborrhoeic but is secondary rather than primary.

Clinical Manifestations

These vary according to the site.

Head   The most common manifestation is a dry scaling of the scalp with greasy hair (dandruff). The scalp feels irritable and occasionally becomes sore. Perifolliculitis occurs and may lead to loss of frontal hair. In severe cases the scaling becomes heaped up to form thickened plaques which are greasy looking. At the hair margin an erythematous band may occur and eventually acute inflammation with secondary infection. The fine branny scaling occurs on the face particularly on the eyebrows and around the external auditory meatus.

Blepharitis occurs with slight scaling, there may be loss of eye lashes. Weeping eczema and infected eczematous fissures occur around the nose, mouth and ears. The beard area may be affected by a superficial folliculitis.

Flexures   Usually the axilla, groin, genital area and in women the area beneath the breast are affected.

Trunk   A fine eczematous form is produced which is a yellowish/red colour and paler in the centre. Examination of the edge shows a fine scaling. On the sternal area the lesions are often grouped together to produce a petuloid arrangement.

All the above lesions are prone to infection, particularly the scalp and flexures, impetiginization may occur.

Differential Diagnosis

On the scalp seborrhoeic eczema must be distinguished from psoriasis, but the psoriatic lesion is palpable, localised and not greasy looking. Infectious dermatitis can be separated from seborrhoeic eczema in the same site by the absence of signs elsewhere. Seborrhoeic eczema of the flexures has to be differentiated from psoriasis where there are not usually outlying papules and there are signs of psoriasis elsewhere. It must be noted that often psoriasis is associated with seborrhoeic eczema.

Ringworm and Candida infections can be separated by microscopical examination of skin scrapings. Pityriasis rosea is sometimes mistaken for seborrhoeic eczema of the body but there is an absence of the herald spot in seborrhoeic eczema and the lesions do not follow the lines of the ribs or are as widely distributed.

General Management

As yet there is very little that we can do to help the underlying seborrhoeic state; stress may play a part and should be relieved by rest and sedation. The wearing of light loose clothing should be advised. There is higher instance in alcoholism, diabetes and Parkinson's disease and these should be treated. A low carbohydrate diet and administration of vitamin B complex are thought to be helpful.

Nummular Eczema (Discoid Eczema)

Nummular eczema is probably multifactoral in origin and is often associated with xeroderma. It presents as disc shaped erythematous papules and vesicles, which may be single or multiple. In many forms the papulo-vesicular lesion is not obvious and the presenting lesion is of an erythematous area which eventually becomes affected by a brownish pigmentation with micro-vesicles.

Differential Diagnosis
Differential diagnosis is easy if associated with other obvious eczematous lesions. In some cases it can be confused with ringworm but unlike this it has no active edge and vesicles if they occur, are found in the centre rather than at the edge. It may follow chrome and nickel sensitivity.

General Management
Management of nummular eczema is not easy. There are no specific features which assist in the treatment and these lesions tend to be more chronic than other eczemas. The aim is to relieve the itching and dryness using local steroid creams and avoiding soap and water.

Pompholyx Eczema

This is an eczema of the palms and soles. Hyperhidrosis is commonly associated and many cases show a relationship to stress. Secondary infection is often present.

A few cases appear to be associated with fungus infection of the feet and mould allergy.

Differential Diagnosis
Contact eczema is found on the dorsal aspects of the hands and feet and only rarely on the palms. The vesicular type of dermatophytosis has to be differentiated; it usually presents initially as athlete's foot. It is important in all cases of eczema of the hands to examine the feet also.

General Management
Rest and sedation are important and attempts should be made to find any underlaying psychological factors as these are often important.

Asteotic Eczema (Senile Eczema)

This is a common form of eczema in family practice in the elderly and one which is often unrecognised for what it is. It occurs in people where there is a diminution of the superficial lipid layers of the skin. This produces loss of moisture and subsequent dryness.

Clinical Features

Clinical findings are variable. It may present initially as a pruritus in a dry skin with few clinical signs, and later as a dry eczema which has a crazy pavement appearance due to fissuring. On the hands the fissuring is much finer and there is loss of dermoglyphia (finger prints).

General Management

Frequent washing with soaps or detergents removes lipids and should be avoided in the asteotic skin. An emollient cream applied in the water or after washing helps greatly. I use 30 g of emulsificans ointment emulsified in hot water and added to a bath. Emulsificans ointment can also be used instead of soap.

    Like the atopic patient they are irritated by wool or nylon next to the skin and this should be avoided. The environment should be corrected. Many elderly people use electric fires which are very drying and some form of humidifier is often necessary. The patient should be advised to take baths infrequently.

Pityriasis Alba

This is an infrequent condition in hospital practice but frequently found in family practice. It is found between the ages of 3 and 16 when it may occur in as many as 30—40 per cent. Its aetiology is unknown although exposure to wind and sun appears to play a part. It is less common in the autumn and worse in summer and winter.

Clinical Features

The presenting feature is a depigmented area which is discoid and two or three centimetres in diameter. Lesions are restricted to the face in 81 per cent of cases.

    Clinical examination may reveal a very fine scaling, initially there may be erythema. There is an absence of symptoms. Although the lesions are usually confined to the face they may occur on the body. In my practice I find that a spell of sunny weather usually produces a crop of these lesions; this is due to the fact that the depigmentation then becomes more obvious and is the presenting sign.

Differential Diagnosis

The site of the lesion plus the lack of symptoms help to separate it from nummular eczema. Vitiligo does not scale.

General Management

Most cases are helped by a simple face cream which acts as a barrier against the elements. Explanation that the depigmentation is not permanent together with advice to avoid exposure to the elements are all that are required. Steroid ointments do not appear to give any substantial benefit over simple creams.

Primary Irritant Dermatitis

This is produced by the irritant acting directly on the epidermis. If the irritant is very strong a burn is produced (*toxic dermatitis*), if less strong a chronic eczema is produced (*cumulative insult dermatitis*).

Housewife's Dermatitis

This is the common form of presentation of primary irritant eczema in adults, it is due to repeated maceration and damage to the skin from frequent washing and imperfect drying and contact with soaps, solvents and cleaning solutions.

The eczema presents as dryness and roughness of the skin, with erythema and fissuring, especially at the flexures. Eventually a full eczematous picture is produced. Several years may elapse between stages. Both plantar and palmar surfaces are affected and on occasions the forearms. A common site of presentation is underneath a ring on the finger.

General management is by the avoidance of prolonged immersion of the hands in washing liquids. Rings should be taken off before washing-up and the hand dried before reapplying. An emollient cream such as Boot E45 applied after washing is invaluable.

Napkin Dermatitis

This is a common skin disorder in infants and is produced by the irritant action of faeces, urine and ammonia, the latter is released by the proteus bacillus acting on urine. The rash presents as an erythematous moist area which spares the areas of skin between skin folds; it extends around the genito-anal area to the lower abdoman and inner thighs, vesicles may develop and ulceration occurs. Babies with atopic eczema and seborrhoeic eczema are particularly prone to this eczema.

Napkin psoriasis

Recently there have been reports of psorisiform lesions appearing on the napkin area; there is a high association of infection with candida.

General management is by keeping the areas as dry as possible and well ventilated. Excess heat and humidity should be avoided and also plastic pants. The child should be changed immediately if wet or soiled and the buttock cleaned with olive or corn oil in the very acute stages, later it may be possible to use just warm water. The napkin should be used either as a skirt or discarded and the buttock exposed to air. Gentian violet and brilliant green 0.5 per cent in zinc paste is useful in napkin psoriasis.

Allergic Contact Dermatitis

This is produced by an allergic response to a sensitizing substance (allergen) applied to the skin. Only minute traces of allergen are necessary to produce a reaction. In some cases they only become active after exposure to ultra violet radiation. It may not be possible to determine whether a purely allergic process occurs or merely a toxic reaction. They are known as photo allergic or photo toxic dermatitis. It has been shown that the most common cause of allergic contact dermatitis is occupational dermatitis and the second common cause is equally divided between clothing and medicinal dermatitis. Allergic contact dermatitis may account for 30 per cent of eczemas in family practice.

Diagnosis

Diagnosis is not difficult if the possibility of allergens are kept in mind. Initially the dermatitis is related to the site of exposure. Eventually, if the exposure is continued it will spread all over the body. It is therefore important to ascertain where was the original lesion and what it was like. A detailed history is always very important. It is also useful to enquire if any workmates are known to have any similar lesions. The patient should be asked if he has any idea what has caused the condition, and it is important for the patient to realise that substances which sensitize are those which have had long usage and that only rarely can substances which have been used for a few days sensitize the patient. The patient should be asked questions about his hobbies, occupation, clothing and previous treatment as these are common sources of allergens. He should also be asked if the rash improves at the weekends or holidays (industrial dermatitis improves then) or if the seasons affect the rash (actinic dermatitis occurs in summer, seasonal dermatitis in spring and autumn). Examination of the whole body is vital as it is one of the peculiarities of contact dermatitis that the primary lesion may be tolerated for many years and a complaint made only when it has become generalised.

Further methods of value in identifying possible allergens are:

1. removal from suspected allergen;
2. re-exposure to suspected allergen;
3. experimental exposure to allergen (Patch Tests[5]).

In many cases the eczematous imprint left by the sensitizing substance is clear and the diagnosis is self evident. In others the diagnosis is not obvious and it is necessary to patch test, a procedure which is best left to the hospital.

It is useful in practice to be aware of the common presentations.

Photo-allergic dermatitis affects only the light exposed areas. In its initial phases it spares the upper eye lids and the V beneath the chin. Porphyria must be excluded.

Cement dermatitis (due to chromium) presents as a dry scaling eczema of the hands and a discoid eczema of the body. The dust often collects on flexures and around ankles which are often affected.

White metal dermatitis (due to nickel, chromium or cobalt) is extremely common. It is nearly always directly related to white metal objects such as clasps, suspender fasteners, rings, zip fasteners and jewellery.

Rubber dermatitis (due to chemicals used in manufacture) occurs from rubber in shoes, boots, clothing and not infrequently from rubber gloves. When the hands and wrists are affected, there is usually a sharp mark of demarcation at the wrist. It often complicates housewife's dermatitis.

Textile dermatitis (due to dyes or formaldehyde) occurs in the axillae where the high degree of humidity accelerates sensitization. Usually a small area at the apex is left free. Trouser dermatitis affects the thighs and the popliteal fossa.

Stocking dermatitis (due to azo dyes) affects the dorsum of the feet first followed by behind the knees and then the middle of the thighs (stockings dyed with non azo dyes can be obtained from Swan and Edgar, London).

Shoe dermatitis (due to chromium, rubber or adhesives) occurs on the dorsum surface of the feet, the interdigital space being spared, rarely the soles may be affected by chronic eczema.

Cosmetic dermatitis (due to dyes, ointment bases, perfumes and nail varnish) is usually confined to the face and often affects the eye lids first. Where oil of bergamot in perfume is used a photo allergic reaction is produced, it is known as Berloque dermatitis which produces bizarre patches of erythema followed by pigmentation.

Applied medicaments   Neomycin, lanolin, dettol and C.T.A.B. in leg ulcers, local anaesthetics in haemorrhoidal preparations, neomycin, framycetin and hydroxyquinolones in eczemas, and bases and stabilizers used in ointments are likely sources of sensitization. It should be remembered that if sensitization occurs whilst the steroid ointment is used, the reaction is rarely severe.

Plants   *Primula obconica* is a common and potent sensitizer in this country. Initially reactions occur on the eye lids; bullous streaks may occur from actual contact. Chrysanthemums and compositae produce a chronic scaling eczema. The thumb and fore-finger are affected by allergy to narcissus and tulip bulbs.

Airborne dermatitis (due to pollens and moulds) is not uncommon in country areas, where it occurs usually in the spring or autumn (seasonal eczema). A chronic scaling eczema results which affects all of the face and neck, the edge is diffuse and extends below the clothing line.

Occupational dermatitis   Workers in the building industry commonly suffer from cement dermatitis; engineering workers suffer from chrome sensitization due to traces of chromium in lubricant and cutting oils; trauma plays an important part; bakers get an eczema of the hands due to sensitization to persulphate; hospital works frequently suffer from contact eczema due to penicillin, streptomycin, chlorpromazine and antiseptics; hairdressers have a primary irritant dermatitis due to caustic solutions and frequent washing and a contact dermatitis due to hair dyes.

The salient features in occupational dermatitis are that usually other workers are affected and that in 80 per cent of cases lesions occur on the hands and forearms. Industrial dermatitis accounts for 1 per cent of all injuries in industry and is a recognised industrial disease for which compensation is allowed[6].

Management

The management of contact dermatitis is often straight forward but on occasions can be difficult. The identification of the allergen is the prime factor and then the removal of the patient from the source. Removal produces an immediate cure, but in a few cases lesions may persist for months or years.

Allergens can be avoided by the replacement of rubber gloves, metal spectacles or suspenders by plastic ones. I advise patients who wear rubber or plastic gloves to choose loose fitting ones and to wear inside cotton gloves which can be washed at frequent intervals. The rubber gloves should be washed before removal. In industry it may be necessary to change jobs. Education of the patient to danger from allergic substances, immediate washing after contact with allergens, regular use of an aqueous cream after washing and regular inspections are important in preventing reoccurrences.

Dermatitis which is secondary to infection is caused by sensitization to a bacteria or by-products of tissue destruction. Treatment should be aimed at controlling the infection and treating the source of the infection e.g., chronic otitis media, leg ulcer.

General Principles of the Management of Eczema

Although there are many varieties of eczemas the treatment of them is basically the same. The basic principle in the treatment of eczemas is the need to vary the treatment according to the pathological state. Treatment which will not be tolerated by an acute lesion is often tolerated by a chronic lesion and that which will be effective in acute stage may have little effect on the chronic stage.

Another bewildering aspect is the multiplicity and variety of medications available for treatment. It is best for the family practitioner to select a few well tried medications and to stick to these until he has gained experience with them before venturing further, if at all. Recently there has been a tendency to treat all eczemas with steroid ointments. These should be used but it must be realised that traditional treatments are still of value.

Acute Eczema

In this stage the eczematous process is in an active and reactive phase, only the mildest of medications are tolerated and secondary infection is common. It is in this phase that lotions are most effective. Linen strips or Regal gauze are soaked in the solution and it is necessary to change or re-moisten at three hourly intervals to prevent drying out and the formation of adhesions. The following lotions are useful:

1. silver nitrate, 0.5 per cent aqueous solution;
2. potassium permanganate, 1 part in 8000;
3. aluminium acetate lotion. B.N.F.

The first two are invaluable where infection is present. Unfortunately they have the minor disadvantage that pigmentation occurs with their use. If not too moist topical steroid creams can be used. Bed rest is helpful where the lesions are extensive.

When the lesions are beginning to dry up shake-lotions such as calamine lotion can be used. If there is infection, gentian violet (0.5 per cent) can be added.

Sub-Acute Eczema

It is in this and in the chronic type that topical steroids are most effective. If moist and in the flexures, cream is most probably the better; in drier areas the ointment is more suitable. At least three main levels of activity exist. In ascending order of potency they are:

1. hydrocortisone 21-acetate, 1 per cent;
2. triamcinolone acetonide, 0.1 per cent, fluocinolone acetonide 0.025 per cent;
3. betamethasone 17-valerate.

These are all that are required in family practice. When infection is present clioquinol, aureomycin or neomycin can be added. Framycetin, graneodin and bacitracin can also be used.

Tar preparations are helpful, they tend to promote epithelization and reduce irritation and are useful in the sub-acute and chronic phases of eczema. It is best to start with calamine and coal tar ointment. If this is tolerated well a coal tar paste B.P.C. can be used.

Chronic Eczema

This responds best to tar preparations such as the above and also topical steroids. Areas which are lichenified respond well to tar paste bandages such as 'Coltapaste'. These are applied directly onto the skin and covered by crepe or Elastoplast bandages after covering with stockingette. They are of particular use in children where they are of help in breaking the scratch reflex.

It should be remembered that eczematous patients tolerate water badly and removal of the ointment should be by cleaning off lightly with liquid paraffin instead of washing with water.

When the lesions are beginning to clear it is as well to remember that Lassar's paste by itself or with an equal part of soft paraffin provides protection to the newly formed epidermis.

Exfoliative Eczemas

Rarely an eczema may become completely generalised with erythroderma and exfoliation. Hypothermia may occur and may mask infections such as pneumonia by the failure of the body to show a rise in temperature. High output cardiac failure may occur due to diversion of blood to the skin and hospital admission and management is required.

Seborrhoeic Eczema

Seborrhoeic eczema is usually associated with secondary infection and the use of antibiotic or chemotherapeutic agents with the steroid is essential. Seborrhoea is controlled by the use of selenium sulphide in a 2.5 per cent shampoo. It is shampooed into the hair and scalp twice weekly for two to three weeks. After this period I find that the scalp becomes greasy and irritated, but by this time control has usually been achieved. I then advise the use of a centrimide shampoo and this should be applied twice weekly. Synalar gel and Betnovate scalp lotion help to control the minor forms of erythema and itching in the early stages of seborrhoea.

Sulphur is also effective in seborrhoea of the trunk and this can be applied either as 2 per cent precipitated sulphur in calamine lotion or as a stronger preparation in salicylic acid and sulphur ointment B.P.C.

Systemic Therapy

1. *Sedation* is important to all cases of eczema. For children I use elixir promethazine, for adults amylobarbitone and in the elderly chlorpromazine. The dose is adjusted to produce relief without producing drowsiness, both children and adults will often tolerate doses which would be soporific in healthy people. Nitrazepam can be used as a soporific in adults.

2. *Antibiotics* should be used if there is very extensive secondary infection and lymphadenitis. Swabs for culture and sensitization to antibiotics should be taken first.

3. *Systemic Steroids* are not recommended for atopic eczema as the condition tends to flare up when therapy is discontinued. In hospital practice they are of occasional value in exfoliative dermatitis and severe contact dermatitis.

PSORIASIS

Nature and Condition

Psoriasis is a genetically determined condition of the skin in which there is an abnormally high epidermal turnover resulting in well defined salmon pink lesions of the skin with a characteristic silver scaling. The lesions usually progress from an acute to a chronic phase and there may be intermittent attacks.

The concept of psoriasis being a purely epidermal condition is superficial and the truth lies deeper. It has been shown that patients with psoriasis have a folic acid deficiency. In generalised psoriasis there is a low serum albumen and an increase of globulin, mainly IgE. Eight per cent of psoriatics have a normochromic anaemia with an associated low serum iron. In some psoriatics malabsorption from the gut can be shown to be the cause of the low folic acid levels.

Psoriasis affects between 1 and 2 per cent of the population. It is common in the caucasian, less common in the coloured and rare in the negro. The mean age of onset is 27.3 years[7]. It is rare in infancy and old age, it commonly starts between 5 and 15. It is affected climatically, improving with sunlight in 78 per cent. Hot weather improves it in 77 per cent and cold weather makes it worse.

Although a chronic disease the outlook is not a poor one as many physicians and patients were led to believe. In 38.5 per cent psoriasis will completely disappear at some time or other; in 10—25 per cent it clears for long periods of life[7]. The majority have recurrent attacks of months or years.

Pathology

There is a high epidermal cell turnover with imperfect keratinization and an absence of the kerato hyaline later. The keratin has mucous like qualities. Closely set micropustules are found in the upper epidermis together with hyperkeratosis and elongation of rete ridges.

Clinical Features

The characteristic lesion in psoriasis is that of a hyperkeratotic plaque which is well defined at the margin. The colour is salmon pink but as the hyperkeratosis becomes more pronounced, a silvery white colour is produced on the surface, gentle scratching of the lesion produces fragmentary silvery scales. Continuous scratching denudes the surface of scales and reveals an erythematous base with pin point bleeding points. The lesions are non-itching except in moist infected areas.

In acute forms the silvery scaling may not be so prominent and the lesion be more erythematous. As the lesion progresses scaling occurs but an erythematous margin may still be present. If the plaque is in a moist area such as the axilla or groin, the hyperkeratosis may not be obvious and presents instead as a moist fissured erythematous plaque. Scaling may also be absent in some flexural and penile lesions.

Three other features are important in psoriasis.

1. Attacks often follow specific instances of stress.
2. Attacks often follow tonsillitis.
3. Lesions often develop at the site of injury (Koebner phenomenon).

Variants of the Basic Epidermal Lesion

According to how the basic lesion develops, certain clinical pictures may develop. It is as well to be aware of these variants although amongst them there is nearly always a typical basic lesion which helps in diagnosis.

Guttate The lesions are small, from a few millimetres to a centimetre in diameter. It is a common form of presentation in the young and is the presenting form in 14—17 per cent of psoriatics. Scaling is not often obvious initially unless searched for.

Nummular This is the common form of presentation. Discoid plaques are formed usually several centimetres in diameter. If several plaques coalesce, large areas of irregular shapes will be covered, some of which are gyrate. The silvery scaling is obvious.

On the nails, hands or scalp the lesions are not typical of the basic lesion and present as follows:

Nails Pitting of the nails occurs and is diagnostic of psoriasis. The pits are about the size of a pinhead, although more rarely, larger pits may occur. They occur in approximately $\frac{1}{3}$ of patients. Where psoriatic arthritis occurs the association is as high as $\frac{2}{3}$.

Scalp Here the lesions present as palpable, hyperkeratotic, white, scaling plaques. The plaque is dry and may involve part or the whole of the scalp. In some cases there may be loss of hair.

Hands and Feet Two types are seen on the hands and feet. In one there is a dry scaling eczematous like eruption which may eventually become a hard plaque of keratin like tylosis. In the other a pustular form of psoriasis occurs, which presents as small lakes of pus beneath the epidermis; the lesions are sterile. The pustules eventually abort at the surface and leave brown scales. The skin has a glazed appearance. Pustular bacterid used to be differentiated but it is now believed that they are the same condition.

It should be remembered that psoriasis is usually symmetrical and that the commonmost site of occurrence is the elbows and knees, where it often commences as hyperkeratotic plaques which are slightly silvery. Lesions are less common on the face.

Two other forms may occur which are rare but serious in their prognosis.
Generalised Erythrodermic Psoriasis Here the psoriasis presents as a severe erythema which covers most or the whole of the body. It usually occurs in a patient with existing active psoriasis which has been overtreated and when steroids are withdrawn, scaling is not marked. The thermoregulatory mechanism is lost and high output cardiac failure may occur.
Generalised Pustular Psoriasis Crops of pustules develop on the skin and on psoriatic lesions. Fever or constitutional changes occur. It is of serious prognosis and as in generalised erythrodermic psoriasis it indicates a highly eruptive flare. The withdrawal of steroids may precipitate it.

Psoriatic Arthropathy

In addition to the epidermal changes, articular changes may occur which affect the distal interphalangeal joints, and there is swelling between the joints producing 'sausage fingers'. It is more common in females and is particularly associated with nail changes. Rheumatoid factor tests are usually negative.

Diagnosis

Of all the dermatological conditions, to diagnose this is one of the easiest as a careful general examination usually reveals several of the typical lesions. It is as well to remember that in hospital, most of the cases seen have been present several days or weeks and are fully developed. In family practice earlier lesions are seen where the characteristic hyperkeratinisation may not have developed. Observation over two or three days will usually find typical lesions. To search is to find; in all dermatological conditions where there is doubt, completely undress the patient.

When looking for psoriasis always examine the nails, elbows, knees and scalp. Lesions here are often overlooked but are diagnostic.

Differential diagnosis

Seborrhoeic dermatitis is easily confused in the scalp if no other lesions are present but in seborrhoeic dermatitis the plaque is moist and a greeny yellow colour. Itching is often marked. At the edge there are erythematous margins and outlying papules. Pityriasis rosea is not uncommon in family practice and may be confused with early psoriasis. The scaling is not marked and is powdery rather than flaky. The lesions follow the line of the ribs and a herald spot is often seen. Tinea circinata may mimic psoriasis in the acute phase. Examination of the edge of tinea circinata with a hand lens should reveal the presence of tiny vesicles which are pinpoint size in diameter. Eczema of the palm imitates the hyperkeratotis form but itching is usually present. Secondary syphilis and lichenplanus must also be considered.

Finally remember that psoriasis may occur in association with eczema, seborrhoeic dermatitis and lichen planus.

Assessment

Psoriasis only accounts for about 7 per cent of patients with skin conditions in family practice. Its importance however, is greater than its percentage because of its difficulty in management. The psoriatic tends to be a regular attender. The management of such patients is therefore of importance, or else a feeling of despair will be instilled in doctor and patient alike. The patient must be seen not only in his dermatological but also in his social and psychological context in order to treat and help him.

The problem therefore of the psoriatic is also psychological, and stress may not only precipitate but perpetuate it. Socially the disease may be unacceptable.

The family practitioner also has a role in the education of the psoriatic to let him know clearly the nature of his condition and its management. It is important throughout that a positive approach is maintained. Ingram[8] paints a pathetic picture of the psoriatic. 'There is nothing so sad as the despondancy of the psoriatic who has been informed that his ill is incurable'. It may be incurable in the sense that we cannot affect the genetic defect of its chronicity but it certainly can be treated and cleared. It is a sad reflection on management today that there are still a multitude of patients in family and hospital practice who have been told that they are incurable. It is the role of the family practitioner to prevent a recurrent condition becoming chronic.

In the UK a society exists to help and educate those who have psoriasis.

> Psoriasis Association,
> 7 Milton Street,
> Northampton N.W.2 7JG

Treatment

It is important to realise that psoriasis occurs in two phases, the acute and the chronic. In the acute phase the erythema is marked and the lesions are spreading. In the chronic phase the hyperkeratosis is very evident and the lesion relatively stationary.

In the acute phase, strong ointments will be poorly tolerated. It is often best merely to apply vaseline and later coal tar and salicylic acid ointment, B.P.C. In the chronic stage stronger ointments will be tolerated.

Coal tar and salicylic acid is probably the best treatment for guttate psoriasis, but dithranol may be required on resistant areas.

Dithranol Preparations and Regimes

Dithranol has been the mainstay of treatment for many years. It probably acts by inhibiting cell production thereby reducing faulty epidermal turnover. Ingrams treatment has been the standard treatment for many years but is not easy to use in family practice. I find that the following regime using a stiff dithranol ointment described by Seville[17] more acceptable.

Stiff dithranol ointment: Dithranol 0.5 per cent, salicylic acid 0.5 per cent, chloroform 2.5 per cent, hard paraffin B.P. and white soft paraffin B.P. in equal quantities to 100 per cent.

This ointment has the advantage of being easy to apply, one strength only is used and control is achieved by lengthening or decreasing the interval between applications. If the ointment spreads onto the surrounding skin, slightly smaller quantities of ointment should be used. Spreading is restricted by lightly covering the application with talc and then applying 5−10 cm stockinette to the limbs and 25−35 cm stockinette to the trunk. Old nylon stockings covered with crepe bandages or old cotton under-clothes can be used when stockinette is not available. A bath should be taken between treatments to control the reaction.

Treatment should be stopped if moistness, cracking or soreness occurs and if the psoriasis spreads whilst producing any of these symptoms. Yellow soft paraffin B.P.C. should be applied and after an interval treatment can be recommenced on a few thickened areas. Flexures are easily inflamed but the following preparation is usually tolerated: dithranol 0.25 per cent, salicylic acid 1.0 per cent, emulsificans ointment to 100 per cent. It is an excellent preparation for the scalp as it can be washed out easily. A coal tar shampoo should be used 2−3 times weekly.

The treatment must be continued until the skin is entirely clear, that is, when there is nothing to feel with the fingers and the texture is normal. The dithranol stain can then be seen peeling off leaving the skin a normal colour. The depth of stain that occurs is an indication of the effectiveness of the treatment and the patient should be advised of this.

White's tar paste should be used on the face. White's paste is also useful after the termination of dithranol treatment as its application assists in the removal of treatment stains. (Goekerman's treatment involving tar paste is too complex and messy for family practice).

Topical Fluorinated Steroids

Although a popular treatment dermatologists have been having second thoughts about its use. Writers are beginning to warn about the dangers of frequent relapses occurring two to three weeks after treatment. If large areas are treated when relapse occurs it may extend even more so that the patient becomes caught up in an 'iatrogenic whirlpool'. Once the patient has got used to the elegant steroid preparations it is difficult to get him to change. Change over to tar ointments should be made before dependence occurs. Unfortunately dithranol reacts violently with the skin when steroids have been applied and an interval of at least one month should be allowed.

Systemic Treatment

Amytal in doses of up to 100 mg three times a day in the young adult and Vallium (5 mg) in the elderly are often beneficial. Extra sedation at night may also be necessary. The aim should be to give a dosage which will relax the patient but will not make him soporific.

Methotrexate, arsenic and steroids used systemically have serious side effects; they should be reserved for hospital use.

In conclusion two important factors in the treatment of psoriasis should be remembered:

1. treat until the skin is completely clear.
2. treat as soon as possible.

If this is done the prognosis is improved.

BACTERIAL INFECTIONS

Nature and Condition

From the moment we are born the skin is colonized by many bacteria and some fungi. Control of bacterial populations on the skin is by the acid mantle produced by liberation of free fatty acids from sebum, dessication and desquamation. In addition to these factors bacteria have an inhibitory affect on other bacteria, an effect which is known as bacterial interference. There is also a direct relationship between the gram negative and the gram positive populations.

The dermatological pattern of bacterial populations is therefore one of ecological harmony, the resident ecology changing with the ages of man and disturbed only by intermittent attempts at colonisation by other bacteria.

Infection may occur when either the 'soil or the seed' is altered. Alteration in the soil occurs when the trauma produces breaches in the epidermis allowing bacteria to penetrate. Alterations in the general health of patients can decrease resistance. Diabetes, alcoholism and nutritional deficencies produce conditions which are more susceptible to skin infections. Alterations in the immunological process has a similar effect and recurrent infections occur in hypogamma-globulinaemia and prolonged administration of steroids. Changes in the seed occur when there is either heavy innoculation or a change in the virulence of the organism.

Staphylococcus aureus can occur in heavy concentrations on the skin in a number of people who then become carriers, bacteria being dispersed in airborne micro-flakes of skin. The infection is usually present in the external nares and perianal areas. As many as 20 per cent of patients are carriers. Such carriers are also more liable to infection.

Impetigo

In impetigo the cocci infect the superficial and epidermal layers, the granular layer is usually left intact and forms the base to any vesical or bulla. The disease is contagious.

The infection is usually due to a pure staphylococcal infection, less common a streptococcal infection and more rare a mixed staphylococcal and streptococcal infection. The infection spreads onto the skin and when fully populated clinical lesions occur.

Clinical Features
The epidermal infection rapidly produces vesicles and bullae. In infants spread is rapid and the bullae predominate to produce pemphigus neonaturum. In children and adults the bullae rapidly burst to form and exude serum and produce honey coloured crusts. Only rarely are the bullae obvious unless fed by fluorinated steroids.

An inflammatory edge is present which gives on occasions, a circinate appearance. In haemolytic streptococcal infection there is often a marked inflammatory halo and lymphadenitis. In bullous impetigo the bullae do not burst so readily, and lymphadenitis is rare. The crusts are a light brown in colour. Beneath the crusts a raw erythematous base is observed.

Streptococcal impetigo is not common but there is a relationship between impetigo and acute glomerulonephritis.

Treatment

The first priority is the removal of the crusts followed by application of an antibiotic or chemotherapeutic ointment. Crusts can be removed by bathing with saline. Cetrimide cream is also a useful way of removing the crusts and should be applied several times a day. After removal of the crusts an antibiotic ointment should be applied which should be non-sensitizing and not used generally internally. A proprietary preparation combining neomycin, bacitracin, framycetin and gramicidin can be used, with a change to oxytetracycline after three days, if there is no response.

Oxytetracycline is preferable as it has a low sensitizing preparation. It has been found that some patients are resistant to tetracyclines[9] and chlomamphenicol cream or fucidin gel can be used as alternatives.

Aqueous gentian violet 0.5 per cent lotion is an old remedy but is a useful one where supervision of treatment is required and where co-operation of the patient is doubtful.

In streptococcal infection and where lymphadenitis or constitutional disturbance occur systemic antibiotics should also be given. Swabs should be taken for culture prior to administration. Erythromycin is the drug of choice in staphylococcal impetigo and penicillin in a streptococcal infection. It is important to realise that impetigo is often secondary to other conditions and these will require treatment if control is to be obtained. Pediculosis capitis often presents as impetigo at the nape of the neck or the hair. Scabies can present as a generalised impetigo, particularly in children. More rarely it can occur with eczema and or with seborrhoeic dermatitis.

Furunculosis (Boils)

Aetiology

In furunculosis staphylococci or streptococci infect the hair follicle and abcess formation occurs with necrosis. Eventually there is a discharge of pus and a central necrotic plug.

Furunculosis is common and single furuncles are frequently treated at home without reference to the doctor. The incidence is higher than generally recognised. Occasionally they become recurrent or infect whole families, and it is in this form that they are brought to the attention of the family practitioner. Although not common in early childhood the incidence increases after puberty. In children impetigo is a more common skin infection than furunculosis. They are common in allergic patients and children who are atopic.

Furunculosis is also associated with seborrhoea and diabetes. The urine should always be tested for sugar in cases of recurrent furunculosis.

Trauma is a factor in the production of furunculosis and points of friction are sites for furuncles. The most common site is the nape of the neck, followed by the forearm and the buttocks. Boils are most frequent in winter.

Clinical Features

The lesion presents as an erythematous papule surrounding a follicle. There is often an outer zone of erythema. The lesion may itch initially but this rapidly changes to pain. The lesion rapidly extends over 2 to 3 days to form a painful swelling 1–2 cm in diameter. Pustules occur at the centre of the swelling and gradually extend and soften. Eventually the furuncle bursts and discharges pus. The central necrotic plug is present and is eventually discharged. Healing follows, leaving a pale violet mark and eventually a permanent white scar. The lesions are painful until the pus has been released. In the nose and external auditory canal, pain may be severe. They usually occur singly, there may however, be occasions when they are multiple and in certain people they may be recurrent and they may occur in an epidemic form in hospitals or families. Furunculosis of the external auditory meatus is discussed in Chapter 10, page 126.

Diagnosis

Diagnosis is not difficult. In the early stages they may be confused with superficial folliculitis but in the latter the lesion is only 1 or 2 mm in size and it is usually present in its tens or hundreds rather than ones or twos. Boils in the axillae must be differentiated from hidradenitis. In the latter the presence of nodules, sinuses, its chronicity and absence of acute pain and tenderness helps to separate the two.

Treatment

Local Treatment of Non-recurrent Boils   The aim is the alleviation of pain, the release of pus and the reduction of the spread of infection. The first two can be controlled by the application of kaolin poultices. Saline soaks can be applied to the nasal passages. As soon as the lesion discharges pus, change the application to Pasta magnesium sulphate B.P. Smaller lesions can be treated merely by the application of an antibiotic ointment on and around the boil. Neomycin or aureomycin ointments are probably the most effective. Antibiotic ointments help to prevent the spread of infection. Fucidin is claimed to have a direct action on the boil itself.

General Treatment   Elimination of any underlying factors which affect or pre-dispose to boils is important. Systemic therapy is rarely required and there is little evidence except in the case of Lincomycin to suggest that it reduces the life history of the boils unless given early in the condition. Antibiotics should be given if there is lymphadenitis and if the boil is present on the upper lip of the face. If antibiotics are given, bacteriological swabs should be taken preferably from pus. Swabs if taken over the boil tend to be frequently negative and even if positive one cannot be certain that it is not one of the staphylococci normally found in 20 per cent of individuals and of a different strain. Reduction in the source of infection can be helped by the use of chlorhexidine cream B.P.C. applied to the nasal and peri-anal areas.

Recurrent Boils   These present a more difficult problem in their treatment and management. After treating the individual lesion as outlined for single boils, efforts must be made to reduce and change the reservoir of infection. The reservoir may be in the individual himself, the family or the community. Predisposing medical conditions should be eliminated. Swabs should be taken from the peri-anal and nasal areas of patient and contacts and chlorhexidine cream B.P.C. antibiotics applied to these areas. Patients presenting with boils after discharge from hospital may harbour more virulent strains and antibiotic resistant organisms.

Prior to the use of medications a bath should be taken using an antibacterial soap, followed by a body rub with surgical spirit; nose picking is prohibited and paper tissues used; long cotton underwear should be worn and changed daily.

Some resistant cases have responded to inoculation with nonpathogenic strains[10].

Erysipelas and Cellulitis

Nature and Conditions

Although erysipelas is often described at length and cellulitis only briefly mentioned, in family practice erysipelas is rare and cellulitis is not uncommon. Both are streptococcal infections of the skin and sub-cutaneous tissue; rarely other bacteria may be the cause. The distinction between the two is not always clear and they may alternate with each other. In cellulitis the subcutaneous tissue is infected, in erysipelas the more superficial tissues.

Clinical Features

Both present as extending erythematous areas with the following features:

Erysipelas	*Cellulitis*
Prodromal symptoms	
Severe Toxic changes	Mild toxic changes
Palpable well defined edge	Diffuse edge
Solid oedema, blisters and vesicles	Soft pitting oedema
Lymphangitis and lymphadenopathy	Lymphangitis

Both usually follow breaches of the epidermis, from fissures or ulcers. In erysipelas permanent lymphatic damage, chronic lymphoedema and recurrence are not uncommon. Erysipelas occurs mainly on the face and legs. Cellulitis is a common complication of leg ulcers.

Differential diagnosis

Angioneurotic oedema occurs suddenly and pain is absent. Superficial phlebitis is easily palpated. Contact dermatitis can be severe and bullous, but the history is usually obvious.

Treatment

Treatment is by injection of penicillin in full dosage for 7 days, together with gentian violet (0.5 per cent aqueous) or chlorhexidine cream B.P.C. applied topically to any fissures.

VIRAL INFECTIONS

Warts

Nature and Condition

Warts are produced by infection of epidermal cells by a virus. The infection is transmitted by contact. Moisture and trauma play a part in increasing the susceptibility to infection. The use of swimming baths and gymnasiums has been associated with peaks in incidence.

The incidence of warts in the population is between 7 and 10 per cent but in institutions may rise as high as 25 per cent. Two-thirds will involute within two years. The highest incidence is found between the ages of 11 and 20. It is uncommon under the age of 8 and not common in adulthood. The number of warts in an individual is not only related to the incidence of infection outside the host but also the incidence of infection on the host and new warts will occur three times as frequently in the infected.

New warts can appear as old ones disappear. Manning and Epstein[11] showed a linear regression rate. This is against the probability of antibodies being the main factor in healing and suggests the possibility of an abiotic change in the virus. It is probable however that both antibody production and abiotic changes play a part in elimination of the virus.

Pathological Changes

These mainly consist of hyperplasia of the epidermal layers. There is marked hyperkeratinisation and in some areas parakeratosis. Below the granular layers are vacuolated cells.

Clinical Features

Warts present in several forms:

Common Warts   These usually affect the hands and they measure up to 1 cm in diameter although many larger ones may occur. They are short circumscribed papillary growths which are flesh coloured at first but may become discoloured brown or black with dirt and age.

Plane Warts   These are usually smaller in size and are only slightly elevated. They are common on the face, neck and arms; large numbers may be present.

Filiform and Digitate Warts   Here the height is greater than the breadth, the thread-like lesions presenting either singly or in groups. The papilloma may or may not be separated at the base. They are rarely more than 0.5 cm long and occur most frequently on the face and neck.

Plantar Warts   These occur on the soles of the feet. Due to pressure they do not present clinically as a papilloma but as a circumscribed area on the skin with a clearly defined edge of keratin. The colour is that of the skin. Gentle lateral pressure with a scalpel shows that the central roughened area is formed by multiple papillae which can be separated. Capillaries can be seen coursing between the papillae, and are seen as pin-points of pigment. They are painful.

Plantar warts may be multiple and form mosaic warts which present as a plaque. Some may be soft and others keratinous and hard, simulating corns. However, paring off the keratinous layer displays the typical wart beneath.

Condyloma Acuminata (Acuminate Warts)   These occur mainly around the genital areas but they can also occur in other moist areas. They present as a soft moist, pink, papillomatous lesion, several of which may group together to form cauliflower like masses. They may be from a few millimetres to several centimetres in diameter. They are usually multiple and are often sexually transmitted. Antigenically they differ from common warts.

Diagnosis

Diagnosis is not difficult. The tendency of the warts to be multiple and occur in the young distinguish them from a verrucous squamous cell carcinoma, which usually have an undurated base. Peri-ungual warts can be differentiated from peri-ungual fibromata of adenoma sebaceum by the fact that they arise from the nail folds rather than from the sides of the nails. Fibromata are usually smaller. Plane warts have to be distinguished from lichen planus. Plane warts unlike lichen planus do not itch and Wickhams striae can usually be distinguished in lichen planus. Acuminate warts have to be differentiated from secondary syphilitic condylomata. Routine seriological tests for syphillis and gonorrhoea are advisable.

Assessment and Management

Although the incidence of warts is high in the community (7–10 per cent), the number attending family practice is not as high. Many family practitioners find that very often the population accept warts as a part of normal infection that

children go through. Patients attend more frequently with verrucae because of
the pain involved or with filiform and digital warts because of the deformity.
Occasionally small epidemics of infection occur when new schools or bathing
pools open. The question of transmission from bare-foot gymnastics is still
debatable.

Treatment
Treatments for warts are legion and the fact that spontaneous cure can occur
makes the evaluation of treatment difficult. Barr[12] in a survey of banal warts of
the hand analysing 16 different popular methods of treatment found that in
most cases cure rates only averaged 59.8 per cent which is less than if left alone.
He comments that, 'there is no doubt normal life span of the wart is the friend
of both the patient and of the therapist'. It has been said that the best way of
managing warts is to let them manage themselves.

The treatment of common warts should therefore be conservative, and this is
especially so in children where painful procedures may be psychologically
harmful. Too vigorous treatment can also result in scarring. Treatment should be
aimed at reducing the reservoir of infection and this can be achieved by treating
whole members of the family and by regular inspection at schools followed by
the holding treatments.

I have found the following methods useful:

1. Cover with waterproof adhesive strapping and reapply daily. This softens the
wart and helps to reduce the spread of infection to other parts of the hand.
2. Accurate application of moistened silver nitrate stick; this is an effective
anti-keratolytic. Black pigmentation from the deposited silver occurs.
3. 40 per cent acid salicylic plaster which is cut accurately to fit the wart, is
then covered with adhesive strapping and re-applied after 5–7 days interval.
4. Salicylic acid collodion B.P.C. is applied accurately to the wart twice daily.
Plane Warts   These rarely cause anxiety on the patient's body but can occur on
the face where they may be cosmetically unacceptable. They can be treated by
the application of 3 per cent salicylic acid in aqueous cream applied twice daily.
Plantar Warts   Because of their common association with pain and discomfort
to the feet they require effective treatment. Fortunately since Vickers paper in
1961[13] we have a method which gives a high rate of cure and with his method
he achieves a cure rate of 93 per cent. A very important factor in the treatment
is that the procedure is painless.

Dead tissue and scales must first be removed with a nail file or the side of a
blade of a pair of scissors each evening. Then soak the wart-bearing portions of
the sole of the foot for 15–20 minutes in 3 per cent formaldehyde solution. The
strength of this formalin should be increased by 2 per cent each fortnight (up to
9 per cent) until the skin around the wart is dry and cracked. The application of

petroleum jelly to soften the areas of the skin nearby and the surrounding area of normal skin, prevents fissuring and cracking of normal skin during the treatment. Two or three points are of importance in this form of treatment. Firstly, after several days of treatment, a hard keratin layer will form over the wart unless paring is effective. I find in my own experience that paring is best done with a small hand emery board. Providing pressure is applied laterally and not vertically, little discomfiture is experienced. Secondly, application of the lotion is by pouring the solution into a saucer or flat dish then placing the foot upon it. It is important, however, that the wart itself should not be pressed against the dish beneath, and free access of the solution allowed. Occasionally plantar warts become inflamed with secondary infection and Castellani's paint applied locally and a course of antibiotics is indicated.

Occasionally, requests are made for immediate treatment of warts, such requests should be resisted except in a few rare cases in adults where for social reasons or persistant pain the request may be justified. Curettage will give between 60 and 80 per cent cure rate but the patient should be warned of the possibility of scarring occurring afterwards. Liquid nitrogen, almost equally effective, is unfortunately, not readily available in family practice. However, CO_2 snow will give an almost similar cure rate.

Curettage The area of the skin is sterilized and an injection of local anaesthetic made beneath and around the wart, the skin is then snipped with scissors just external to the outer margin of the wart. If this is not done when curettage occurs there is a tendency to tear pieces of normal epidermis away. A spoon curette about the size of the wart is used, and the whole of the wart scooped out. Attention should be particularly paid to the base of the wart to remove as much of the wart as possible, the small bits that are left can be cauterized by the application of a little liquor phenol applied on an orange-stick. A deep crater is left which should be trimmed flat with scissors. It is also important to remind the patient that this is not an obsolute cure. No wart treatment is.

Carbon Dioxide Snow CO_2 snow can be purchased in small cylinders together with an expansion chamber. CO_2 is rapidly released and the evaporation of the liquid produces cooling and the production of a solidifed CO_2 which is collected in the expansion chamber and then pressed with the small tool supplied. The resultant CO_2 is then pressed with the small pencil-shape and applied firmly over the wart. The pencil should cover the whole of the wart and contact be maintained until a slight ring of frosting appears around the wart. This usually takes approximately 15 seconds, after several days a blister forms which separates within about 7 days. It should be noted that the above procedures are not without some degree of discomfort either through injection of local anaesthetic or due to the freezing process. Their use in children, therefore, is not advised.

Condyloma Acuminata   The treatment unlike that of other warts, is much more specific and podophyllin is effective in the following preparations and method. Podophyllin however, is an antimitotic drug and treatment should therefore be carried out by the doctor or nurse, as severe inflammation and ulceration can occur. Wipe the parts clean, paint the surrounding skin with petroleum jelly to protect it and then paint with 30 per cent podphyllin in acetone using a cotton wool tipped applicator.

Allow to dry and then powder with talcum powder. Leave for six hours and then wash with soap and water. Repeat in 7 days if necessary. For several hours or days the area becomes inflamed and painful in some cases. The pain can be controlled by the application of 5 per cent lignocaine ointment.

Herpes Zoster

Aetiology
The condition is an infection of the skin and nervous tissues by the virus *Herpes varicellae* in a patient who has previously had chicken pox. Chicken pox is considered to be the primary infection and herpes zoster a reactivation of a latent infection along a particular nerve distribution.

Pathological Changes
The epidermis is infiltrated with polymorphonuclear leucocytes, giant cells may be found and there are balloon cells containing intranuclear inclusions. Intracellular oedema occurs and produces vesicles. Inflammatory changes also take place in the basal ganglia and posterior nerve roots; more rarely there may be an extension to the anterior horn and the other parts of the brain. Necrosis and scarring may occur in nervous tissue.

Clinical Features
Ninety per cent of cases occur in those over the age of 45. There is often a preceding history of trauma. Pain is often the presenting symptom and occurs in about 60 per cent. Hyperaesthesia, occasionally paraesthesia, slight malaise and fever may also occur two or three days before the eruption of an erythematous papular rash which usually follows the line of a dermatome. Within 12–24 hours the papules become vesicles approximately 2–4 mm in diameter with a surrounding inflammatory zone, which becomes purulent and eventually forms a crust. The crust separates after about 2–3 weeks and leaves a depigmented scar. Characteristically the vesicles develop at different times.

Occasionally herpes zoster is severe and the vesicles may become bullous and haemorrhagic. Constitutional symptoms with fever may occur and the older the person the greater the likelihood of the condition being severe. Encephalitis is a rare complication. The condition is usually unilateral and not recurrent. A generalized form may occur in patients who are debilitated or who have been on steroids for prolonged periods or where the autoimmune process has been diminished.

In 10 per cent pain can be severe and may be prolonged for months or years (post herpetic neuralgia) especially in the elderly.

The trunk is the site most frequently affected but involvement of the ophthalmic branch of the trigeminal (fifth) cranial nerves is not uncommon occurring in 10–15 per cent. If the nasal branch is involved there is also involvement of the eye. Conjunctivitis, corneal ulceration, ocular and facial palsies may also occur. If the geniculate nerve is affected lesions appear on the pinna and external auditory canal and there may be associated deafness and vertigo; it is of importance as it is a cause of facial palsy (see Chapter 10, pages 125 and 126).

Differential Diagnosis

This is not difficult when vesicles develop. Herpes simplex is the most likely lesion to be confused with it. Herpes zoster is usually much more extensive and the dermatome pattern usually followed. As in herpes simplex a smear taken from the base of the vesicle shows the presence of giant cells and helps to separate it from other causes of vesicles.

Early recognition of onset is particularly important where there is involvement of the ophthalmic division of the trigeminal nerve. Here corneal involvement is heralded by herpetic vesicles on the affected side of the nose and when this is observed a specialist should be consulted as the use of corticosteroids is of major importance in preventing serious eye complications.

Treatment

Treatment during the pre-eruptive phase should be confined to simple analgesics. For many years treatment of the eruptive phase has merely involved the administration of analgesics and the application of calamine lotion to the lesions, but more recently antiviral agents have been introduced. Liberal dusting of the lesions with talcum powder is helpful, though the grounds for its use are equivocal.

Antiviral Chemotherapy   Idoxuridine inhibits DNA formation by competing for thymidine. Providing it can reach virus infected cells and is used in the *early* eruptive phase, it is an effective antiviral agent. Idoxuridine has been used in clinical trials as a 40 per cent solution in dimethyl sulphoxide with encouraging results. It is available commercially as a 5 per cent solution which the manufacturers recommend should be used as a paint applied four times a day, but good results have been reported when it is used as a wet dressing changed frequently. Application of the lotion should not be for more than four days since further use results in whealing maceration and ulceration of the skin. The solution stings on application and a garlic like taste may occur. It should not be used in pregnant women as its teratogenic effect is not known.

Analgesics   Pain may be severe and prolonged and a suitable and adequate analgesic must be given at frequent intervals, those analgesics that are addictive should be strictly excluded. If pain is severe and persists for longer than three months a local anaesthetic block of the affected nerve may be tried. If this proves successful permanent destruction of the nerve, by alcohol injection or surgical division should be considered.

Herpes Simplex

Nature and Condition
The condition is an infection of the skin and nervous tissue by *Herpes hominis*. It is one of the commonest infections but it's symptoms are generally so trivial that the doctor is rarely consulted unless the condition becomes recurrent.

Pathology
The early lesion shows as a thin walled vesicle deeply situated in the epidermis with spongiosis and ballooning. There is an infiltration by polymorphonuclear leucocytes and the presence of multinuclear giant cells.

Clinical Features
The characteristic lesion is of a group of small vesicles. Each vesicle is approximately 1—2 mm in diameter and the group measures approximately 3—4 cm in diameter. The vesicle has a slightly erythematous base, and is filled with clear fluid which become purulent after several days. Vesicles may coalesce to form bullae and eventually become ulcerated. The lesions rapidly heal and the total life of a lesion is approximately seven days. Mild burning and itching are the main complaints. The main sites of occurrence are on the lip, mouth and after this the nasal area.

The primary infection usually arises on the buccal mucosa and the secondary on the lips. Primary infections usually have constitutional changes with fever, lymphadenopathy and leucocytosis; the reaction can be particularly severe in young adults. The recurrent infection is marked by the absence of constitutional symptoms and by the smaller size and closer grouping of the lesions. According to the site there may be slight differences in its presenting features as follows:

Herpetic Gingivo Stomatis   This occurs mainly in young children. The vesicle presents as a white plaque and then as an ulcer with a yellow base, there is enlargement and tenderness of the regional glands. In children there is salivation and dribbling of saliva from the mouth.

Herpetic Vulvo-vaginitis   The lesions of the mucous membrane are as described above, but ulceration frequently occurs with adhesion of the neighbouring surfaces, considerable oedema of the prepuce and labia may occur.

Herpetic Kerato-Conjunctivitis   Oedema, dendritic ulcers and punctate and marginal keratitis may occur. The pre-auricular node is enlarged.

Inoculation Herpes Simplex (Herpetic Whitlow)   This occurs when the virus is implanted deep into the skin, usually on the finger. Vesicles are deep and have a honeycombed appearance; the condition usually occurs in doctors and nurses.

Generalised Herpes Simplex   This occurs in the very young and in the undernourished. Lesions are larger and umbilicated; rarely the primary lesion presents as an influenza- or infectious monoclueosis-like infection.

Differential Diagnosis

Herpes simplex is differentiated from herpes zoster by the lack of pain and the localised form of lesions. Vesicular eczema is differentiated by the itching and the absence of cropping. Diagnosis can be confirmed by the examination for giant cells of the base of the blister as described in herpes zoster. Samples can be taken for viral culture. In the genital area napkin rash is separated by its wide-spread nature and the absence of small vesicles. Steven-Johnson's syndrome has to be separated from herpes simplex of the lips which may occur with cold or pneumonia. In the Steven-Johnson's syndrome the patient is usually much more ill and skin lesions of erythema multiforme are often present. It is well to remember however that erythema multiforme may follow herpes simplex infection.

Treatment

Idoxuridine is used against herpes simplex in lower concentrations than those required for herpes zoster. Concentrations of between 0.1 and 5 per cent have been found to be effective.

Wet dressings of aluminium acetate lotion at the moist stage and surgical spirit dabbed on when the lesions are drying are helpful.

Antibiotics may be necessary if secondary infection occurs or there is lymphadenitis.

Infection in neonates has a high mortality especially in premature children. Wheeler and Huffner advise the administration of gammaglobulin to the mother and caesarean section[14]. The child should be given gammaglobulin for ten days.

Molluscum Contagiosum

Aetiology

Molluscum contagiosum is an infection by a virus of the pox group; it occurs only in human skin. Unlike the herpes viruses, it reduplicates itself within the cytoplasm and not the nucleus. It is spread by contact and by fomites; outbreaks have occurred in association with swimming pools. In England it usually occurs between the ages of 10 and 15 years. Little is known about its occurrence in the community and there is room for investigation.

Clinical Features

After an incubation of 14–50 days a small papule occurs, which becomes a waxy white in colour, there is a central depression from which gelatinous material can be extracted. The lesions reach 5–7 mm after several weeks and persist for several months or, in a few cases, 2 or 3 years. The face, arms and genital regions are the areas of prediliction. Itching may occur.

Pathology

Cellular growth produces pear shaped bodies in the epidermis. The papules are compressed to form fibrous strands between the bodies, at the centre of the lesions cells are destroyed to leave molluscum bodies which are collections of eosinophilic inclusion bodies.

Differential Diagnosis

Diagnosis is easy if multiple lesions occur. Doubtful ones are confirmed by extrusion of molluscum bodies and examination under the microscope.

Treatment

Castellani's paint is applied as a holding treatment in children. In older children extrusion of the molluscum bodies is carried out by gentle pressure after perforating with an hypodermic needle or carbolic acid is applied to the contents of the lesion on a pointed orange stick.

FUNGAL INFECTIONS

These present a problem and a challenge to the family practitioner, little is known about their true incidence in the population, as most of the figures have been obtained from hospital clinics. There are therefore excellent opportunities here for research in family practice. Only recently has it been shown that *Trichophyton rubrum* is not the most common ringworm infection of feet and nails, instead it is *Trichophyton interdigitale*. The error has arisen because *T. rubrum* is more likely to be referred to hospital clinics.

The incidence and type of fungus infections vary widely with the geographical area.

Identification, if not obvious, may need microscopical examination and culture for confirmation; often the laboratory will obtain the specimen for you.

If this is not so, or the practitioner wishes to examine them himself, then it is important to observe the following points when collecting samples. Scrapings from the skin should be taken from the active edge of the lesion or base of the nail and smeared on a slide. On the scalp or beard, dead, lustreless broken hairs should be chosen. A drop of 10 per cent potassium hydroxide solution is added to the smear and the slide is warmed gently for 10 minutes. The specimen is then examined for spores and mycelia. If too bright a light is used with the microscope and the condensor is not adjusted the details of semitranslucent fungi will not be seen.

The culture and microscopical examination for fungi is not always easy and a negative result does not always mean that fungus is not present. Culture takes about 4 weeks.

Candidiasis (Thrush, Monilia)

Candidiasis is due to infections by a yeast, usually *Candida albicans*. It is present in the gut and mouth as a saphrophyte. Infections occur internally only when there is systemic disease or debility, or use of antibiotics. It occurs on the skin where there is excess of moisture, warmth, maceraction or diabetes.

Clinical Features
Oral   In the mouth there are soft, white curd like lesions which on removal leave a raw area (unlike milk curds). It is common in infants.
Perleche   Chronic fissuring with whitened edges occurs at the angles of the lips, often due to poor fitting dentures, a high proportion are infected by candida, a few have a vitamin B deficiency.
Intertrigo   Pink, polycylic areas with white overlapping edges, affect areas beneath the breast and in the axilla, umbilicus or perianal areas. It must be differentiated from seborrhoeic dermatitis and psoriasis in these areas by its appearance and culture.
Erosio Interdigitalis   This is a not uncommon infection of the web and interdigital spaces; usually the fourth space is affected. It presents as a red itching area with macerated white skin.
Chronic Paronychia   The nail fold becomes inflamed and separated from the nail to form a deep pocket, from which pus may be extruded. The nail becomes discoloured brown and ridged. It is differentiated from bacterial infection by culture.

Differential Diagnosis
Candidiasis must be differentiated from other fungal infections, intertrigo, contact dermatitis and, on the mucosa, lichen planus and leukoplakia. In culture *Candida albicans* will grow on both dermatophyte test medium and Sabouraud's agar and will not respond to griseofulvin.

Treatment
Excess heat and perspiration must be prevented and skin folds should be separated, by means of a good brassiere or avoidance of tight corsets. Gentian violet 0.5 per cent aqueous paint is extremely effective in all cases, but due to staining Nystatin ointment may be preferred. Both should be applied three times daily. Chronic paronychia is treated by packing the open nail fold with nystatin ointment and then sealing with nail varnish to prevent moisture entering. The varnish is removed by a cleaner next day and the process repeated, until the cuticle entirely regrows.

In recurrent or extensive candidiasis it is important to exclude underlaying systemic disorders, especially diabetes.

Treatment of Griseofulvin-sensitive Dermatophytes

Before a description is given of the various manifestations of griseofulvin-sensitive infections those general principles of management common to them all will be described.

Topical Treatment
Topical treatment should be given in all cases even when griseofulvin is given.

Solution potassium permermanganate BNF, one part diluted in seven parts of water to make a 1/8000 solution, is useful in infected, weeping lesions when stronger preparations are not tolerated.

Benzoic acid compound ointment (Whitfield's ointment) is a very effective fungicidal, it can be used as either quarter- or half-strength ointment where the lesions are inflamed.

Magenta paint is useful in moist areas such as the groins and interdigital spaces.

There is also a wide range of proprietary preparations containing a variety of antifungal agents, although cosmetically more acceptable they have no great pharmacological advantage over the simpler preparations.

Systemic Treatment
Griseofulvin has revolutionised the treatment of fungus infections especially in tinea capitis where complete depilation was often necessary to effect a cure. It should be administered preferably in the fine particle (F.P.) form which is equivalent to half the dose of normal griseofulvin tablet. The tablets should be taken in association with a high fat meal as this increases absorption. It is given in the following dosage:

adults — 125 mg (F.P.) i.q.i.d.
children — 125 mg (F.P.) i.b.d. or i.t.d.s.

Acute inflammatory reactions will heal themselves and unless treated with griseofulvin in the first few days systemic treatment is not required. Toxic effects of griseofulvin are usually mild but headaches, skin rashes, gastro intestinal disturbances, angioneurotic oedema, exfoliative dermatitis, leucopenia and porphyria may rarely occur. Griseofulvin should not be given in porphyria.

Variations in dosage of griseofulvin may be required and these will be indicated under the descriptions of specific fungal infections given below.

Tinea Pedis

Aetiology

This fungal infection of the skin of the feet or toes is due to either *Trichophyton mentagrophytes*, *T. rubrum*, or *Epidermophyton floccosum*. The first two produce most of the infections and those produced by *E. floccosum* are much rarer. Infection is more prevalent in closed communities where there are communal swimming and washing facilities, consequently there is a very high incidence in mining communities. Although considered a trivial condition by many, it must be remembered that there is often infection of the nails a condition which is disfiguring and very difficult to treat.

Clinical Findings

The infection presents as a scaling or macerated area of skin, usually between the toes and only later spreading onto the rest of the feet. In the macerated phase the skin becomes white; rarely the condition may become inflammatory, vesicular and pustular. *T. rubrum* may present as hyperkeratotic, dry, scaling areas. The acute inflammatory stage may be associated with an 'ide' reaction, an antigenic reaction to the fungus presenting as a vesicular rash between the fingers or as a generalized erythematous eruption.

Differential Diagnosis

Tinea pedis must be differentiated from simple maceration of hyperhidrosis by culture. In hyperhidrosis there is bilateral lividity. Pustular psoriasis is difficult but in fungus infections the 'glazed look' is absent and psoriasis is usually bilateral. Contact eczema usually occurs on the dorsum of the foot.

Management

Prevention is better than cure. Three basic practices are recommended:

1. don't walk barefoot;
2. don't exchange footwear;
3. don't use communal bathrooms.

Stockings can be sterilized by boiling and it is probably best to change for new after the commencement of treatment. Shoes can be sterilized by 12% lotion formaldehyde. Zinc undecenoate dusting powder, B.P.C. can be applied after possible exposure (e.g., baths). It is important to check families.

Tinea Unguium (Onychomycosis)

This infection of the nail plate is usually by the same three fungi that are involved in tinea pedis. *T. rubrum* is the worst offender. The infection occurs at the side of the nail plate and the fungus may be dead by the time it reaches the end of the nail.

Clinical Findings
Initially the nail becomes discoloured becoming white or yellow and occasionally becomes brown. Thickening of the nail plate occurs and the nail becomes lifted up by a heap of keratin. The nail frequently splits longitudinally and may disintegrate into a friable yellow mass.

Differential Diagnosis
Psoriasis of the nail is the condition most likely to produce confusion, fortunately signs of pitting and psoriasis are found elsewhere. Nail dystrophies associated with eczema and lichen planus occur, but there is repeated absence of fungus on culture.
     Culture of fungus from nails is often negative but there is often a tinea pedis associated and this is more likely to give positive findings.

Management
There is a very high association of tinea pedis, onychomycosis and fungus infections elsewhere; these should all be treated as well as the nail infection. Long term treatment with griseofulvin is required but results are poor even following therapy for as long as 6 months for the hands and 12 months for the feet. Better results can be obtained by administering griseofulvin and then removing the nail. Before advising surgery I usually observe the response to griseofulvin for 3 months.

Tinea Capitis

This is produced when the hairy parts of the head (excluding the beard) are infected by fungus. Different fungi predominate from country to country. Transference of infection is by direct or indirect contact. In England *Microsporum canis* and *M. audouinii* are the most common causes. *M. audouinii* produces small epidemics whilst *M. canis* produces only a few cases at a time.

Trichophyton schoenleinii (favus) has been reported as a common cause in Northern Ireland.

Tinea capitis is a disease of the growing hair and mainly occurs in children usually between the ages of 6 and 10 years, but occasionally earlier. It usually cures itself spontaneously at puberty. It has been shown to occur in a carrier form.

Pathological Features

Three main forms of infection may occur:

1. *Ectothrix*   Hyphae are present both inside and outside the hair shaft. On the outside arthrospores form a mosaic pattern.
2. *Endothrix*   Hyphae and arthrospores are present only on the inside. The spores are large.
3. *Favus type of invasion*   The inside only is affected, air spaces are present and arthrospores are rare.

Clinical Features

These vary with the species of fungus involved. Ectothrix infections of *M. audouinii* produce a lustreless, balding, grey scaling patch of the scalp containing many hairs which are broken about 3 mm from the skin surface.

Occasionally the lesion itches. Rarely it is very inflammatory with boggy oedema and pustules; the lesion is then known as a 'kerion'. In endothrix infections the hairs are broken off at the level of the skin and the lesion presents as a balding patch with or without black dots. Inflammation may occur in some forms of infection, varying from mild to its severest form when it presents as a kerion. In *T. schoenleinii* there may be yellow cup shaped lesions (scutulum).

Differential Diagnosis

The characteristic broken hairs help to distinguish it from alopecia areata which has exclamation mark hairs. In trichotillomania the hairs are broken at different levels. In seborrhoeic eczema the hairs are not broken and scaling is very obvious. A carbuncle may be confused with a kerion but symptoms are marked.

Diagnosis can be confirmed in *M. audouinii* and *T. canis* by Woods light when the affected hairs fluoresce. Not all fungi fluoresce and in these cases microscopy and culture of affected hair is required. Where large numbers are involved the use of hair brushes or plastic scalp massagers are useful to collect samples.

Management

Griseofulvin should be given in normal dosage for six weeks. Where it is beneficial to supervise treatment closely the following regimes may be followed with success:

1. griseofulvin (F.P.) 25 mg/Kg bodyweight as a single dose given once weekly for four weeks.
2. griseofulvin (F.P.) 2.0 g as a single dose in adults.

Tinea capitis is infectious and it is essential to eliminate contacts by screening using the methods listed above. After treatment with griseofulvin the affected hairs become very brittle, easily breaking off and spreading infection. The affected hair should either be clipped short or a cap worn and the scalp should be washed frequently.

Tinea Cruris (Dhobie Itch)

This is a dermatophyte infection of the skin of the groins. The infection is usually transmitted from the foot and *Epidermophyton floccosum* is the most common cause of infection. The infection can also be spread by fomites. It is uncommon in women.

Clinical Features
The lesion presents as a brown erythematous patch with a well marked edge and slight scaling. It affects the groin and particularly the thighs. Classically it is supposed to spare the penis and scrotum; detailed examination however usually reveals minute involvement. Fading in the centre of the lesion may not be as obvious as in tinea corporis (see below).

Differential Diagnosis
Seborrhoeic eczema and psoriasis usually have signs elsewhere and seborrhoeic eczema usually has outlying papules. Erythrasma is not quite as active as tinea cruris and there is only mild scaling.

Management
The feet should always be checked and treated if necessary. Griseofulvin should be administered in normal dosage.

Tinea Corporis

This is ringworm of the glabrous skin, affecting the limbs, trunk and face. *Trichophyton verrucosum, T. mentagrophytes, T. rubrum* and *Microsporum canis* are the usual causes, *T. verrucosum* and *M. Canis* being the most common. Cattle are the main source of infection of *T. verrucosum* although small mammals may play a part. The highest incidence occurs in January, February and March when cattle are indoors and there is also a rise in June when the byres are cleared out. Transfer of infection is by direct contact or by fomites. Smaller mammals such as hedgehogs (*Trichophyton, Erisacei*) and Voles (*Microsporum persicolar*) may all pass on infection. The degree of virulence of the fungus determines the epidermal reactions. *T. rubrum* produces a mild chronic scaling reaction. *T. canis* may produce an inflammatory one.

Clinical Features

Here the characteristic finding is of a circinate macular, scaling lesion with an active edge which is slightly raised. The lesion tends to fade in the centre. It may be either slow or rapid in its spread. When the spread is rapid extensive areas may be involved, these lesions are more erythematous and close examination of the edge with a lens reveals micro pustules. In the slow form the colour is often more brown with less tendency to fade in the centre.

Differential Diagnosis

In its less acute forms it has to be separated from nummular eczema, psoriasis, seborrhoeic eczema and pityriasis rosea. At times differentiation is difficult and *all* scaling lesions of which there is any doubt should have scrapings taken for examination.

Management

It is important to find the source of infection if possible and eliminate it. The patient should be completely examined to see if there is fungus elsewhere on the body.

Tinea Barbae

Ringworm of the beard is not very common and is usually due to infections by *T. verrucosum* and *T. mentagrophytes*. It is caught from animals and is invariably inflammatory.

Clinical Features

Two types are produced: inflammatory, kerion like lesions and superficial crusting, pustular lesions with broken hairs.

Differential Diagnosis

Sycosis barbae affects the upper lip and chin usually and scaling is absent. Cocci are cultured from the pustules and nares.

Management

The beard should be shaved and griseofulvin given for 6 weeks.

INFESTATIONS

Scabies

Aetiology

Scabies is an infestation by the mite *Sarcoptis scabeii var. hominis*. The female measures on an average 0.4 mm in length and 0.3 mm in breadth; the male is half the size of the female. The body is oval and contains four pairs of legs. The female burrows in the stratum corneum producing a tunnel or burrow. Along the length of the tunnel she deposits faeces and eggs which gives the burrow a brownish pigmentation in parts. The burrow is about 1 mm in diameter and is made by the females. The burrow measures several millimetres in length and is slightly serpiginous.

The incidence of scabies varies greatly, either presenting as sporadic minor outbreaks or as severe epidemics. Closed communities, proximity and insufficient public health inspection play a part, but other unknown factors are also involved. Despite public health and medical care the incidence of scabies has been rising in recent years.

Clinical Features

The Burrow   This is pathognominic of scabies and occurs on certain selected sites which vary slightly according to age. On initial infestation burrows may occur generally, but after sensitisation has occurred the burrows are confined to selected sites. In adults these are the flexures of the wrist, the under borders of the hands and the interdigital spaces dorsally. The next common site is the extensor surface of the elbows together with the feet and penis. Mites may also live in the nipples and natal clefts. In children the lesions may also occur on the soles of the feet and palms of the hands.

After about one month sensitization occurs and severe itching is produced. It is thought that sensitization is probably to the mite but secondary invaders such as staphylococci may also play a part. Sensitization is followed by the production of vesicles, these usually occur beneath the burrow just behind the mite but may occur elsewhere, in particular the hands and feet. In children and infants vesicles may be very prominent and on occasions may be bullous. Papules also develop followed by ezematous lesions. Secondary infection by staphylococci occurs and impetiginous lesions are frequent and may be the presenting symptoms. Unlike the burrow these lesions occur all over the body. In adults the head and face are usually spared but in some children however the head and face may be involved. The eczematous and secondary infection may be severe with oedema, lymphadenitis and constitutional changes. On the penis very often erythematous nodules may occur.

Itching   Severe itching is characteristic of scabies and occurs after sensitisation. The itching is usually worse at night. In a small proportion of patients itching may not be complained of although excoriation may be present and in a few cases there is no itching and an absence of excoriation as well. Many cases have been previously treated with steroids and as a result signs and symptoms may be masked.

Diagnosis

Diagnosis is made conclusively by identification of the burrow and isolation of the mite. This is best done by the insertion of a hypodermic needle to open up the burrow and then to tease out the mite. The mite usually adheres to the point of the needle. It is just visible to the naked eye as a dark speck.

Treatment and Management

Most people are incredulous on being told that they have scabies and I find it invaluable to show the patient the mite if possible. In my experience insect phobia has not occurred from this procedure. This also helps in explaining to the patient that they have caught it from someone, as the mite can only be caught by close contact or occasionally from the use of bed sheets which have recently been vacated; some tact may be required in identifying the source of the infestation. Failure to do this explains many failures in treatment, as treatment does not prevent reinfestation from the previous source. Laundering of clothing and bed sheets is sufficient to remove the mite.

Secondary infection is common and may be severe. Impetiginous forms should be treated as outlined on page 420 but lymphadenopathy is common and systemic antibiotics are often required. It is important however to treat the scabies first, or control of the infestation will not be achieved.

Benzyl Benzoate   This has been the classic treatment of scabies. It is applied as an emulsion in a concentration of 25 per cent. Approximately 60 ml are required for each application. A warm bath should be taken before the emulsion is applied and the body scrubbed with a nail brush, especially over the areas where burrows are present. The patient then dries himself, paints on the emulsion, completely covering the body but excluding the face and scalp. The lotion should be allowed to dry and this takes approximately 30 minutes. Fresh change of clothing is given and the worn articles of clothing are sent to be laundered. The family should all be treated at the same time and disinfestation of clothing and bed clothes also performed at the same time. The procedure should be repeated in 48 hours and a bath can be taken 24 hours after treatment. The itching will not stop immediately but usually occurs within 7 days later, although on rare occasions this may be even later. Unfortunately benzyl benzoate has the disadvantage of being irritant and in many patients suffering from severe eczema and excoriation the treatment is not always pleasant and may be resisted in children.

Gamma Benzene Hexachloride In the concentration of 1 per cent this is an effective acaricide. It has the advantage of not irritating and is the treatment of choice especially in children and excoriated lesions. No previous bathing is required and it can be applied as a lotion or cream, the latter being preferable as no drying time is then required. Lower concentrations are not so effective. A single application is all that is required and this should be left 24 hours before removing or washing. A tube of 50 g is usually adequate.

Crotamiton This is effective as a 10 per cent cream or lotion; preliminary bathing is not required.

Monosulfiram This is effective as a 25 per cent solution which is diluted with two to three parts water immediately before use.

Pediculosis

Two sucking lice infest human beings, *Pediculus humanus* and *Phthirius pubis*. They have three pairs of legs which are attached to the anterior third of the body. *Pediculus humanus* measures 2—4 mm in length and has a grey-white elongated body which may become reddish after ingestion of blood. *Phthirius pubis* measures only 1—2 mm in length but is almost as broad as it is long, and has the appearance of a small crab. It is yellowish grey and difficult to detect with the naked eye. Eggs are laid on cases attached to hairs; they are whitish grey, about 1 mm long oval and are attached to the hairs completely. It should be remembered that *Pediculus humanus* can transmit typhus, trench and relapsing fever.

Clinical Features

Pediculosis Capitis Infestation of the head is not quite as common as it was but its incidence can still be as high as 17 per cent. There is therefore no room for complacency. It tends to occur in children, especially when there is long hair which is neglected. Itching is a common symptom followed by scratching, excoriation and impetiginization. Examination usually shows excoriation from the nape of the neck and between the shoulder blades. Only occasionally do people present with lice, the main complaint being one of itching or impetigo. Impetigo may occur on the scalp where it forms a septic, mattered offensive mass and enlargement of cervical lymph glands occurs frequently. Examination with hand lenses shows the characteristic egg capsules or nits and also the lice.

Pediculosis Corporis Infestation of the body is much rarer than capitis and I have only seen it a few times in a rural practise over thirteen years. It occurs where there is bodily neglect and used to be known as Vagabonds Disease when it was associated with malnutrition, lack of washing, severe infestation and was marked by pigmentation. It is transmitted in clothing or bedding and produces irritable papules, excoriation of the back is a common presenting sign. The louse is rarely found on the body but can be found together with the eggs on the seams of under garments, where it should be searched for with a lens.

Pediculosis Pubis   *Phthirius pubis* is usually sexually transmitted. It lives on the pubic hairs but may occur on other hairy areas of the body nearby. It may also occur on the eye brows and the hairs of the arm-pits. Blue grey macules 0.5 cm in diameter, known as maculae caerulae may appear on the body especially on the inner aspects of the thigh and the sides of the trunk. There is intense irritation.

Treatment

DDT   This is still the most effective remedy. It is obtainable as a 2 per cent solution of which about a table-spoonful is worked into the hair of the scalp and allowed to dry. The hair is washed after 24 hours. For pediculosis corporis 10 per cent powder should be dusted on the body twice daily for two weeks and 2 per cent powder can be dusted on the clothing. Clothing can be sterilised by boiling the under garments and pressing the outer garments with an iron. Particular attention should be paid to the seams. DDT will kill both lice and eggs. Unfortunately resistant strains are developing and its use in the future may be limited.

Gamma Benzene Hexachloride   This is effective as a 0.2 per cent solution, 10 ml of which is required for massage into the scalp and hair. It should be washed out after 24 hours. A 2 per cent shampoo is also effective and is applied to the hair and scalp for 4 minutes. It may be necessary to repeat this 2 or 3 times at intervals of 4 days. It is available as a lotion and as a shampoo.

The powder is effective in a concentration of 0.6 per cent. Gamma benzene hexachloride will only kill lice; it does not affect eggs unless it is combined with a detergent.

Malathion   This is an effective pesticide and ovicide for the scalp and is less irritating than the others. A 0.5 per cent lotion is massaged into the hair and scalp, allowed to dry and left for 12 hours. The process should be repeated 7 days later.

Unfortunately the lotion is inflammable and not suitable for use by untrained people. It has the advantage that the health visitor or doctor can treat the patient immediately. It should be kept away from the eyes. Each application requires 10 ml of the lotion.

ACNE VULGARIS

Aetiology

Acne vulgaris is defined as a chronic inflammatory disease of the pilosebaceous follicules. Although an extremely common condition a great deal still remains to be determined about the exact aetiology and to some extent treatment is therefore empirical. It may occur in the first few weeks of infancy and then does not occur until puberty when it is common. It is rare in adults, but occurs occasionally in women aged twenty to thirty five when it is often related to menstruation.

The pilo-sebaceous glands are under the control of several hormones. Androgens are the main stimulatory hormones controlling sebum production. The androgens may be of ovarian, testicular or adrenal origin. The adrenal cortex releases glucocorticoid hormones which act in a permissive capacity to the release of androgens which then stimulate the sebaceous gland. Pituitary secretions also facilitate the response of the sebaceous gland. Oestrogens and progesterone have an inhibitory effect.

Corynebacterium acnes and *Staphylococcus albus* occur as dominant colonies in acne-form lesions. A decrease in sebum flow occurs which is due to hyperkeratosis around the neck of the canal and also possible qualitative changes in sebum, in which there is an increase in squalene and wax esters. The hair is prevented from extruding itself and together with the sebum acts as a foreign body to the pilo-sebaceous apparatus producing an inflammatory reaction when the contents rupture the gland. Heredity is known to play a part and the condition is improved by sun light and aggravated by cold. In tropical areas however a severe cystic form may occur. The part of the diet is not proven although many dermatologists advise dietary restrictions. Acne is aggravated by bromides, iodides, sodium phenytoin, phenobarbitone, steroids and ixonicotinic acid. Stress has long been considered a factor but the evidence for this is equivocal. Mineral oils applied topically will produce acne form lesions.

Pathology

Hyperkeratinisation of the neck of the follicule occurs, the sebaceous gland fills with keratin and an abscess may develop in the follicule so that an inflammatory infiltrate forms nearby.

Clinical Features

Acne vulgaris occurs on the face, anterior chest, upper arms and dorsum of the chest, particularly between the shoulder blades. It does not occur normally elsewhere. It is often preceded by seborrhoea. A variety of lesions are produced.

The Comedone   This is a horny dark plug which fills a sebaceous follicule, it can be extruded on light pressure, usually they are less than a millimetre in diameter but on occasions may be larger.

Papules   These also occur at follicules and may be flesh coloured or slightly erythematous, they measure one to two millimetres in diameter.

Pustules   These occur at the site of follicules with or without the presence of comedones or papules.

Nodules   These are flesh coloured and may measure up to one to two centimetres, they are associated with deep inflammatory changes.

Cysts   Fluctuant cysts may measure up to two centimetres in diameter.

Scarring   Severe lesions are followed by scarring which is often keloidal.

The course of the condition is very variable and polymorphic. Acne may affect one part more than another. Scarring is often precipitated by squeezing and scratching which occurs when neurosis is present.

Differential Diagnosis

The diagnosis is not difficult if comedones are present. Peri-oral dermatitis can produce pustulation around the muzzle area. It is well to remember that acne can be produced by chemicals other than the drugs mentioned above. Chlorinated hydrocarbons (used in making conductors and insulators) cutting oils, crude petroleum and asbestos may all produce such lesions.

Treatment

As yet there is no cure for acne. It is possible however to control it and due to the introduction of antibiotics this can be done much more easily than before. It is important to stress the normal course of the disease to the patient, particularly its physiological nature and the period over which it extends. During the adolescent period an individuals consciousness of his appearance is much greater than ever and casual inadequate attention and treatment of a patient's condition only confirms his impression of cosmetic and social inferiority. Initial impressions are important and I have always found it well worth while to spend a short time with these patients and their parents discussing their condition and its management. Such an approach facilitates treatment and gives confidence in the doctors management of the condition which may extend over many months and years.

The various treatments which are available can be divided into four main groups; general, topical, systemic and physical.

General Measures

It is often noted that when the hair is allowed to cover the face, as with a fringe, there is an increase in the number of acne-form lesions. Keeping the hair in place by means of clips or ribbons often prevents these lesions occurring. Washing is another important factor in treatment as it removes excess sebum. I find detergents preferable to the use of soaps as rather stronger concentrations can be used. I find that one teaspoon of Stergene to 2/3 pint of hot water adequate; the face should be rinsed thoroughly afterwards. Alternatively 1 per cent Cetavlon Cetrimide lotion or, if the detergent is preferred in a toilet soap form, Genatosan skin bar can be used. Any foods which appear to aggravate the condition such as chocolate, solid fats and nuts should be avoided. Greasy preparations on the skin should not be used. Cosmetics can be used for special occasions and should be as non greasy as possible.

If the patient wishes for some cosmetic covering the use of flesh coloured proprietory preparations such as Eskamel are all that is required. The patient should be cautioned about squeezing or picking the lesions as this produces inflammation and secondary infection. Disfiguring comedones can be removed after washing several times with hot water and then applying a comedone extractor directly over the lesion, only slight pressure is then required to extract the comedone. This should not be performed on comedones which look inflammatory.

Topical Treatments

Are mainly dependent upon the exfoliative effect of sulphur, resorcinol, benzyl peroxide and beta napthol. It is important to realise that to be effective a mild degree and sometimes severe degree of peeling and erythema is required and unless this is obtained results will often be disappointing. The treatment should be carried out at night and the application washed off in the morning.

Sulphur is cheap and effective in most mild cases of acne. A variety of lotions can be prescribed and all are equally effective. Using calamine lotion and 5—15 per cent sulphur precipitans the sulphur content can be increased to obtain an adequate reaction.

Zinc sulphide lotion, B.P.C., has a stronger action and is useful when the acne is more pustular.

Resorcinol has a much more powerful action than either of the above. It is useful in the more resistant case. Patients should be warned that it may be necessary to rest the treatment for two to three days as the reaction is more severe. It is used as recorcinal and sulphur paste B.P.C. Strong reactions may occur with this. Resorcinol has toxic effects and is absorbed through the skin where it can produce myxoedema; it should not be used for prolonged periods. Some proprietary brands containing resorcinol are flesh tinted and are therefore cosmetically very acceptable.

A variety of other preparations containing benzyl peroxide, beta napthol and retinoic acid have also been used from time to time. Their reaction tends to be much stronger and in the case of retinoic acid which was hoped to be very effective, the reaction has often been found to be too irritant for general use.

Topical steroids will suppress the inflammatory reaction. I find the following preparation excellent for day-time usage: 10 per cent sulphur precipitate, 2 per cent hydrocortisone, crem. brulidene add 100 per cent. Proprietory steroid preparations for the treatment of acne are available. In acne prolonged use of steroids may produce a gram-negative infection.

Systemic Treatment

Antibiotics The tetracycline group of antibiotics has been shown to be very effective in the pustular inflammatory and nodular forms of acne. It is important to realise that for antibiotic treatment to be effective it must be continued for at least two or three months and even longer. It may be necessary to repeat the treatment at intervals. It is not justified in mild non-inflammatory cases.

Oxytetracycline is the cheapest and most effective antibiotic and it should be given in doses of 250 mg twice daily. The dosage can be doubled in severe cases for the worst first week, but when control is obtained it can then be reduced to 250 mg daily. Diarrhoea may be a complication in a few cases, but this can often be prevented by advising the patient to eat live, not pasteurised, yoghurt. Where oxytetracyclines fail the following alternatives can be used.

Clomycline is more expensive than oxytetracycline. It is given in a dosage of 170 mg twice daily. Erythromycin is given in the same dosage as oxytetracycline.

Hormones Oestrogens are effective but have to be given in doses which produce feminisation. 'Enovid', a contraceptive pill, can be used in women who have finished adolescence.

Systemic Steroids These have an anti-inflammatory reaction which can be useful in the nodular, acute form and very severe cases. Its use however is not justified in family practice. Local injections of steroids can be very useful and the injection of triamcinolone in a dose of 0.2–0.4 ml of a suspension containing 5 mg/ml, into cysts will rapidly reduce inflammatory reaction and reduce the cyst size. Persistent injection will produce atrophy.

Physical Treatment

Ultra-violet light can be given twice weekly, in mild erythema doses. It is not as effective as sun light and the effect soon tends to wear off, it is useful as a temporary measure.

Dermabrasion is reputed to be of assistance in cases where scarring is profound and the opinion of a plastic surgeon may be advisable in the severe cases of scarring.

It is important to remember that the majority of patients respond to simple regimes and treatments without resource to more expensive forms of treatment. In a condition which requires treatment over several years it is as well not to rush in with all the most expensive forms of treatment, but to reserve these for periods of exacerbation.

ROSACEA

Aetiology

Rosacea is an affection of the face characterised by persistant facial erythema, telangetasia and hypertrophy; it is often associated with acneform lesions and is sometimes called Acne rosacea although there is no pathological relationship with Acne. Unlike acne vulgaris which occurs in the young, rosacea tends to occur in the middle age group. Several factors appear to stimulate its production and persistence, but whether they are the cause or have just aggravated it is as yet unknown. Although a great deal has been postulated about its cause, all that we can say at the moment is that something renders the facial area very sensitive to a variety of stimuli which appear to play a part in the production of rosacea.

Psychological factors have long been regarded as important in the aetiology of rosacea as the condition affects the flushing area of the face which is under nervous control. Alcohol and strong stimulative drinks such as hot coffee and tea have been incriminated, together with gastritis, but the evidence is inconclusive. Rosacea is usually worse at the menopause and there is an association with gynaecological disorders. Local sepsis is often associated with the pustular variety. Sepsis usually arises in the teeth and sinuses and these should be checked.

Exposure to the elements aggravates rosacea; wind, heat and light can all be factors. There is an increase in its incidence in spring, especially if the weather is turbulent.

Desmodex folliculorum is a mite 0.4 mm long, present in the sebaceous glands and its numbers are increased in rosacea but whether its presence is primary or secondary is unknown.

Pathology

Initial changes are those of capilliary vasodilation which eventually becomes permanent and low grade inflammatory changes around the vessels and sebaceous glands, followed by hypertrophy of the sebaceous glands and fibrosis of connective tissue.

Clinical Features

Rosacea may present in several forms of varying severity. Vasodilation is the earliest manifestation. It occurs as a transient flushing of the face, particularly affecting the nose, cheeks forehead and chin. The changes are usually symmetrical but occasionally they may be unilateral. It is followed by telangectasia with papules and pustules. The vasodilation becomes permanent and with the hand lens dilated vessels are seen in the skin which gives it a reddish purple hue. Follicular papules and pustules occur, there is some oedema and the sebaceous glands have dilated orifices. A nodular cystic form may follow in severe cases and the skin becomes thickened and its surface irregular. Some of the cysts may discharge. Crusting may occur in some forms. Ocular changes may occur which presents as a blepharitis or a conjunctivitis. Keratitis, iritis and epeiscleritis may also occur.

Rhinophyma is thought to be a form of rosacea. It occurs commonly in association with it but may also occur without it. The nose becomes gradually hypertrophied and irregular.

Differential Diagnosis

Acne vulgaris is distinguished by the presence of comedones and the absence of telangectasia. Steroid induced rosacea tends to be much more florid.

General Management

Rosacea has social implications because of its disfiguring nature and its old association with alcohol (often unwarranted) which may provide a source of fun for friends but acute embarrassment for the patient. There is no doubt that psychological strains and stresses are imposed upon the patient by his condition and these in themselves often make the patient withdrawn and more easily prone to react to stress.

Treatment

Treatment should be aimed at eliminating those factors which appear to be aggravating the condition. It is worth while spending a little time going into the history of these patients. Detail is important; although one small factor may have no great effect by itself, a summation of many factors may.

Topical Applications
Sulphur has a place in treatment, especially where there is slight scaling which is sometimes associated with the Desmodex mite. It can be applied as a 2 per cent

suspension in calamine lotion, or as a stronger preparation of salicylic acid and sulphur cream.

Cortisone ointments produce a vaso-constrictory effect which is beneficial in rosacea. Unfortunately this is followed, in the case of fluorinated and more potent steroids, by permanent dilation and eventually a rosacea like condition can be produced by the steroid itself. I have not noticed the above effect with the use of hydrocortisone which I find useful in the following preparations applied twice daily: 1 per cent hydrocortisone powder, 1 per cent aureomycin, emulsificans ointment to 100 per cent.

Systemic Therapy
Tetracyclines have been shown to be effective in rosacea. Sneddon[15] showed an improvement which was maintained in two thirds of patients for over six months. Both pustulation and erythema were controlled. The dosage of tetracycline was 250 mg twice daily continued for several months. Ampicillin is useful in patients intolerant to tetracycline but is not quite as effective.

Physical Treatment
Facial massage from the bridge of the nose to the cheek is useful, particularly where the skin feels oedematous. Liquid paraffin can be used as a lubricant. The use of CO_2 slush and in severe cases plastic surgery by shaving techniques can be of value in rhinophyma.

TUMOURS

Most malignant tumours of the skin are rarities. The following are chosen because of either their frequency or malignancy.

Seborrhoeic Keratoses

Seborrhoeic warts or basal cell papillomas are common in family practice. They may occur in two's or three's, or they may be present in hundreds and they are found on most people over the age of 50.

Pathology
Seborrhoeic keratoses show branching dermal papillae and immature epidermal cells. Focal keratinization produces spherical, lamellated cysts. Melanocytes and pigmention are found.

Clinical Features
The lesions may be *superficial*, flesh coloured, velvety areas with an abscence of skin creases. Tiny 'birds' foot imprints are seen on the lesion. The *papillomatous*

type is like a soft, greasy, friable wart. Two other forms are found more rarely. The *mèlano-acanthotic* type is rounded with focal points of keratinization visible on the surface (like a currant bun). The *pedunculated* type has features of the last two and has a pedicle. The sizes vary from a few millimetres to several centimetres. The colour varies from pink to black.

Differential Diagnosis

This is not difficult due to their friability. Inflamed lesions may itch and, if pigmented, simulate melanomas. An antibiotic ointment will rapidly improve the lesion. Basal cell carcinomas are harder and gelatinous beneath the crust.

Treatment

Currettage removes the lesions. A method that I prefer is to paint the lesion sparingly with trichloroacetic acid after covering the surrounding area with vaseline. The wart sloughs off after a few days. Treatment can be repeated if necessary, superficial types respond to sulphur and salicylic acid ointment.

Basal Cell Carcinoma

Basal Cell Carcinoma is the most common epidermal malignant tumour but is not seen all that frequently in family practice. It is more prevalent in white fair and freckled people. It spreads slowly over months and years but does not metastasize. It is usually found on the face.

Clinical Features

Classically it presents as a rodent ulcer which has a pearly rolled edge, is semitranslucent with blood vessels seen in the substance. The ulcerated centre has a crust which on removal reveals a gelatinous base. Other types are sometimes found; pigmented, adenoid, cystic, button like (dome shaped), morphoeic (flat cicatricial, ivory colour) and superficial pagetoid (eczematous with a fine rolled edge). The lesions when first seen measure a few millimetres to a few centimetres but if left extensive ulceration occurs. Growth is very slow.

Differential Diagnosis

Keratoacanthoma and squamous cell carcinoma extend rapidly. Removal of the crust does not reveal a gelatinous base. Melanocytic naevi are not as hard and often have hairs.

Squamous Cell Carcinoma

Squamous cell carcinoma is rare. It extends rapidly and metastasizes. It arises from unhealthy skin as an indurated tumour that ulcerates and bleeds easily. It is common on light exposed areas.

Malignant Melanoma

Malignant melanoma is extremely rare in family practice, one third arise from pigmented naevi and there is often a history of trauma. Usually black, dark brown, or red (amelanotic), it arises as an itching bleeding tumour. From the periphery streaks of black pigment may extend. It is extremely malignant and metastases occur early. Whenever suspected urgent consultant opinion should be obtained.

Treatment
Treatment of basal cell carcinoma, squamous cell carcinoma and malignant melanoma is by surgery, radiotherapy or chemotherapy. Consultant opinion is required to decide which to select.

PREMALIGNANT CONDITIONS

Are much more likely to be met with than tumours and prompt treatment may prevent malignancy.

Senile, Actinic and Arsenical Keratoses   These are knife hard flakes of skin which are very adherent and a few millimetres in diameter. The first two arise on the face, forearms and hands, the latter on the hands and feet. When they become inflamed, malignancy often follows.

Intraepidermal Neoplasm   Also known as Bowen's disease this is a chronic eczematous like patch which is resistant to treatment including steroids.

Cutaneous Horn   This rock hard tumour, which has a horn shape, varies from only a few millimetres to centimetres long.

All the above lesions may give rise to squamous cell carcinoma.

Malignant Lentigo   This flat, irregular pigmented lesion of the face occurring in the elderly, measures several centimetres in diameter and may give rise to a malignant melanoma.

CUTANEOUS MANIFESTATIONS OF SYSTEMIC DISEASE

More and more skin conditions are being related to either systemic diseases or systemic poisons. The following are some of the common associations that a practitioner should know.

Systemic Diseases

Xanthomas   These are yellow red plaques or tumours of the elbows, knees, or eyelids. They are occasionally generalised and are associated with hyperlipaemia, hypercholesterolaemia and reticuloses.

Necrobiosis Lipoidica Diabeticorum   Paper thin atrophic plaques with visible blood vessels are common on the legs in association with clinical and preclinical diabetes.

Erythema Nodosum   The painful, reddish, purple nodules of the legs are toxic changes associated with streptococcal, tuberculous and sarcoid infections.

Dermatitis Herpetiformis   Grouped small itching vesicles, which leave pigmentation, occur on the shoulders and sacral area in association with enteropathy and ulcerative colitis.

Sarcoid   One third of patients with the red or purple infiltrated plaques or nodules have associated systemic sarcoid, particularly in the lungs.

Lupus Erythematosis (L.E.)   Twenty five per cent of patients with systemic L.E. present with a rash on the skin such as erythematous 'butterfly' distribution, discoid L.E. (follicular plugging, telangectasia, scaling) or purpura.

Gout   Yellow nodules occur on the rim of the ears and distal interphalangeal joints.

Scleroderma   (*hard skin*) Digital calcifications and Raynauds disease are associated with systemic sclerosis; in 3/4 the oesophagus is involved.

Systemic Malignancy

Dermatomyositis   Fifteen per cent of patients with dermatomyositis — muscular weakness and a skin rash with toxic changes — have a carcinoma.

Acanthosis Nigricans   Warts, pigmentation of axilla and groin, thickening of the skin of palms, soles and tongue occur. Severe manifestations of this condition often have an internal malignancy.

Annular Erythemas   Annular erythemas with bizarre patterns may be associated with internal malignancy.

Pruritus   In the young pruritus may be associated with Hodgkins disease, and in the elderly with neoplasms, (it may also indicate liver disorder, gout and renal disease).

Exfoliative Dermatitis   Neoplasia may precipitate exfoliative dermatitis, especially in the elderly.

Systemic Allergens

Drug Eruptions

Drug eruptions are common and may mimic any skin rash; rather than attempt to give a detailed list it is more important for the practitioner to restrict himself to a few well known drugs and to be aware of their possible skin manifestations. Literature is supplied by drug firms and there are references in Rook[16]. A drug eruption should be always considered in the differential diagnosis of a rash.

Urticaria

Urticaria is an allergic reaction with the release of histamine which produces itching white wheals with a surrounding erythema, usually about 1 cm in diameter but they may be larger (giant urticaria) and severe (angioneurotic oedema). The distribution is general but in papular urticaria, which is due to insect bites and is common in children, there is a central punctum and the lesions are grouped. Urticaria is usually transitory and due to ingested foods such as strawberries and shellfish. A few cases are familial due to exercise or stress (cholinergic). Many cases of urticaria become chronic and increasing numbers are being shown to be due to drugs and infections, e.g., penicillin traces in milk and cheese, phenolphthalein (in red colouring and pink icing), aspirin, quinine (found in bitters), food dyes and preservatives, bacterial infections, helminths and drugs.

Treatment

An attempt to identify the cause and eliminate it should be made. Mild cases respond to antihistamine treatment in tablet form. Severe giant urticaria may require injections of antihistamines and severe angioneurotic oedema may require injections of adrenaline (0.2–0.5 ml of 1/1000), especially if there is respiratory obstruction.

References

1. Milne, J. A. (1970). *Practitioner* 205, 452.
2. Gill, A. K. and Baxter, D. L. (1964). *Arch. Dermatol.* 89, 734.
3. Fievrel, M. (1969). *Brit. J. Dermatol.* 81, 113.
4. Sneddon, I. B. (1974). *Prescribers J.* 14, 1.
5. Boardman, H. J. (1969). *Triangle* 9, 26.
6. Ingram, J. T. (1968). In *Industrial Dermatoses and the Industrial Injuries Act* (London: Churchill, J. & A. Ltd).
7. Farber, E. M., Bright, R. A. and Nall, M. L. (1969). *Arch. Dermatol.* 98, 248.
8. Ingram, J. T. (1953). *Brit. med. J.* 2, 1951.
9. Gonnor, B. L. (1972). *Brit. J. Dermatol.* 86, 48.
10. Maibach, H. I., Strauss, W. G. and Shinefield, H. R. (1969). *Brit. J. Dermatol.* 81, Suppl. 1 69.
11. Manning, M. A. and Epstein, W. L. (1963). *Arch. Dermatol.* 87, 306.
12. Barr, A. and Coles, N. B. (1969). *Trans. St. John Hospit. dermatol. Soc.* 55, 69.
13. Vickers, C. H. (1961). *Brit. med. J.* 2, 743.
14. Wheeler, C. E. and Huffner, W. D. (1965). *J. amer. med. Ass.* 191, 445.
15. Sneddon, I. B. (1966). *Brit. J. Dermatol.* 78, 649.
16. Rook, A., Wilkinson, D. S. and Ebling, F. J. G. (1969). In *Textbook of Dermatology* p. 362 (Oxford: Blackwell Scientific Publications).
17. Seville, R. (1975). *Brit. J. Dermatol.* 93, 205.

19

Diabetes Mellitus

E. Wilkes

EPIDEMIOLOGY

There are about the same number of unknown diabetics in the community as known cases. Various surveys with different standards and techniques all have tended to confirm this[1,2] and the incidence in the United Kingdom population is likely to be rather more than 1.5 per cent.

Such a figure includes purely biochemical diagnoses in patients who may be asymptomatic. In an elderly population abnormalities of carbohydrate metabolism may approach an incidence of about 10 per cent but many of these will not fulfil the World Health Organisation criterion[3] for the diagnosis of diabetes — a blood sugar of more than 120 mg per 100 ml 2 hours after a standard glucose loading. However, many of these patients will be operating throughout the day at a far higher blood sugar level than the common physiological range of 80 or 90 mg per 100 ml, and may not be producing glycosuria only because of the higher renal threshold associated with increasing age. Clearly therefore, many with glycosuria may not be diabetic and many diabetics may not show sugar in their urine. The attainment of the diagnosis in an asymptomatic elderly patient may well end only in dietetic advice. This may not even be particularly helpful, since some authorities[2] doubt if early diagnosis does much to alter the clinical course.

Screening for diabetes in practice populations is thus best restricted to those with a family history of the disease, the obese, those over fifty years of age, and women with a suggestive past obstetric history — such as babies weighing at birth over 10 lb (4.5 kg), stillbirths, or repeated miscarriages, large families, or excessive weight gain in pregnancy.

TYPES OF DIABETES

The diagnosis of diabetes mellitus possibly includes a small group of rather different diseases. This would account for the variation between the well—

preserved state of many long—standing diabetics compared with recent cases diagnosed with retinopathy or nephropathy already established or rapidly progressive. The British Diabetic Association has recommended the following classifications of the disease:—

> The *potential diabetic* has a normal glucose tolerance test but has either both parents diabetic, a diabetic identical twin, or an equivalent strong family history of the disease, or has given birth to a child of over 4.5 kg birth—weight or a stillbirth with hyperplasia of the pancreatic islets without associated rhesus incompatibility.

> The *latent diabetic* has a normal glucose tolerance test which becomes abnormal under a stress such as pregnancy, infection, or obesity.

> The *asymptomatic* or *chemical diabetic* has a diabetic type of glucose tolerance test but random blood sugar levels will be below 130 mg per decilitre. Such cases, like the overt diabetic, can have their diabetes induced or exacerbated by the use of common drugs such as steroids, thiazides or oestrogens, including the oral contraceptives.

CLINICAL DIABETES

Rarely the disease may be associated with local pancreatic damage. Chronic pancreatitis, haemochromatosis, pancreatic tumour or surgery, or a history of acute pancreatitis — perhaps after mumps — are examples of this. Diabetes may be associated with other endocrine disorders such as thyrotoxicosis, aldosteronism, phaeochromocytoma, Cushing's syndrome, Addison's disease, or acromegaly. It may be associated with chronic renal failure or severe liver disease such as cirrhosis. Virus infections such as with Coxsackie B4 may also be implicated[4].

An autoimmune factor may be associated. There is a well—established clinical association between pernicious anaemia, thyroid disease and diabetes and this is linked, for example, with the finding of antibodies to thyroid and gastric parietal cells more commonly in diabetics than in non—diabetics.

In family practice however the vast majority of our problems come under the heading of idiopathic diabetes as it affects three main groups — the juvenile type diabetic, the maturity onset diabetic, and the diabetic woman.

The Juvenile Type Diabetic

In the juvenile or insulin-dependent diabetic we may have a clinical presentation of the most acute onset, proceeding from apparently normal health to ketosis and coma over a few hours. Although normally less dramatic than this, the onset is usually more acute and less insidious than in the maturity onset case.

The presenting features of diabetes to the well-informed layman are, correctly, thirst, polyuria and weight loss. These common symptoms may be exacerbated by anxiety and may be temporarily allayed by tranquillisers even in the presence of obvious diabetes. The thirst will be made worse by sugared drinks or foods and the polyuria may be associated with a white staining of clothing, boots or even water closets, as the glucose crystallises out of drying drops of urine.

The feeling of tiredness may be marked and may occur in the hypoglycaemic state known sometimes to precede the onset of diabetes. Monilial infections of mouth, penis, vagina or intertriginous areas, and urinary infections are common. Pruritus vulvae is frequently associated. Furunculosis and boils, almost always mentioned in orthodox textbooks, do not in fact seem to occur more often in diabetics but when they do will tend to be more severe, proceeding perhaps to frank abcess formation, and so further exacerbating the clinical state.

The disease may also present as any of its acute or chronic complications, so covering a wide range of systems and symptoms.

Acute Complications

The most important of the acute complications, perhaps, is diabetic keto-acidaemia or ketosis. This may come quite unheralded or may be preceded by an infective illness or errors in insulin dosage over a few days or hours. The patient tends to become more drowsy and dehydrated, and shows the deep and rapid respiration of 'air-hunger'. There is marked ketonuria and usually of course glycosuria also, but not necessarily any other helpful physical signs. A sweet ketone-scent may be smelt on the breath of severer cases. Abdominal pain and vomiting may mimic an acute abdominal emergency. Such a clinical situation merits of course immediate transfer to hospital, since water and electrolyte deficiencies must be corrected and hour by hour laboratory control of the response to therapy may be essential. If the journey to hospital will take some hours, blood should be taken for glucose and electrolytes and a drip of normal saline set up. Soluble insulin in a dose of 50 to 100 units (half intravenously and half intramuscularly) should be given, dosage varying with the severity of dehydration, the depth of coma, and the weight of the patient. A rough guide as to blood sugar level may be obtained quickly at the bedside by the use of Dextrostix (Ames). Any possible hypoglycaemia is to be countered by the administration of intravenous glucose. The full regime with monitoring of blood glucose, potassium, pH and pCO_2 can then be started soon after arrival in hospital.

Although chronic nervous lesions are more common, acute neuropathies also occur. The diabetic neuropathies seem to be the group of complications most clearly associated with poor control and as such at least partly preventable. Usually one finds a mixed motor and sensory involvement of the lower limbs, with pain, weakness, paraesthesia and loss of reflexes. More rarely this can affect all four limbs. A motor disorder usually of the legs, with the signs of an upper motor neurone lesion yet with muscle wasting, is described as diabetic amyotrophy[5]. Cranial nerve palsies are of such sudden onset that they are likely to be of vascular origin.

These problems merit careful symptomatic treatment whenever possible combined with strenuous attempts to achieve better diabetic control. Physiotherapy can be helpful in maintaining independence and mobility and the pain may be helped by diphenylhydantoin or carbamazepine if simple analgesics prove unhelpful.

Chronic Complications

Although presenting a far less dramatic need for therapeutic intervention, it is the chronic complications of diabetes that cause by far the greater volume of suffering and disability.

Atherosclerosis occurs both earlier and more severely in the diabetic. Increased incidences of strokes, myocardial infarction and peripheral vascular disease are well documented. Gangrene of the lower limb often may be the result of combined vascular disease and sensory and trophic impairment. Atherosclerosis in the diabetic also may affect specifically the small vessels of kidney, nerves and retina.

Proteinuria is noted in 4 per cent of recently diagnosed diabetics[6], this figure rising to 16 per cent in longer-standing cases. There may be associated pyelonephritis. The proteinuria may be massive in the later stages (more than 3 g per 24 hours), and hypertension may add further complications.

There is no specific treatment available for the nephropathy other than to try and improve diabetic control and any associated pyelonephritis. Cyclophosphamide may prove to be of value. Heroic measures such as dialysis or renal transplants cannot often be considered seriously in the management of what must be thought of as a diffuse lesion affecting also the retina and the myocardium. Slowly progressive renal failure may have to be observed over many months.

Atherosclerotic changes in the vasa nervorum may not correlate well with the degree of chronic neuropathy encountered, but is likely to be relevant in older patients who so often present with a picture of pain and paraesthesiae in the feet and with absent ankle jerks. Vibration sense is so often impaired in the elderly that this sign is not usually helpful. The loss of pain occurs at a more advanced stage and may well be associated with involvement of the autonomic nervous system in the formation of trophic ulcers. This autonomic involvement in turn can lead to less obvious symptoms such as impotence (said to be common in diabetic males), nocturnal diarrhoea, or urinary incontinence. Leg oedema, reduced or abnormal sweating, postural hypotension and pupillary changes may be helpful confirmatory signs.

The ophthalmic complications of diabetes are the most distressing of all. Cataracts in the younger diabetic may require earlier extraction. In badly controlled young diabetics, the deposition of glycogen in the pigment epithelium precedes a network of new blood vessels, haemorrhagic glaucoma and blindness. The commonest ophthalmic problem, however, is the diabetic retinopathy.

The venous changes here are dilatation proceeding to microaneurysm, while the arteries reflect atherosclerosis and hypertension. Haemorrhages and hard exudates also occur and cottonwool spots – retinal infarcts consequent on arterial occlusion – may if numerous indicate the imminent onset of proliferative retinopathy. Macular damage by exudate, haemorrhage, or oedema from nearby vascular disease is the main cause of blindness, and diabetic cases make up 7 per cent of new blind registrations in England and Wales.

An attitude of reasoned optimism must be maintained, since only 50 per cent of diabetics have evidence of retinopathy after 15 years, and stationary periods or remissions can occur for long periods. Treatment by light coagulation seems to be the most helpful. Hypophysectomy for the severer, and drug therapy (heparin, clofibrate) for the milder cases may still have a place in management.

Patients recently diagnosed as diabetic may suffer temporary visual disturbances for a month or so because of local lens changes consequent on treatment. Such patients merit urgent reassurance for they may think that they are going blind.

Skin Lesions

Cutaneous Candidiasis and pyogenic infections have already been mentioned. Other non-specific dermatological lesions commoner in diabetics are necrobiosis lipoidica and granuloma annulare. Scattered skin xanthomata can occur in hyperlipidaemic cases. Pseudoxanthoma nigricans – dusky, pigmented hyperkeratoses in skin folds especially of axilla and groin – are benign lesions that sometimes involute after excess weight has been lost. Pigmented scars on the skins of diabetics with neuropathy are common after slight trauma and are dignified sometimes by the name of diabetic dermopathy.

Foot Lesions

Foot lesions are common and if neglected may lead to the demoralisation of the patient and to the disruption of the established life-style. This is inevitable in an elderly patient should admission to hospital over many weeks be indicated. Such foot lesions are usually preventable and are the result of badly fitting shoes, minor trauma or infection, or amateur chiropody. With impaired sensation, a poor blood supply, indifferently controlled diabetes, a low standard of hygiene and poor supervision, the stage is set for the paronychia, the cellulitis or the trivial skin defect to develop into an indolent deeply penetrating ulcer or gangrene that may well need many weeks of in-patient treatment. It is just as important — but far rarer — for the family practitioner to look closely at the feet on routine follow-up than to organise blood sugar estimations. Soon after the diagnosis has been established, the patient should be carefully and repeatedly briefed about the care of his feet. He should know that absence of pain is not reliable and that frequent visual inspection of the feet is indicated — daily when sensation is known to be impaired. Shoes should be comfortable and of good quality. The feet should be washed thoroughly, frequently but gently, and not rubbed vigorously when being dried. Talcum powder should be used, and well-fitting socks changed daily. These precautions and the rapid reporting of trivial problems would save much needless expense and human suffering. Both consultant diabetician and family practitioner have perhaps tended to understate the importance of this simple regime.

The Maturity Onset Diabetic

The more advanced age of such cases naturally implies a greater incidence of atherosclerotic complications: but on the whole the later the age of onset, the milder the diabetic state and the complications, so the maturity onset diabetic is not usually to be treated in any way as an invalid. Clearly the presence of a chronic cough in an elderly diabetic makes a chest X-ray mandatory because of the increased incidence of pulmonary tuberculosis known to be associated with the disease; and the justifiably relaxed attitude of the doctor must not be allowed to become slack and over-optimistic. That this is a less dangerous form of the disease however is exemplified by the negligible danger of diabetic ketoacidosis in such cases, and the presence of marked ketonuria will transform the management to that of the juvenile type.

There is one form of diabetic coma, however, both dangerous and peculiar to the maturity onset diabetic — the so-called hyperosmolal non-ketotic diabetic coma. This rare condition occurs typically in the obese mild diabetic. The blood pressure is maintained and there is no ketosis. There is however profound dehydration, abnormally viscous blood with the threat therefore of arterial or venous thrombosis, hypernatraemia, severe hypokalaemia, and blood sugars often over 1000 mg per 100 ml. Precipitating factors include infection in an elderly and debilitated patient, diabetogenic drugs — especially thiazides, and a disturbance of the osmoregulatory system consequent on the gross hyperglycaemia. Over 20 per cent of cases will die. Treatment is by insulin, potassium replacement, and hypotonic saline.

Normally however the maturity onset diabetic is not insulin-dependent and can be managed either by diet alone or by diet and oral hypoglycaemic agents.

The Diabetic Woman

Diabetic women may have menstrual irregularities, may be comparatively subfertile, and their babies have a higher mortality rate of about 10 per cent. They have also a higher incidence of foetal abnormality. The maternal mortality rate should be as for the non-diabetic in experienced centres.

Diabetic women in pregnancy should be managed by soluble insulin given twice daily and should be carefully supervised, usually by a joint obstetrician-diabetician team to whom they should be referred as soon as pregnancy is diagnosed. Insulin requirements remain unaltered during pregnancy in about 25 per cent of cases but normally fall slightly in the first trimester and then increase. Since excessive weight gain, pre-eclampsia, polyhydramnios, ante-partum haemorrhage and large babies may help produce the higher foetal mortality near term, usually a planned Caesarean section or induction takes place at about 37 weeks. The child should be treated as premature and as especially susceptible to the respiratory distress syndrome or hypoglycaemia.

The improved maternal mortality figures stem from the frequent and strict supervision of diabetic control imposed over the months and including routine admission for several weeks before delivery is planned.

Diabetic women who wish to take the oral contraceptive pill can usually do so with the appropriate increase in their insulin dosage.

The majority of paediatricians have a rather tolerant attitude in the management of the older diabetic child or adolescent and may be more interested in a normal growth rate than normal blood sugars. The enormously variable levels of physical activity and the dietetic indiscretions characteristic of the age-group make acceptable a range of blood sugar levels not greeted as uniformly satisfactory by orthodox diabeticians. When they take charge of the rather older age-groups the family practitioner may need tact and diplomacy to smooth out the difficulties of this transition, perhaps especially in supporting the mother.

TREATMENT OF DIABETES

Diet

The basic treatment for all types of diabetes is carbohydrate restriction. Cases showing hyperlipidaemia and hypercholesterolaemia may also require restriction of animal fat intake.

The Exchange or Portion System* established by the British Diabetic Association seems by far the simplest method of giving a standardised yet varied diet. Each portion listed consists of a 10 g portion of carbohydrate and the patient is told that he or she may have a certain number of such portions daily. An average normal carbohydrate intake would be about 30 10 g portions daily. A young active diabetic would be allowed about 20 10 g portions. A maturity onset diabetic would be permitted some 15 10 g portions, and an obese diabetic not on insulin might have to struggle along on 10 10 g portions. The age and morale of the patient, the degree of obesity and the rate of weight loss, and, most important of all, the degree of glycosuria charted on routine testing will influence the amount of carbohydrate permitted. It is not recommended that patients should routinely weigh out their diet. Such advice would be unrealistic. Although 80 per cent of obese maturity onset diabetics can be controlled by diet alone, only about one third of diabetics keep strictly to their diet.

Insulin

The juvenile-onset diabetic, the patient liable to ketosis, and the maturity onset diabetic whose diabetes cannot be adequately controlled by oral hypoglycaemic agents need insulin as well as their diet. Maturity onset diabetics may temporarily need insulin during stressful periods of intercurrent illness or surgery.

The aim of the treatment is to maintain as closely as possible a normal level of blood sugar throughout the 24 hours. This is best done by the twice daily injection of shorter-acting insulins and this routine is indicated for diabetics in their teens or younger, and for all diabetics during periods of stress such as pregnancy or illness, or who cannot attain adequate control by longer acting preparations.

Many authorities believe that neuropathy and retinopathy can be prevented, improved or delayed by long periods of control of the blood sugar to as nearly normal levels as possible. Even with two injections a day however this is not easy to achieve. Many labile or brittle diabetics — and these will include almost all cases under twenty years of age as well as some older patients — will be pushed into hypoglycaemia if too tight a control is attempted. Such patients have a lower level of insulin antibodies and a lower insulinogenic reserve than the more stable diabetics and moderate hyperglycaemia and glycosuria will have to be accepted.

There are three commonly used short-acting insulins. Soluble Insulin B.P. has an acid pH. 'NUSO' Neutral Insulin is neutral with a pH of 7.2 and is said to be more stable and less irritant at the injection site. Otherwise the two are identical. The third preparation is Actrapid Insulin. This is a porcine insulin and seems more effective than the commoner bovine insulin against which a high

* Obtainable from the British Diabetic Association, 3—6 Alfred Place, London W.C.1.

titre of antibodies may be developed. Thus hypoglycaemia can be produced by a change not of dose but of insulin source and this possibility must always be kept in mind.

By a mixture of short— and medium—acting insulins it is often possible to maintain very satisfactory control. The old combination was of a soluble-protamine zinc insulin mixture given once daily but this is being less often used now. This is partly because many believe these insulins should not be mixed in the same syringe and partly because of the tendency to produce hypoglycaemia late at night or in the morning. Isophane insulin (NPH) with a duration of action of 12 to 22 hours is now more often used with soluble insulin and in a twice-daily injection is probably the regime of choice for most insulin-dependent diabetics. A biphasic insulin — Rapitard — is a mixture of 25 per cent porcine and 75 per cent bovine insulins. This has a duration of action of 12 to 20 hours and a mixture of Actrapid and Rapitard given twice daily gives equivalent results to the Soluble-Isophane combination.

Once-daily injection regimes may be possible by the use of more modern long-acting insulins than protamine zinc. Ultralente with a duration of action of 36 or more hours, lente with a duration of action of up to 30 hours, and made up of 3 parts of semi-lente to 7 parts of ultra-lente are used for this purpose. Globin zinc insulin may also be used since it has a duration of action of 18 to 24 hours.

Such once-daily injection schemes should not be used in brittle, adolescent, pregnant or ill diabetics or in those who need 40 units or more of insulin daily. Mild diabetics can probably be well controlled, however, by once daily mixtures of lente and semi-lente insulins or by the soluble and isophane combination.

It is unhappily true that many diabetics are not properly briefed in detail about the routine involved in their insulin injections. The injection sites should be used in rotation, and the upper arms, upper thighs and lower abdominal wall are all suitable areas. This rotation will reduce the likelihood of fat atrophy. Cleanliness of the skin must be important yet local cellulitis is surprisingly rare.

Many patients become confused over the strength of their insulins. Their attention should be drawn to the colour codes and to the fact that soluble insulin is available in a strength of 20 units per ml as well as, like all the other insulins, 40 and 80 units per ml. They should be supervised in drawing up their insulin since the British Standard Insulin syringe is calibrated for 20 units per ml.

Patients should be encouraged, if they are sensible and experienced, slightly to modify on their own initiative their insulin dosage, if this is clearly indicated. Increases in dosage are indicated if glycosuria is marked and a decreased dosage should be used if energetic pursuits are being undertaken or mild hypoglycaemia is being experienced. Such minor alterations are usually done in increments of 4 units and more large-scale alterations probably require some medical involvement. Any illness may require a major increase in insulin and this clearly demands medical supervision.

If disposable syringes are not issued to diabetic patients unless they buy them, they should be encouraged to boil their glass syringes frequently and to keep them clean in syringe holders in spirit cases. In the UK disposable needles may be prescribed by hospital doctors but not by family practitioners. Syringes should be checked frequently to see that there is no leakage. If the patient's sight gradually deteriorates, the dosage injected may vary to a dangerous degree and cause mysterious difficulties in the maintenance of adequate control.

Oral Hypoglycaemic Agents

The main value of these drugs is in stabilising the maturity-onset diabetics who are not adequately controlled by diet alone. They are of less value in juvenile-type diabetes.

The two main groups of drugs are the sulphonylureas and the biguanides. The sulphonylureas act by stimulating the β cells of the pancreas to produce more insulin.

Tolbutamide was the first of these to be used widely and is given usually three times daily in doses of 0.5 g. Reports from the USA and Belfast[7,8] have shown that diabetic patients treated with tolbutamide or other hypoglycaemic agents sustain more frequent myocardial infarcts than those treated by diet alone. These findings are by no means universally accepted and clearly diabetics who do not diet conscientiously may well constitute a self-selected group at greater risk. The studies at the least however serve to remind the clinician that this group of powerful drugs should not be used for maturity-onset diabetics merely to permit a more liberal regime. They are to be given only when the poorly controlled diabetic state gives firm indication for their use.

Other side-effects are either comparatively unimportant (rashes, indigestion) or rare (abnormal liver function tests, blood dyscrasias).

A longer-acting sylphonylurea is chlorpropamide, popular since it can be given in a once-daily dosage of 100 to 500 mg. The prolonged action makes hypoglycaemia even more than usually dangerous and deaths have been reported. Cholestatic jaundice can be caused by this drug and severe facial flushing after alcohol is more frequent and troublesome than with other sulphonylureas such as tolazamide.

Glibenclamide is the most recent and potent of the sulphonylureas, and is given once or twice daily in doses of 2.5 to 20 mg. This drug seems to attain its maximal hypoglycaemic effect within a few days of starting treatment while other sylphonylureas may take a few weeks. Glibenclamide seems to stimulate insulin synthesis as well as release, but the choice of sulphonylureas is still a matter for the personal preference of the physician, who is bound also to bear in mind that the hypoglycaemic effect may be potentiated by common drugs like salicylates, phenylbutazone, β-blockers and monoamine oxidase inhibitors, and also by less common drugs such as dicoumarol, probenecid and sulphaphenazole. The hypoglycaemic effect may be diminished by steroids, oral contraceptives, thiazides and adrenaline.

In overweight maturity onset diabetics the biguanides should be exhibited first if diet alone has proved insufficient. They cause a weight loss that is helpful and is not merely due to anorexia. If the biguanides fail on their own they should be supplemented by a sulphonylurea since some cases respond well to the combination. Occasionally the biguanides are used with insulin in the management of obese insulin-dependent diabetics and this combination may produce a major reduction in insulin requirements.

The biguanides should be avoided in the presence of a tendency to ketosis or important liver, kidney, cardiac or pulmonary disease, in pregnancy, or if the patient is dehydrated or ill. In these circumstances phenformin can cause lactic acidaemia and the patient may become shocked and hyperglycaemic. The most popular biguanide nowadays is probably the sustained-release phenformin capsule — given in a dose of 50 mg twice daily. Alternatively metformin is given, when used alone, usually in a dose of 0.5 g to 2 g three times daily, but smaller doses will be required if it is used in conjunction with insulin or a sulphonylurea.

The American study showed that this group of drugs also might possibly be associated with an increased incidence of coronary disease. Less important side-effects are nausea, vomiting and anorexia and these symptoms will be less prominent if the drug is taken during a meal. Diarrhoea, malaise, vitamin B_{12} malabsorption and liver and kidney damage may also occur. Both phenformin and metformin also have a fibrinolytic effect.

Hypoglycaemia

Any moderate alteration in insulin requirements, as may often happen with the brittle diabetic, or after strenuous exercise, a missed meal or an accidentally excessive injection may all cause acute hypoglycaemia. Early symptoms include hunger, sweating, pallor, tachycardia, or headache, while anxiety, obstinacy and aggression may be prominent. Patients may behave as if they were drunk and become voluble and confused, with slurred speech, delirium and coma.

All patients must be warned to take heed of their own usual early symptoms of hypoglycaemia — a tingling or numbness around the mouth seems quite common — and to take the sugar in an easily portable form (usually sweets) that must always be carried against just such an emergency.

Nearly every practice will have one or two diabetics who are liable now and again to present in a hypoglycaemic coma too deep for oral treatment; and it must be one of the more routine but satisfying triumphs of general practice to convert the unconscious patient back in seconds to normality by the intravenous injection of glucose. Since convulsions, brain damage, or death may occur if treatment is delayed, this sort of episode is always to be treated as an emergency. Milder but frequent episodes can lead to permanent intellectual deterioration and myocardial damage.

Islet cell tumours are the commonest cause of spontaneous hypoglycaemia and other causes include gastric surgery, liver disease and poisoning by alcohol, salicylates, antihistamines or monoamine oxidase inhibitors.

Iatrogenic hypoglycaemia is however easily the commonest group and prolonged supervision is essential if hypoglycaemia supervenes after the administration of a long-acting insulin or sulphonylurea. Mildly arteriosclerotic patients may become chronically confused with even mild but long-continued hypoglycaemia and this can be difficult to diagnose unless the possibility is borne in mind.

The beta-blockers are now widely used in therapeutics, so it is important to remember that they may potentiate the dangers of hypoglycaemia, and the patient may with surprising suddenness sink into coma.

Every diabetic should carry a card giving details of his name and address, his doctor, his diabetic state and a simple first aid procedure.

GENERAL MANAGEMENT OF DIABETES

Routinely, and if neither age nor disability render this inadvisable, the daily management of the diabetes should largely be left to the patient. Once the diagnosis has been established, perhaps just by a random blood sugar of over 200 mg per 100 ml, or a two-hour post-prandial level of more than 140 mg per 100 ml, or by a full glucose tolerance test, then the diagnosis should be followed by the thorough briefing of the patient. As well as routine medical consultations the briefing should ideally include sessions with the dietician, perhaps advice concerning employment or extra allowances from a social worker, and certainly suggestions for the care of the feet from a chiropodist especially experienced in diabetic foot problems.

If the patient is insulin-dependent he should be instructed in the technique of self-injection and in the timing of his diet. A small meal three or four hours after a soluble insulin injection, for example, is advisable and the characteristics of the particular regime, and any possible problems, should be carefully explained.

Routine pre-prandial urine testing with Clinitest (Ames) may at first be carried out two or three times daily but after a while, if the tests show only occasional 1 per cent glucose or frequent negative results, this can be reduced to once daily and then once or twice a week. The frequency should be increased if there is any malaise and if glycosuria becomes consistently more marked than usual, the patient must report.

If there is ketosis (most susceptible patients can be taught to test for this but the district nurse or health visitor can speedily become involved in any episode of poor control) then again the doctor should see the patient. Minor modifications of treatment within agreed limits can be initiated by the patient if he feels well but shows rather more glycosuria than usual. Many patients become experts in the management of their own case.

It is perhaps relevant here to mention that false negative tests for glucose may result from the concurrent administration of levodopa or ascorbic acid. False high results may also be caused by these drugs and also by aspirin, tetracyclines, nalidixic acid and isoniazid. In practice this seems to matter comparatively little.

There are many administrative methods by which the expertise of the specialist can benefit the diabetic patient without at the same time depriving him of the variety and continuity of care offered by the family practitioner. In one city in the UK a well-trained family practitioner acts not only as part of the hospital-based clinic team but also as a liaison officer discharging back suitable cases to the care of their own doctors. This helps prevent dangerous over-loading and depersonalisation of the hospital diabetic clinics. The specialist diabetician then has time to concentrate on new or difficult cases whilst the patient benefits from a routine of care from his family doctor instead of from a harrassed stranger. In other cities 'miniclinics' have been set up in health centres that are visited regularly by the consultant physician. Elsewhere special trained practitioners may take over this role.

Whatever the local arrangements may be, the routine management of diabetes is a fascinating and long-term responsibility that should remain mainly, but not exclusively, within the province of primary care.

In the UK one of the most successful of all patients' associations is the British Diabetic Association, located at 3–6 Alfred Place, London W.C.1. All younger patients should be advised to join this association. A local representative may attend the local hospital diabetic clinics and the association can offer a range of services from suitable recipe books to a distinguished medical section.

References

1. Redhead, I. M. (1975) In *Screening in General Practice* (Hart, C. R. ed.), (Edinburgh and London: Churchill Livingstone).
2. Malins, J. (1968) *Clinical Diabetes Mellitus*, (London: Eyre and Spottiswoode).
3. World Health Organisation (1965) Technical Report Series No. 310.
4. Gamble, D. R. and Taylor, K. W. (1969) *Brit. med. J.* 3, 627.
5. Garland, H. (1955) *Brit. med. J.* 2, 1287.
6. Hall, R., Anderson, J., Smart, G. A. and Besser, M. (1974)*Fundamentals of Clinical Endocrinology*, 2nd edition, (London: Pitman Medical).
7. University Group Diabetes Program (1970). *Diabetes* 19, 747.
8. Hadden, D. R., Montgomery, D. A. D. and Weaver, J. A. (1972) *Lancet* i, 335.

20

Common Thyroid Disorders

E. Wilkes

INTRODUCTION

The three common disorders of the thyroid are non-toxic or simple goitre, hypothyroidism and hyperthyroidism. These conditions can merge one into another. The term Graves' disease is reserved for the syndrome of goitre, hyperthyroidism and eye signs. Myxoedema, from the mucinous polysaccharide deposited in certain tissues, is synonymous with thyroid deficiency. Since these disorders or their sequelae may be long-lasting and associated with a high local incidence or a familial pattern, the family practitioner must be implicated not only in the initial diagnosis but also in follow-up and management.

There have been major advances in recent years in our knowledge of thyroid disease. For example, thyroid antibody estimations are now highly relevant to clinical management and diagnosis. A high antibody titre in a case of non-toxic goitre indicates an important autoimmune component, such as might be expected in Hashimoto's disease. A lower antibody titre is found in hypothyroidism, and typically a still lower level in most cases of Graves' disease.

Most physicians would now agree that an autoimmune element is generally involved in thyroid disorders, possibly in conjunction with genetic and environmental factors. For example, the long-acting thyroid stimulator (LATS) may well be a thyroid antibody produced by lymphocytes and yet with thyroid stimulating properties. Although its discovery has prompted so far more questions than answers, LATS is becoming slowly part of the elucidation of clinical problems. Other recent research activities concerning thyrotrophic releasing hormone (TRH) are becoming even more speedily incorporated into clinical management, and typify our increased interest not only in the target-organ and the pituitary but also in the hypothalamic nuclei.

SIMPLE GOITRE

Aetiology

Certain endemic goitre areas have been known for centuries. These are associated with iodine deficiency, and this still remains the commonest cause of goitre today, probably accounting for over 90 per cent of cases.

Half a century ago 10 per cent of schoolgirls in the Derbyshire Peak District of Britain were goitrous[1]. More recent investigations[2] there have demonstrated an incidence of 66 goitres per 1000 patients, but in the most isolated areas surveyed the figure rose to 18 per cent. Some 10 per cent of those with goitres had a positive family history.

These figures are about twice as high as the 34 goitres per 1000 found in Sheffield[3]. Many areas, especially in the South of Britain, will have a far lower incidence but in North-East England 9 per cent of women and 1 per cent of men have some degree of thyroid enlargement[4]. Characteristically females are from 3 to 9 times more frequently affected than males, the maximum incidence being in middle life, but in the Derbyshire survey some 28 per cent of all thyroid abnormalities occurred in subjects less than 40 years of age. Children, however, were only rarely affected.

Many patients in endemic areas will have small goitres occurring in adolescence or pregnancy and these may well subside spontaneously without treatment. The goitres are formed through excessive secretion by the anterior pituitary of thyroid stimulating hormone (TSH) in an attempt to maintain a euthyroid state despite what may be only a marginal iodine deficiency.

The situation may be exacerbated by the extra physiological demands of pregnancy and the increased renal clearance of iodide that also occurs at that time.

Enzyme deficiencies causing dyshormonogenesis, mostly inherited as a Mendelian recessive, form a very small proportion of goitres. These characteristically start in childhood and will be reduced in size, like the adult goitre, by the use of thyroxine. The commoner iodine-deficiency can be prevented by the routine use of iodised salt. If the goitre is of fairly long-standing it may respond to thyroxine but the longer the history and the more nodular the goitre the less responsive it will tend to be.

Diagnosis and Investigation

If a small goitre in a child is noted on routine examination, the child should be referred for full assessment. In an adult it may be more helpful to ignore the finding, especially if the patient is clinically euthyroid, is well, has none of the stigmata of the rare thyroid cancer, and is part of a community or family subject to simple endemic goitre. Periodic review of goitre size and function and reassurance may well be all that is needed.

The commonest indication for some investigation is that the patient is conscious of the enlargement; in the Derbyshire survey there were two thyroid abnormalities left untreated to every one that was treated.

Carcinoma of thyroid is a rare disease but recent asymmetrical enlargement, a hard thyroid nodule — especially one associated with a diminished radioiodine uptake, some tenderness or pain, local pressure effects, such as a mild stridor or hoarseness usually absent even with very large goitres, or cervical lymphadenopathy are all valid indications for referral.

Thyroid pain is usually, if it is well localised, due to haemorrhage or, if it is diffuse, to autoimmune thyroiditis. A family history of goitre or associated autoimmune disorders such as pernicious anaemia, make this latter diagnosis more likely. Abnormal flocculation tests, a raised level of IgG, a high ESR, and high antibody titres are confirmatory investigations.

Acute generalised thyroid pain is likely to be due to De Quervain's thyroiditis — probably a viral infection associated with fever and systemic upset and running a variable clinical course. This settles with simple analgesics and without long-term sequelae although 10 mg prednisolone three times daily for a week or so, gradually tapered off, may be needed to control the more severe cases.

It must be remembered that occasionally goitres are drug-induced. Antithyroid drugs such as carbimazole, and iodides, phenylbutazone and tolbutamide may act as goitrogens. Goitrogens in food do not occur to any significant degree in the Western diet. Apart from iodine deficiency demonstrable by raised radioidine uptake, low plasma inorganic iodide and diminished iodide urinary excretion, the simple goitre should be associated with a euthyroid state, with a raised level of Thyroid Stimulating Hormone (TSH) and low levels of thyroxine (T4). Raised serum triiodothyronine (T3) can be seen in euthyroid goitre cases and iodine depletion can cause an increased serum T3/T4 ratio. In those goitrous subjects with a nodular or cystic goitre and with no evidence of iodine deficiency or autoimmune thyroiditis it is postulated that the goitre is due to a previous iodine-deficiency state that lasted long enough to make the goitre irreversible.

The clinical examination of the neck should be by inspection and then palpation. The patient should be asked to swallow with the head back and the thyroid — both lobes and isthmus — is felt with the patient sitting. The goitre may be soft, firm or hard and its consistency smooth, finely nodular or nodular. Calcified areas are rare and can be felt in some large and long-established goitres. The isthmus is felt as a firm band. Cystic enlargements restricted to the midline above the thyroid, are likely to be thyroglossal cysts. The lobes of the thyroid, as a very rough guide to the normal, should be no bigger than the terminal phalanx of the patient's thumb. Auscultation may demonstrate increased blood supply to the gland, especially if there is hyperthyroidism or the patient is on antithyroid drugs.

Management

Although individual cases may sometimes cause difficulty, the general management of simple goitre is straight-forward.

Hard or large nodules, especially if also a cold area on scan, should usually be subjected to surgery. Larger goitres are also best removed for cosmetic reasons unless the patient is unwilling or is for some reason unsuitable for surgery. Any associated thyroid dysfunction should of course be corrected. Large goitres are more often associated with toxic change but are so much rarer now than small goitres that these are more usually associated with thyrotoxicosis.

For all that most small simple goitres do not need any treatment save observation, thyroid function should usually be investigated as the euthyroid state may be less obvious in the presence of associated anxiety. Advice to take iodised salt to those living in endemic areas is especially important for poorer households not likely to eat adequate quantities of milk and fish; and this should form part of the family practitioner's routine antenatal advice for all that some commonly prescribed vitamin tablets contain potassium iodide in adequate dosage.

HYPOTHYROIDISM (MYXOEDEMA)

Aetiology

Hypothyroidism is the thyroid deficiency that can arise *de novo* or in association with endemic goitre, with dyshormonogenesis, with the use of goitrogens, or rarely with prolonged lithium therapy, with a history of autoimmune thyroiditis or Graves' disease, or as a consequence of thryoid maldevelopment, irradiation or surgery. It occurs yet more frequently iatrogenically as a complication of treatment since the introduction of radioactive isotopes, and also results from either therapeutic attacks on the pituitary gland or from primary pituitary disorders.

Data concerning the incidence of hypothyroidism is still fragmentary and unreliable. It is, like the other common thyroid disorders, most likely to affect females in middle or later life. There is a familial tendency. In the Derbyshire survey[2] hypothyroidism was diagnosed in 3 per cent of cases of past or present goitre and in a quarter of these cases it was a complication of treatment. This figure is probably too low; by how much we do not know.

Diagnosis

The clinical presentation varies, as with other thyroid disorders, from the gross and obvious to the subtle diagnostic problem or the subclinical case.

In the obvious case, the patient looks older than her years and moves and thinks slowly and clumsily. The voice is hoarse and its lack of modulation mirrors the emotional flatness of the patient. Tongue and vocal cords may be infiltrated by myxoedematous tissue, as may the skin, when typically it produces a non-pitting puffiness around the eyes. The skin is rough and has a characteristic yellowish tint. The hair is coarse and dry and often thin. This may be especially obvious in the eyebrows, and pubic and axillary hair also may be scanty. The patient does not like the cold, has gained weight and is constipated. The mental changes can be mistaken for arteriosclerosis or depression, but the occasional episodes of noisy aggression or frankly psychotic behaviour ('myxoedema madness') are well recognised in this disease. Less well recognised, perhaps, is the normal cerebration and the sense of humour retained in some quite severe cases.

Menses are heavy in the middle-aged but amenorrhoea is common in the younger patient. Vascular disturbances show as a tendency to angina, peripheral cyanosis, a liability to suffer from Raynaud's phenomenon, cardiomegaly, bradycardia, and a low voltage electrocardiograph — although a considerable minority will show normal tracings. Nervous signs may include perceptive deafness, carpal tunnel syndrome, non-specific aches and pains, or more rarely swollen tender muscles, epilepsy, drop attacks, cerebellar ataxia and peripheral neuropathy. Delayed relaxation of the Achilles tendon reflex may be a helpful and easily elicitied sign, but is most obvious in the severer cases. Pernicious anaemia may be an associated diagnosis, as may a straightforward iron-deficiency picture. Hypothyroidism must always be thought of in cases of coma, and this is especially so if hypothermia is also present.

Clearly, in a mild case presenting perhaps as fatigue, depression and faecal impaction it is helpful to have known the patient prior to the illness. Relatives and family doctors may both be handicapped by seeing the patient too frequently, so that the gradual transformation tends to be diagnosed late or by a stranger.

In children, too, the gross case may be obvious enough: delayed clearance of neonatal jaundice, failure to thrive, drowsiness, the protruding tongue and the umbilical hernia are classical but rare. More often one is faced with an underweight, short child who is not as bright as other members of the family. X-rays may show retardation of ossification and permit the date of onset of the hypothyroidism to be estimated. When in any doubt a paediatric opinion must be sought.

Investigations

Since lifelong replacement therapy will usually be indicated, all necessary investigations must be undertaken to confirm the clinical diagnosis. The protein bound iodine (PBI), T4 and T3 will typically be low and the serum TSH will be high. In borderline cases thyroidal radiodine response to TSH stimulation may be normal: but Thyrotrophin-Releasing Hormone (TRH) given in a dose of 200 μg intravenously after blood has been taken for basal TSH, PBI, T4 and T3 estimations will show no change in circulating hormone levels after three and six hours but an abnormally great elevation of TSH after 20 and 60 minutes. This is diagnostic and has made interesting phenomena such as the inverse ratio between thyroid activity and levels of cholesterol or creatine phosphokinase of little clinical significance.

Management

The treatment of hypothyroidism is to give l-thyroxine permanently in appropriate dosage. In patients with ischaemic heart disease this treatment may initiate or increase angina or cardiac decompensation. Older patients need lower doses than younger adults. A good routine is to begin therapy with 0.05 mg once daily and to increase the dosage by that amount every four weeks up to a usual maximum of 0.2 mg daily. Many patients are well controlled on 0.1 mg daily. A satisfactory clinical response should be associated with a normal serum TSH and this is used to monitor treatment. Pre-treatment photographs will demonstrate the effectiveness of therapy after six or twelve months.

L-triidothyronine has a more rapid and short-lived action and is useful intravenously in the management of myxoedema madness or whenever the rapid correction of myxoedema is necessary. Such emergency measures are dangerous however and should usually be carried out in special hospital-based units.

Myxoedema coma associated with hypothermia, and sometimes with pneumonia and pancreatitis, is still a very serious emergency with a high mortality.

HYPERTHYROIDISM

Aetiology

Hyperthyroidism has been found[5] in 0.3 per 1000 men and 1.9 per 1000 women. The Derbyshire Peak District Survey reported an overall incidence of

1.6 per cent and stated that thyrotoxicosis accounted for 20 per cent of all thyroid abnormalities. In the same population some form of thyroid surgery (for all causes) had been experienced by 1.4 per cent yet the medical treatment of thyrotoxicosis was commoner than surgical.

In iodine-deficiency areas some 15 per cent of cases of hyperthyroidism, although clinically identical, may be due to elevated levels, not of thyroxine (T4), but of circulating triiodothyronine (T3). This T3 toxicosis is especially liable to occur in patients with a past history of partial thyroidectomy or radioactive iodine therapy or with autonomous thyroid nodules.

When iodine therapy is given to goitrous subjects in an iodine-deficiency area, occasionally hyperthyroidism will ensue. This is known as the Jod-Basedow phenomenon.

Clinical Features

The clinical picture of thyrotoxicosis is well known but bears repetition. The condition occurs mainly in women and characteristically in early middle-age. The patient complains of nervousness, fatigue, palpitations, sweating and tremor. She eats voraciously and yet is losing weight. Her stools are unusually frequent. She tolerates warm weather badly. She cannot keep still. The periods are scanty or absent. There may be some thinning of the hair. There is some change of personality, usually emphasising irritability, fear, loss of confidence, obsessional traits, anxiety or depression. Latent diabetes may be made manifest and rarer presentations include a proximal myopathy, myasthenia gravis, osteoporosis and hypercalcaemia.

Very occasionally the overwhelming fatigue predominates to produce an apathetic thyrotoxicosis in which the laboratory tests confirm hyperthyroidism yet the patient more resembles the hypothyroid state.

The cardiovascular system, especially in the elderly patient, can bear the brunt of the toxic changes with angina, cardiac failure, sinus tachycardia, and atrial fibrillation, either paroxysmal or permanent, and difficult to control with the standard digoxin dosage. All such cases demand urgent investigation of thyroid function.

On examination the patient is flushed, warm, sweating and restless. The doctor's palm placed on the out-stretched finger-tips of the patient is the best way of feeling the fine, rapid, hyperthyroid tremor. The pulse is fast and bounding and the systolic pressure is somewhat raised.

The thyroid may or may not be obviously enlarged and nodules may or may not be palpable. A systolic bruit, accompanied sometimes by a thrill, may be heard by lightly placing the stethoscope on the thyroid isthmus. This sign may be absent and, as so often, may be present only in the more florid case.

Eye signs may be absent but are important enough to be described in some detail.

The eyes can be more prominent than in any high myope. The exophthalmos may be asymmetrical or unilateral in ophthalmic Graves' disease, in which eye signs are unaccompanied by any other clinical manifestations of hyperthyroidism; but in the usual case of Graves' disease exophthalmos, when present, is symmetrical. The sign is caused by the infiltration of the orbital contents by lymphocytes, fat, water and mucopolysaccharide, and so can be mimicked by any orbital space-occupying lesion.

The eye signs may persist long after the successful exhibition of effective treatment for the thyroid disorder.

Lid retraction is diagnosed when the patient looks straight ahead and sclera can be seen between the corneal limbus and the upper lid. This is characteristic of Graves' disease when present at all angles of gaze.

Lid-lag can be seen when the patient's eyes follow the doctor's finger as it moves vertically downwards and sclera again is visible between corneal limbus and upper lid.

Lid retraction may prevent full lid apposition and so lead to corneal ulceration, keratitis, or other serious complications. Such complications may be further associated with ophthalmoplegia – diplopia due to extrinsic muscular palsy – or to malignant exophthalmos in which the ophthalmoplegia is combined with pain, conjunctival chemosis, lid oedema, and visual impairment that can proceed to blindness. Such cases merit urgent admission to hospital.

Rarer signs of hyperthyroidism include pretibial myxoedema – a localised thickening of skin and subcutaneous tissue typically on the shins but possibly also on the face – occurring in some 5 per cent of cases of Graves' disease.

Thyroid acropachy (resembling clubbing but without any increased blood supply, and with a characteristic soap-bubble X-ray appearance denoting new bone deposition in affected phalanges and metacarpals), splenomegaly, thymic enlargement, generalised lymph-node enlargement and vitiligo can also be associated.

Diagnosis

It is clear that in diagnosing mild cases of thyroid dysfunction many factors are involved and computerised diagnosis has successfully competed against the acumen of experienced clinicians. It is hardly surprising that among family practitioners' referrals of possible cases of thryotoxicosis a substantial number are found to be suffering solely from anxiety or other psychiatric states[4]. Hyperthyroidism and psychiatric disorders can closely resemble each other but the thyrotoxic patient tends to be older and to lack a significant past psychiatric history.

As a diagnostic aid the Newcastle Thyrotoxicosis Index has been found helpful and is reproduced in Table 20.1.

Table 20.1   Newcastle Thyrotoxicosis Index
Reproduced with permission from Hall, R. *et al.*, (1974)[4]

Item	Grade	Score
Age of onset	15—24	0
	25—34	+4
	35—44	+8
	45—54	+12
	55 and over	+16
Psychological precipitant	Present	−5
	Absent	0
Frequent checking	Present	−3
	Absent	0
Severe anticipatory anxiety	Present	−3
	Absent	0
Increased appetite	Present	+5
	Absent	0
Goitre	Present	+3
	Absent	0
Thyroid bruit	Present	+18
	Absent	0
Exophthalmos	Present	+9
	Absent	0
Lid retraction	Present	+2
	Absent	0
Hyperkinesis	Present	+4
	Absent	0
Fine finger tremor	Present	+7
	Absent	0
Pulse-rate	Over 90 per min	+16
	80—90 per min	+8
	Under 80 per min	0

Euthyroid range −11 to +23.   Doubtful range +24 to +39.
Toxic range +40 to +80

The diagnosis of thyrotoxicosis in pregnancy can be difficult but the condition usually remits, and relapses only when the pregnancy is over. If treatment is indicated, this should probably be by carbimazole. Over-treatment may produce a neonatal goitre. Under-treatment may permit neonatal Graves' disease. This is a rare condition typically associated with a euthyroid mother who recently has had a partial thyroidectomy for a hyperthyroid state associated with high levels of LATS. As LATS is an IgG molecule it has the characteristic half-life of some four weeks and the disease will tend spontaneously to remit after that time as the transplacental passage of LATS has ceased. In spite of this anticipated remission, more severe cases who are thriving badly and may show restlessness, tachycardia, cardiac failure and some eye signs should be treated by half (approximately) of the adult dose of carbimazole. In confirming the diagnosis it is to be remembered that in the first week or so of life the PBI is abnormally high so other tests must also be used and indeed the whole situation calls for expert paediatric management. These cases are usually born to mothers whose Graves' disease was associated with localised myxoedema, since these are the patients who tend to produce the highest LATS levels.

Laboratory Investigation

The laboratory investigation of thyroid function has changed over the last few years. It is now possible to diagnose far more precisely the actual stage of dysfunction that is producing the clinical disorder.

The natural tendency is for physicians to use the more recent, elaborate and expensive tests and to use less enthusiastically the inexpensive and longer-established procedures.

It is perhaps pertinent to remark that this is not always justifiable. The simple, often automated estimation PBI can be a major help in the confirmation of the great majority of cases of thyrotoxicosis. There are limitations to the accuracy of the test. Iodides, ingested perhaps with cough mixtures, or incorporated in shampoos or handcreams, or as a result of radio-opaque investigations months before, can cause a false high reading. Certain drugs such as phenytoin or salicylate or prolonged phenothiazine therapy may compete with thyroxine for the protein-binding sites and so produce a false low PBI reading. The protein level is raised by oestrogens or pregnancy, and lowered by androgens or in patients with defective renal or hepatic function (hypoprotein-aemic states). The commonest drugs affecting the PBI level are the oral contraceptives. But when these facts are remembered, the PBI is still one of the most valuable tests routinely available to the family practitioner.

To confirm the diagnosis of Graves' disease a second and confirmatory test of thyroid function is highly desirable. A frequently used routine investigation is the free thyroxine index, commercially available as Thyopac-3 (Amersham).

The thyroxine-binding plasma proteins allow only tiny amounts of thyroid hormone to circulate in the free or unbound form. The major protein with the greatest affinity for thyroxine is known as thyroxine-binding globulin (TBG). The residual binding capacity is a measure of unoccupied binding sites on TBG and allied proteins. When labelled T3 or T4 is added to serum the amount bound by the protein will be proportional to the level of the previously circulating thyroxine. Addition of a resin or other substance that adsorbs the residual unbound thyroid hormone permits this to be measured. In the commercially available Thyropac-3 test low values will be observed in Graves' disease and high levels in myxoedema. To avoid misinterpretations due to plasma protein fluctuations the product of serum PBI or T4 and the residual binding capacity gives us the Free Thyroxine Index — one of the most reliable simple tests of thyroid function and correlating well with the Effective Thyroxine Ratio which similarly combines serum thyroxine levels and Residual Binding Capacity.

Massive steroid dosages, major endocrine disorders, and severe illnesses such as acute porphyria, can gravely affect thyroid function tests.

Other well-established tests such as the T3 suppression test may well become obsolescent because of the value of newer investigations using TRH — a synthetic form of the hypothalamic thyrotrophin releasing hormone. Although the TRH test may be affected by oestrogens, thyroid or antithyroid substances, steroids, theophylline and levodopa, this substance seems likely to provide a major advance in thyroid investigation. For example, a normal TSH response after the intravenous injection of 200 μg of TRH effectively excludes hyperthyroidism and its value in the diagnosis of hypothyroidism is mentioned in that section.

The laboratory investigation of ophthalmic Graves' disease is another valuable field for TRH and has shown that this syndrome can be associated with a euthyroid state, or hyperthyroidism, or hypothyroidism that may require treatment[6].

Many patients with ophthalmic Graves' disease who have an impaired or absent response to TRH have high triiodothyronine (T3) levels and may have therefore the condition of subclinical T3 toxicosis. This can be a relatively stable state which does not necessarily need treatment. More usually, it will be remembered, high T3 levels are associated with clinical hyperthyroidism and in hypothyroidism T3 levels are low or normal. T3 levels can thus be helpful in monitoring the effectiveness of antithyroid therapy but accurate T3 estimations are not routinely available from all laboratories yet.

Other conditions with an absent or impaired response to TRH include euthyroid (treated) Graves' disease, some nodular goitres, pituitary disorders or patients under treatment for Parkinson's disease with levodopa.

Management

Once the diagnosis of clinical hyperthyroidism has been made, the appropriate therapy should be started. If in elderly patients the laboratory diagnosis of hyperthyroidism is clear but the clinical condition does not bear this out, some doctors will tend to defer treatment and keep the patient under observation. This can be dangerous. Routine investigations may rarely reveal a high PBI level months before the clinical diagnosis catches up with this, and the patient may then present as gravely ill with uncontrolled cardiac failure. It is perhaps more appropriate to delay therapy, if we must, in less vulnerable, younger patients. The dangers of cardiac failure in the older patient make it desirable to treat the laboratory diagnosis and to forestall the development of the clinical state.

Surgery

It is extraordinary that such a crude procedure — in physiological terms — as partial thyroidectomy should be so successful. To cut out part of the thyroid gland because it is over-active still gains very good results, even in an age of such medical sophistication as to permit the treatment of acromegaly by oral medication. In many areas partial thyroidectomy is the treatment of choice for all who are good surgical risks.

Patients should be rendered euthyroid before surgery by antithyroid drugs and rested for a week or two before surgery while potassium iodide 5 mg three times daily is taken. This routine has made virtually extinct the dreaded complication of earlier decades — the thyroid crisis. This presented with hyperpyrexia and an acute hyperthyroid state early in the post-operative period. It was commoner in less well-managed patients or those who had an acute infection. Anti-thyroid drugs, iodides, sedatives, intravenous fluids, antibiotics and sympathetic blocking agents such as propranolol will usually control this serious, but now very rare, condition.

Tetany may occur shortly after the operation and is due to surgical interference with the blood supply of the parathyroid glands. Calcium salts may be needed for a short time, but adjustment often takes place over the months and only in rare cases is lifelong treatment with calcium required.

A husky voice due to recurrent laryngeal nerve trauma is also a most uncommon complication.

It may well be, however, that the fine reputation of this surgical procedure is due in some small part to the poor quality of long-term follow-up. A recent report[7] on patients treated by partial thyroidectomy showed 6 per cent with recurrent thyrotoxicosis and 36 per cent as hypothyroid. Post-operative hypothyroidism is commonest in those with a high titre of microsomal antibodies, so that this investigation should be part of the routine in the selection of surgical cases. Since 25 per cent of these patients will be hypothyroid within a year of effective surgery, alternative modalities of treatment should be preferred.

Surgery will remain for some time the treatment of choice for thyrotoxic patients with large goitres, for those who have had relapses, poor control or other problems with antithyroid drugs, and who are too young for radioiodine, and for those who are fit and prefer surgery to prolonged drug therapy.

Radio-active Iodine

The most trivial and comfortable treatment, so far as the patient is concerned, is with the radio-active iodine isotopes. The dangers of consequent malignant disease have not been confirmed in older patients and the treatment is cautiously avoided in younger patients. A major problem with this treatment is the overriding need for long-term follow-up. Despite increasing refinements in technique, we must still cater for 10 per cent of myxoedema one year after treatment and no less than 40 per cent a decade later. Replacement therapy with thyroxine is simple but is far more dangerous when myxoedema is well-established and associated with angina. The long term follow-up, investigation and diagnosis must be part of the interest and responsibility of the family practitioner even if computerised hospital follow-up is arranged.

Anti-thyroid Drugs

In the majority of hyperthyroid patients under 50 years of age many physicians would recommend treatment with anti-thyroid drugs and at the moment the drug of first choice is carbimazole. Potassium perchlorate is not suitable since it can produce aplastic anaemia or a nephrotic syndrome, and because of its iodine-blocking action it must not be employed before thyroid surgery. The thiouracils seem to be less popular than carbimazole.

The routine dosage is to give 40 mg of carbimazole in 3 or 4 divided doses each day for a month or two and then gear the future dosage to the clinical response. Daily maintenance dosage is usually in the 15—20 mg range. Marked thyroid enlargement means over-treatment, failure to respond means a wrong diagnosis or an unreliable patient who is not taking the medication as prescribed. Treatment if effective can be gradually phased out after some 18 months and the patient kept carefully under review. Some physicians use sympathetic blocking agents like propranolol if symptoms like sweating or tachycardia are troublesome. A dose of 40 mg three times daily is usually appropriate and will help with symptomatic control while thyroid investigations are being pursued, without of course affecting thyroid function tests.

Patients on carbimazole should be instructed to report any significant malaise, sore throat or rashes. Some clinics use thyroxine concurrently since this makes the carbimazole dosage less critical in avoiding hypothyroidism.

Only about half of patients who respond well to carbimazole will remain in permanent remission. These figures need to be compared with the 25 per cent of spontaneous remissions and indeed the 10 per cent mortality encountered before the days of antithyroid drugs. Myxoedema also has been recorded after antithyroid drugs and this emphasises yet again the need for lifelong follow-up.

Eye Symptoms

The treatment of eye symptoms is in most cases simply that of the underlying thyroid disease. Grittiness can be helped by methyl cellulose eyedrops, conjunctivitis by local antibiotics, and oedema by diuretics. For severe lid retraction one drop of 5 per cent guanethidine eye-drops night and morning is helpful, but resistant cases may have to come to tarsorrhaphy also. For resistant congestive ophthalmopathy 60–80 mg of prednisolone daily should effect rapid improvement or the surgical decompression of the orbit will be necessary.

Skin Myxoedema

Localised skin myxoedema responds well to high-potency steroids under polythene occlusive dressings but the intralesional injection of steroids will give more rapid but more localised results.

Acknowledgment

I am most grateful to Professor D. S. Munro who kindly looked over, with many helpful suggestions, the preliminary version of this chapter.

References

1. Turton, R. H. J. (1933). *Proc. roy. Soc. Med.* **26**, 33.
2. West Derbyshire Medical Society (1966). *Lancet* ii, 959.
3. Kilpatrick, R., Miln, J. S., Rushbrooke, M., Wilson, E. S. B., Wilson, G. M. (1963). *Brit. med. J.* 1, 29.
4. Hall, R., Anderson, J., Smart, G. A. and Besser, M. (1974). *Fundamentals of Clinical Endocrinology* 2nd edition. (London: Pitman Medical).
5. Logan, W. P. D. and Cushion, A. A. (1958). *Morbidity Statistics from General Practice* Vol. 1 (General). (London: H.M.S.O.).
6. Alexander, L. (1974). *Update* 9, 813.
7. Hedley, A. J., Ross, I. P., Beck, J. S., Donald, D., Albert-Recht, P., Michie, W., and Crooks, J. (1971). *Brit. med. J.* 2, 458.

21

Anaemia

J. Fry

INTRODUCTION

Anaemia is but a symptom or sign of some other underlying disorder. It may be the result of obvious or hidden blood loss. It may be due to a fault in blood formation or it may result from destruction of blood cells in the body. Whatever the underlying cause, the discovery of anaemia, or its suspicion by the physician, is the signal for prompt action to investigate and probe further to determine the true nature and causes of the condition. It is bad medical practice to treat merely the end product, the anaemia, without establishing the correct diagnosis and putting right, where possible, the cause.

A sense of perspective is necessary. Anaemia is a common condition. It is likely that in a family practice of 2500 persons, the physician may expect to discover 25—40 new cases of anaemia each year, providing that he is alert to its possibilities and is prepared to investigate likely cases and to take steps to screen persons who may be particularly 'at risk'.

Of these 25—40 new cases almost all will be iron-deficiency hypochromic anaemias. Most will be associated with some obvious or hidden blood loss from the female reproductive tract or the gastro-intestinal tract in both sexes. Other types such as megaloblastic and hyperchromic anaemias or haemolytic anaemias will be rare.

In the same practice the physician may expect to diagnose a new case of pernicious anaemia or some other type of megaloblastic anaemia only once every 5 years or so and to discover a haemolytic type of anaemia only two or three times in his whole professional lifetime. Of course if he works in an area where there is an increased prevalence of some genetic abnormalities of haemoglobin, such as sickle cell anaemia, then the proportion of these will be greater.

Leukaemia is rare and in the same size practice population only one new case will occur every ten years. Myelomatosis is even less common and Hodgkin's disease (lymphadenoma) will also occur about once every decade.

It is necessary to state at this stage, and it will be referred to again later, that anaemia is one of the conditions that exist undiagnosed in most communities. In other words, although the physician may be alert and active in his approach and pick up those cases of anaemia that present themselves to him, it is likely that there are as many undiagnosed and untreated in his practice community who do not seek medical advice or who, if they do, have not yet been diagnosed. This deficit of undiagnosed cases is an argument for intensive screening of populations for anaemia.

The *effects* of anaemia are those of both the anaemia and of the underlying causal condition. The classical symptoms of pallor, tiredness and irritability are so non-specific and common in so many other non-anaemic patients that they should not be accepted as specific for 'anaemia', but should merely act as alerters for investigative action. It is a disappointing experience for the physician to find that having had the satisfaction of diagnosing and correcting anaemia in a patient to be faced still with some symptoms of tiredness, irritability and depression in the same patient.

EPIDEMIOLOGY

Three special periods of incidence should be noted. First, in infancy 'anaemia' is not uncommon and it is interesting to note that it is only in this age period that the incidence is higher in males than in females. In the second period, in women between 20–50, anaemia is particularly frequent. Thirdly, in both sexes, anaemia is frequent in the elderly.

CLINICAL GROUPS

There are many classifications of anaemia depending whether an aetiological or haematological viewpoint is taken. In practice the most useful classification is one based on the presenting clinical picture. I find that it is helpful to define five groups in which the clinical approach is somewhat different.

1. Anaemias in infancy and childhood.
2. Anaemias in pregnancy.
3. Anaemias in women in active reproductive period (20–50 years)
4. Anaemias in the elderly.
5. Special types.

In each group there may occur a variety of specific types of anaemia.

Infancy and Childhood

The physiological variations in the blood findings in infancy must be appreciated and understood before a diagnosis of anaemia is made.

The normal infant has a high level of haemoglobin at birth (17 g/100 ml). The level falls after the first week and by 3 months of age it is approximately 11.5 g/100 ml. This is a normal fall and is uninfluenced by iron therapy. The haemoglobin level remains low during the first year of life (below 12 g/100 ml) and then rises slowly to reach 14 g/100 ml by the age of 10 years.

However, true anaemia does occur and is not infrequent even in developed and affluent societies. Anaemia in infancy and childhood is very frequent in developing societies and is more prevalent in the lower social groups in a developed state.

Iron deficiency anaemia is the most common form of anaemia in infancy and childhood and at this period the most likely cause is not blood loss but a defect of blood formation. The diet is deficient in iron. This is particularly likely in bottle-fed babies, but it will occur in breast-fed babies whose mothers are anaemic and low in iron reserves. Premature and small babies are a special at-risk group.

The next most frequent type of anaemia is the anaemia associated with haemolytic disease of the new-born from the presence of Rh antibodies. It is a condition that is preventable and one that the physician should be prepared for with sound antenatal care and supervision.

Rare are the other types of anaemia in childhood. Leukaemia must be mentioned because the child often presents with pallor and anaemia is found. Hereditary spherocytosis, thalassaemia (Cooley's anaemia), sickle-cell anaemia and other hereditary haemoglobinopathies are very rare. So are glucose-6-phosphate dehydrogenase deficiency, lead poisoning and iatrogenic aplastic anaemias.

Less uncommon are those secondary anaemias associated with general poor health, anorexia, malnutrition and renal and respiratory diseases. Blood loss from trauma, infestations and haemorrhagic disorders are other possible causes.

The clinical presentation is most often a non-thriving infant, although sometimes he may be plump from over-feeding with carbohydrates or even starved with kwashiorkor. Pallor is the striking feature and should lead to a blood investigation. It should be recalled however that many healthy and normal children with fair complexions are pale but not anaemic.

Anaemia in Pregnancy

Anaemia in pregnancy is fully discussed in Chapter 16, page 312.

Anaemias in women in 20—50 age group

This is the most frequent clinical group of anaemias in practice. They come on quietly and without warning. There are no specific symptoms but traditionally they are associated with the 'one degree under feeling', with general malaise, tiredness, irritability, breathlessness, sore tongue, pallor and even oedema of the legs. However, many women who are found to be anaemic present no symptoms and the finding is often incidental.

It is surprising what severe degrees of anaemia, below 5 g/100 ml, may be compatible with the normal duties of a mother and housewife, providing that the progression of the anaemia has been gradual and prolonged.

Anaemias in these women are most likely to be the result of some excessive blood loss. The usual cause is menstrual bleeding, but bleeding piles, a bleeding hiatus hernia or peptic ulcer, or regular aspirin consumption also may be responsible. An additional factor is the poor iron-deficient diet that many of these women take.

An important feature of these anaemias is the tendency for them to recur after successful therapy. The reason is that the underlying cause persists, and the usual cause is menstruation. The lesson to learn is that these women need to continue extra iron supplement until well past the menopause.

Anaemia in the Elderly

The elderly are particularly liable to anaemia. There is a mixture of multiple causes, as with most diseases in this age period.

As at all other ages, iron deficiency anaemia is the most common type secondary to blood loss from the gastro-intestinal tract and to deficient diet. In addition there are many diseases that may lead to anaemia that become more likely in the elderly. Thus cancer of all types may lead to cachexia anaemia, urinary infections, malabsorption from rare causes, aspirin and other drugs such as phenyl butazone and the anticoagulants may cause bleeding from the gut. Rheumatoid arthritis and other collagen diseases, liver diseases and hypo-thyroidism are other causes. Pernicious anaemia, myelomatosis and leukaemia, are more common in the elderly than at other ages, but are still very rare in normal practice. Then as part of a deficient diet scurvy and folate deficiency may lead to anaemia and in certain areas gut infestations and malaria are other causes.

Even more than at other times the diagnosis of anaemia in an old person must lead to a full social and personal assessment as well as clinical investigations to decide on the cause and management of the anaemia.

Anaemia in the elderly is also discussed in Chapter 24, page 588.

Special Clinical Presentations

This group is an artificial one but is useful as a reminder of certain clinical situations that should require extra care and attention from the physician.

The *sudden and unexpected faint* in an apparently healthy person may be an early feature of a sudden and severe internal haemorrhage. This may occur with a bleeding peptic ulcer, a ruptured ectopic pregnancy or a spontaneous rupture of a pathological spleen.

Angina on effort has been the first feature of anaemia in a number of men and women in my experience. The angina often disappears once the anaemia has been corrected and does not recur for many years. It is important to check the haemoglobin levels of all new cases of angina.

Post gastrectomy patients and those with small gut resections must have annual blood checks because anaemia, from malabsorption, is common in this group. Most of these are iron deficiency anaemias but some may be megaloblastic anaemias from vitamin B12 or folic acid deficiencies.

In this group should be included patients with a past history of hiatus hernia, duodenal ulcer and even bleeding piles. They are at risk to develop anaemia.

Overseas travellers particularly the young who travel rough to the Far East and Africa may return with a malabsorption syndrome and steatorrhoea, gut infestations or chronic malaria that may cause anaemia.

'Odd persons' such as the vegans on deficient diets, recluses of all sorts, self-medicators with aspirin are others at risk.

DIAGNOSIS AND ASSESSMENT

Suspicion of the possibility of anaemia must be confirmed by measuring the haemoglobin levels and the red-cell indices. In addition the appearance of the blood cells on a smear is necessary and this should include the white-blood cells and platelets. The levels of these cells is now part of the standard blood report from any good laboratory.

Unless the practitioner works alone and away from any medical centre it is now most economical and most reliable to carry out blood tests in a laboratory equipped with modern machines. It is no longer possible for the practitioner to carry out his own haematology unless he is an unusual enthusiast or research worker.

The practitioner should from the blood report be able to make a diagnosis of anaemia and the most likely type. For a more definitive diagnosis of a macrocytic or haemolytic anaemia or one that is non-responsive to treatment the patient should be referred to a haematologist. It may be necessary to measure vitamin B12, folic acid, serum iron levels and to carry out a bone marrow examination.

As noted, the diagnosis of anaemia is a first step and once made a full clinical examination of the patient is required including a pelvic examination. In addition it may be necessary to carry out barium contrast media radiological examinations of the upper and lower gastro-intestinal tract, a chest radiograph, urine examinations, tests for occult blood in the faeces.

In summary the modern practitioner must have access to a reliable laboratory. With this facility he should by well able to confirm the diagnosis of anaemia and to treat the great majority of the common types. He must however be certain of the complete and full diagnosis in clinical, social and community terms. The patient may require much more help and follow-up than the mere prescription of pills or injections. He or she may need assistance with food and diet and help with life in general.

TREATMENT

The primary treatment of anaemia is to treat the primary cause wherever and whenever it is discovered. It must be stated honestly that in about one-third of the cases of anaemia in our practice we have found no obvious cause, but that response to oral iron has been satisfactory.

The specific treatment of the anaemia depends on the type. Thus, iron is given for iron deficiency anaemias, folic acid when such deficiency is proven and vitamin B12 when this deficiency has been established. Blunderbuss poly-pharmacy is not only bad practice, it leads to considerable confusion in further assessment and follow-up.

Failure of treatment is usually the result of failure to continue with the treatment once the patient feels better. As noted, it may be necessary to continue with iron, folic acid and certainly with vitamin B12 in pernicious anaemia, for long periods and even for the patient's lifetime.

Iron Preparations   Oral iron is best and simplest when iron therapy is required. Ferrous iron is better absorbed than ferric iron. Effective doses should contain 200 mg of ferrous iron per day.

There are many oral iron preparations and the physician can select his own choice on his own experience. It is always wise to start with the cheapest, namely, ferrous sulphate tablets.

Side effects are not infrequent. They affect the gastro-intestinal tract with symptoms such as nausea, vomiting, colic, constipation or diarrhoea.

Iron must be given until the haemoglobin level returns to normal and if the primary cause has been corrected therapy can then stop but follow-up is essential to detect relapse.

Parenteral iron is rarely necessary. Intra-muscular injections are painful and intravenous injections may cause alarming local and general reactions. Parenteral iron is indicated only when there is proven malabsorption of iron.

Blood Transfusion   Transfusion may be required with severe anaemia and especially when it is of recent and acute onset.

Vitamin B12 This is indicated only for pernicious anaemia and other rare types of malabsorption. It must be continued for life. Given in the form of hydroxocobalamin, once established a maintenance dose of 1000 µg every 2—3 months is adequate.

Folic Acid This is specific therapy for proven folate deficiency. Folic acid in 5—15 mg dosage is adequate for maintenance.

FOLLOW-UP

Once therapy has commenced a regular follow-up programme must be organised with frequent blood tests until the blood picture returns to normal.

In most cases a twice a year blood test is sufficient but defaulters must be contacted.

At Risk Register

It is important to have an 'at-risk' register of patients who have been diagnosed as anaemic and who are under therapy or have ceased therapy, in order to ensure their regular attendance for supervision.

In addition there are patients with certain conditions that should be added to the register since they are specially at risk to develop anaemia. These are any who have had a gastrectomy or small gut resections, chronic renal disease, hypothyroidism, premature infants, rheumatoid arthritics, and social isolates and food fadists.

SCREENING

In theory there appears to be a good case for regular mass population screening for anaemia but in actual practice it is much better to be aware of the possibility of anaemia and to concentrate on selected known cases at follow-up and on special at-risk groups.

22

Emotional Disorders

C. A. H. Watts

NORMAL EMOTIONAL RESPONSES

Life is full of problems, and the art of living is to find solutions for difficulties, or ways and means of circumventing them. The healthy man enjoys working on a problem, hence the popularity of bridge, crosswords and jigsaw puzzles. One important aspect of the doctor's job is to help people to develop this outlook. There are at least three main points of contact between the patient and the doctor when it is easy and natural for the family practitioner to assume the role of teacher. Premarriage guidance has much to recommend it. At no time in life are young people more receptive, and it is important for them to recognise that the doctor is there to consult on problems other than those of healing. Instruction can be carried out in groups, especially if there is a cooperative clergyman in the area, who can both collect the class together, and share in the teaching. The second point of contact is the antenatal clinic. Childbirth can be made easier for the mother by her understanding of what is going to happen when she comes into labour, and how she can best cooperate with the nurse or doctor who will be attending her. Many unnecessary fears and difficulties raised by 'old wives' tales' can also be dealt with, and a defence against such stories created for the future. Well baby clinics are the third meeting point where doctor and mother can discuss problems rather than diseases. This kind of contact can be extended to other groups of people, for instance by courses on retirement, or well geriatric clinics. All this work is a very useful part of preventive medicine. In such meetings the objective should be to make the patient more independent. People should be encouraged to air their problems and be shown ways in which they can solve them for themselves.

The time factor, of course, imposes a limit on the hours we can spend in this kind of exercise, or indeed in our dealings with the psychoneurotic patients who, in spite of our best educational efforts, will appear in large numbers at the surgery. We all get anxious and depressed at times, and the family doctor just cannot be a parent figure to console every time there is an unkind twist to fortune. Happily the public can and do carry a lot of this burden themselves. Never the less one of the functions of the family practitioner is to be available to patients with problems, both psychic and somatic. He is in a position to decide whether the matter is in fact serious or trivial, although it must always be remembered that problems which appear trifling to the doctor may be a heavy burden to the patient. In this situation care must be taken to see that the patient does not lose face, and this is not always easy. A good deal of tact may be needed in explaining the situation and in allaying the fears of the patient, if he is not going to be made to feel foolish. Doctors who have all been taught anatomy, physiology and the basic sciences of the job, need to remind themselves that often the layman is completely unaware of what is normal. The sight of tastebuds on the back of the tongue can frighten the life out of a young woman with a hangover as, after a heavy night, she gazes at her tongue in the mirror and sees them for the first time. The young husband who during sex play discovered his wife's cervix caused considerable consternation. He was sure that she had a lump in her pelvis. Such minor problems are common and the only treatment necessary is reassurance, but once again this must be given without loss of face.

Emotional upsets are still viewed by most people as inferior to clear cut organic disease. Our patients have got this message loud and clear, and they usually present us with a respectable physical symptom. It is so much easier to complain of some ache or pain, rather than feelings of anxiety or depression which are often very hard to describe. Traumatic situations can be just as upsetting as the first sight of taste buds, and once more the layman can be unaware of this. A young childless woman came to see me because of a headache. After a very brief discussion it turned out that another pair who were close friends, had been given indefinite accommodation until their own house, a bit further down the road, was completed. The situation was far more stressful than the patient had allowed for, and the love-hate relationship with her friends was the real problem. To learn that such feelings were really within normal limits came as a great relief, and this was all the treatment she needed. Like the lower animals man has his basic instincts of foodseeking, sex, aggression and flight from danger. All these have become so modified and disguised that often normality goes unrecognised. Sexual problems can cause a great deal of unnecessary suffering. There are young people, widows and widowers whose consciences are tortured by guilt feelings over masturbation, because they do not appreciate that this is a normal response to certain situations. The young man who is shy of women, but enjoys mens' company, may be plagued by the idea that he is a homosexual, that he is going to miss out in life. The fact that we are all bisexual animals, able to appreciate the attractions of our own sex as well as enjoying the satisfying differences between the two can come as a surprise and a relief. It is very bad advice to tell such a person to get married and that this will solve his problems, but it is sound advice to urge him to seek mixed company, so that he may well put himself in the way of finding a bride. An open ear to problems such as these can save the patient much suffering, take up little of the doctor's time, and it prevents the escalation of small troubles into significant illness.

ANXIETY

Every illness carries with it a quota of anxiety. This may be a very minor problem such as whether it is wise to go to the office with a streaming cold which could infect others, or it may be a serious worry as when the sufferer has a fear of cancer hidden away. All illness carries with it two diagnoses. The patient usually has his own idea as to what is wrong. If the doctor's diagnosis confirms what the patient thinks, and the problem has no serious implications, then the consultation will be straight forward and successful. If, on the other hand the two diagnoses are very different, there will be little progress until the patient's fears have been uncovered and dealt with. If the patient fears he has a cancer, he is most unlikely to reveal this directly, or to use that word which is too terrifying to mention. He may admit to having thought 'there was something serious the matter with him.' It is of little use to brush this idea aside casually by saying he has nothing to worry about, or worse still, by telling him there is nothing wrong. He must be encouraged to reveal his fears so that they can be discussed before he is specifically reassured. After a very short time in practice a doctor can tell intuitively the organic case from the psychoneurotic. He must also learn to detect when the patient is satisfied with the interview in much the same way as an actor knows when he is holding his audience.

There is a strange paradox evident in modern medicine. As our tools become more efficient and powerful, our patients tend to become more, not less, anxious than they used to be. Just because we have so many potent and helpful remedies, man seems far less tolerant of pain and more prone to anxiety. The dental surgeon is a frightening person to the majority, in spite of the fact that most of the pain and discomfort has been taken out of dentistry. Thirty years ago there was always that fearful agony of suspense for all concerned while the family waited for the crisis in a case of pneumonia. This delay was accepted and endured by the doctor and the relatives as a painful but normal part of life. Today if an illness lasts for more than a day, anxiety tends to emerge and it may become excessive. The victim of glandular fever or a painful herpes zoster can become quite a problem because there is no rapid cure for the symptoms. The fact that the illness can go on for weeks or months may give rise to incredulous concern in the patient or his family. Modern man almost demands an instant cure. Thanks to the mass media, people today know a lot more about medicine than they did 50 years ago; they want to know what is going on and they have a right to question their doctors. On the whole they are very reasonable people and are willing to accept that the doctor has no crystal ball in which he can divine an accurate diagnosis every time, but they resent being hurried, hoodwinked or humiliated. Every patient should leave the surgery feeling that his problem has been taken seriously. A very good safeguard against resentment is to ask the patient at the end of the interview 'And is there anything else?' The doctor must be prepared to exert himself to win the confidence of the patient. To undress for a physical examination is embarrassing for most people, and it is just as difficult and unpleasant for a patient to unburden himself of worries. He cannot be expected to trot out all his fears and problems without a good deal of encouragement.

Diagnosis

Once it has been decided that the patient has a significant emotional problem, then it is important to take a detailed history. The story of the first attack is important, and the date should be noted. The symptoms should be recorded in detail, care should be taken to see nothing is missed out. The patient should be questioned about possible sources of worry in the home, at work, financial difficulties, sex problems and a note should be made of the family history. Here the family practitioner working in the community has a great advantage over any consultant in that he often starts off by knowing a lot about the patient and his background. There is a man in the village who is doing well in life. His mother is a strange character who is so afflicted with body odour that the shops all serve her first, and she is excluded from the public houses. This obviously imposes a strain on him; he has a problem which he would be reluctant to reveal to anyone. However when the subject was raised by one of my partners he was very relieved to know that others understood and sympathised with his difficulties. The process of history taking will occupy a complete session, and if the doctor has acquired the confidence of the patient, the examination can usually be left until the next consultation. Patients rarely resent this if it is suggested that everything possible has been done in one session, and that the sick person must make another appointment for a check up. He is asked to bring a specimen of urine which is passed after the big meal of the day. Occasionally an immediate examination is necessary if the patient is so obviously worked up about his problems. I was called out one Sunday morning to see a young woman who complained of pelvic discomfort. She had a vaginal discharge, and it was obvious to me that she felt she had a cancer or something terrible. When I put it to her bluntly she admitted to this fear. I told her husband to bring her along to the surgery that afternoon where I could do a cervical smear and a much better pelvic examination than at home. In fact I found that she had lost a tampax swab in her vagina, and I was able to produce an instant cure, something which happens all too rarely in medicine. The patient was profuse in her apologies for having been so negligent and stupid, and she needed a good deal of face-saving reassurance that her fears in the circumstances had not been unreasonable, nor her call unjustified. I told her that the incident had in fact made my day, as it was rarely possible for a family practitioner to cure 'a cancer' so easily!

The intensely anxious patient is an emergency and every effort should be made to solve the problem, or at least relieve the tension of the situation as soon as possible. Usually, as has been said, the examination can be delayed, but when it does happen it must be thorough covering every possible system. A normal ESR is reassuring. The attitude of the patient during the process is of interest. The anxious patient tends to keep asking questions, and cranes her neck to try and see what the blood pressure machine is recording. If any special investigations are necessary, these must be carried out before the diagnosis can be finalized. If in the end all is negative, the patient should be told that there is no organic disease, and that the symptoms are due to stress. This statement must be made in a positive way so that it sounds respectable and reasonable. The patient must be made to feel that she was right to see the doctor about such troubles. If she is obviously upset by the suggestion, and says such things as, 'So there is nothing wrong, I am just imagining it all,' or if she shows signs of indignation, then the lines of communication have been inadequate. It is probably the fault of the doctor, but it is also possible that the patient is paranoid and lacks insight. Usually the diagnosis is accepted, often with relief, and then a further session should be arranged at which all possible sources of stress are investigated. These should have been noted in the history, but if there is a good rapport, the patient may well disclose troubles she had hidden away in the first place. For example, at this stage one woman told me that the real problem was that she had had a poison pen letter about her husband. She was quite sure that there was no truth in the allegations, but the whole incident had upset her a great deal. She had felt that she must get it off her chest to some one, but she needed to develop a good deal of confidence in her doctor before she was prepared to reveal the situation. It is incredible how loath some people can be to discuss a problem which is making them ill with worry. Linda married and left our practice. She was clearly suffering from a severe emotional upset when she consulted her new doctor, but he was unable to help her so he passed her on to a psychiatrist who was equally unsuccessful in solving the problem. In the meantime her mother developed lumbago and was seen by a member of our firm. She had spinal metastases which were causing the pain, and the primary was a large malignant mass in one breast. This was really the basis of Linda's trouble, but the problem was such that she found herself unable to divulge her worries to anyone. In spite of our modern permissive society, there are still people who find it very difficult to talk about sexual problems, and sometimes the greatest tact is needed in the approach to this subject.

Management

If anxiety in one form or another is the basis of the patient's trouble, this can usually be solved in a few short sessions which include discussion, explanation and reassurance. If the patient is not a lot better after six such interviews, then the diagnosis should be reconsidered. A few people are helped simply by being able to get their troubles off their chests to a sympathetic listener. Others don't feel this is enough, and they make it clear that they need some medicine or pills to take home. To some, the bottle of medicine is 'the doctor sitting on the mantle piece.' It also proves to the world that the patient is ill, and that the doctor is taking her condition seriously. I usually give such people a placebo in the form of vitamin tablets. Tranquillizers such as the diazepine group of drugs, or the barbiturates we used to use before chlordiazepoxide was made, have only a limited use in the treatment of anxiety. They are no substitute for helping the patient to face up to, or to solve their problems. There is no denying that they can be very useful in an emergency, but the patient can become addicted, and if possible long term treatment with these drugs should be avoided. They should be treated with the respect we accord to steroids and opiates, and prescribed only with equal care and circumspection. If the psychoneurotic patient does not respond to simple measures such as I have outlined, then an alternative diagnosis must be made. Some are cases of endogenous depression, and this subject will be dealt with later. Some are inadequate personalities who are unable to cope with life. Every practice has a few of these people. They usually have fat files.

PATIENTS WITH THICK FILES

This is the group of people which has been described as the heavy burden patients. They have very thick record files, and they attend or send for medical help far more often than the average patient. They fall into three main groups. A few of them are worn down by the sheer multiplicity of their physical ailments. One such patient is a cardiac invalid from longstanding rheumatic heart disease. She has a chronic back problem which can be very troublesome, and she always sleeps with a board under her bed. She has extensive and disfiguring psoriasis and, a lover of children, she is infertile. She has been ill in one way or another all her life, but she finds it hard to accept illness, and she remains an anxious person always expecting the worst to happen. To maintain a reasonable level of health she seems to need constant support and reassurance from her doctor. She has a ten minute consultation every month. If she did not get this organized attention, she might well use up far more of the doctor's time and nervous energy by sending for him at awkward hours. As it is we have between us settled on this routine, and it works pretty well for both parties.

With the second group there is no serious medical problem, but the patient is readily bowled over by the least upset. It may be because of some problem in the home, or the patient feels she has collected 'a dose of "flu".' She tends to have a low pain threshold and is often accident prone. The patient seems to need some one to lean on. Some manage tolerably well as long as the prop is there, but remove that support and the patient's world falls to pieces. The doctor may for a time have to be a kind of substitute for the lost love object. This kind of person is not easy to handle, and it is all too easy to hate the sight of her as she walks into the consulting room. In family practice, however, we cannot get rid of patients like this as can the hospital services, by discharging them back to the care of the family doctor. Every practice has a few of these patients, and we must find ways of coping with them, or face years of irritation and frustration as they turn up again and again, only to be rejected in a fruitless if brief interview. No one can solve their problems, or change them into placid carefree types, but they do need help to carry the heavy burden of their own inadequacies. They urgently need a guide, protector, philosopher and friend who is prepared to make them feel welcome and who will support them; with such help they are often able to cope after a fashion. This means that the patient has to be seen at regular intervals, and I try to make the interval as long as possible, but they can rarely go beyond a month. At such sessions they are encouraged to talk, reassured, congratulated on any achievement and generally supported. The consultation must be strictly limited in time; one cannot, and in my view should not, spend long hours in psychotherapy. Ten minutes is usually quite long enough. Such an approach helps the patient and is not frustrating for the doctor. This kind of relationship can go on for years. Sometimes the patient crosses what Willi Mayer-Gross used to call 'the golden bridge', and they then seem to be able to manage on their own, as long as the stress of life is not too hard for them. Ivy was emotionally immature and over attached to her mother. Even when married with a family she told me that her mother was the centre of her life. She knew this was wrong but could not alter it. Her mother had a coronary death and Ivy was thrown into a state of great distress. I had to carry her along as described above for a number of years. She was an intelligent woman and had considerable insight. 'It was not for nothing my mother called me Ivy,' she once said. After a long period of time she came to see me less and less, and in the end found she could cope. She had crossed the bridge!

The third group in this category is the patient with a built in depressive temperament. Some people are born to be Hamlets or Jonahs. They are very like the last group, immature sensitive people who are easily hurt and react by becoming miserable and depressed. They are always in trouble and tend to be the odd man out. They find it hard to settle down and do a job of work, and if they get the sack, it is always the employer who is at fault. They may find it hard to get a mate, and if they do marry the union is rarely a tranquil happy one. Depressions are common, suicide may be attempted, but neither drugs nor ECT improve the patient. Once again long term supportive treatment, with regular short sessions is probably the best form of management. A young woman of 17 left home because she could not get on with her family. She fared no better with landladies, but in the end married a patient longsuffering man who seemed able to help her. She became pregnant and at once acquired a sense of tranquillity she had never enjoyed before. After the birth of her son she became so depressed and miserable she had to be admitted to a psychiatric hospital. She improved, but she never regained the happy poise she had enjoyed in pregnancy. The ECT removed the psychosis, but it did not change the congenital pessimist into an optimist. Her puerperal psychosis was such a fearful experience, she never dared risk another pregnancy.

Family practice owes a great debt of gratitude to the late Michael Balint. He realised how much psychiatry there was in our work as family doctors, and he felt that if the problem was to be tackled at all, then the family practitioners were the right people to do most of the work. He rightly emphasised the need for family physicians to have training in the subject, and by his writings and seminars, he showed that this was a practical possibility. His book[1] is a medical classic which should be read by all medical students and doctors. It is not that every one will be able to accept his approach, but he does compel one to think beyond the presenting symptom, and even beyond the physical diagnosis. Not only does he help the doctor in the art of psychotherapy, but he also encourages one to be interested in the problem cases with fat files I have just described, instead of taking the easy way of complete rejection.

There is no bold highway in the treatment of the psychoneurotic patient. Each one is different, and each doctor develops his own technique. Medawar[2] concluded that any successful form of psychotherapy has certain clearly defined characteristics:

1. there must be assurance of regular sympathetic hearings;
2. the patient must be made to feel that his problem is being taken seriously;
3. the patient must be made to realise his problems are shared by many other people;
4. some attempt should be made to explain the mechanism of the illness.

All this kind of treatment depends upon the patient developing a good rapport with his physician, who helps by his understanding, sympathy, his explanations, reassurance and interpretation of symptoms. The sense of empathy is an essential ingredient of the situation. Lord Platt[3] stated that he had never been able to develop an attitude of aloofness or detachment, and he stressed the importance of being able to share and understand the emotional stress of patients under his care. This kind of attitude is, surely, the basis of all good medicine, and does not just apply to the treatment of the psychoneuroses. The patient who has become a diabetic or who has a coronary occlusion, needs much the same kind of help if he is going to accept his disability, and learn how to live with it.

DEPRESSION

Nature

We all know what it feels like to be depressed. Some people feel a bit down every Monday morning, at the thought of facing a new week of work. Many of the disappointments and frustrations of life induce a sense of depression. Illness and death in the greater family is a part and parcel of normal life, and these situations induce both anxiety and sadness. Sudden death from a road accident or from a coronary thrombosis naturally puts the surviving spouse into a state of acute depression. This type of response which is dependent on circumstances is called a *reactive depression*, and it is a form of anxiety state. The patient must be encouraged to find ways and means of dealing with the problem. If it cannot be solved, she must learn to live with it. A young woman came to see me very angry and distressed. Her husband had been referred to hospital with purpura, and they had told her he had leukaemia, and this implied his days were numbered. The news of this disaster at first seemed overwhelming, but she adjusted to the situation well, and when he came home she was able to do a splendid job, nursing him herself through a long and painful terminal illness. After the first shock she learned to accept and live with the problem.

  Depression can be a symptom attached to any type of illness. Virus diseases such as influenza or hepatitis are prone to make the patient feel depressed, and this state of melancholy can persist long after the precipitating fever has gone. In the same way certain drugs are liable to make the patient feel depressed. Reserpine, which was one of the earliest agents to be used to combat hypertension, had this great disadvantage. In susceptable subjects it could produce a profound state of depression, which lingered on weeks after the drug had been stopped. The same thing can happen with modern drugs such as methyldopa. Hormone upsets can have the same effect, and this must be a factor which produces such a high incidence of depression at the menopause. The syndrome was so common at this stage in life it earned the name involutional melancholia. Some women for a similar reason, have a mini-depression every time they menstruate. The contraceptive pill can cause depression in young women, and it is a not uncommon cause of frigidity. Happily in most cases of this kind, the depression clears as soon as the pill is stopped. Deficiency diseases like diabetes, pernicious anaemia and pellagra can cause depression, and it is common in upsets of the thyroid gland. Any organic brain disease such as arteriosclerosis, Parkinsonism, injury or tumour can cause a profound state of melancholy. The treatment of this type of case is, wherever possible, to remove the cause.

The third type of depression, the *built-in neurotic type of melancholy* has already been described in the section on the thick file patient. It is mentioned here for the sake of completing the list of depressions.

The fourth type is called *endogenous depression*. The patient with this type of depression cannot be talked out of his unhappy state, but the condition can be corrected by means of drugs or electroshock. Often but by no means always, it appears to come out of the blue, to have no apparent cause. The middle aged woman will tell the doctor that she has a good husband, three lovely children, a beautiful home, everything indeed to make her happy, but she feels utterly miserable. After a few weeks on treatment with antidepressant drugs she feels quite different.

Depression in as it were, a pure culture, is rare, it is far more often a mixture of the various types. A woman who has been widowed is depressed as a normal response to adverse circumstances. She may cope well until she gets influenza which makes her so dejected and ill she becomes a case of endogenous depression in need of physical treatment. In some cases of endogenous depression the cause is obvious. It can come on after the sudden unexpected loss of a mate, or even the threat of such a loss. It differs from a reactive depression in that it is irreversible, even when there is a change of fortune. A young man was very proud of his newborn son, and he felt on top of the world. On the third day after the birth, his wife nearly died from a pulmonary embolus, and for days she was in an intensive care unit. This sudden and unexpected reverse of fortune pushed the husband into a severe state of depression, which did not clear even after his wife had made a good recovery and returned home with the baby. The husband remained tense and apprehensive, and the horror of what had happened kept going round and round in his mind. This unpleasant circular type of thought was only eased when he took full doses of an anti-depressant drug. Another example of reactive depression turned endogenous is that of a woman of 70 who along with her husband came to live in the village to be close to her daughter. The patient had never had any illness, physical or mental, and she was working until the time of her move. The uprooting brought on a severe depressive reaction, and the old woman wept as she told me she wished she had never come to the place. Discussion of the problem gave no relief, but two weeks after she was put onto drugs for depression she began to adjust to the situation, joined the old peoples association and enjoyed becoming a member of the new community. The drugs had helped her to adjust, although the basic cause of her depression remained. After six months the treatment was stopped, and within weeks she was back to square one with her depression, but a second course of drugs cleared the symptoms again.

Aetiology

It seems likely that depressive symptoms, however they occur, are caused by the same basic underlying mechanisms, but the precise nature of such mechanisms (in either physiological or biochemical terms) is still unclear. A number of suggestions have been put forward, but all have been modified as a result of later investigations. Schildkraut[4] suggested that depressive mood represented a relative lack of neurotransmitter effect at central nervous synapses, either as a consequence of reduced transmitter release or impaired post-synaptic receptor function; such a mechanism would lead to lowered central nervous responsiveness and would be reflected in the lack of reactivity so characteristic of retarded depression. However, analysis of the mechanisms whereby antidepressant drugs, and in particular the tricyclic compounds and monoamine oxidase inhibitors, produce their effects has revealed the hypothesis to be, at best, an approximation to what actually occurs in the nervous system during depression. The picture is confused by the fact that many biochemical and physiological systems undergo changes concomitant with mood swings: cationic metabolism, amine and carbohydrate metabolism, hormonal and fluid balance, all show variations, and their full significance is yet to be assessed.

Any biochemical or physiological model of depression has to take into account the common observation that, in some cases of reactive depression, and certainly where depression follows a change in a person's circumstances — financial loss, personal disappointment, etc., a reversal of mood may be brought about equally suddenly by a second environmental change without the intervention of physical methods of treatment. Individual differences in responsiveness to events likely to precipitate depression and the fact that what may cause a mood swing on one occasion may be without effect on a second occasion, even in the same individual, cause further difficulties for any simple, unified hypothesis of depressive mechanisms.

The toxins of hepatitis and vitamin B deficiency both precipitate depression. Time alone usually clears the sad mood of post-hepatitis depression, while pellagra, 'mal de la misère' as the French call it, is rapidly cured by giving large doses of vitamin B. Endogenous depression is caused by some genetic metabolic predisposition. This basis is most obvious in the manic-depressive psychosis where for no apparent reason some form of biochemical upset gives rise to the violence of mania, or the utter dejection of melancholia. This is a classical example of the illness 'in pure culture.' Both of these states are impervious to psychotherapy, but they can be reversed by physical methods of treatment.

In 1934 Lewis reviewed a series of depressed patients who were ill enough to have been admitted to the Maudsley hospital. He used every art short of the analyst's couch to discover the cause of the depression. In 15 per cent the basic cause was beyond dispute. In 69 per cent of cases there were precipitating factors, and in a mere 16 per cent of the patients he could find no possible cause for the depression. He commented that because he had found no cause, this did not mean no such cause existed. I reviewed a series of 148 cases. Only severe types were included in which the diagnosis was as certain as it can ever be in psychiatry. In 33 per cent I could find no basic cause, but in 67 per cent there was either obvious trauma or a precipitating factor. Like Lewis I feel sure that in the patient with no obvious cause, there may well be concealed worries, fears or problems which may well be searing the conscience. Linda (p. 492) was depressed because she thought, not without good reason, that her mother was concealing a cancer. Neither her family practitioner nor a psychiatrist could extract her haunting fear from her, and there must be many people like Linda. It is also possible that the patient just does not recognise the cause of the depression, and may well have repressed the idea or just considers that the vital clue is irrelevant and not worthy of mention.

The Evolution of Endogenous Depression

The onset of endogenous depression is usually slow and insidious. The end product of a depressive psychosis is rarely seen today as modern treatment has usually modified the symptoms before that point is reached. Various stages can be described. Ennui is the first phase. For no apparent reason the patient feels indescribably tired, and has lost her drive and sparkle. The housewife who is usually quite capable of 36 holes at golf, finds to her dismay, even going upstairs a real effort. The keen gardener who always looks forward to an hour of two of pottering about outside after his day's work, hasn't the energy to get out of his chair. At first this distressing sense of exhaustion is explained in simple terms. The patient feels he is run down, and he tends to boost his flagging morale by suggesting that it is due to overwork. If hypomania has preceded the depression, this may well be true. However such a facile conjecture does not satisfy the patient for long. After a while he begins to think that either he is 'becoming neurotic,' or that he is developing some serious disease like cancer. Either of these rationalizations gives rise to anxiety which is often intense. The stage of anxiety is the second phase of depression, and severe irrational or inexplicable anxiety is very suggestive of endogenous depression. If the patient is worried because his nerves are going, this in layman's language means that he is going mad, and he can see himself ending up in a psychiatric hospital. If his fear is that of cancer, reassurance from his doctor gives him no comfort. He reasons that either the doctor is trying to shield him from the dreadful truth, or that he is just not skilled enough to detect it. This phase of anxiety ends when a depressive threshold is passed, and the patient becomes frankly depressed. It should be noted that in phase two a paradoxical situation is possible in that the depressed patient will deny feeling depressed. Periodic anxiety is often a mild form of endogenous depression. When anxious the patient fears he may die. Once the depressive threshold has been passed, he wishes he were dead. He would rather be dead than face the ignomony of going mad, or if cancer is his dread, he may as well die now as wait for the agony of his inevitable fate. His ability to sleep gets worse so that he worries by night as well as by day. If able to work it is only by driving himself to the limit and he is painfully aware that his standard of efficiency is well below his norm. It has been said that whereas the anxious patient stops work, the depressed patient gives up his pleasures. He tends to keep on at work as long as he can. The final stage is one of psychosis. The patient may be so retarded that even to speak or move is a real effort, or if anxiety remains a dominant factor, he paces the room like a captive animal, muttering to himself until he collapses from sheer exhaustion. He may well have delusions such as that he has committed the unforgivable sin, or that he has venereal disease and is infecting all who visit him. Visual or auditory hallucinations may add to his misery. He readily misinterpretes his environment. A doctor who was depressed, dropped a newspaper off his knee as he sat before the fire. It became alight and his immediate reaction on seeing the flames was that he was in hell. He felt that at last his fears had been vindicated. I saw him soon after the incident and his violent reaction of horror and alarm was pitiful to witness. No illness known to man is more painful than a severe depression. Even a mild episode can be a devastating experience. The sense of misery is intense, and the victim feels isolated from his group. He thinks that no one understands him or can help him, and he is completely without hope. The fact that not infrequently these people kill themselves is a measure of their wretchedness.

Diagnosis of Endogenous Depression

The symptoms of this illness can be collected into five main groups. The patient may not admit to symptoms from each group, but three or four of such symptoms are very suggestive of the diagnosis.

1. *Tiredness*   The first symptom has already been mentioned. It is an inexplicable falling off of energy and drive. This may show itself in a general inefficiency. The house-proud wife becomes slovenly in her organization. The patient finds himself too tired for sex, or normal social activities.

2. *Sleep Disturbance*   There is an upset of the normal sleep rhythm; usually this is insomnia in some form. Early morning waking is very typical, but if anxiety is a prominent feature, difficulty in dropping off may occur, or sleep may be fitful and unrefreshing. Hypnogogic hallucinosis may occur for the first

time in life and cause alarm, and sleep itself may be disturbed by horrific dreams. A minority of patients find they sleep too much. They can drop asleep at any time, but they feel even more exhausted when they awaken. They tend to go to bed earlier and earlier but even if they sleep for 12 to 14 hours, their sleep has been completely unrefreshing. Morning lethargy is a feature common to those who sleep too much or too little.

3. *Mood Swings*   There is a much more violent swing of mood than is usual for the patient. No other illness produces this symptom to the same degree. This may assume the diurnal pattern of morning lethargy which clears as the day progresses, ending in near normality by bedtime. It is often associated with early morning waking which gives the patient plenty of time to contemplate the horror of yet another day. This swing of affect is very distressing, as hope alternates with fears and dreads in an endless succession. The symptom is one of the factors which tends to keep the patient away from the doctor. When ill she has'nt the energy to take her to the surgery, and when well, she bluffs herself that her troubles are over, arguing that she has no problem to explain to her physician, and so excuses herself from a consultation.

4. *Habit Changes*   There are habit changes which are much more noticable to the family than to the doctor, and if the patient is prone to attacks of depression, these warning signs are readily picked up by close relatives. The lustre goes from the eyes, or mannerisms such as hair twisting, or playing with the teeth are recognised as prodromata. The man who regularly has a pint at the local drops the habit. Maybe he hasn't the drive to get down to the pub, or he cannot face the remarks of his friends who keep asking him what has gone wrong. Alternatively he may start taking double whiskies instead of the regular pint, and he becomes an alcoholic. One man became a compulsive gambler with a one armed bandit, a woman may start to run up debts. The victim may become over religious. One woman who was a Catholic, had married a Protestant in a registry office. In depression, after twenty years of happy married life, she was overcome by feelings of guilt and insisted on getting remarried in church.

5. *Overt Symptoms*   There are overt symptoms of depression. The patient looks sad, and if questioned may burst into tears or admit to crying bouts for which there is no reason. There is the odd case of the smiling depression who can mislead the unwary, as she can in fact, be very suicidal. As a rule the patient readily admits to feeling low and miserable. Life seems to have lost all meaning and purpose.

Estimating Suicide Risk

With any patient who is depressed it is most important to estimate the suicidal risk. This is easy to do, and is always helpful to the patient. *There is no risk of putting ideas into the patient's mind if the proper technique is used.* My method is as follows. I ask the patient, 'Do you feel depressed?'. The answer is usually yes. I then go on to ask 'Just how depressed do you feel?' This generally evokes no reply, and the patient may look puzzled. 'Do you feel fed up and browned off?' Again there is a positive response, but the reaction to the next question, 'How fed up do you feel?' produces no reaction. I then ask, 'Do you sometimes feel that life is not worth living?' This always prompts a reply. The patient may say that he is not as bad as that yet, or he may agree that he often feels that way. If the reply is negative, there is no need to go further, the suicidal risk is negligible. If he has agreed that life is not worth living, then I go on to ask him, 'Have you ever thought of killing yourself?' This may be met with a firm denial, 'I'm not as bad as that,' or he may admit that the idea has been on his mind. If he replies in this way, ask him if he had ever made any plans of how to do it. If he agrees that he has, and reveals what he had in mind, then his life is really in danger from suicide. My response to such admissions is to tell the patient that I realise just how bad he must have felt, that for some time he must have been going through hell, and I tell him what a wise chap he has been to come and see me. All his symptoms confirm my opinion that he is suffering from a depressive illness, a disease as real as pneumonia or a broken leg, only far more distressing. I tell the patient that it is fortunate that today this is a treatable illness, and I ask him to try and be patient with himself and with me, and that in a couple of weeks or so he should be feeling a great deal better. This sort of talk makes the patient feel a bit better almost at once. It eases him to share the guilty secret of his death wish, and it comes as a pleasant surprise to find that instead of being shocked, the doctor seems to understand just how he feels, and for the first time in weeks he may see a glimmer of hope. The doctor has told him it is a real illness for which there is a remedy. He is not just being a stupid neurotic.

Disguises of Depression

Endogenous depression is not only one of the most unpleasant afflictions of mankind (and it should never be forgotten that even a mild depression can be a devastating experience) but is also very common and frequently overlooked. It is missed because so often in the early stages it is heavily disguised. Anyone can diagnose the severe psychotic type of case, the patient who is retarded, agitated, or clearly deluded. By far the most common disguise for depression is that of anxiety. I have already shown that a phase of anxiety often precedes the onset of depression, and it is all too easy to accept the symptoms at their face value. Thirty years ago, I used to spend hours trying to help people like this with long therapeutic sessions. Endogenous depression is a self limiting illness which usually remits in time. If the patient was having psychotherapy when the remission occurred, then the treatment got all the credit for the result. Over the years many of these patients have relapsed, and the diagnosis of depression became obvious. Anti-depressant drugs were far more rapid in effecting recovery than the psychotherapy.

The emotional control centre in the hypothalamus is very close to the autonomic centres, so that it is not surprising to find that malfunction in one area affects other centres. Autonomic upsets are very common in endogenous depression, causing palpitations, bowel upsets, sweating and many other symptoms, which can in fact dominate the picture. The second disguise is thus that of an organic lesion. Physical disease can be closely simulated; for example, bowel atony can look like intestinal obstruction. If there is any doubt as to the basis of the illness, organic disease must be carefully excluded. The differential diagnosis can be very difficult indeed. I have had three cases of cerebral tumour which in the first instance presented as typical cases of endogenous depression, and one of these was so convincing in her symptoms of melancholy that she had a course of E.C.T. before the organic lesion was discovered. A man of 60 came along to see me with a cough and sputum. He had a tachycardia and so was referred to a chest clinic for a check up. There was a suspicious shadow at the left apex and a lung carcinoma was suspected. The man took to his bed and in a short time he was quite cachectic. After one visit his wife told me that before he took ill he went through a strange period. Normally an indolent man, he had been getting up at five in the morning to garden. At 60 he was full of fanciful ideas such as adopting children or taking in boarders. 'I thought he was getting the mania,' his wife told me. With this clear history of hypomania, I had a recheck of his chest. The physician decided that the lesion was unaltered and benign. He was transferred to a psychiatric hospital where he had ECT and made a good recovery. But for his wife's story of the hypomania he would have certainly died, as I had assumed he was going downhill with carcinomatosis.

Confirmed organic disease confers no immunity to depression. This condition can be grafted on to any illness, acute or chronic. If a patient is failing to make the progress one would expect, the symptoms of depression should be sought. A hospital sister who broke her femur was making very heavy weather of the illness. The surgeon decided she was depressed and gave her amitriptyline. She was at first very upset by the diagnosis, as she herself felt that anyone who took psychotropic drugs was a confirmed neurotic, and she resented this implication. After a couple of weeks she was quite astonished to find how much better she felt, and she was certainly an easier patient to cope with on the ward. In spite of her views on the subject she improved, and it was clear that she had been suffering from a depressive graft. The same kind of thing can happen with a chronic illness. Any case of senile dementia should be assessed for depression. It is not uncommon for the family to assume that the absentmindedness of Granny and her eccentricities are due to 'softening of the brain,' whereas in fact the old lady is labouring under the burden of a depression, and adequate treatment can give her a new lease of useful life.

The final disguise of depression is that of the behaviour problem which is out of keeping with the normal way of life of the patient. The middle aged housewife is caught shop lifting, the respected church warden becomes an exhibitionist, the young wife and mother has an affair. Many worthy citizens do the most stupid things, they become drunkards, run up debts, or kick over the traces sexually, they adopt a behaviour which is quite foreign to their normal demeanour. Cynics will say they become depressed because they have been caught out, but a careful history from the patient or the spouse will often reveal convincing evidence that they were depressed before the offence. They may even describe a period of hypomania which occurred before the depression, and this puts the diagnosis beyond doubt. However, it is small comfort for the patient to be treated and restored to normal, when she has been through the courts and her reputation is in ruins. The importance of an early diagnosis in minor depressions, cannot be stressed too much.

Management of Endogenous Depression

The treatment of this illness is made up of two parts, supportive psychotherapy, and physical measures. Most people depressed for the first time, are bewildered by how they feel. They are only too willing to blame themselves or accept that they are becoming introspective hypochondriacs. They don't feel that their illness is medical, and after advice from friends and relatives, to pull themselves together, they don't really expect much help from the doctor. An aquaintence of mine who became depressed was very reluctant to see a psychiatrist. However after the interview he was quite elated. He told his father that the doctor knew exactly how he felt and the consultant had described the patient's symptoms far better than he was able to do himself. He came away convinced for the first time that he was suffering from a genuine illness, and what is more, that the medical profession seemed to know all about it. The average depressed patient cannot understand himself, and he does not expect others to understand him. To establish a good rapport is the first step in any treatment. The second is to assess the suicidal risk; this subject has already been dealt with on page 501. The third measure is to initiate physical treatment.

There are three kinds of drug which help the depressed patient: tricyclic antidepressants, monoamine oxidase inhibitors (MAOI) and lithium carbonate. *Tricyclic Drugs*   These are indicated for patients with insomnia. My choice is amitriptyline. The safest plan is to use one type of drug only until one is really familiar with it. Use the pure drug and avoid tablets which contain mixtures of medicaments. Any of the drugs prescribed must be given in adequate doses; small homeopathic measures are useless. As a rule on full dosage, the patient feels a little better in a week or ten days, much better after three weeks, but it takes six weeks to get the full benefit. I usually see my patients twice a week until they are really on the mend. Easy and regular access to the doctor is a great comfort to such people. Once the patient is feeling better, weekly sessions are adequate, and once back to normal, a monthly consultation is enough. Patients who are suicidal or severely depressed are best referred to a psychiatrist for treatment, but this is not always possible or convenient. The next of kin must then be informed of the risks, the importance of keeping the patient under constant surveillance, and he should be given the tablets so that he can be sure that the right number are taken at the correct time. The patient needs to keep on the drug for a long time. As a rough guide, those under 30 need to take the tablets for three months and those over 30 for twice that time. *Underdosage and failure to persist in the treatment long enough, are the two most common mistakes made in treatment.*

If possible I like to start with a full dose of amitriptyline, that is 25 mg thrice daily and 75 mg at bedtime. This large dose usually ensures sleep without having to give a hypnotic. On this regime the patient is likely to feel sedated, and the day time dose may need to be modified. If the patient has to go to work, drive a car, or care for young children, then I would give 10 mg thrice daily and 50 mg at night, gradually increasing the dose up to 10 mg four times a day and 100 mg at bedtime. The side effects are unpleasant. They include a dry mouth, blurred vision, constipation, postural hypotension and drowsiness, but they usually pass if the patient has the courage to carry on with the treatment. Many people have pointed out to me that while during the first week they could not keep their eyes open, after ten days they feel invigorated and quite different. Some people just cannot tolerate the drug, and then it is worth switching to imipramine in the same dosage, or dothiepin (Prothiaden). The latter is said to have less side effects. If after three weeks on a tricylic drug at full dosage there has been no relief of symptoms, review the diagnosis. If it is still considered to be endogenous depression then try a course of the MAOI drugs.

Monoamine Oxidase Inhibiters   There are two main indications for these drugs. The first is when the patient presents with symptoms of hypersomnia. He says he can drop off to sleep at any time, but he is constantly tired. He tends to go to bed earlier and eariler and can sleep the clock round, but when he awakens he is completely unrefreshed. This type of patient often feels worse when given a tricyclic drug, but he improves on an MAOI. As with amitriptyline one usually has to wait for a week or two before an improvement sets in, and when it does come the patient is often surprised and mystified by his feeling of well being. A man once told me that he only had one worry left, and that was what would happen when he left off his tablets! After a week or so of treatment, hypersomnia gives way to insomnia, and I treat this by giving 50 to 75 mg of amitriptyline at bed time. In spite of all that has been said about the dangers of mixing these two types of drugs, I have never had any adverse reactions. If amitriptyline upsets the patient, I give nitrazepam 5 to 10 mg, but if it works I prefer the tricyclic drug.

The second indication for MAOI drugs is failure to respond to tricyclics, and here again I have found it unnecessary to wait for a few weeks before starting the new treatment. If the patient has already had three weeks on amitriptyline, and has to wait two more weeks before the new drug works, one does not want to try his patience too long. William Sargant has always maintained that there is no risk in mixing these drugs, and I agree with him.

In my view isocarboxazid is the safest of the MAOI drugs, tranylcypromine is the quickest acting, and phelelzine is about half way between the two. Iproniazid is the most potent of all. It is also the most toxic, and is not recommended. Liver damage is the big danger. Hypertensive crises can occur if the patient on any of these drugs eats foods containing tyramine. Every patient on these drugs should be given a card stating the name of the drug they are on and a list of the dangerous food items. In addition opiates and anaesthetics are contraindicated, and any patient visiting a hospital or a dentist should carry a letter to indicate the antidepressant drug he is taking. Adrenalin should be avoided in patients on the tricyclic group. Having pointed out the danger of these drugs, it is important to stress that *they can be most useful*. Many family practitioners and even psychiatrists have been scared off using them, and this is a pity because they certainly have a place in the treatment of depression. I have had more really dramatic recoveries on MAOI drugs than on the tricyclic group. If proper precautions are taken, these drugs are quite safe to use in family practice.

Lithium Carbonate   It has long been recognised that lithium is the drug of choice in the control of mania and over the last 20 years its value as a prophylactic agent against manic-depressive illness has been established. Patients liable to recurrent attacks of depression can be a real therapeutic problem, and continuous lithium therapy is well worth a trial.

When lithium is prescribed it is important to consider the principles described by Kerry[5] so that it may be used safely and effectively. The management of patients on lithium therapy requires careful control of dosage by measurement of blood lithium levels as the therapeutic level of lithium is very close to the toxic level. Also very low serum lithium levels may indicate that the patient is not taking his tablets. Accurate methods of estimating serum lithium levels are now routinely available. The test requires 10 ml of whole clotted blood and the patient should not have taken any lithium tablets just prior to the test. It is best to begin with a low starting dose, e.g., 400 mg at night, with serum lithium estimations about twice a week, gradually building up the dosage until the serum lithium is in the range of 0.8–1.4 mEq/1. In a normal healthy adult 20–30 mEq of lithium ion daily are needed to obtain a serum lithium concentration of 0.8–1.4 mEq/1. Thus about 1000 mg lithium carbonate (27.2 mEq lithium ion) will be required daily in divided doses. However, the precise dosage must be tailored for each particular patient since it is possible for one patient to require twice as much lithium as another to maintain the same serum lithium concentration. It is useful to monitor the serum lithium every week for the first month, every two weeks for the next month or two, and then, depending upon there being a series of satisfactory serum levels, every month for a further six months. Once the patient has been stabilised the blood tests should be repeated every three months. The occurrence of physical illness or states which are likely to disturb electrolyte (especially sodium) balance will make extra care and more frequent serum lithium estimations necessary again. Any condition involving sweating or diarrhoea can lead to dangerous increases in the serum lithium level.

The side effects may be classified into mild, moderate and severe depending upon the extent to which they impair the general functioning of the individual and are fully reviewed by Vacaflor[6]. The commonest side effects are fine tremor of the hand, which may be enough to prevent the holding of a cup of tea in comfort, and gastro-intestinal irritation, which occasionally may include nausea, vomiting and diarrhoea. If this should happen the drug should be stopped and then started again after a few days at a lower level.

Kidney disease contraindicates the use of lithium so that if the family doctor is initiating treatment he should first test the urine and have a blood urea estimation carried out to check kidney function.

It is perhaps opportune at this stage to emphasise the futility of giving minor tranquillizers of the benzodiazepine group, such as chlordiazepoxide (Librium), to treat the melancholic patient. *These drugs are useless in the treatment of depression.* Today there is a tendency to put patients who seem anxious onto a minor tranquillizer. If there is any doubt about the diagnosis, I think it is wiser to treat the case as one of depression. This will do no harm to the anxious patient. Anti-depressant drugs like amitriptyline have a tranquillizing effect, and I have often found that persons on such drugs may well be prepared to discuss problems which were worrying them, items they declined to talk about at an earlier interview. On the other hand, if the depressed patient is treated as a case of anxiety, he may well decide that all attempts to help him are useless, and may kill himself.

Diazepam (Valium) may be useful in suppressing the fits which can occur in the depressed epileptic on antidepressant drugs, otherwise the minor tranquillizers are contraindicated. The fact that they are quick acting and virtually have no unpleasant side effects makes them highly habit forming, and unlike the anti-depressants, it is often very difficult to stop the patient from taking them. The basic effect of a minor tranquillizer is not unlike that of a double whisky. It is, however, much cheaper for the patient, but not for the taxpayer.

Specialist Referral

Drug treatment has certainly revolutionised the treatment of endogenous depression in family practice, but there are still some cases we are unable to help on our own, and I feel that the psychiatrist should be called in to help under the following circumstances.

1. If the patient is mentally very disturbed with obvious retardation, agitation or overt delusions. Generally patients like this are safer in a psychiatric hospital.
2. Patients with suicidal ideas should be referred to a psychiatrist. This should not be done with such rapidity that the patient feels either rejected, or that his family practitioner is in a panic. A domiciliary consultation can make the hand-over very much easier for the patient.
3. If the patient has failed to respond to drugs, or if he has only climbed half way up the hill, and is in an arrested depression, ECT is indicated, and I feel this is better given at a psychiatric clinic.
4. If the diagnosis is in doubt a second opinion is indicated.
5. Chronic depression remains a problem, especially for the family. A psychiatrist may sometimes help by taking the patient in to hospital to give the family a break, or to let them get away on holiday.
6. The depressed patient who lives alone is in a very vulnerable position, and should be referred to a psychiatrist for possible hospital care.

The outlook for patients suffering from depression is a great deal better than it was, but there is no room for complacency. There is still a hard core of patients who fail to respond to any kind of treatment, and we still don't know how the various forms of treatment work. The problem of depression certainly has not been completely solved. Today it is largely the job of the family practitioner to treat the illness, and he can do so in about 90 per cent of cases. It is important that he should do this as far as possible. The psychiatrist is still a frightening figure, hence all the jokes about him which are so much more common than about other members of the medical profession. It is unfortunate that this prejudice is augmented by certain undeniable disadvantages that can follow even a consultation with a psychiatrist. In the UK the fact that a man has had such a consultation is enough to exclude him from the police force, to load his insurance premium, and may prevent his emigration. The history of a stay in a psychiatric hospital can make a childless couple ineligible for adoption, even if their state of infertility is the basis of the illness. This sort of prejudice may be deplored, but we live in an imperfect society, and because of this real if unworthy bias, it behoves the family practitioner to practice as much psychiatry among his patients as he can. To have suffered a depression which recovered under the treatment handed out by the family practitioner carries with it far less stigma than reference to a psychiatric clinic or hospital, and such treatment by the family doctor can be of the greatest possible service to the patient.

HYPOMANIA AND MANIA

Hypomania occurs in about 6 per cent of people who suffer from depressive episodes. It may precede or follow the depression, and it can be precipitated by antidepressant drugs, especially the MAOI agents. If it is due to drugs, the condition usually subsides rapidly if the dose of the drug is lowered. Hypomania is a productive state of elation, and is more than the euphoric relief most patients have when a depression has receded. The syndrome is pleasant and harmless unless it is the prodrome to true mania. This is a much more serious problem, but it is a rare condition. I have had only 8 cases in a practice of 8000 patients over some 28 years. When it does arise it is a devastating experience for the whole family, and as it is very liable to recur, the prospect of a manic episode is viewed with considerable alarm.

Management of Mania

Most cases of overt mania need to be treated in a psychiatric hospital, both to protect the family from the great inconvenience of an elated, sleepless, overactive individual who never stops talking, and it is even more important for the protection of the patient from himself. The respected parson may start living with prostitutes to convert them, or the family savings may be squandered in spending sprees on a lot of useless objects or ideas. Admission is not easy as the victim has no insight into his illness, and to be housed in a psychiatric ward is the last thing he wants to happen. These patients have to be signed into hospital under section 25. To persuade the patient to go quietly may demand a great deal of patience and skill, but he must never be deceived as to what is happening. Deception may make an admission easier in the short term, but in the long run it produces a very resentful patient, who may well have to be supervised as regards his illness for years.

The sheet anchor of mania prevention is continous lithium therapy and this has already been described (p. 506). Patients may resent the periodic blood check, but such an inconvenience is a small price to pay if the major disaster of a manic episode can be prevented. Lithium has the advantage of apparently acting 'directly on the underlying manic process, whereas the major tranquillizers merely suppress overactivity and restlessness, leaving the patient drugged and drowsy but still with the fundamental manic mood and ideation' (Peet[7], p. 37). In highly active or disturbed patients in whom rapid control is desirable lithium can be initiated in combination with other drugs, such as chlorpromazine or haloperidol, which will contain the patients' behaviour until the lithium acts on the underlying manic process. This takes about 6–10 days at which time the dose of tranquillizer can be reduced (Peet[7] p. 38).

THE SCHIZOPHRENIAS

Schizophrenia is not a single disease, but a collection of syndromes which tend to have a familial basis. The family with the worst record in our practice had four simple schizophrenics, one schizoaffective case, and three florid schizophrenics in the greater family, spread over two generations. Schizophrenia is still the most serious form of mental illness, although the prognosis is better than it used to be. According to my observations[8] over a quarter of a century, some 18 per cent had made a complete recovery. This may take a long time to come about. One man had a fixed delusion which took over 20 years to burn itself out. Another 46 per cent were at home and working efficiently, but the disease had left its mark. Many of these were on continuous drug therapy. Twenty five per cent were living at home but they were unemployable, and the remaining 11 per cent were permanent long stay hospital residents. A small proportion of this series, about 8 per cent were able to survive in the community without any medical attention. They were odd eccentric people, but they were able somehow to carry on living in the community. Times are changing, fifty years ago most schizophrenics were admitted to the asylums for observation and custodial care. They deteriorated as much from the dreary routine of the wards to which they were committed, as from the schizophrenic illness, and the outlook was bleak indeed. Today most cases can expect an early discharge to the community. This more progressive attitude, as well as the advent of drugs, has gone far to improve the prognosis. However this more enlightened regime does mean that cases come back to the care of the family doctor, and the modern family practitioner has a role to play in the care of this type of illness. Compared with depressive syndromes, schizophrenia is a rare disorder. With a list of 3000 patients, the practitioner should expect to find one new schizophrenic every year. The responsibility is however, rather greater than this low incidence implies as these people need help over many years and for 4 cases out of 5 it is a permanent afflication.

Types of Schizophrenia

Simple Schizophrenia

Simple schizophrenia occurs more among males. The patient has no gross psychotic symptoms, but has lost his drive and he is completely unable to compete in the rush and bustle of modern life. Roger gave up working at 23. He was admitted to a mental hospital for a short spell so that his problems could be investigated, but he has never done an honest days work since he was discharged 22 years ago. Helped by an aging mother he potters about at home. He seems completely unable to apply himself or keep going at any job. In some ways he is

like the first stage of depression, the phase of ennui, but the patient seems
content with his empty life and does not get depressed. Thomas has never
worked since I have known him. He lives alone and paints lurid pictures no one
wants to buy, but this way of life satisfies him. Norah walks the country lanes
with her little dog, summer and winter. She is tanned a dark brown by the sun
and is as thin as a lathe, but she never comes to see the doctor or complains of
anything. In previous generations before the days of the welfare state, such
people would have been tramps and vagrants. Today they can, if they choose,
live in greater comfort. The onset of the illness is slow and insidious, and there
appears to be no treatment. The patient as a rule is content with his lot, it is the
family which suffers. Norah's only child is a university graduate, and she finds it
very hard to accept her mother's eccentricities.

Schizophrenia Vera

Three categories are described in the text books, hebephrenia, catatonia and the
paranoid type.

Hebephrenia and Catatonia   Today it is rare to see florid cases of these two
categories; this may well be because of earlier diagnosis and treatment which
prevent the evolution of the gross symptoms. Sudden onset cases are easy to
diagnose, and the family usually call for help at a very early stage of the illness.
This type of case tends to carry a good prognosis. Few illness are more
distressing to a family than a sudden unexpected mental breakdown, especially
in a young person. It is a comfort to realise that these acute cases usually do
well, although some may become arrested schizophrenics, with clear marks of
mental deterioration. Leonard was a bright boy at the grammar school. At 17 he
became schizophrenic and a great problem to his family. The disease has burnt
itself out, and now at 47 he is an eccentric batchelor living alone, but he is a
conscientious worker in a local quarry. The slow onset case is more difficult to
diagnose. Relatives often hang on too long, hardly knowing how to put their
troubles into words. Quite often the patient is equally reluctant to see a doctor,
and he may actively resent medical intervention. Some of these recover in time,
or make a partial recovery, and others go relentlessly down hill so that in the end
medical aid becomes inevitable. A good rapport and drug treatment helps most
of these cases, but others deteriorate no matter what one does. It seems that a
few schizophrenics, even today, must remain permanent residents in psychiatric
hospitals. The big majority make better progress in the community, although
some of these need continuous help and supervision.

Paranoid Schizophrenia   I have suggested that the clinical picture of hebe-
phrenic and catatonic cases had modified in my life time. This does not apply to
the paranoid type of case. Their behaviour is much the same as it always was.
These patients do not readily seek medical advice as they have no insight and
they always blame others for their troubles. The family doctor is in the best

position to help this type of case. The family practitioner starts off by being a familiar figure in the community, and he must bend over backwards to get and keep the confidence of the patient. The paranoid person is reluctant to admit he is ill, but if only he can be persuaded to take phenothiazine drugs, he may be much easier to handle. If possible it is better to manage without a psychiatrist; such a consultation would offend the patient, and if an admission to hospital was arranged, this would be clear evidence that the doctor as well as the family was ganging up against him. Katie was a middle aged woman who transferred to my list because she felt that her own family practitioner had bewitched her. She was completely obsessed by hatred against him. If she looked to the left she could often see the devil himself complete with a knot in his tail and this was all the fault of her old doctor. I persuaded her to take phenothiazines and antidepressant drugs, and soon the heat had gone out of her symptoms. Asked about her previous doctor she still reacted against him, but without any great feeling, and the devil which she could still see at times had ceased to worry her. The doctor who is handling such a case has to befriend the patient, he has to try and see things from her angle so as to get her confidence, and persuade her to accept treatment. If the paranoid ideas involve the doctor himself, he is unlikely to be able to help her.

The sheet anchor of treatment in schizophrenia is the phenothiazine group of drugs, of which chlorpromazine was the first to be used in this way. In patients who are liable to default in their treatment, long acting forms like Modecate can be given by injection. All drugs have their snags. It should not be forgotten that phenothiazines and prochlorperazine can produce fits in susceptible subjects. In known epileptics they should be given with caution. Mary was such a case, and she began to get ideas that her husband had another woman. Her fears were unfounded, and her suspicions disappeared when she was given chlorpromazine, but the dose of anticonvulsants had to be increased. In a few cases long term treatment can produce irreversible choreiform or athetoid movements. This is a tragedy, but the illness is so serious it is a risk one must take.

The schizophrenic group are usually quiet withdrawn people, but they do appreciate the understanding and friendship of their doctor or anyone who is interested in their welfare. They seek someone to talk to who is prepared to listen to their most bizarre symptoms without surprise or alarm. They are unlikely to abuse the opportunity offered to them and with the illness in a state of arrest they are far less troublesome and time consuming than either the chronic neurotic or depressive. Most people would agree that long term custodial care in a psychiatric hospital is undesirable, and there is an urgent need for hostels in the community for these patients. With a safe sheltered background and a little supervision, especially as regards drug taking, many more schizophrenics could hold down jobs and make a contribution to the community as well as improve their own condition. Hostels are also needed when the home appears to be the wrong environment for the patient. Recent work has shown that the less communications the schizophrenic makes with relatives in the home, the happier he seems to be. It is as if he wants peace and quiet for his state of detachment, as well as security, and it is possible that a hostel would be, under these circumstances, better for these people, and for their families than living at home.

THE PSYCHIATRIC EMERGENCY

Nothing is more alarming to the ordinary layman than a sudden mental breakdown which comes on out of the blue, and is completely unexpected. The acute confusional state, which usually comes on in the aged, comes into this category. Granny goes to bed with a cold, but by nightfall she is talking incessantly, and seeing things (see Chapter 24, page 628). In common parlance she has gone stark staring mad, and this produces great concern in the family. One can detect the anxiety in the voice of the person putting in the call. In my experience most of these people can be dealt with in the home. The first step is to reassure the family, both by an attitude of unhurried calm, and by the promise of rapid help. The patient needs to have a careful examination as she may have an infection which has precipitated the breakdown. This may mean antibiotics, but the mental confusion needs liberal doses of vitamins and a sedative such as diazepam, 10 mg by injection and 20 mg to take at bedtime. The second dose can be taken by mouth. Delirium tremens is a similar reaction. It should usually be dealt with in hospital where adequate supervision is always on hand, but I have coped with the odd case at home, with the treatment described above. Sedation by a diazepam injection and parenterovite by injection in massive doses should be given on the first day and vitamins by mouth thereafter. Recovery from a condition such as this is usually quite rapid. By the next day the patient is calm and all the hallucinations have gone. In the elderly this is far better than an emergency admission to hospital which is likely to add to the disorientation and confusion of the patient, and the rapid recovery in the home gives great satisfaction to all concerned.

Compulsory Admission to Hospital

The schizophrenic emergency may present difficulties. One patient of mine had a loaded shotgun ready for the next doctor or welfare officer who called, and not unnaturally, his family were terrified of him. If violence is likely, it is a good plan to take more help than you are likely to need. In this case I contacted the police, and the welfare officer and I went to the house with no less than six

police officers in two cars, the ambulance was concealed round the corner. I
went to the door between a sergeant and a constable and the rest stood on the
road. With such a show of force his aggression crumbled. His one request, which
was granted, was to go to hospital in a police car. If, as happens very
occasionally, the patient has to be overpowered, once he has been downed, first
remove his footwear, and then give a powerful sedative by intramuscular
injection. I have always used Omnopon (a mixture of soluble salts of the
morphine alkaloids) 20 mg and scopolamine 0.4 mg, but 20 mg of diazepam
would probably do just as well. In 28 years I have only twice had to sedate a
patient in this way, and I have undertaken some 104 compulsory admissions.
When a patient has to be 'certified' the most important item is time. This is a job
that should never be tackled in a hurry. The first step is to see that the family
support the idea of admission to hospital. Once this is clear one must take time
to argue with and persuade the patient to accept the idea. If necessary it may be
spelled out to him that in the end he has no choice, but that it is far better to go
willingly. A social worker who knows his job is a great boon. The old time
mental welfare officers in this area were dedicated experts who were prepared to
come along at any hour, and they would often take the patient to hospital
themselves. On rare occasions the impasse has been solved by my taking the
patient along to hospital myself. A compulsory admission is a very traumatic
experience for the patient and the family. Any step which will make it easier for
the patient to accept the decision and go quietly, should be given serious
consideration. The only plea to which a deaf ear should be turned, is the
patient's request to put the admission off until the morrow. Once the course of
action has been decided it must be carried out the same day. Doctors need to be
familiar with the legislation concerning compulsory admission in their respective
countries.

SUPPORT FOR THE FAMILY

The doctor's main function is that of the healer, but the family practitioner's
role extends far beyond attempting to cure disease. This is particularly valid in
times of crisis. The problem of bereavement is commonplace in our work. I was
never told in my medical training anything about how to handle this important
subject, but that was a long time ago when many useful subjects were omitted
from the curriculum. However it is only ten years since I heard of a young house
physician being told to break the news to parents that their child had leukaemia.
So even a decade ago in some quarters the most junior doctors were supposed,
by the light of nature, to be able to deal with this most traumatic situation.

   If the family practitioner has maintained a good relationship with the
patient and the family, his job when death strikes may be painful, but he can do

a great deal to help. He suffers with the family and this sense of empathy helps those in trouble. He can assist in a very practical way be ensuring that the family get sleep at nights by way of hypnotics, and maybe some sedation by day. This is one of the rare occasions when I feel that the minor tranquillizers and hypnotics are useful, but I make it clear from the outset that they are to be used only for a limited time. I am prepared to use such drugs for a week until the anniversary day has passed. If a sleeping drug is given care must be taken to see that an adequate dose is prescribed. Half sleep broken by troubled dreams is worse than no sleep at all. A couple lost two children in a drowning accident. I gave them both 400 mg of sodium amytal and 800 mg of meprobamate. They slept for 12 hours and were far better able to cope with the painful days which lay ahead. It is ideal if one can cut out the tranquillizers at the end of the week, but this is not always possible. Many a childless widow living alone derives great comfort from the nitrazepam she has to take every night. One of the inevitable results of widowhood is that not only is there great sorrow, but the woman is deprived of the very person in whom she usually confides in time of trouble, and also of male company. Short periodic sessions with an understanding male family practitioner can be a great help to her in this period of readjustment. As a rough guide, I try to get the family back to a normal routine in two weeks, and the agony of despair should have eased in six weeks, but of course there are great individual variations. Torrie's book on widowhood[9] is excellent reading for such a patient, and I am prepared to lend my copy to suitable patients.

Bereavement is only one of the major crises in life. The tumultuous times of late adolescence cause a great deal of parental anxiety, each set of parents tending to feel that their own problems are unique and worse than those in any other family. A mental breakdown in some member of the family creates a great crisis, and at no time in life can the support of the family practitioner be more useful. He can explain what is going on, and he should paint the best prognosis compatable with the truth. When things like this go wrong in the family, there is a great sense of guilt. The parents ask themselves, 'How much of this is our fault?' More often than not it is nature and not nurture that is to blame, and reassurance from the family doctor on this score can be a source of great consolation.

PSYCHIATRIC PROBLEMS IN CHILDHOOD

Serious psychiatric problems in childhood are rare. I have never recognised a case of autism in the practice. Hyperkinetic children can be a great problem to parents, and cause more distress than mental subnormality. Any serious upset should have the benefit of expert opinion, but many minor problems can be dealt with by the family doctor. Habits such as nail-biting, nose picking and tics are best ignored, but time should be taken to question the parents about possible problems, and reassurance should be given. The same thing applies to infantile masturbation. I am always surprised how few cases of this are reported, as the phenomenon itself must be very common. The habit is both striking and at times embarrassing. Cases I have followed up over years, have come to no harm. Parents are rarely surprised by the label of masturbation, and I tell them that it is an unsocial habit like nose picking. In private it should be ignored, but not allowed in public. Like many habits, they usually pass given time. Two of the major traumata of childhood are sibling rivalry, and starting at a new school. Every child deposed from being the baby in the family feels jealous, but conceals his feelings as he knows they will meet with parental disapproval, but they remain there, loaded with guilt. The deposed child must be compensated by being made in every possible way to feel important. He should always go to bed after the younger child, and his mother can, after bedding the baby, say how much she has been looking forward to having the older child to herself. A quiet game or a read with one or other parent should be more or less routine. The older child should get pocket money before the younger, and his status is enhanced if he gets more cash than his sibling. He must be encouraged to look forward and feel that growing up is worth while. It is all too easy for him to wish to regress, to lie in the babies cot, borrow the dummy or start wetting the bed after good bladder control has been established. Discussing the problem with parents often reassures them, and they may well produce ideas of their own. One small girl derived obvious satisfaction when her height was measured and she was found to be taller than her tiresome and uncooperative sister who was difficult to measure.

Next to being born or getting married, going to school for the first time is one of the major status changes in life. The surprising thing is that so few children are really disturbed by the experience, and it suggests that the technique of infant teaching must be very good. However, school phobias are not uncommon and they demand the concerted attention of teachers, parents and sometimes a member of the medical team. The health visitor is probably better than the family practitioner himself. In retrospect I have found that the odd case has been an infantile depression. One patient who had a severe depression at 19 gave a history of school phobia at 7 and again when she went to grammar school. She remembered these episodes and felt they were the same phenomenon.

CONCLUSIONS

Anxiety and depression are very common problems in any practice. The patient, in part because of the nature of the complaint, in part because the family and friends have been at pains to point out to her that 'it is *just* her nerves', feels inferior and hardly expects to be welcome at the surgery, no matter how ill she feels because of her symptoms. Starting out in practice many doctors feel disconcerted by such people, and they are uncertain how to handle them. The thick file brigade are always a problem, but apart from these patients the majority can be helped considerably. The doctor should learn to accept such cases as interesting people with a problem. They present a challenge to his therapeutic skill, and in the end they can prove most rewarding. He will be a much better doctor to all his patients if he can help these people. It does not require great skill to treat patients who have simple diagnosable conditions which respond rapidly to treatment, especially if the patient is sensible, cooperative and grateful. The people who give a poor history and have vague complaints, who panic readily and seem never to be satisfied, these folk are a greater challenge. They are there in every practice and can either be dodged or dealt with. Any doctor who tries the latter course in all honesty and sincerity will find it a very gratifying part of his work.

References

1. Balint, M. (1964). *The Doctor, His Patient and the Illness*, (London: Pitman Medical).
2. Medawar, P. B. (1968). *The Art of the Soluble*, (London).
3. Platt, Lord (1972). *Private and Confidential*, (London: Cassell).
4. Schildkraut, J. J. (1969). *Neuropsychopharmacology and the Affective Disorders*, (Boston: Little Brown and Co.).
5. Kerry, R. J. (1975). The Management of Patients Receiving Lithium, In *Lithium Research and Therapy*, (editor, Johnson, F. N.), p. 143, (London: Academic Press).
6. Vacaflor, L. (1975). Lithium Side Effects and Toxicity: The Clinical Picture. In *Lithium Research and Therapy*, (editor, Johnson, F. N.), p. 211, (London: Academic Press).
7. Peet, M. (1975). Lithium in the Acute Treatment of Mania. In *Lithium Research and Therapy* (editor Johnson, F. N.) p. 25, (London: Academic Press).
8. Watts, C. A. H. (1973). *Brit. med. J.* 1, 465.
9. Torrie, M. (1970). *Begin Again*, (London: Dent).

23

Care of Children

S. Carne

INTRODUCTION

Children differ from adults, not only in that many of the illnesses from which they suffer are different, but also in their response to disease, both physically and emotionally. Equally important are the social problems involved in the care of children, ranging from major items, such as baby battering, to relatively minor problems of intra-family life.

Preventive medicine in children is at least as important as the therapeutic aspects. Disabilities – potential or actual – ignored in childhood can lead to a life time of invalidism. Every child has the right to be offered full facilities to achieve his or her maximum potential. Doctors involved in child health have a major responsibility in this respect.

Much of the care of children, both in health and disease, falls within the province of the family doctor. His duties encompass both the provision of care for the ordinary illnesses from which children suffer and a full preventive health service including developmental assessment of the pre-school child and the maintenance of a full immunisation schedule.

The family doctor has a unique opportunity to understand the needs of his child patients in relation to the needs of the family.

In many group practices one or more of the physicians have a special interest in child health problems. In the United States the pattern is usually for the doctor doing this to confine his medical practice to children but in Britain, and many other countries, it is more usual for every primary care physician to look after his own list of children for ordinary problems but to leave the prophylactic care of all the children in the practice to those members of the group who have a special interest in this field. The attachment of health visitors to family practices has considerably extended the facilities which the practitioner can make available to his patient, especially in the fields of preventive and social medicine.

Examinations

Children do not usually initiate a consultation with their doctor. That decision is taken on their behalf by a parent or guardian who also proceeds to act as interpreter for the child's history. What then happens in many instances, is that the history is presented as the adult perceives it, with embellishments culled from his own interpretation of the facts. Even if the physician asks a direct question of the child, all too often it is the mother (or father) who answers. This happens so frequently, that the doctor may not realise its significance.

When examining a young child, the first essential is to gain his confidence. There are various ways of restraining a child so that he can be examined; very occasionally these may be necessary, for example, to look at the throat. Usually, however, if the child comes to regard his doctor as a friend, no restraints whatsoever are needed and the child will permit almost anything to be done to him. The family practitioner, of course, has one major advantage over other doctors. Most of his young patients will already know him and be accustomed to the equipment he uses. The auriscope has no fear for them, nor the stethoscope. Tongue depressions are best avoided. The child will usually open his mouth wide enough, particularly if he has done this at every consultation — which is an added reason for carrying out a full examination every time.

It is often easier to examine a young child's ears while it is resting on its mother's shoulders. To avoid any misunderstanding I usually ask the mother to hold her baby in the 'winding position'.

If the child is frightened — which is most likely to happen when he meets a new doctor for the first time — some of his fears may go if he is allowed to wander round the consulting room while the history is taken. When it comes to the physical examination, the child should be allowed to first play with the stethoscope and auriscope (blowing out the light is a good introductory game) before they are used as diagnostic instruments. Until they are accustomed to its use, the sight of a thermometer may often be associated with a syringe. It should be inserted very gently, preferably into the axilla. Rectal examinations are always uncomfortable, even to adults: to children they are also frightening. If the patient is tensed up, the initial digital insertion will itself be painful and the value of any subsequent probing is probably minimal. In spite of the well-known dictum about not putting one's finger in, the doctor must decide whether the information he is going to derive warrants the assault.

Note-keeping

Every doctor knows that proper records must be kept. The difficulty is in deciding what constitutes a proper record. The more we write in our records, the less we subsequently read.

It is very important to keep a list of all the vaccinations a child has had, and probably also the infectious illnesses. (If for no other reason, this data will be useful when later the mother seeks details before a regular school medical check up). Because much of the illness seen in children is relatively minor, it is easy to discard this data from the notes, but considerable diagnostic information can be culled from a knowledge of the frequency and timing of recurrent coughs, colds and otitis media.

Prescribing

The response of children to drugs varies according to (a) the age, the weight and body surface area of the child and (b) the drug used (for example, children are especially sensitive to the morphine group, atropine and salicylates but require relatively large doses of digitalis and its derivatives).

There are no simple rules for determining the correct dose, only guide-lines. The dosage of each drug should be checked whenever there is any doubt.

Most of the drugs administered to children are in liquid form. In Britain it is now standard procedure for these to be given in multiples of 5 ml. There are available standard 5 ml spoons and parents must be encouraged to use these at all times. Domestic teaspoons vary considerably in size from 2.5 to 6 ml. If the quantity of active drug in the 5 ml measure is too great for the child (e.g., it is being administered to a small baby) the entire quantity of the medicine dispensed should be diluted by the pharmacist with an appropriate diluent so that each 5 ml dose contains the desired quantity. One exception to the rule is the paediatric digoxin elixir (in both the BNF and proprietory forms). This must not be diluted but each dose given, if necessary, in a smaller quantity than 5 ml. To facilitate this, digoxin elixir and other drugs falling within the same 'not to be diluted restriction' are dispensed in a bottle with a measuring pipette.

Where a drug requires to be diluted so that the correct dose is in a 5 ml measure, it is usually unnecessary for the doctor to identify the diluent. The pharmacist will do this if requested, for example:—

> Elixir triclofos 2.5 ml
> Diluent   2.5 ml
> Sig 5 ml nocte

Both the BNF and MIMS indicate a dose range for children, usually by age. The literature available from the manufacturers will also give the appropriate variations in dosage. Help in deciding the correct dose should also be available from the pharmacist.

The fewer medicines prescribed for any patient, the more likely are they to be taken regularly. This applies even more to children than to adults. Every mother knows how difficult it can be to get a child to take one spoon of medicine. Trying to get several different mixtures into the child at the same time is asking the impossible. In the treatment of upper respiratory tract infections, for example, most experienced practitioners select one symptomatic remedy which they prescribe if and when reassurance alone is insufficient. If an active remedy is being prescribed (e.g., an antibiotic) it is not usually necessary to prescribe a symptomatic remedy, such as a cough linctus, at the same time.

Where antibiotics are used, it is important to stress that they be taken regularly. Only an obsessional mother will wake her child during the night to maintain a 6-hourly dosage schedule, which is not necessary. Four times daily gives just as satisfactory an antibiotic response in most cases. With many of the antibiotics, to achieve the best blood levels, each dose should be given at least 15 minutes before meals. The drug should be continued until all the prescribed quantity has been consumed. Loose stools are a possibility with most antibiotics and need not prevent the course being finished. Live yoghurt will often prevent the occurrence of loose stools and may also relieve the pruritis ani, while enabling the antibiotic course to be finished. If diarrhoea is troublesome, and if other side-effects occur, the doctor should be consulted before stopping the drugs. These facts should be explained to the mother every time an antibiotic is prescribed though, naturally they should be put into lay language. There is no need for vitamin supplements when a short course of antibiotics is given. Rashes are common with ampicillin and do not necessarily imply a hypersensitivity to all penicillins.

The Child as a Symptom of Family Illness

The child may sometimes be the presenting symptom of family illness. He is taken to the doctor because of a cough, loss of appetite, or many other non-specific symptoms. Careful clinical examination reveals either a lack of objective evidence of disease or the presence of some minor disability, such as catarrhal rhinitis. It is tempting to leave it at that; reassure the mother, and perhaps offer her a symptomatic medicine to give to the baby. If, however, the doctor listens carefully to the whole history, using his 'third ear' to grasp the innuendo, he may often detect the notes of discord which indicate that all is not well within the family. Sometimes he will recognise the mother is depressed and/or the father an alcoholic. The variety of factors causing family discord is endless and many mothers — and fathers — are ashamed to consult their doctor about what they feel to be personal domestic problems. Instead they translate their anxieties into a worry over some minor symptom manifested by the child.

Frequent night and emergency calls to the same family are almost diagnostic of this syndrome. Indeed, in such families the child is often the only member who is healthy.

HOUSE CALLS

With the increased pressure on the family doctor's time, coupled with travelling and parking problems in most urban areas, the possibility of the child being brought to the doctor's consulting room must be considered as an alternative to making a house call. There are no firm rules to guide the mother or the doctor in making this decision. Each case must be assessed on its merits. 'Illness travels well in children'. Provided the mother and her feverish child are not expected to stay in the waiting room, and provided there is no difficulty in getting the child to the surgery, there is no reason why this should not be done. Children can be brought to the doctor with almost any of the infectious fevers; indeed, an increasing number of exanthemata are appearing at the surgery.

The difficulty sometimes lies in ensuring they are separated from others in the waiting room. Provided there are spare consulting or examination rooms, and the reception staff are trained to understand the difficulty, no problems need arise. On the other hand, if the mother is unwilling, for any reason, to bring the child to the doctor, then the child must be visited at home. Prescribing over the telephone is never a safe procedure.

The frequency with which follow-up house calls or surgery attendances need be made will depend on a multitude of variables; the nature of the illness, the presence of complications or the possibility of their developing, and the social circumstances.

Admissions to Hospital

The main clinical factor determining admission is the need for specialised treatment facilities, for example, an oxygen or steam tent, the need to monitor blood gases, or surgery. Any infant in respiratory distress will almost certainly need hospitalisation and the need may be urgent. In these cases I ask the mother to wrap the infant in a warm blanket and take the pair of them in my car direct to the hospital. I have taken this action about five times in twenty years of family practice. On each occasion I have rung the hospital Casualty Department and informed them in advance of the action being taken. The same action may be used in cases of status epilepticus and status asthmaticus.

In less urgent cases the most frequent reason for admitting a child to hospital is the presence of adverse social factors — mainly inadequate parental support (e.g., one-parent families) poor housing, etc. Also influencing this decision are anxiety and general emotional immaturity on the part of the parents, which is as common among the wealthy as it is among the poor, coupled with a lack of faith in the ability of their doctor to cope with their problem. This probably explains, at least in part, why admission rates for acute respiratory infections are much greater when a call service doctor has attended a child at home.

NORMAL GROWTH AND DEVELOPMENTAL ASSESSMENT

In the past two decades considerable advances have been made in our knowledge of the normal pattern of maturity of a child. Previously the physician noted the appearance of a few 'milestones' in a child's life: the age at which the child sat up, crawled, walked, and began to talk. We now know a lot more about the development of the central nervous system and, in particular, the special senses, motor activity and co-ordination. There are a wide variety of tests for the assessment of a child's physical development but the controversy over their value remains to be settled. They are time consuming and some will argue that the information to be derived does not warrant the expenditure of that amount of time. Others are convinced that the time devoted to developmental assessment is at least as valuable as the time spent on other prophylactic procedures in family practice.

The emotional development of a child is equally important but techniques for measuring this have not yet been adequately refined, and recognition of psychological problems depends primarily on the identification of behaviour disturbances in the child or the family.

Descriptions of the tests of child development are available in many text books devoted exclusively to this topic and will not be elaborated here. However, a few important points will be emphasised.

Which tests are selected must be the decision of the individual practitioner. In the case of a number of disabilities remedial action is possible and their early identification is very important: for example, the recognition of a squint before amblyopia develops (see p. 549). There is a dangerous myth held by some mothers that nothing can be done for a squint until the child goes to school; but at this stage it is usually too late to preserve binocular vision, and irreversible amblyopia may have developed. Every child must be examined at the age of 7 months to see if he is squinting and the tests should be repeated at every subsequent routine examination.

Equally important is the recognition of a hearing defect (see Chapter 10, p. 114). Even though it may not be possible to restore the hearing to normal, the provision of a hearing-aid before the child is 1 year old will lead to vastly improved speech development compared with that in a child whose hearing defect is ignored.

The search for a congenitally dislocated hip must continue until the child is seen to be walking normally. While most will be identified at the immediate post-natal examination, in some cases the dislocation may not be apparent until the child is older, or it may have been missed. Talipes should also be identified at the first examination but it, too, may have been missed.

Congenital heart diseases are considered on page 579. Auscultation of the chest and examination of the femoral pulses are easy to carry out if performed routinely and do not take more than a few seconds of the doctor's time at each examination.

Many other congenital anomalies can readily be identified on inspection but minor defects may require careful examination and may be missed unless, for example, a defect in palatal closure is specially sought.

Testicular development should be noted. In infancy, if there is any doubt whether the testes can descend into the scrotum, it may be reasonable to delay referral until the child is 5 years old (see p. 394). Genital anomalies in girls are extremely rare and most will not be manifest until puberty.

The management of umbilical and inguinal herniae are considered on page 544.

The early recognition of cerebral palsy is very important in order that appropriate treatment can be arranged, but whether the early recognition of children with minor motor disabilities is of importance is open to question. Unless the examiner is well experienced in carrying out these tests, it is easy to misinterpret the findings.

It is very important not to sow seeds of doubt in the minds of the parents about the child's development, unless the doctor is sure of his findings. The exceptions are those cases where urgent action is required. For example, every child suspected of having a squint or hearing defect should be urgently referred to a specialist, but the suspicion in infancy of a possibly mentally retarded child is less important and referral may be delayed until the doctor is a little more sure that there is a doubt. At that stage of life no therapy is available and if the diagnosis should prove to be wrong, untold harm may be done to the child's psychological development by implying that something serious was amiss ("There's no smoke without fire").

Rate of Growth

The growth and development of a child from conception to maturity is a continuous process. However, growth does not proceed at a steady pace: at certain times it is far more rapid than at others.

There is no one 'normal' weight, nor 'normal' height, for a child. It is important to recognise the considerable variation within the range of normal. Many perfectly healthy children have been dragged by anxious mothers to be 'checked up' because their weight did not match that on a standard chart. Now that emphasis is being placed on obesity, many others are having medical care because they fall within the upper ranges of a centile chart. It is inherent in the concept of such charts that there shall be a range above and below the mean.

There are various weight charts and graphs available giving the range above and below the mean (usually the 3rd, 10th, 25th, 50th, 75th, 90th and 97th centiles). There are important geographical and racial variations but at present separate charts are not available. For example, West Indian babies tend to weigh more, and the mean weight of Indian babies is less than that of white British babies.

Far more important than the fact that a child is on one of the high or low centiles for his age, is a record that he has moved up or down the scale. A child progressing steadily on the 50th centile, who is suddenly found to be on the 25th or 75th line, warrants further investigation to see why this change should have taken place, though the explanation is usually simple.

Skin fold thickness is sometimes used as a measure of obesity but unless it is done regularly the data can be misleading. Obesity can be seen almost as accurately with the eye and confirmed by pinching the skin. Skeletal maturity is a guide to the age of a child's development in relation to its actual age and will also serve as a guide to growth potential. However, the value of the information derived from this measurement has always to be weighed against the hazards of irradiation, as well as the technical difficulties in accurately positioning the part to be X-rayed. Dental maturity may also be used as a guide.

Teething

In theory, cutting teeth should be asymptomatic. Cutting the second dentition is certainly relatively painless, as can be vouched for by most 6 to 12 year olds when they go through this stage of development.

Babies cut their primary dentition between the ages of 6 months and 2 years and a multitude of disorders which occur at this time have been blamed on the erupting teeth. Most children are irritable at times coinciding with the eruption of at least some of the deciduous teeth.

In past centuries 'teething' was a frequent recording in parish mortality registers and the same diagnosis is still being blamed, both by doctors and parents, for many non-fatal attacks of pyrexia, convulsions, diarrhoea, bronchitis and otitis media, in young infants.

There is no satisfactory proof that any of these disorders can be directly attributed to cutting teeth. The author has, however, noted in many babies the appearance of an eczematoid rash on the cheek overlying an erupting tooth. The prognosis for this rash is invariably excellent; it is not a precursor of eczema. Apart from this rash on the face and a degree of irritability, he agrees with Illingworth who remarks: 'Teething produces nothing but teeth'.

Should the child be fractious, extra cuddling may be all that is needed. A small dose of aspirin (e.g., paediatric soluble aspirin tablets) may be helpful but teething jellies are almost certainly little more than a placebo.

Walking

The first propulsive movements made by babies is a crawl; there are different varieties. The majority crawl on their hands and knees, usually forward, but some tend to go backwards much of the time. A few babies, in spite of using all four limbs, kick themselves forward from a crawling position using one leg to provide the force. There are also some babies who make their first movements by sitting on their buttocks and jumping forward.

Children learn to stand and then to walk at some time between the ages of 6 months and 2 years. There is a considerable variation in the age at which they start to do this. Some very intelligent children are late starters and many children who are not so bright start to walk at an early age.

The natural stance of a child who is learning to maintain his balance is for the feet to spread apart and turn out (*metatarsus varus*). In addition, the distribution of fat in an infant's legs is not the same as that in an adult. In a healthy child both the thighs and calves are relatively plump and the medial metatarsal arch is filled with a fat pad. The effect of the fat distribution on the posture is to give the child the appearance of flat feet, knock knees and bow-legs. At various stages in the development of normal posture, all three are physiological.

Flat Feet

A persistent true flattening of the medial longitudinal arch of the foot is very rare. In *normal* infants and young children, the medial arch is filled with a pad of fat which creates the appearance of a flat foot and this is aggravated because of the natural stance at this age. Many children also walk in such a way that the heels of their shoes wear down maximally at the outer side. Indeed, many children continue to do so until puberty, without there being any evidence of mechanical or other disability.

True flat feet can be readily recognised by getting the child to stand on tip toe without his shoes and socks. A normal arch can then be clearly seen on the medial side of the foot. It can be further confirmed if, after the child is asked to walk a few paces, the sole of the foot is inspected. The area over which the body weight is applied will show up very clearly as a dirty half-moon, with the medial metatarsal arch still clean.

No treatment at all is needed for a pseudo-pes planus. Many children, unfortunately, have been condemned to months and even years of unnecessary exercises and considerable sums of money have been needlessly spent in building up the heels of childrens' shoes when all they are suffering from is a normally developing foot. (Not infrequently, the author has seen a heel raised on the wrong side of the foot!).

Knock-knees (Genu valgum) and Bow-legs (Genu varum)

These 'disabilities' are considered together because they are the two ends of a normal spectrum of growth of the legs. Because of the distribution of fat in the legs of young children and their normal stance, the legs of a baby appear to be bowed when he starts to stand up and then to walk. The straightness of both tibiae can be confirmed by holding a ruler against the shin to demonstrate that the bone is quite straight. It is the distribution of fat which gives the bowed appearance, and this is absolutely normal.

So, too, is the subsequent appearance of knock-knees. Up to the age of 6 or 7 years, most children continue to maintain their balance by keeping the feet slightly apart and everting the heel, giving the impression of knock-knees.

Almost all the knock-knees and bow-legs seen in infants in Britain today are physiological. No treatment is needed. In the physiological 'pseudo-knock-knee' the gap between the medial malleoli of many children may be as much as 2 to 3 inches.

True bowing of the bones in the legs — the tibiae and fibulae and usually both femurs as well — is due to pressure being put on the bones when they are too weak to carry the load. The commonest cause is rickets and surgical correction may be necessary. Since most infant milks and cereals have Vitamin D added to them, rickets has become a rarity among children in Britain. It is still seen in children deprived of adequate sunlight, and cases are reported from time to time in coloured immigrant children, mainly those from the Indian sub-continent.

Overlapping Toes

In children the tendency for one toe to overlap another — often bilaterally — is usual. There is no evidence that spreading the toes to keep them straight makes any different to the prognosis. Usually no action is necessary but if the overlapping toe is a nuisance or is being constantly rubbed on the shoe, a surgical correction may be necessary.

BABY AND CHILD BATTERING

Nature

All parents chastise their children from time to time — some more frequently and some more violently than others. At one end of the scale there is evidence that it may be positively harmful not to punish a naughty child by either smacking or admonishing him. At the other end, there are instances of children being killed, permanently maimed or very severely injured in one or a series of attacks made on them by their parents or guardians.

The term 'battered baby' was introduced by Kempe in 1962 to describe a 'clinical condition in young children who have received serious physical abuse generally from a parent or foster parent'. Later the phrase 'child abuse' was used to soften the effect of a diagnosis. Recently 'non-accidental injury' has found more favour as many people feel that the use of the word battered arouses a punitive response in the reader and further alienates the battering parents, thereby adding to the difficulties of promoting a trusting relationship with the family.

The nature of battering varies greatly from mild bruises to such injuries as lead directly to the death of the child. Besides having bruises and broken bones the child may have scratches, burns, scalds and/or visceral injuries. The term 'battered' also includes emotional abuse, since there is considerable evidence to show that the battered child is also the victim of mental cruelty. Indeed in some instances the nature of the abuse may be exclusively psychological. Many believe that the meaning of the term should be extended to include those cases in which the parents' unconscious hostility places the child in a situation in which he is 'accidently' injured. Another category which is sometimes included in the syndrome is 'failure to thrive' where an infant is starved of food or love or both, sometimes to the point of death, though some workers prefer to distinguish these infants as victims of a more passive 'rejection' syndrome.

Incidence

It is possible to so extend the criteria for defining this type of assault that every child who suffers any injury, however minor, as a result of parental action is described as a battered baby. Were this so, more than half the children in the country would be labelled 'battered babies'.

Because the definition varies, it is difficult to be precise about the extent to which battering actually occurs. Recent reports indicate that some 3000 children are battered in Britain each year, of whom about 15 to 20 per cent die as a direct consequence of their injuries. These figures suggest that the average family practitioner will see about one case in nine years. However there are geographical pockets, scattered around the country, in which this problem is very much more common than elsewhere. The full explanation for these variations is not yet known, but it does mean that some family practitioners see one or more new cases every year, while others may never see a case.

Aetiology

A variety of studies have been conducted which were aimed at isolating the psychological and social factors which might be common amongst battering parents. Certain characteristics have emerged, a combination of which may greatly increase the risk of a battering incident. The parents of battered children tend to be young, the maximum incidence occurring in parents in their early twenties, and have often had 2 or 3 children in rapid succession. Sometimes there is a history of premarital, unplanned or unwanted pregnancy and often the mother is pregnant again or has recently been delivered. The maximum incidence is in children under the age of 6 months so that it is possible that unrecognised post-partum depression plays a part in the syndrome by its effects, either directly on the mother-child relationship or indirectly on the husband. However, no age is exempt.

Whilst battering parents have many emotional and social problems, many do not fall into any specific psychiatric category. In some cases one or both parents is suffering from alcoholism, epilepsy or schizophrenia but in many of the studies where epilepsy was said to be more common amongst battering parents the epilepsy has not been substantiated by medical evidence.

There is a group of parents associated with this syndrome who are said to be habitually aggressive in all their personal relationships and may show a long history of violence and a readiness to enter into conflict with authority. These parents may have difficulty in coping with stress and in controlling themselves in stressful situations. Some studies demonstrate a higher incidence of criminal convictions in battering parents.

Another group which has been isolated are described as being rigidly controlling. There are reports of some mothers describing feelings of severe agitation when their baby is not clean or manifests behaviour which is not amenable to control such as messy eating and which is perceived as naughtiness. Often these mothers have an obsessionally tidy house and their children are physically well cared for.

Not infrequently there is a history of deprivation and rejection in infancy in the parents and it is possible to confirm that in their own childhood they, or one of their siblings, were battered (i.e., they came from a 'battering family'). In childhood they were often given love only conditionally and excessive demands for correct behaviour were made, leading to feelings of worthlessness and lack of self-esteem. They have been described as emotionally immature having un-realistic expectations of love and appreciation from their babies so that when the baby fails to give the required response the parents perceive the baby as rejecting or deliberately frustrating them.

There is a growing awareness that the immediate postnatal period is of crucial importance in the development of the mother-child bond and that some practices in pre-, peri- and postnatal care in hospital obstetric departments can interfere, sometimes avoidably, with this process. For example studies by Kennell and Klans in Cleveland have shown that mothers allowed unhindered contact with their newborn babies were more affectionate with them than those whose babies slept in separate nurseries. This was particularly noticeable in mothers of babies of low birth weight or of babies who were placed in intensive care units immediately after birth or stayed in hospital for prolonged periods.

Anxiety for the welfare of the baby may lead one to forget the need of the mother who has just been delivered to hold and touch her new infant, even for only a few moments, when in some cases a momentary delay in whisking the baby away for special observation or treatment would do no harm. In such a situation the mother is often too shy to ask for the baby and afraid of appearing 'a nuisance'. Indeed, mothers of first babies may not themselves appreciate the importance of this first contact and after an exhausting delivery may feel too emotionally drained to seek it. If separation from the mother for a prolonged period is subsequently unavoidable this early contact may be all the more crucial.

The characteristics outlined above may help in the identification of those families who are specially at risk but it should be remembered that no social class or group is totally free of battering parents. Battered babies have been found in families with a good educational and cultural background and from wealthy as well as poor homes; it has even been reported in the children of professional men and women including doctors. However, where the parents are of above average intelligence the battering is likely to be psychological rather than physical.

Clinical Features

It cannot be too heavily emphasised that any physical or psychological injury in a child could be the result of the deliberate act of one or both parents. The suspicions of the doctor should be aroused if the history of the accident as given by the parents does not quite ring true. Children do not usually break a limb bone in mid-shaft falling off a sofa or playing with father; nor do they burn themselves. Multiple injuries are especially suspicious and so too are recurrent accidents.

Not infrequently there is an inordinate delay seeking advice. A child with a fairly severe injury may not be taken to the doctor till the next day, or even later. It is as though the parents had hoped to hide their guilt, but finally realised that some treatment was essential.

Proportionately there are more head and face injuries than in genuine accidents, when it is the knees, hands and forearms which are most frequently injured. A grazed knee is not likely to be evidence of battering.

Very often the 'innocent' parent will start to defend his or her partner's innocence. This collusion by the parents is an important indication of a disturbed family background.

There is an increase in the frequency with which these episodes occur at certain peak periods of domestic distress — meal times or bed times; weekends when father is home; or school holidays when the children are around to annoy the mother all day. In a family that is well known, the doctor or health visitor may have already recorded the fact that the mother is depressed or father is an alcoholic or either is epileptic. This information may also be elicited in taking the history, though it requires considerable tact and skill not to antagonise the parents and so negate most of the good the doctor can do.

Management

Making the diagnosis, or even suspecting it, is the first stage in the management. A decision has then to be taken whether or not to put the child into a place of safety — which usually means immediate admission to hospital. A request by a family practitioner for admission to a paediatric unit of a battered baby — suspected or proven — should be sufficient grounds for this to be done in every case. In making these arrangements, the family doctor — and the hospital staff who receive the child — must be careful to avoid expressing their fears, if they want the parents to co-operate in the later management. 'I am a bit worried about this bruise. I think Johnny should go to hospital for a few days to get some tests done', is the sort of remark to make, not 'Johnny must go to hospital to find out who did this to him'. Care must be taken to preserve the link between the mother and child either by admitting her as well or by encouraging prolonged daily visiting.

There are conflicting views on what is to happen to the child and the family once the immediate crisis has been resolved. Should the child be later returned to his natural parents? How far are the police to be involved, if at all? What is the role of the family doctor and his team? Does he have an active part to play, or is he merely a referral agency?

In many areas a multidisciplinary approach is adopted and a case conference is called as early as possible involving hospital staff, the local clinic doctor, the family practitioner, the health visitor and a social worker who may already know the family or who may have been asked to make an evaluation of the psycho-social circumstances after the crisis event. Often it is helpful to have a representative of the police with experience in this area present as well. Such a course of action ensures the maximum amount of communication between agencies. In many fatal cases lack of such communication has subsequently been shown to be a contributory factor in the failure to prevent an event which several people were aware could be imminent.

However, we must take great care that our methods of investigating accidents in children do not result in more social harm than good. There is a danger that our natural fears of missing an abused child and of accusations of negligence from the mass media may result in over zealous quizzing of the parents by too many people — often in public. Accidents do happen and, whereas in the past the parents of injured children were met with sympathy and support in their distress, today they may leave hospital feeling that no-one believed their story about the circumstances of the accident because so many people — the receptionist, the nurses, the casualty officer and the ward sister — cross examined them. If only one parent was present at the time of the accident the other may begin to believe that the child's injuries were 'non-accidental'. Parents frequently have guilt feelings when their children are injured, even when the accident was outside their control, and to exacerbate these feelings is cruel.

In some families the battering is repeated either on the same child or another within the family, in spite of warnings and actions by doctors and social workers. The fact has to be faced that there will be a small proportion of cases where no amount of psychiatric and social care will protect the child or other children in the family in the future and it may never be possible to return the child to the care of its parents. Where a child is returned to the family adequate follow-up is essential.

In many cases treatment may be of benefit and sometimes it may not even be necessary to admit the child to hospital (or other place of safety).

The initial injuries may be relatively minor, though unless the domestic crisis is dealt with, further, and probably more extensive batterings are always possible. Sometimes the shame felt by the parents for what they have done will help resolve the crisis, but it is unwise to rely on this alone. The arrival of help, including the family doctor, may break the tension within the family, who can often, in these special instances, be best helped as a unit held together rather than divided.

The swift introduction of a social worker when abuse is first suspected is essential as at this time the parents are likely to be less hostile and resistant to help than at a later stage. The dependency needs of the parents must be met in order to build up a friendly and sympathetic relationship. It is important that everyone involved in the treatment of battering parents is aware of their own natural feelings of aggression towards the perpetrators of the abuse as any perceived criticism on the part of the parents will only increase their anxiety and hostility and may even precipitate further abuse of the child. Battering parents need a sustained relationship with a caring person and this demands a great deal of time and emotion — an important consideration for the family practitioner in deciding on the extent to which he wishes to involve himself in the treatment and aftercare of battering parents.

Prevention

The battering of a baby is not an isolated event but the result of a progressive breakdown of parental care. One important diagnostic feature which has come to light from recent research is the frequency with which these children have been taken to their doctor before the event. The story as told by the mother is that the doctor said: 'There is nothing the matter with your child'. Finally, she 'just had to do something'. Family practitioners recognise 'frequent attendance' as an important diagnostic feature at every age, on a par with any other symptom — though, of course, only rarely is it an indicator of a baby battering family.

The health visitor holds a key position in the early recognition of at risk families since regular visits to mothers of young children are accepted by the mothers as part of her work, giving opportunities for spotting the signs outlined earlier. Sympathetic enquiries before injuries occurred have often revealed a mother's extreme distress in response to her baby's crying. A child may be described as being 'different from the others' and the mother may even admit she cannot love the child. Battering commonly takes place during normal mothering activities such as feeding, bathing, dressing and nappy changing, and tactful enquiry about a mothers feelings at these times may not only be revealing but also help the mother express her feelings about her baby.

Future Research

Much has been written about baby battering but there is still scope for many more studies, especially in family practice where the combined skills of a multidisciplinary team of health care workers may be of immense value. As a result of the information derived from these investigations, we should be able to define more precisely the nature and extent of the problem.

THE ALIMENTARY TRACT

Abdominal Pain

Abdominal pain is one of the most frequently encountered symptoms in family practice; it is as common among children as it is among adults. It is convenient to classify attacks into acute, recurring or chronic. Some acute attacks are the first presentation of what is to become a chronic or recurring problem.

It is an unusual family that does not have in its mind the possibility that the child may be suffering from appendicitis when they consult their family practitioner because the child is complaining of 'tummy ache'. Even though the child may have had several similar attacks previously, this does not lessen the parental fear.

We do not know how many appendices have been removed unnecessarily. Not infrequently one sees a patient, usually an adolescent female, who has already had her appendix out and who will admit that her symptoms before the operation were no different from those now experienced.

Differential Diagnosis

The differential diagnosis of abdominal pain encompasses almost every bodily system. Most diseases of the gut can cause pain. It is not an uncommon occurrence to see a child with an obvious acute gastroenteritis present as abdominal pain without mentioning the diarrhoea or vomiting until asked.

Urinary tract infection is one of the classical differential diagnoses of an acute appendicitis. The other is mesenteric adenitis. The presence of abdominal discomfort in a child with an acute upper respiratory infection has never been satisfactorily explained: why should the mesenteric glands enlarge, and if they do, why should they be painful? Alternative diagnoses include referred pain from the pleura and spine, hypoglycaemia and diabetes, and lead poisoning (now even rarer than it was previously, since the adoption of lead-free paints for children's toys and cots).

Epileptic attacks can sometimes be accompanied by abdominal pain. A number of children with recurrent attacks of abdominal pain come from migrainous families and when they reach their late teens they themselves frequently develop migraine. For this reason some children with recurrent abdominal pain are labelled as suffering from a 'migraine equivalent'. Another diagnostic label — now somewhat less in favour than in former years — is the periodic syndrome, otherwise known as cyclical vomiting. In this condition the child gets recurrent attacks of vomiting and abdominal pain, sometimes accompanied by a fever as high as 40°C. Some clinicians use the terms 'periodic syndrome' and 'migraine equivalent' as synonymous, while others describe minor differences between the two diagnoses.

Girls at the time of the menarche often have their abdominal discomfort attributed to the pending arrival of menstruation.

It is now generally recognised that the majority of children with recurrent abdominal pain are not suffering from any identifiable physical illness and that emotional factors play a large part in the aetiology of their illness. Sometimes the child may be saying he has 'tummy ache' because he finds it difficult to say more precisely what he finds the matter with him. Many of us suffer minor abdominal discomforts from time to time, when also feeling miserable, worried or depressed; the tummy ache may be a convenient and acceptable presenting symptom. Children rarely complain of feeling miserable when they go to the doctor. Though most children are relatively unsophisticated they still prefer to keep misery as a problem to be presented to mother and pain as a symptom for the doctor; or perhaps the parents perform the symptom transformation on behalf of the child coupled with their own image of the problem.

A number of these children are suffering from indigestion, no different from dyspepsia in adult life. Barium meal studies are not usually necessary and are rarely feasible during an attack. (By the time an appointment can be arranged for an X-ray, most acute gastric ulcers which might have been present will have resolved). Where barium studies have been carried out, it has been shown that peptic ulcer is not as uncommon among children as is often thought.

Management

A full history must always be taken. In the case of recurrent attacks it is wise to repeat the history from time to time. At some stage, but not usually on the first presentation, investigations will be needed; full blood count, urinalysis and perhaps a barium study.

Some probing will be necessary into the relationship between the child and his family, the child and his school, and the parents and the school. No one technique for taking this part of the history is more suitable than any other. The doctor's own personality is important in helping him decide which questions to ask; the choice influenced to a great extent by his own attitudes and hang-ups.

Therapy is even more difficult, though the taking of a full history is often a major factor in getting the child and his parents to recognise that the doctor *understands* the problem. No one remedy appears to be any better than any other in the absence of a finite diagnosis. Some doctors prescribe antacids and/or anti-cholinergics; others recommend tranquillizers or laxatives. Many family practitioners prefer to avoid the use of drugs in treating children with recurrent pain, either in the abdomen or elsewhere. This is one of the problems for which the family doctor can be the specialist.

Referral to another specialist (paediatrician, surgeon, gynaecologist or psychiatrist) may nevertheless be desirable at some time, if only to reinforce the original opinion expressed by the family practitioner.

Appendicitis

Nature

It is still not clear what the function of the vermiform appendix is or why it should be so frequently infected. On rare occasions an acutely inflamed appendix will resolve, sometimes with the help of an antibiotic, though this is not usually a recommended form of therapy. In most cases, however, the natural history is for the inflamed appendix to rupture, spreading infected material into the peritoneal cavity.

Incidence

Approximately 4 children per 1000 under the age of 15 are admitted to hospital in Britain each year with appendicitis; relatively more boys than girls. Approximately 8 per cent of youths will have had their appendix removed before leaving school. A practitioner with an average sized list will see about two children a year with this disease, which is very much less than is sometimes thought.

Appendicitis can occur at all ages but it is uncommon before the age of 5 years. It is important to recognise the disease in young children because it is among them that most deaths from appendicitis are reported — the younger the child the greater the risk.

Clinical Features

Every first-aid worker and medical student is aware of the clinical picture of a patient with central abdominal pain radiating in a few hours to the right iliac fossa but in at least 25 per cent of cases the pain starts not in the umbilical region but in the right iliac fossa or one of the other quadrants, usually if the appendix low in the pelvis is to be palpated, but its diagnostic value is feature. The pulse rate is initially raised but then slows, to increase in rate again as peritonitis supervenes. The temperature is raised, but rarely more than 39°C. A higher temperature is one feature against this diagnosis.

Very often there is a story that the child has been awake all night, or keeps waking up with abdominal pain. On this story, irrespective of whether the pain is central or to the right or left, an acute appendicitis must be considered as a likely diagnosis. Some experienced practitioners will admit a child to hospital on this history alone.

There are various physical signs which may be found on palpation of the abdomen. Each has its advocates — none is infallible.

Rectal examination is essential if a rectal abscess or an inflamed appendix low in the pelvis is to be palpated, but its diagnostic value is somewhat over-rated. There is no need to carry out this examination if other evidence points to the diagnosis. The surgeon himself will, anyway, want to put his finger in and every time the examination is carried out it is painful and disturbing to the child.

The classical differential diagnosis is an upper respiratory tract infection with mesenteric adenitis, but the presence of a red throat does not, *per se*, exclude the possibility of an acutely inflamed appendix. If there is any doubt the child should be kept under observation. Urinary tract infection in children very often presents with abdominal pain and vomiting; a urine sample should always be examined before operation. Constipation, too, may cause low abdominal pain and sometimes may even be accompanied by a little pyrexia.

The failure to recognise one of the rarer surgical differential diagnoses such as obstruction associated with intussusception or a Meckel's diverticulum, is less important because in these cases a laparotomy is an equally essential part of the treatment.

'Chronic' and 'grumbling' appendicitis probably do not exist. The evidence on which these diagnoses are made is usually open to considerable doubt. Most doctors will not infrequently see a patient, usually in their teens or twenties, with acute abdominal pain, in whom the appendix has already been removed some years previously. Very often the patient will say that the pain is similar to that they had before the operation, and often that they had had several attacks previously of a so-called grumbling appendix. Rather than invent a new diagnosis to explain the patient's pain, it is usually better to admit the error of our ways in the past and acknowledge that an innocent organ was sacrificed.

When a pathologist examines the specimen removed at operation from a child with a grumbling appendix, his report is likely to show the absence of a true infection. The significance of both faecoliths and hyperaemia is doubtful.

Indigestion is almost as common in children as it is in adults, even if peptic ulceration is less frequently demonstrated. The abdominal discomfort — and sometimes vomiting — may be mistaken for an acutely inflamed appendix. Children with indigestion are usually apyrexial; true guarding is absent. A number of girls, as they approach puberty, have attacks of abdominal pain at intervals. Many later suffer a similar discomfort when they ovulate.

Management

In family practice the problem of the management of a child with acute appendicitis, once the diagnosis has been made, resolves itself. The child must be admitted to hospital.

The difficulty lies in deciding whether the diagnosis is appendicitis. If, for example, the child has mesenteric adenitis, he is almost certainly better observed at home. Every case must be very carefully assessed. The history is almost as important as the clinical examination. If there is any doubt, the family practitioner should re-examine the child after a few hours, and if he is still in doubt, the child should either be seen at home by a surgeon or admitted to hospital.

In some centres day surgery or early discharge is being practised on children with an uncomplicated appendicitis. The family practitioner will then have the responsibility of after-care including, sometimes, removal of the sutures. Most surgeons will indicate their preference for when this is to be done.

Post-operatively there is no need to keep the child in bed. Indeed, inactivity is contra-indicated because of the risk of venous thrombosis, though this is rarer in children than adults. The child may return to school two weeks after his operation and start games a month later.

Mesenteric Adenitis

Nature

The pathology and the significance of inflamed mesenteric glands in children is not clear. A diagnosis of mesenteric adenitis is usually made when a child with an upper respiratory tract infection complains of abdominal pain which is not dissimilar to that of acute appendicitis. Whether these glands form part of the defence mechanism against viral infections is not clear. The age incidence (3 to 8 years) suggests it may be. Indeed, it is not certain that mesenteric adenitis is a true clinical entity, but it is a useful diagnostic label for acute or recurrent abdominal pain with no other detectable pathology.

When tuberculosis was more prevalent in Britain, TB mesenteric adenitis was a not uncommon finding.

Clinical Features

The child is usually pyrexial and will complain of 'tummy ache'. Vomiting frequently occurs. This tends to be less severe than in appendicitis, but this is difficult to assess objectively. There is often also an upper respiratory infection, a rhinitis or pharyngitis (even a follicular tonsillitis). The site of the abdominal pain is usually difficult to locate and the abdomen on palpation is not usually very tender. Youg children may guard at every examination even when nothing at all is the matter.

Management

Once the diagnosis is established there is no need for treatment other than observation.

Meckel's Diverticulum

Though relatively common — it is found in 2 per cent of the population — it rarely causes symptoms in children. Because part of the mucosa may be gastric, it can give rise to symptoms of dyspepsia and intestinal bleeding. If a segment of bowel loops around the diverticulum it can cause intestinal obstruction.

Intussusception

Nature and Incidence

An interssusception is the result of the invagination of a segment of gut into the segment immediately distal.

The incidence of this condition varies in different parts of the world. The disease appears to be much less common in Britain than it was two decades or more ago. It is most frequent in children between the ages of 6 months and 2 years.

Diagnosis

The symptoms are those of acute intestinal obstruction; pain, vomiting and shock. Bloody mucous resembling redcurrant jelly may be passed per rectum or found on the finger-tip of the glove after a diagnostic examination. On gentle palpation of the abdomen, a sausage shaped tumour can be felt.

Treatment

The child should be sent to hospital immediately. Occasionally the intussescep-tion can be reduced by hydrostatic pressure but usually laparotomy is necessary so that the reduction can be carried out manually. Any fluid or electrolytes lost in the vomit or sweat will usually have to be replaced before the operation can be commenced.

Pyloric Stenosis

Nature and Incidence
Hypertrophy of the circular pyloric musculature leads to a variable degree of obstruction. It occurs in about 3 live births per 1000; the ratio of males to females is 4 : 1 and it is relatively more common among the first born. There is often a family history.

Diagnosis
Symptoms do not usually appear until the infant is about 2 to 4 weeks old, when he is brought to the doctor because he is vomiting. This is often, but not always, projectile. The vomiting tends to occur at the end of or just after a feed. If the child has been put back into his cot, the vomit may reach the other side of the room. There is usually a failure to gain weight and a history of constipation.

Gentle palpation of the abdomen during and just after a feed will usually reveal the diagnostic tumour in the pyloric area. Very often visible peristalsis can be seen; this is diagnostic of intestinal obstruction, the commonest cause of which, at this time of life, is pyloric stenosis.

The differential diagnosis is that of vomiting in an infant.

Management
Perhaps most family practitioners will see 2 or 3 cases in their non-hospital professional career. Most will not have the experience to manage such a case themselves. Surgical repair, after the correction of any dehydration or anaemia, is usually preferred to medical management.

Prognosis
The prognosis is excellent. Long-term follow-ups have shown no permanent disability after surgery in infancy.

Gastro-enteritis

Nature
Both diarrhoea and vomiting are extremely common symptoms: there can hardly be a person who has not had either at some time. The diagnosis of gastro-enteritis describes a disease in which these two symptoms are accompanied by a constitutional disturbance of varying severity. Some clinicians apply

the diagnostic label 'infantile gastro-enteritis' to the disease when it occurs in the first two years of life, in which age group it is potentially extremely serious. There is a risk of severe dehydration resulting from the loss of fluids and electrolytes mainly in the watery stools, but also in the vomit. The possibility of severe dehydration is also present in older children and adults but the risks are very much less. Up to the early 1950s infantile gastro-enteritis was a major cause of death among infants in Britain; it still is, in many underdeveloped countries.

Pathology

Various *E. coli* serotypes have been incriminated in different epidemics of gastro-enteritis and sometimes they may be cultured from the stools of older children with diarrhoea. However, not infrequently – particularly in older children – neither pathogenic bacteria nor viruses can be incriminated, in spite of the epidemiological evidence of an infective nature to the illness.

Infection with salmonellae, dysentery and cholera may all resemble ordinary diarrhoea and vomiting in their clinical picture but a stool culture will indicate the difference.

Epidemiology

In Britain diarrhoea and vomiting is endemic but from time to time there are minor epidemics. Major epidemics are most likely to occur, and are potentially more serious, in a closed or semi-closed community, such as day nurseries and the infants' ward of a hospital.

The best prophylactic is a constant vigilance in maintaining absolute cleanliness when dealing with everything possibly contaminated with a stool – whether or not it is known to be infected.

Diagnosis

The diagnosis rests on the history. Vomiting may be minimal or even absent. Sometimes a child may have a temporary looseness of his bowels due to dietary indiscretions. The only way to be sure this is the case is to wait and follow the course of the illness. It is not usually necessary to get a stool culture from every child with diarrhoea but this precaution is essential in infants attending a nursery or in hospital. It is also desirable to get a stool culture from any child who has recently been abroad or is in close contact with someone who has been. Stool cultures will be necessary if the diarrhoea persists more than 48 to 72 hours. Other physical signs must also be sought. In typhoid fever diagnostic rose spots may be seen, but only for a short period during the illness.

The differential diagnosis is that of both symptoms individually. Sometimes an acute appendicitis or other surgical abdominal emergency may present with diarrhoea. So, too, especially in infants, may an acute systemic infection. Otitis media, pneumonia and meningitis are common causes for diarrhoea and/or vomiting in young children. Urinary tract infections can also present in this way and will not be recognised unless a urine culture is obtained.

Dehydration can be identified in its early stages from a loss of skin elasticity. Pinching a fold of skin from the abdominal wall between two fingers will show a slow return to the normal contour if the child is dehydrated. Loss of weight over a short period is also a guide but usually there is no weight record recent enough on which to base this calculation. In a more advanced stage, the anterior abdominal wall flattens out and assumes a boat shape. This contour is normal in healthy adults but is abnormal in infancy. The child, too, is very apathetic and the character of its cry alters.

Management

There is no specific drug treatment for gastro-enteritis. The mainstay of therapy is the correction of fluid and electrolyte balance. Most cases are relatively mild, even in infants, and can be managed as well at home as in hospital. The parents are asked to give the child absolutely nothing to eat or drink, only plain water (first boiled if there is any doubt about its cleanliness). Into each 125 ml is dissolved one sodium chloride compound effervescent tablet BNF. The restriction on food intake includes milk. It is particularly important to stress this to mothers who may otherwise assume it is all right to continue to give it to their baby. Milk is not restored to the diet until the diarrhoea ceases, and then only in limited quantities: quarter strength on first day; half strength the second day; full strength on the third day, unless the diarrhoea returns, in which case milk is again completely omitted.

Antibiotics are only needed if the diarrhoea is due to a systemic infection, such as otitis media. Their use is contra-indicated in ordinary gastro-enteritis, since they are very likely to induce antibiotic resistance. In specific infections, such as one of the dysenteries, antibiotic drug resistance is very common, even in organisms which appear to be sensitive in vitro. Furthermore, the carrier state may be prolonged if antibiotics are used and many antibiotics are themselves liable to cause diarrhoea and so prolong the illness.

If the dehydration has advanced to the stage of being recognisable on ordinary clinical examination, intravenous fluid replacement is almost always essential and the child should be admitted to hospital at once. The younger the baby the more rapidly will the dehydration be manifest and the more harm will it do. If an infant with gastro-enteritis is nursed at home, frequent follow-up is essential. An early sign of impending trouble is a failure to take such liquids as are offered. The mother must be instructed to contact the doctor if this occurs.

Nevertheless, provided dietary restrictions and fluid replacement are started promptly, the majority of children, even infants, improve very rapidly at home. In older children with diarrhoea, one of the standard anti-diarrhoea remedies — a kaolin and morph mixture, diphenoxolate with atropine (Lomotil), or codeine phosphate tablets — may be prescribed. Kaolin mixture may be prescribed for infants and younger children if it is felt that some medicament should be given, though its action is little more than that of a placebo. It is never a substitute for fluid and electrolyte replacement.

Constipation

Most breast fed babies pass a stool less frequently than bottle fed babies; once every other day is a common finding, and sometimes only once a week. The stool is also different in consistency.

Sometimes a baby may have difficulty in passing his stool. If the stool is hard — which is more likely in a bottle fed baby — it may be painful. Hard stools indicate an inadequate amount of water in the diet. If the baby is bottle fed, an extra 25 ml of plain water in each bottle (without adding extra milk powder) will often solve the problem. Extra sugar may also have a laxative effect but there is no evidence that either brown sugar or glucose is more beneficial than white sugar.

Occasionally a hard stool may cause a fissure-in-ano. A gentle rectal examination (using a gloved fifth finger) will indicate the diagnosis. A local anaesthetic cream applied to the anus before the stool is passed will usually relieve the condition. The first application has been known to lead to the passage of quite an accumulation of faeces.

Laxatives should hardly ever be needed at any stage in childhood, except in the management of encopresis and severe true chronic constipation. Mothers should be reassured that while diarrhoea may be potentially lethal, constipation rarely causes any long-term harm — which is more than can be said for laxatives. It is bad enough when mothers buy laxatives over the pharmacy counter without a doctor's prescription, to administer to their children nightly or once weekly ('gives the child a good clear out every Saturday night'). It is quite wrong for the physician to encourage this abuse of nature by prescribing or even recommending a potent drug which is unnecessary.

However common it is, a regular daily bowel action is not the only norm for colonic evacuation.

Hirschprung's disease (primary megacolon) is a rare condition. The absence of autonomic innervation to one segment of the lower colon causes a local failure of the gut to relax so that the passage of stools is obstructed. If the autonomic segment is relatively low, in spite of the rectum being empty on digital examination, removal of the examining finger may be followed by a gush of liquid faeces. The affected infant is not only constipated but also usually shows signs of failure to thrive to a varying degree. The diagnosis of Hirschprung's disease is made by a barium enema. The treatment is usually surgical.

Megacolon can also arise secondarily to rectal obstruction caused by persistent constipation. The gut innervation is normal throughout its length. A rectal examination will reveal the impacted hard faeces. The condition is self-perpetuating. As hard stools are difficult to pass, the longer the bowels remain unopened the harder become the rectal contents.

Encopresis

Sometimes the end product is liquification of the stools above the impacted faecal rocks. The liquid stools trickle out of the anal orifice, giving the spurious impression of diarrhoea. This condition is known as encopresis. Treatment is by evacuation of the rectum. Oral laxatives will rarely be powerful enough and could anyway lead to perforation of the gut. If suppositories or ordinary enemas (administered by a district or practice nurse) fail, manual removal will be necessary. For this procedure a general anaesthetic may be required. Subsequently, regular enemas at gradually increasing intervals will be needed until a regular spontaneous action is restored. Regular does not necessarily mean daily. Bulk in the diet, either as bran or one of the bulk laxatives, will usually be necessary, especially for the first few weeks. The use of laxatives in the management of encopretic children is one of the few occasions on which their use can be justified.

Not infrequently, encopresis is only one manifestation of a severe emotional disorder.

Hernia

Nature

A hernia is a protrusion of the contents of a body cavity through a defect in the wall enclosing it. In children most hernias are congenital in origin.

Hiatus Hernia

Hiatus (diaphragmatic) hernia is not uncommon, especially in its mild form. The oesophagus is relatively short and part of the stomach protrudes through the gap in the diaphragm. Alternative names are 'sliding hiatus hernia' or 'partial thoracic stomach'. It usually presents in infancy, at any time after the first few weeks of life, the main symptom being vomiting. This is often little more than an exaggerated posseting but occasionally it may be projectile and must be differentiated from pyloric stenosis. Weight gain is usually not affected. Thickened feeds may be kept down better than an ordinary mixture and the child may vomit less if he is nursed in a sitting position.

Blood loss is not uncommon. Frank haematemesis is rare but occasionally the vomit can be blood-stained. Usually the main evidence for the blood loss is the discovery of an anaemia or the finding of occult blood in the stools. In practically every case the disease is self-limiting. Spontaneous recovery is usual at any time between the age of 6 months and 1 year. Management is directed at reassuring the mother. Special feeding chairs are available but the need is rarely great enough to warrant the expenditure.

Barium studies are also unnecessary unless there is doubt in the mind of the doctor, or the parents are worried. Most mothers are reassured by an explanation of the aetiology, coupled with the favourable prognosis that the child will stop vomiting by the age of 1 year.

Follow-up studies of gastro-intestinal symptomatology and function in adults who have had a sliding hiatus hernia during their first year of life, have not been carried out.

Only very rarely does the condition not settle, in which case an oesophageal stricture may develop as the child grows older.

There is a rare variety of hiatus hernia in which the gastro-oesophageal junction is normally sited but the fundus prolapses upwards at the side of the oesophagus, through the hiatus in the diaphragm. Because part of the thorax is occupied by the prolapsed stomach, there may be respiratory distress or recurrent chest infections. Obstruction of the gut is also a possibility, presenting as an acute emergency. Straight X-rays of the chest and upper abdomen will indicate the probable diagnosis.

Umbilical Hernia

This is relatively common, especially among black children. In white children they usually close spontaneously by the age of 18 months; a year or two later in black children. Even the most enormous protrusion will usually disappear before the 4th birthday. There are rarely any complications and no treatment is usually needed. When the child cries the hernia will be more prominent and the mother must be reassured that crying is not the cause of the rupture. In previous generations, strapping of the abdominal wall with a crepe bandage or elastoplast was advocated, often with an old sized penny held in place over the gap in the anterior abdominal wall. This is unnecessary and it may even delay spontaneous healing.

Inquinal Hernia

This occurs in 1–2 per cent of infants born in Britain, mainly boys. Very often it is associated with a hydrocoele and/or undescended testes. The mother herself usually notices the swelling which, like an umbilical hernia, is more prominent when the child cries. It also *is not* caused by the crying.

Once the diagnosis is made surgical repair is desirable as strangulation is not uncommon. Some surgeons will even operate if the mother clearly describes the swelling, even though they themselves cannot always identify the hernia pre-operatively. The author worked as a house surgeon to such a surgeon, and confirms this view.

Femoral Hernia
This is very rare in children.

Coeliac Disease

Nature
A defect in the function of the small intestine mucosa is associated with diminished transport of food and electrolytes from the gut lumen to the circulation and an excess passage of water, fat, and sometimes protein in the opposite direction. There is invariably some weight loss and a slowing of linear growth. These are aggravated by the anorexia which is usually present. In 75 per cent of affected children, the most prominent feature is diarrhoea. The rest of the clinical picture is a mixture of the effects of loss of the various essential nutriments, calories, protein, minerals and vitamins.

The severity of coeliac disease varies from the classically malnourished child with bulky offensive stools and prominent abdomen to minimal symptoms in a child who is being investigated because his or her weight is below par.

Clinical Features
The onset is usually insidious. An acute infection or any other stress exaggerates the clinical features and brings them to the attention of the parents or doctor. Abdominal discomfort is a frequent complaint and borborygmi can often be heard. Though abdominal distention is a common feature, the parents rarely notice it until it is brought to their attention. If there is a loss of weight it will usually be mentioned by the parents and if height and weight graphs are available for the child being examined, his decline from a normal or high to a low percentile place on the chart will be evident. The weight loss is often most prominent from the buttocks; this is a useful diagnostic clue.

Other nutritional defects include anaemia, usually hypochromic, but in older children it may be macrocytic due to folic acid malabsorption. Hypoproteinaemia, sometimes severe enough to cause oedema, is common. Rickets is seen in perhaps one child in ten with coeliac disease; it is most likely to occur at a time of rapid growth. Sometimes the presenting symptom is a general irritability and other features of behaviour disturbance, such as excessively bad tempers. Eczematoid lesions are also a feature in some patients. In severe cases hypotonia has been reported, as well as bone pain and tetany.

Diagnosis
In many diseases it is occasionally justifiable in a primary care situation to confirm a suspect diagnosis by means of a therapeutic test, usually whilst waiting for the results of special investigations. Coeliac disease is one of those instances where a therapeutic trial is never justifiable.

Because the treatment is control of the diet, where the diagnosis is obvious and beyond doubt, it might be thought worth trying a gluten free diet in a child with all or some of the features in coeliac disease, but if this is the right diagnosis the diet will have to be continued, perhaps for life, and intermittent relaxation of the dietary restrictions can be positively harmful. Therefore, no alteration should be made in the diet until the tests have been carried out. Referral to a paediatric unit equipped to carry out such a full diagnostic assessment is therefore mandatory. The diagnosis is usually made as a result of evidence obtained from a jejunal biopsy. Other pathology tests include stool examination for steatorrhoea, a full blood count, including folic acid levels, and blood biochemistry. Bone age is measured radiologically and a barium meal may show characteristic changes in the upper part of the small bowel. The height and weight should be plotted on standard charts and these help also in the assessment of subsequent progress.

Pathology

Coeliac disease in children is probably the same disease process as idiopathic steatorrhoea in adults. Where this disease is first recognised in adulthood, it is usually assumed that the pathology had been present in the earlier years of life but had not been recognised. In all cases there is some abnormal sensitivity to gluten. This abnormal sensitivity is found in the mucosa of the small bowel from the duodenum to the upper jejunum, but its nature is not known, nor is the precise part played by gluten, which is a part of wheat, rye, barley and oats.

Management

Total removal of gluten from the diet is essential. Advice from a qualified dietician is desirable and excellent help is available from the Coeliac Society* who can also advise parents how to make the food appetizing. 'Cheating' is not uncommon, either by the child himself or by the parents, and invariably leads to a relapse.

In the early stages of treatment vitamin and mineral supplements may be necessary. Few family practitioners will have enough experience to manage a case in the early stages but once the child is stablised the task is less formidable, mainly because both parents and child should understand what they have to do, and why.

As the child grows older he may develop a tolerance for gluten: perhaps one affected child in three appears to improve. After five years satisfactory freedom from symptoms and biochemical effects, an attempt may be made to gradually introduce gluten into the diet to see if a relaxation of the strict dietary control is possible.

* The Coeliac Society, PO Box 181, London NW2 2QY.

Cystic Fibrosis of the Pancreas

Nature

Cystic fibrosis is also known as fibrocystic disease or mucoviscidosis. It was originally thought to be a disease affecting only the pancreas and lung but it is now known to affect many other organs, including the exocrine glands. The secretion of an abnormally viscid mucus is responsible for most of the clinical features: —

1. Recurrent chest infections which are superimposed onto an obstruction with viscid mucus of the smaller bronchi and bronchioles.
2. Pancreatic deficiency which causes malabsorption and steatorrhoea. The malabsorption is responsible for the child's failure to thrive.
3. Biliary cirrhosis. This is much less common than the other two features.

There is also a high concentration of sodium, potassium and chloride in the sweat. This forms the basis of an important diagnostic test.

Incidence

Approximatley 1 child in 2500 Caucasian children is born with the disease. The incidence is much less in most other races.

There is a strong family incidence of the disease, which is inherited by an autososmal recessive. The gene is relatively common in the community; it is possessed by approximately 1 person in 25 to 50 but heterozygotes do not appear to be affected.

Clinical Features

The three main clinical features are recurrent respiratory infection, an abnormal stool and failure to thrive. Cystic fibrosis should be considered a possible diagnosis in a child with any of these features.

Recurrent respiratory infections are the main presenting symptom. Sometimes, but not always, the infection is severe. Staphylococci are frequently indicted as the causative organism. There is often a harsh cough but adventitious sounds in the chest may not always be prominent. An increased respiratory rate, cyanosis and rib recession indicate the severity of the attack.

The stools are usually abnormal from birth. The disease may present with intestinal obstruction due to meconeum ileus within the first few days of life but this is not very common (5 per cent of cases). The stools are bulky, though not necessarily more frequent. In the first few weeks of life they are greenish in colour but later they become pale with a characteristic odour which lingers in the room*. The stool looks greasy and the mother may notice it is difficult to wash the napkins.

---

* When the author was a paediatric house physician he claims to have recognised that a fibrocystic child had been re-admitted to his ward, because he could detect the smell as he entered the front door of the hospital.

A failure to thrive may be the feature most noticed by the parents who do not recognise the abnormality of the stool, especially if it is in their first child, and regard the frequent coughs as normal. The abdomen is usually bloated and a rectal prolapse is fairly common.

The severity of the disease varies considerably. In a mild case the diagnosis may not be easy. It can, however, be confirmed by the sweat test. This can be done in family practice but the test is not needed frequently enough to warrant expenditure on the equipment, nor to enable the doctor to assess the significance of a border-line result. A child suspected of having cystic fibrosis should, therefore, be referred to a paediatrician.

Because of the relatively high incidence of the disease among siblings, all the brothers and sisters of an affected case should be fully investigated.

Differential Diagnosis

Any child with one or more of the diagnostic features should be investigated. Coeliac disease can be diagnosed by an intestinal biopsy. In a doubtful case both this and the sweat test will be needed. If respiratory signs are prominent the possibility of asthma may have to be considered but in this disease there will be no abnormality of the stools.

Management

The majority of children with cystic fibrosis will be under the regular care of a consultant paediatrician and their diet should be supervised by a dietician. Pancreatic supplements will be needed with every meal.

Some paediatricians recommend that the child be on antibiotics all the time; others prefer to confine their use to acute exacerbations of respiratory infection. Frequent sputum culture is necessary to ensure that resistance has not arisen to the antibiotic being used. Equally important is daily physiotherapy to promote drainage of the secretions. The mother can be taught how to do this so that the child can have his treatment at home.

Whenever possible, respiratory complications should be avoided. The family doctor should make sure the child has been vaccinated against measles.

Prognosis

Formerly few children with cystic fibrosis survived into their teens but with the availability of broad-spectrum antibiotics to reduce the effect of chronic or recurrent chest infections, the outlook has improved considerably. Unfortunately many older children with the disease are still respiratory cripples. The antibiotics have not been available long enough to know the long-term effects.

Many children with a chronic disability, especially those affecting their diet, tend to manifest psychological difficulties, particularly at and after puberty; these will often be brought to the family doctor.

Genetic counselling should be offered to the families of all affected children.

EYE DISEASES IN CHILDREN

Introduction

The examination of the eye is an essential part of a full clinical examination of a child, both to detect local disease and also because the eyes are sometimes involved in other disease processes. At least as important as the examination of the eye is an estimation of visual acuity.

Vision

The normal tests for vision depend on the patient knowing the alphabet. The age at which children master this skill varies considerably, reflecting very often the social pressures to which they are put in learning. Because Snellen's charts cannot be relied upon in most children until they are 7 to 8 years old, alternative tests for assessing distance vision have been devised. The 'E' test has been generally superceded by the Sheridan-Gardiner test, in which the child points to the same letters on a card when presented with isolated letters held at a distance by the examiner. This test can be used in most children from the age of 3 to 4 years.

In younger children the vision may be tested by rolling balls of different sizes — the smallest being about 10 mm in diameter — in front of the child, at a distance of about 3 metres. The child is observed to see if his eyes follow the movement of the rolling ball. This test can be performed at the 7-month routine examination. Using coloured sweets such as Smarties has the advantage that if the child succeeds in the test, he may collect a prize.

Both eyes should be tested together and separately. Considerable patience is required on the part of the examiner and obviously a child cannot be examined whilst he is fractious.

In the first few weeks of life some assessment of vision can be made by observing the child's eyes when he follows a torchlight and later when he stretches out his hand to grasp an object.

Strabismus (Squint)

Nature
Strabismus is a failure of the visual axis* of the squinting eye to be directed at the object being viewed by the other (non-squinting) eye. The second image, usually the weaker, is at first suppressed; the child uses only one eye. If the

---

* The visual axis runs from the fovea to the object being looked at.

squint remains untreated for any length of time the suppression becomes permanent and irreversible. This condition is known as amblyopia.

Binocular vision starts to develop in infants at a variable age, but always by the time the child is 6 months old. Many children with normal eyes have an alternating squint during the first few weeks of life but this should disappear spontaneously before the infant is 6 months old.

The presence of a broad bridge to the nose may give the impression of a squint (pseudo-squint) even though the eyes are straight, particularly if epicanthic folds are present, causing more temporal than nasal sclera to be exposed.

In some children the squint is vertical. These are very much less common than horizontal squints. Sometimes a child with a vertical squint will hold his head on one side, giving the impression of torticollis, in order to balance the two visual images.

Most squints in children are of the non-paralytic (concomitant) variety. All the ocular muscles function normally but binocular vision does not develop properly. This can occur if the vision in one eye (or both) is not normal. The child may be long-sighted (hypermetropia is the commonest cause of squint in children) or short-sighted; astygmatism may be present or the child may have a congential cataract. Paralytic (non-comitant) squints are much rarer in children; they are most frequently due to trauma, as in birth injuries and battered babies. They can also follow an encephalopathy, such as those complicating the exanthemata; they may also result from a brain tumour.

Diagnosis

A squint may be obvious. Sometimes it is the doctor or health visitor who first recognises it; sometimes it is the mother, who may complain that one or both eyes 'turns in' from time to time. Every child should be examined for squint at the age of 7 months. A simple test is to observe the position of the light reflection in both eyes when a torch is shone into them from at least 18 inches away. A pseudo-squint may be differentiated by the cover test but if there is the slightest doubt that a squint exists, it must be fully investigated.

Cover Test   The child is asked to look at an object (e.g., a pencil or the ophthalmoscope light) held at least 18 inches from the eyes. If one eye appears not to be looking in the direction of the object, the other eye (the 'good' one) is covered with a card held by the examiner but not pressed into the child's orbit. The squinting eye will then move in the opposite direction to its squint in order to view the object. In the case of a convergent squint the eye moves laterally and with a divergent squint it moves medially. Not infrequently the squint alternates from one eye to the other and the cover test must be used for each eye in turn.

In older children the squinting eye may be 'lazy' as a result of amblyopia and be unable to take up the fixation. The cover test will be negative, but in these children the convergence or divergence is usually so gross as to be beyond doubt.

Sometimes the degree of ocular imbalance is so slight that in normal circumstances the binocular function can compensate for this. Such a latent squint can be identified by the alternate cover test.

Alternate Cover Test   This consists of rapidly covering each eye in turn, asking the child to fix on an object. The eye being uncovered is carefully observed and any movement to take up fixation indicates a latent squint.

Latent squints are usually asymptomatic but occasionally they may be responsible for headaches. In the presence of other severe illnesses, a latent squint may become manifest.

In some practices the initial cover test is left to the health visitor or nurse, who can be trained to do this. If the squint is latent it may be much harder to recognise. Many family practitioners find it difficult to be sure whether or not this is present. No ophthalmologist should object to being asked to see a child suspected of having a manifest or latent squint.

Management

It is essential that every child with a true squint is seen as soon as possible by an ophthalmologist; certainly before the child is a year old. Treatment will depend on the cause and extent of the strabismus. Refractive errors can be corrected with glasses; the normal eye may have to be occluded with a patch or darkened lense; orthoptic exercises may be needed. Sometimes one or other of the extra-ocular muscles may have to be re-aligned surgically.

A squint which is still present when the child has his 7-month routine medical examination warrants further investigation; certainly before the child is a year old. If an infant, however young, has a fixed squint, he should be referred to an ophthalmologist even earlier.

After referral to a specialist, it is important that the family practitioner assures himself that the child is carrying out the treatment advised. Many children dislike wearing glasses and some mothers are at first unwilling to insist that the child wears them at all times. Some children may even deliberately lose or break the glasses.

Prognosis

It is not always possible to guarantee the successful cosmetic outcome of treatment but most cases of amblyopia due to strabismus ought to be preventable provided every child with a squint is diagnosed early enough in life and treatment is properly carried out.

Refractive Errors

These are common in children. Usually the defect is relatively minor and easily correctable with properly prescribed glasses. Minor degrees of refractive error may not require correction. It is therefore preferable for every child who might need glasses to first see a consultant ophthalmologist.

There are very few symptoms of a refractive error. The most significant is a squint in an infant or young child. Many children – adults as well – tolerate a not inconsiderable refractive error without being aware of it until they are routinely tested at school or for a job. When prescribed glasses at the age of 9, a nephew of mine commented that he had not realised the kitchen linoleum at home was patterned!

Some children with a refractive error may be brought to their family practitioner because they blink, but the vision in most children who blink is normal.

Conjunctivitis

Nature

Conjunctivitis is inflammation of the mucous membrane lining the eyelids and the globe of the eye. Sometimes the cause is chemical or traumatic and, especially in older children, a number are allergic in origin. Most, however, are due to an infection, usually bacterial but sometimes viral. A conjunctival inflammation is also part of certain systemic viral infections, such as measles.

Epidemics of conjunctivitis are not uncommon in closed communities, especially day nurseries.

Clinical Features

The eye feels sore and the child will want to rub it. Often there is some photophobia. On examination the lining of the eyelids and the whites of the eyes are red. There is epiphora (excess tearing) and, if the infection is bacterial, the discharge is purulent. In a severe case the eyelids may be swollen and difficult to open, or dry pus may stick the lids together.

Differential Diagnosis

The inside of the eyelids must be inspected for a foreign body, especially if the conjunctivitis is unilateral. Some children with sore eyes rub both and a foreign body may present as a bilateral conjunctivitis. The other causes of a red eye in adults are uncommon in children.

It should always be remembered that if a child is crying when examined, the eyes may well look red and watery.

The seasonal incidence will indicate the possibility of an allergic conjunctivitis. Itching is a frequent complaint and often there is a history of asthma, eczema or hayfever.

Management

The management of conjunctivitis depends upon its cause. A mild chemical or traumatic conjunctivitis will usually recover spontaneously; local antibiotic eyedrops may be used prophylactically. Allergic conjunctivitis will often respond to a local or systemic antihistamine. Local steroid eyedrops may be necessary but these should be carefully supervised, preferably by an ophthalmologist, as there is a major risk of inducing steroid glaucoma.

Bacterial conjunctivitis is best treated by the frequent instillation of a wide-spectrum antibiotic in the form of eyedrops. Chloramphenicol eyedrops, which do not produce the adverse haematological side-effects of the systemic administration of this drug, should be used hourly during the day. An antibiotic ointment may be prescribed in addition to the drops for use at night. If improvement has not occurred within 48 hours the organism is not sensitive to the antibiotic, or the diagnosis of bacterial conjunctivitis is incorrect. Some mothers are afraid they may damage the eyes. This hardly ever occurs but it sometimes inhibits the mother from using the drops. In babies a short intensive course may be administered by the practice nurse: one drop into the conjunctival sac every minute for 15 minutes, and then every 5 minutes for 2 hours.

Hygienic measures are also important. The eyelids may be gently bathed with clear water and the child should use his own flannel and towel, particularly at a nursery or school. When an epidemic occurs in a school, a conjunctival culture is advisable; in sporadic cases this is seldom necessary or practical.

Styes (Hordeolum)

Nature

An abscess of an eyelash follicle.

Epidemiology

The causative organism is usually a staphylococcus. Styes are especially common in teenagers. They tend to occur when the child is under stress, such as facing examinations. Frequently one stye is followed by another, presumably because the child rubs his eyes and spreads the infection. However, it is unusual for a stye to pass from one patient to another.

Clinical Features

A painful red swelling can be seen on the edge of the eyelid. Left to itself the stye will point and discharge the purulent contents with complete resolution.

Management

The use of antibiotics either locally or systemically is unnecessary unless there is a spread of infection beyond the follicle. Eye ointments of any kind tend to encourage a local spread to neighbouring follicles. Pulling out the hair from the infected follicle may encourage more rapid healing, as will the local application of heat, which is also very soothing.

Meibomian Cysts (Chalazion)

Meibomian cysts are less common in children than adults. In the acute stage they may be mistaken for a stye unless their situation within the eyelid and not at the edge is recognised. Sometimes the infected cyst bursts and this leads to resolution, but usually the cyst becomes chronic and will need to be curetted. It is sometimes possible to leave the operation until the child reaches his teens and is old enough to co-operate in an outpatient procedure under a local anaesthetic.

Blocked Tear Duct

Nature

In about 2 per cent of infants the naso-lacrimal duct in one or both eyes may not be patent at birth. In the majority of these children the cause is a simple blockage due to mucus or debris which almost always clears spontaneously at some time within the first 6 months of life. Very rarely the duct may be obstructed at the nasal end by a membrane.

Clinical Features

When tears start to appear in the eyes at around the age of 3 weeks, they will be seen to be excessive. The epiphora may then develop into a mucoid or muco-purulent discharge. Very often an infected blockage of the tear duct is mistaken for a conjunctivitis and vice versa. Sometimes there is an acute local infection (dacryocystitis).

Management

The natural history is for the duct to unblock itself spontaneously. There is usually no need for active intervention unless there is a superimposed infection, in which case local antibiotic eyedrops may be prescribed. Eye ointments could further block the duct. In an uncomplicated case the eye can be kept clean by bathing twice or thrice daily with moistened sterile cotton wool or gauze swabs. Massage of the tear duct may be helpful.

The results of conservative management are at least as good as those from active intervention. It is only necessary to refer the child to an ophthalmologist if the duct fails to open spontaneously by the age of 6 months, which is not a very common occurrence, or unless there is an acute superadded infection which fails to respond to treatment.

Blepharitis

Nature
Crusting of the eyelids is common, especially among school children — adolescent boys in particular. It may be mistaken by parents and teachers for conjunctivitis. Very often it is accompanied by seborrhoea of the scalp (dandruff). It is not usually contagious. Bathing the eyelids may be helpful. In persistent cases the use of aureomycin eye ointment twice daily for 1 to 4 weeks will help but the condition is likely to recur. Alternatively, steroid eye ointment may be used but the prognosis is no better.

VACCINATION AND IMMUNISATION

There are several ways of controlling the spread of infectious diseases. The most satisfactory method is to eliminate the source of infection from the community, as is done in the case of rabies and psittacosis by controlling the import of animals and birds and, in the case of cholera, by maintaining a clean supply of water. A second method of control is to isolate every infected person, which is still done in the case of smallpox and certain other potentially lethal infectious diseases. Isolation was also the standard procedure until the late 1940s for many other common infectious diseases, such as diphtheria and scarlet fever.

The third method of controlling the spread of infectious diseases is by vaccinating all, or the majority, of the population against that disease so that they become immune to it. When a large proportion of the population is uninfectable, transmission of the disease is restricted.

As none of the vaccines is completely free from side-effects, and as not all of them guarantee complete immunity, careful consideration has to be given to the advantages and disadvantages of each vaccine. In Britain a specialist committee appointed by the Department of Health and Social Security — with representatives from family practice — constantly reviews the problem and from time to time offers guidelines from which have been drawn up a schedule of vaccinations to be offered to every child (Table 23.1). The vaccines used may be either live or inactivated. Live vaccines utilize an agent related to the causative organism of the disease, such as the use of cowpox vaccine against smallpox, or an attenuated form of the disease organism, such as the Sabin oral polio vaccine. Examples of inactivated vaccines are pertussis and the Salk injectable polio vaccine.

Each of the vaccines available in this schedule will be described in turn.

Table 23.1   Schedule of vaccinations for children

Age	Interval	Vaccine	Notes
6–8 months		Triple antigen* Polio	Omit pertussis if history of convulsions or allergy
8–10 months	6–8 weeks	Triple antigen* Polio	
1 year		Measles	
14–16 months	6 months	Triple antigen* Polio	
5 years		Diphtheria and tetanus; Polio	Or school entry if earlier
11–14 years		BCG	Both sexes – TB test first
11–14 years		Rubella	Girls only
15–19 years		Tetanus toxoid Polio	On leaving school

* Diphtheria, tetanus and pertussis.

Diphtheria

The fall in the mortality rate from diphtheria in Britain, a disease which, at the turn of the century, had been the commonest cause of death among children aged 5 to 10 years, began before the introduction of immunisation, but the rate of decline accelerated rapidly in the early 1940s when diphtheria toxoid vaccine was actively sponsored by the government. It had fallen equally rapidly 20 years previously, when it was introduced in the USA and parts of Europe. The decrease in morbidity has been equally dramatic, so that today most family practitioners in the UK may never see a case.

For the primary course a greater degree of immunity is achieved by the use of an adsorbed toxoid: purified diphtheria formal toxoid with either aluminium hydroxide or phosphate as an adjuvant. This is generally given in combination with tetanus and pertussis (see Table 23.1 for schedule) and *must* be administered intramuscularly. Injected sub-cutaneously there is a strong possibility of producing a nodule in the sub-cutaneous tissue, which may persist for many years.

For the pre-school and subsequent booster doses, the plain formal toxoid vaccine is preferred. It is injected intramuscularly, deep sub-cutaneously or intradermally*.

The plain formal toxoid may be combined with tetanus toxoid: pertussis vaccine is not given after the age of 3 years. The unadsorbed vaccine is

* *Adsorbed* vaccine must *not* be administered intradermally.

unsuitable for a primary course of immunisation, particularly in younger children.

Children who are unwell at the time should not be immunised; nor should children with a history of convulsions or atopy. Adverse reactions to the diphtheria component are usually mild; a local erythema may persist for a few days. Severe allergic reactions are rare.

Tetanus

As tetanus is not a notifiable disease, the true incidence is not known; less than 50 cases a year have been reported in the past two decades. Nevertheless, in spite of the rarity the benefits are considerable, not least an avoidance of the need to give anti-tetanus serum with all its hazards.

Tetanus toxoid is usually administered to infants (see Table 23.1 for schedule) in combination with diphtheria and pertussis. The adsorbed vaccine (see 'Diphtheria' above) gives a better immune response.

Adults and older children who have not been previously immunised should be given a primary course if their occupation puts them at risk. The injection of the adsorbed vaccine should be intra-muscular or, alternatively, plain fluid toxoid 0.1 ml may be injected intradermally over the age of 10. Reactions to tetanus toxoid are uncommon.

Pertussis

The argument for and against routine pertussis immunisation is not yet resolved. The side-effects of this component of the triple antigen may be severe; in particular the long-term results of an encephalitis can be disastrous. Less severe reactions are not uncommon; an irritability lasting 12 to 48 hours has been reported in as many as one child in five given pertussis vaccine. Elixir promethazine 5 ml three times a day is sometimes helpful in reducing the severity of this side-effect. Whenever the first or second injection of triple antigen produces an adverse reaction, future injections must always omit the pertussis component.

Many parents are reluctant to agree to their children being immunised unless they can be assured that the pertussis component has been omitted from all the injections. It is, anyway, never given after the age of 3 years.

Smallpox

In the UK routine smallpox vaccination has not been recommended since 1971, because the risk of complications is now greater than the risk of contacting the disease. It is no longer given routinely in the USA and most other western countries.

Alternative methods, including the selective vaccination of contacts, exist for the control of an epidemic should a case of smallpox be introduced into the country.

Measles

Because of the persistence of maternally transmitted antibodies to the fetus, it is better to delay measles vaccination until after the child is 9 months old and preferably until the second year of life (see Table 23.1 for schedule).

The vaccine at present used is freeze-dried. It should be reconstituted *within* 1 hour of use with 0.5 ml water. Like all other vaccines it should not be given to children who are ill at the time. As the vaccine is produced in chick egg tissue culture, it should not be given to those who are allergic to eggs. It is absolutely contra-indicated in children with a reticulo-endothelial disease, such as Hodgkin's disease. It should not normally be given to children with a history of convulsions, but if the harmful effects of an attack of measles are thought to be great (for example, a child who also has chronic heart or chest disease), prophylactic anti-convulsant cover with phenytoin should be given for 2 weeks, starting 24 hours before the measles vaccine is administered.

Rubella

The only reason for rubella vaccination is to protect the unborn fetus from maternal rubella. It is, therefore, offered to all schoolgirls between their 11th and 14th birthdays. It should also be offered to women of childbearing age, who are found to be sero-negative, and all nurses and those who work in maternity units. It is essential to caution the patient against falling pregnant within 3 months of the vaccination, as the effects of the vaccine on the fetus are identical with those of an attack of rubella. 0.5 ml of freshly reconstituted vaccine is injected subcutaneously. Side-effects are minimal. Attacks resembling a mild rubella may occur. They are more common in adults than children.

Poliomyelitis

The killed virus vaccine, discovered by Salk and administered by injection, has been replaced almost totally by Sabin's live attenuated virus vaccine which is given orally. The live vaccine mimics the natural infection and confers the same quality of immunity, as well as producing a local resistance to infection in the gut.

The three strains of polio virus are present in both types of vaccine. Though theoretically one dose should achieve immunity to all three strains, it is safer to complete the primary course with two further doses of vaccine, as shown in Table 23.1. The antibody levels should be boosted at school entry and school leaving, and it is also wise to give a further booster to anyone travelling to any of the countries where polio is still endemic.

Bacillus Calmette-Guerin (BCG)

BCG is an attenuated living bovine strain of *M. tuberculosis.* The vaccine at present in use is freeze dried. It is reconstituted with the special diluent provided and injected intradermally. The dose is 0.1 ml and the usual site is over the deltoid.

The effect of the vaccine is to produce a local controlled primary focus in the form of a papule 4 to 6 weeks after vaccination. The main benefit of the vaccine is the almost total elimination of the disseminated (post primary) foci of tuberculous infection in vaccinated children (TB nephritis, arthritis, etc.). The vaccine also reduces the risk of contacting the adult form of infection — pulmonary TB.

Where the child is at a relatively great risk, for example, where there is a family history of TB, it is usual to offer the vaccine almost immediately after birth. In the UK, where TB is relatively rare in the community children, other than those at risk, are offered BCG at the age of 11 to 13 years, though in some areas it is offered to every child at birth.

It is usual to TB test (Montaux, Heaf or Tine) every child before vaccination, to ensure he has not already been infected (see p. 104). The vaccine is usually administered by those who have attended a special course; however, the only skill is that of giving an intradermal injection. The appearance of a papule is taken by many as an indication of a successful vaccination but some prefer to check the result by repeating the TB test and doing so again annually. Sometimes the papule ulcerates and the family practitioner, who probably did not himself do the vaccination, will then be consulted. Local hydrocortisone and antibiotic cream applied twice daily usually leads to rapid healing, with no loss of the effectiveness of the vaccination.

INFECTIOUS FEVERS

In western countries few children reach adulthood without having had one or more of the common infectious fevers:

Chicken Pox	Poliomyelitis
Diphtheria	Roseola Infantum
Glandular fever	Rubella
Measles	Scarlet Fever
Meningitis	Whooping Cough
Mumps	

Some of these are now relatively harmless, especially in children, and the public rightly takes a phlegmatic view of their occurrence. The exceptions are diphtheria, meningitis and poliomyelitis, which must always be regarded circumspectly.

With measles, rubella, chicken pox and mumps, it is not unknown for parents to make their own diagnoses and not bother to ask the doctor to see the child. This habit is much more common in the USA, where the doctor has to be paid a fee. The doctor is telephoned to be informed that the child is ill; his advice is sought without his actually examining the child. This practice can perhaps be defended where the affected child is the second or subsequent sibling to get the illness. However, the parental diagnosis could be wrong and it is the author's view that this practice is unwise. Whilst an infectious fever is hardly ever an emergency — very often the first time the mother sees the rash is when undressing the child for bed — every child should be medically examined to confirm the diagnosis and exclude complications.

The volume of work engendered by the infectious fevers can rarely be sufficiently great to warrant the family practitioner not seeing the child at least once during the illness.

Many of the infectious fevers can now be prevented, or the incidence reduced by vaccination. The arguments for and against vaccination in individual cases is dealt with under the specific infections.

Chicken Pox (Varicella)

Nature
A highly infectious, usually benign, illness caused by the varicelle-zoster virus (*Herpes varicellae*). The virus is identical with that found in herpes zoster. Whilst adults with shingles can transmit the virus to a child who then gets chicken pox, the reverse is not the case. The incubation period is usually 16 days but it varies between 14 and 21 days.

Incidence
The disease is world wide and practically every child in the western world gets chicken pox before reaching adulthood, though data on the number who avoid infection is not available. No age is immune; neonates who have been infected in utero are not unknown. The maximum incidence is between 2 and 8 years.

Infectivity
One attack usually produces life-long immunity. The virus, however, remains dormant in a dorsal root ganglion and may later be re-activated in an attack of herpes zoster. Transmission is by direct contact, droplet or airborne spread, and is maximal in the early stages of the illness. By the time the crusts appear the disease is no longer infectious.

Clinical Features

The characteristic feature of chicken pox is the skin rash and this is usually the first sign of the presence of the infection. A few children have a prodromal malaise and sometimes fever.

The initial rash is a red macule which becomes raised and papular. In turn this becomes vesicular and then pustular. Finally, when the pustule bursts or is scratched open it crusts. The change from one stage to the next is rapid: 2 to 4 days from macule to scab. The lesions appear in groups and at any one time separate groups will be at a different stage of development. Thus macules, papules, vesicles, and pustules may be simultaneously recognised on adjacent areas of the body.

The distribution of the rash is typical. The spots are more profuse on the trunk, especially the back, than the limbs and face, but no part of the body is exempt. Lesions are often found inside the mouth, where they can be most uncomfortable for the child.

The whole disease process is fairly rapid and within 7 days almost all the spots will have crusted. The vesicles and pustules usually irritate and the child is tempted to scratch, which may lead to a secondary infection. Any subsequent scarring is attributed to this and not to the primary lesions.

Differential Diagnosis

The lesions of smallpox are distributed peripherally rather than centrally and all are at the same stage of development at the one time. A patient with smallpox is usually very ill but, especially in those previously vaccinated, this may not always be the case and cannot be relied upon as a diagnostic feature. If there is any doubt whatsoever, a smallpox expert must be consulted. In Britain lists of smallpox consultants are available from the area Health Authority. Reliance must be placed on microscopic examination of the vesicular fluid to identify the virus.

Whilst smallpox is the classical differential diagnosis referred to in most textbooks on chicken-pox, the diseases more likely to give the family practitioner difficulty are papular urticaria and erythema multiforme, especially in the first day or two of the eruption. Papular urticaria usually appears in linear groups on the trunk and limbs, rather than groups all over the body. The mouth is always exempt and it is not possible to simultaneously identify all four types of lesion. Erythema multiforme is unlikely to cause confusion if the characteristics of chicken-pox are carefully checked.

It may be necessary at the beginning of the illness to delay making a diagnosis until the appearance of further groups at different stages of development confirm the picture.

Management

There is no specific treatment. Calamine lotion is the traditional application to sooth the itching spots but it can be messy and the author personally recommends a simple talc (baby powder) liberally applied. If sleep is disturbed, promethazine may both sedate and act as an anti-pruritic. A larger than usual dose is often required and provided it is only given at night, a 25 mg tablet may be administered to a 2—5 year old child, and double that dose if the child is older. 5—10 ml of the elixir can be given to infants. Aqueous gentian violet 0.2 per cent as a mouth wash can be messy, but it is soothing if the oral lesions are painful. In most cases the mother and child are content with the doctor's reassurance that no harm will ensue. The child should be advised to avoid solids, especially brittle foods such as toast, and rely on liquids for nourishment.

Prevention
Such is the high degree of infectivity of chicken pox and so relatively mild the illness, there is no point in attempting to prevent an attack. Exceptions should be made in the case of patients on steroids and, in particular, cyto-toxic drugs. These patients themselves may have to be isolated rather than an attempt to isolate the patients with chicken pox, as new cases will be constantly appearing in the community.

Diphtheria

Nature
An acute infectious disease in which there is a) production of a surface membrane at the site of infection and b) generalised toxaemia. The *Corynebacterum diphtheriae* produces a powerful exotoxin which is responsible for both the acute symptoms in the pharynx and the distant effects on the heart and other organs. The incubation period is between 2 and 7 days.

Incidence
Diphtheria has become a rare disease in western countries since the introduction of routine diphtheria immunisation using toxoid to provide immunity to the diphtheria toxin. It is still very prevalent in many underdeveloped countries, where it is a major killer.

Clinical Features
Invasion by *C. diphtheriae* leads to the local destruction of the superficial epithelium and the appearance of a membrane which is very adherent to underlying tissue. The extent of spread of the membrane varies with the severity of the infection. It is not uncommon for the larynx to be obstructed, necessitating a tracheotomy. If the nose is involved rather than the throat, the membrane may not be visible; instead there is a bloody discharge.

Meanwhile the exotoxin is carried by the bloodstream to distant organs, including the myocardium. At this stage the child is usually very toxic and often hallucinating.

Diagnosis

The history and clinical findings will indicate the possibility of diphtheria and a throat swab will confirm the diagnosis. The differential diagnosis is an ordinary tonsillitis and glandular fever.

Management

In the rare event of *C. diphtheriae* being cultured from a nose or throat swab, it would be a wise precaution to first check with the bacteriologist that it is not a harmless diphtheroid. The main part of the treatment of diphtheria is the administration of antitoxin in an adequate dose; the administration of penicillin or erythromycin is of secondary importance. In most cases admission to a fever hospital will be necessary.

Infectious Mononucleosis (Glandular Fever)

Nature

Infectious mononucleosis is characterized by the presence in a blood film of abnormal mononuclear lymphocytes and a positive heterophil antibody titre (the Paul Bunnell reaction). The incubation period is 4—14 days.

Infectivity

The degree of infectivity is usually low: epidemics are rarely reported outside closed communities. Sporadic cases rarely give rise to subsequent cases within the same household.

Clinical Features

There are several distinct clinical features: rarely are all present in one patient. In an epidemic, different signs may be present in different patients, suggesting that they are, in fact, all part of the one disease and not manifestations of separate diseases. The disease is most common in teenagers, but no age group is exempt. Most sufferers, but not all, feel ill and have little or no appetite. Sleeping difficulties are common.

The temperature is invariably raised (38—40°C.) at some time in the illness and frequently may swing up and down. Investigations of a pyrexia of unknown origin (PUO) not infrequently show the cause to be glandular fever. Sometimes the raised temperature is the only physical sign, other than the diagnostic haematological picture. In the anginose variety of glandular fever, the tonsils are large and covered with a white membrane which may persist for several weeks. There may be petechial spots at the junction of the hard and soft palate but these are also seen in other viral infections.

Lymph node enlargement is very common, especially those in the anterior cervical chain, the sub-occipital area, the axilla, the groin and the elbow. Pain is not a prominent feature of these swollen glands but if there is a mesenteric adenitis there may be some abdominal discomfort. The spleen is palpable; some reports quote this in over half the cases, but palpation of the spleen is an art which not all doctors have acquired! Jaundice occurs in about 5 per cent of cases; the liver function tests are indistinguishable from those in infectious hepatitis. A maculo-papular rash occurs in 10 to 15 per cent of cases, usually in the second week. Urticarial and other skin rashes, including purpura, have also been described.

Complications include encephalitis, asymptomatic meningitis and an acute polyneuritis (the Guillain-Barré syndrome). Myocarditis may also occur. The clinical and ECG findings are similar to those found in a coronary thrombosis or pericarditis.

Pathology

Whilst the various physical findings of both the disease and its complications can produce a wide variety of pathological changes, the most significant features in glandular fever are, first, presence in a white blood film of a large number (up to 20 per cent) of atypical lymphocytes of a characteristic appearance. In small numbers these cells may also be found in other viral infections.

Second, the presence of sheep red cell agglutinins can be identified by the Paul Bunnell reaction. This test may also be positive in other conditions. It can be made more specific by repetition after absorption, separately, with guinea pig kidney and ox erythrocytes. (Infectious mononeucleosis antibodies are not absorbed by guinea pig kidney but are absorbed by ox erythrocytes). Not infrequently the Paul Bunnell reaction is negative for the first 1 to 2 weeks after the onset of the illness and repeated tests may be necessary to confirm the diagnosis. The reaction may then remain positive for a long time after the initial infection. This may sometimes be misdiagnosed as a re-infection.

In about 10 per cent of patients the Wasserman reaction may also be temporarily positive. Raised transaminases are also found and indicate some hepatic involvement.

Differential Diagnosis

In a teenager with any of the following symptoms or signs, glandular fever must always be considered:

1. PUO.
2. Tonsillitis with abnormal features. For example, no causative bacterial pathogens can be cultured from a throat swab, or there may be no response to an antibiotic.
3. A rash resembling rubella, measles, or sometimes scarlatina or urticaria.
4. Jaundice.
5. Symptoms of meningitis or encephalitis.
6. Pericarditis or myocarditis.

Though less frequent, the diagnosis must also be considered in other age groups with similar presenting features. However, the interpretation of the haematological findings must be considered carefully and equated with the present and previous history, because the Paul Bunnell reaction may indicate a previous and not the present infection.

Management

There is no specific treatment. The management is symptomatic.

Antibiotics are unnecessary. Ampicillin, prescribed perhaps when tonsillitis is diagnosed or as a blunderbuss therapy for a PUO, is very likely to cause a rash in a patient with mononucleosis. It is important to recognise that the rash is not due to a penicillin allergy because it will be quite safe in most cases to use ampicillin or other penicillins in subsequent infections that are due to a penicillin sensitive organism.

Steroids may relieve most of the symptoms and signs, but relapses are likely after the course is finished. These drugs should be reserved for those patients with serious complications of mononucleosis, such as airways obstruction, when the steroids may be life-saving.

Prognosis

Life threatening complications are rare, and the outlook is usually excellent. Children recover normally but adults often feel depressed long after an attack. This is a particularly frequent occurrence among teenagers. Indeed, students often self-diagnose an attack of depression as glandular fever.

Measles (Morbilli, Rubeola)

Nature

Measles is a highly infectious viral disease. The causative organism resembles the para-influenza virus. Transmission is by droplets from an infected person, mainly at the time the skin rash appears, or a day or two before.

The incubation period is usually around 10 days but it varies from 8 to 14 days.

Infectivity

Isolation of an infected child in a hospital setting is usually essential to protect other children in the ward, some of whom may be severely debilitated. In the home it is neither feasible nor necessary to isolate the sick child from other siblings. One attack of the disease will almost always produce a life long immunity: it is hoped that a single vaccination will achieve the same effect.

With measles it is particularly difficult to achieve complete isolation of infected cases, because the infectivity is maximal before the disease is usually diagnosed. It is, therefore, unnecessary to keep contacts of an infected child away from school, unless and until they show signs of the disease. Cough and coryza are usually the first warning.

It is, however, wise to try to protect a child who is debilitated. It is rarely possible to prevent him coming into contact with other children who have the disease and reliance is better placed on vaccination. Indeed, the availability of a satisfactory vaccine has converted most of the above issues to academic questions.

Incidence

During the first 3—4 months of life most children retain sufficient antibody acquired from the mother to protect themselves from this infection, assuming the mother herself has had a previous attack of measles. Thereafter the incidence increases rapidly, and this is especially true in large towns where the possibility of contact with an infected child is greater.

There is a biennial periodicity in the appearance of epidemics, which is attributed to the effect of previous epidemics upon the degree of immunity within the community.

Though morbidity is high, mortality is low in the countries of the western world but in Africa the death rate from complications is high.

Where the risk of contact is reduced, for example in rural areas, the disease may not occur until the child is a lot older.

The introduction of a vaccine has radically altered the pattern of the incidence of infection, though it is too early to be dogmatic about the success of the campaign and its affect on the individual or the community.

Clinical Features

A mild illness at the time of infection has been reported but this is unusual. The first indication of the disease in most children is the prodromal stage. The child is feverish, with a running nose, sore eyes and an unproductive cough. He is very irritable and miserable. The temperature continues to rise and, in those who are susceptible, there may be febrile convulsions. Two to four days later a rash appears on the buccal mucosa (Koplik's spots). They are most easily seen at the junction of the lower gum and the cheek. In appearance they are like tiny white spots on a bright red background. Similar spots can be seen on the palpebral conjunctiva, especially of the lower lid. It is even easier to recognise them there than in the mouth. Koplik's spots are diagnostic of measles. Within 24—48 hours of the appearance of Koplik's spots, and at the height of the fever, the main rash appears. It is composed of dusty red maculo-papular lesions. Initially discreet, they later coalesce to form large blobs. The rash first appears behind the ears and on the forehead, and then spreads down the face and body. It is as though someone had splashed the child with red paint from the head down. As the rash fades it may leave a brownish skin staining.

Very occasionally there are petechial spots on all or part of the morbilliform rash — haemorrhagic measles.

The temperature remains elevated for the first 2 to 3 days of the rash; the respiratory element, the running nose and cough, continue throughout the illness. Catarrh is the first symptom to appear, and usually the last to clear in measles.

Attenuated forms of measles also occur, mainly in some of the children who have been vaccinated against the disease or who have recently been given gammaglobulin to protect them.

Complications

Moist sounds in the chest are heard so frequently they may be regarded as part of the general infection. Sometimes bronchopneumonia supervenes, especially in children who are already debilitated. The adventitious sounds in the chest are localised, but even more diagnostic of pulmonary congestion is the presence of respiratory distress: dilated alae nasi, rapid respiratory rate, rib recession and sometimes cyanosis.

Otitis media is found very frequently. Slight redness of the drum without earache may be regarded as part of the catarrhal element of measles but acute pain and a bulging red drum indicate secondary infection in the middle ear cavity. Sometimes, too, there is a secondary infection in the inflamed conjunctiva, causing a purulent conjunctivitis.

Post-measles encephalitis appears some 5 to 7 days after the rash, in about one child in 1000 infected. The features are similar to those of other forms of encephalitis. The prognosis from this complication is poor: some 15 per cent die, and a further 25 per cent are permanently disabled.

Differential Diagnosis

Inexperienced practitioners sometimes have difficulty in knowing whether a rash in a child is due to measles, rubella, infections mononeucleosis, or urticaria, or whether it is one of the non-specific eruptions which are often found with other virus infections. Roseola infantum should cause no difficulty in diagnosis: the history is quite different even if the rash is not entirely dissimilar. By the time the rash of roseola appears, the child is usually fairly cheerful, while characteristically a child with measles looks 'measly' — sad and miserable, coughing, and with sore eyes. With measles, too, the child will still be pyrexial when the rash appears.

To the experienced practitioner the main diagnostic difficulty is the occurrence of attenuated forms of the disease. The presence of Koplik's spots may be regarded as diagnostic and this will be confirmed by the history of 3 to 4 days fever and coryza. The classical measles rash will be just discernible behind the ears when the child is first seen.

It is never easy to be certain about the diagnosis of a rash in artificial light. It is much better to view it in daylight or, if necessary, fluorescent light.

Management

Hospitalisation is only rarely indicated, and then almost always for social reasons The occurrence of encephalitis or severe bronchopneumonia are the clinical exceptions.

The child need only stay in bed as long as he wishes. Often this will depend on the cultural pattern of the parents.

Most children with measles want to stay in bed for part, if not all, of the day. There are some, however, who appear to prefer to be up and about.

Occasionally a child with measles is brought by his parents to the doctor's consulting room but if a house call is requested, one should be made. Equally, if the parents bring the child to the doctor and ask if it is all right to do so, no harm will ensue, provided that arrangements can be made for the child to be segregated from others in the waiting room (e.g., a different consulting time, or the child is taken straight to a spare consulting or examination room).

There is no specific treatment for the disease. Linctuses have little more than a placebo effect and there is usually no benefit to be gained from trying to bring the temperature down with aspirin. Some doctors routinely administer a prophylactic antibiotic – usually penicillin V or a sulphonamide; others consider them unnecessary. However, if there are ear or chest complications, an antibiotic should be given for five days. If the bronchopneumonia is particularly severe, the possibility of a staphylococcal infection must be considered and, if possible, sputum cultured. Cloxacillin may be prescribed without waiting for the pathologist's report, once the sputum has been collected.

Prevention

Measles vaccination is now routinely offered to all children in Britain. Where this has not been given, and where the child is thought not to have previously had a natural attack of the disease and prevention or alternation is desirable, human gammaglobulin may be given (250 mg). Supplies are very scarce and should be preserved for essential cases such as severely debilitated children and those about to sit a major examination.

Meningitis

Nature

Meningitis is an inflammation of the meninges mainly as a result of bacterial or viral infection.

Almost all pathogenic bacteria can cause meningitis. In younger children that caused by *H. influenzae* is the most frequent but in older children, and especially adolescents, meningococcal meningitis is the most common form. Viral agents cause aseptic (lymphocytic) meningitis.

The incubation period varies with the causative organism.

Clinical Features

In older children headache and pain at the back of the neck are the main symptoms, often accompanied by a photophobia, nausea and vomiting. Convulsions may occur and the child may lapse into coma.

In young children the symptoms are less specific. The infant is unwell and feverish, and the cry is often high-pitched. Convulsions are more likely to occur than in older children. The fontanelle is bulging; it is important to estimate this when the child is not crying.

Neck stiffness will be present and Kernig's sign is positive. These tests may not be easy to carry out, especially if the child is fractious. It may be possible to elicit his co-operation by asking him to sit up and kiss his knee. When there is neck stiffness and Kernig's sign is positive, the child is unable to do this exercise and will sit up supporting his spine by putting his hands behind his back (the tripod sign).

Diagnosis

This depends on the examination of the cerebro-spinal fluid. Whenever the diagnosis is suspected, a lumbar puncture has to be performed. The most important differential diagnosis is meningism, usually accompanying an upper respiratory infection, very often follicular tonsillitis. Clinical differentiation between meningitis and meningism is important. Meningitis is by far the more serious of the two. If the child has meningitis immediate hospitalisation is necessary so that a lumbar puncture can be performed. Antibiotics must not be given as they can mask the diagnosis.

On the other hand, if the child has tonsillitis with meningism, hospitalisation and lumbar puncture can both be avoided and an antibiotic may be administered. If there is any doubt about the diagnosis, the worst must be suspected and a lumbar puncture performed before an antibiotic is given.

Management

It is usually preferable to treat meningitis in hospital, where there are better facilities for lumbar puncture.

Prevention

In the case of meningococcal meningitis, all contacts may be given a prophylactic course of sulphonamide.

Mumps (Epidemic Parotitis)

Nature

Mumps is an acute infectious disease in which there is a non-suppurative enlargement of one or more of the salivary glands, in particular the parotids. In post-pubital children and adults, the ovaries or testes may also be involved. The incubation period varies between 14 and 21 days.

Infectivity

In Britain mumps is endemic in most urban communities but from time to time there are epidemics. The degree of infectivity is moderate; many adults, though frequently in contact as children, do not get an attack until they reach adulthood, at which time there is a risk of involvement of the gonads.

The period of infectivity probably starts 2 days before the first glandular enlargement appears and continues until the glands return to normal size. It is typical of the spread of mumps within a household for the children to be infected one at a time, and not for all the siblings to be infected at the same time from the first case, as usually happens, for example, with measles.

Pathology

The responsible agent is the myxovirus parotidis. The portal of entry is probably the respiratory tract. One attack usually produces life-long immunity.

Clinical Features

There is usually a prodromal period of 24 to 48 hours in which the child feels unwell; the temperature varies from near normal to 40°C. Earache is often the first symptom of swollen parotids. If the glandular enlargement is not obvious, the ear lobe on the affected side should be gently pulled upwards. This is painless in otitis media. In mumps and otitis externa, pulling the ear lobe backwards may be painful. Not infrequently only one parotid swells, but when both glands enlarge there is often a considerable interval, up to a week, between the two sides. Swelling of one or both sub-mandibular glands is not uncommon but sub-linguinal glandular involvement is rare. In about 30 per cent of cases it is reported that none of the glands are enlarged, even though the child is unwell. Sometimes the only clinical features are the complications. This is especially true in adults.

In about 20 per cent of post-pubertal males, one testicle — rarely both — may be swollen and exquisitely tender. The prognosis is usually much better than the patient fears; sterility is rare though a temporary impotence may occur, probably due to the discomfort of the orchitis and the fear of the possible outcome.

Oophoritis appears to be much rarer. Pancreatitis, too, is uncommon. Involvement of the myocardium, liver, and other organs, has also been reported.

In about half the cases of mumps there is in the cerebro-spinal fluid (CSF) an increase in the number of white cells, mainly lymphocytes, though signs of meningeal involvement (headache, drowsiness and stiff neck) are uncommon.

Routine CSF examination is, of course, not necessary in mumps unless there is evidence of brain involvement. In some patients the only signs are those of a meningo-encephalitis without any parotid or other gland involvement. The diagnosis in these cases depends on culture of the CSF for the virus.

In a doubtful case of mumps antibody titres may also be estimated.

Differential Diagnosis
In children suppurative salivary adenitis is rare but when it does occur it may be recurrent. The main difficulty in diagnosis is to be sure that the swellings are in the salivary and not the adjacent lymphatic glands. A dental infection is also a possible cause of a local swelling. In adults parotid swellings may also be due to calculi, tumours, sarcoid and Mikulicz's syndrome.

If the presenting feature is orchitis, encephalitis or meningitis, without a preceding history of salivary glandular involvement, reliance may have to be placed on the antibody titres, though a history of contact with another case of mumps is helpful.

Management
There is no specific treatment. The need for bed rest will depend upon the severity of the illness, the extent of the complications and the age of the patient. Young children often neither want nor need to stay in bed. An adult with complications will almost certainly be unable to stay out of bed for any considerable length of time. It is traditional to advise a liquid diet with slops (milk puddings, lightly boiled eggs, etc.) but this is often an unnecessary restriction, except perhaps for the first day or two.

Analgesics may be necessary, especially in older children or adults, to relieve the discomfort of the swollen parotid. If there is an orchitis, the scrotum may be supported with a suspensory bandage.

Steroids given systemically (prednisone 10 mg qds for 2 to 3 days, then reducing by 10 mg daily) often produces a dramatic relief but there is no evidence that this influences future sterility. Alternatively, phenylbutazone 100 mg qds may relieve the testicular discomfort.

Prophylaxis
Live mumps vaccine is now available. Its routine use is still under debate.

Pertussis (Whooping Cough)

Nature
The characteristic feature of pertussis is the cough. It comes in spasms in each of which the cough becomes more and more explosive as the child unsuccessfully

attempts to clear his respiratory passages of a thick tenacious mucous. The spasm ends with a loud inspiration – the whoop. The incubation period varies between 7 and 14 days.

Pathology

The disease is caused by *Bordetella pertussis* and *B. parapertussis.* The latter is usually a milder infection. There is evidence that some virus infections can produce a disease closely resembling pertussis.

Culture of *B. pertussis* and *B. parapertussis* is difficult. A culture is most likely to be positive in the first two weeks of the illness, at which stage the clinical features may be less prominent and the diagnosis not suspected. Pernasal swabs or cough plates are the most likely to give successful results but the experience of the laboratory in culturing the organism also seems to affect their ability to get a positive culture.

At the same time there is usually a considerable increase in the white blood count, especially of the lymphocytes. Counts of 15 000 to 25 000 are not uncommon; sometimes it may be as high as 100 000, which may give rise to the suspicion of a leukaemia (though the symptoms are quite different). However, in the past two decades, the high white count is less prominent a feature in children with the characteristic whoop. A number of cases of whooping cough have been seen in children who have been immunised against the disease and this may explain why their white blood count is not so high.

Clinical Features

The disease starts with a catarrhal phase lasting 2 weeks, resembling an ordinary upper respiratory infection with an associated cough, most prominent at night. It is at this stage that the child is most infectious and bacteriological cultures are most likely to be positive. However, except in an epidemic the diagnosis may not be suspected.

The paroxysmal cough starts at the end of the catarrhal phase. The severity of the cough and the frequency of the paroxysms vary considerably. In a mild case the cough begins to ease 3 to 4 weeks from its start (i.e., 5 to 6 weeks from the onset of the illness) but in others the cough and whoop may continue for months.

A secondary infection is not uncommon in the lower respiratory tract, with a superimposed bronchitis or pneumonia.

Bronchiectasis used to be a complication but, at least for the present, it has virtually disappeared, presumably because of the use of antibiotics to deal with any secondary infection.

Management

The mainstay of treatment is the nursing. A humid atmosphere may ease the paroxysm of cough but steam kettles create their own hazards. Feeds should be small and frequent. They should be given a few minutes after the paroxysm, when the child is relaxed. Dry foods which may irritate the pharynx and set off the cough should be avoided. A sedative given to the child at night may be as important for the mother as it is helpful for the child. Phenobarbitone elixir 5 ml (equivalent to 15 mg) in infants under a year and 10 ml for older children is usually effective. Alternatively, elixir diazepam: 2.5 to 10 ml (1 to 4 mg) may be given. Cough syrups are usually little better than a placebo.

Hospitalisation is not usually necessary, except on social grounds. Bed rest is not essential unless the child is very ill; usually this is only in infants. *B. pertussis* is partly sensitive to tetracycline but usually only during the first 2 weeks of the infection which, in most cases, is before the diagnosis is made. Chloramphenicol is even more effective but because of its haematological side-effects it should only be used in a severely ill child, when the risk can be justified. Penicillin (or erythromycin in those who are sensitive to penicillin) will cope with most of the secondary invaders in children; ampicillin is an alternative. For children who have had paroxysms of cough for more than a month, providing there is no superimposed secondary infection, 15 minutes in a decompression chamber will produce a lasting cure in about 50 per cent. The explanation for this is not known.

Prevention
Pertussis immunisation has proved neither as successful nor as safe as was originally hoped. It is not yet known why the pattern of the illness altered at the time the vaccination was introduced in the early 1950s, and what part, if any, immunisation played in this change. Because of the poor antibody response in young babies, it is not usual to start pertussis immunisation until the 4th or 5th month of life. However, the most severe forms of illness occur in infants under that age.

Poliomyelitis (Acute Anterior Poliomyelitis; Infantile Paralysis; Polio)

Nature
In poliomyelitis there is an acute viral infection of the brain stem and spinal cord, which sometimes leads to paralysis. The incubation period lasts for up to 3 weeks. There are three sub-types of the virus, with little antigenic overlap, so that vaccination must include all three types.

Epidemiology
From time to time over the past centuries, epidemics have been reported of infectious illnesses resembling that which we now call poliomyelitis. In the Western world the disease assumed major proportions in the second quarter of

the present century. The spread is by the faecal and oral route. Improvements in
the general standards of hygiene often lead to the appearance of a large number
of cases in older children and young adults, which suggests a decline in the rate
of sub-clinical infection in infancy.

The availability of an adequate polio vaccine has radically altered the
epidemiological pattern, but it would be unwise to assume this is an immutable
situation and that further epidemics will not occur again some time in the
future.

Clinical Features

In its minor form the disease is like other ordinary viral infections. The
symptoms are non-specific: fever, headache, lassitude, nausea and sometimes
vomiting or diarrhoea. It is unlikely to be recognised for what it is, except in an
epidemic or if viral studies are carried out. The majority of minor cases recover
completely without complications (abortive poliomyelitis).

The major form may arise *de novo* or follow immediately after the minor
variety, sometimes with a brief interval of apparent recovery between. The
headache is severe and there are other signs of meningeal irritation, such as a
positive Kernig's and tripod sign.

Limb pains and muscle tremors have been reported but are found in only a
small proportion of cases. The CSF may show a pleocytosis and some elevation
of protein. Many patients recover completely over the next 7 to 10 days without
further complications (non-paralytic poliomyelitis). A variable proportion go on
to develop paralysis. Involvement varies from weakness in a small part of one
muscle group to an extensive flaccid paralysis affecting muscle groups in one or
more limbs as well as those involved in respiration (paralytic polio). In paralytic
poliomyelitis there is sometimes difficulty in swallowing and the patient may
drown in his own saliva. In this form the respiratory centre itself may be
affected.

Differential Diagnosis

The minor form is indistinguishable, except by virological studies, from many
other viral infections. The major form must be differentiated by virological
studies and lumbar puncture from other varieties of meningitis and meningism.
If paralysis is present, a polyneuritis due to other infections or toxins must be
considered. An illness resembling polio can be caused by other entero-viruses,
including Coxsackie A7 and ECHO type 3. Virology is therefore desirable in all
cases, if only for epidemiological purposes.

Management

There is no specific treatment. The minor and major non-paralytic forms are
treated symptomatically. Hospital admission is highly desirable if there are any

complications and obviously essential if there is any weakness of the muscles involved in swallowing or respiration because of the need to maintain the airway by means of suction and the use of a respirator.

The long-term management of the complications of muscle paralysis is best dealt with by a team, including an orthopaedic surgeon, paediatrician and physiotherapist, as well as the family doctor.

Prevention
Salk's killed virus vaccine is administered by injection sub-cutaneously and the Sabin live attenuated virus by the oral route. The oral Sabin vaccine usually gives a higher degree of immunity and, in addition, it probably gives a local immunity in the gut.

Polio still occurs in many parts of the world. The risk of the importation of new cases still remains and the campaign to maintain a high degree of polio immunisation cannot be relaxed.

Roseola Infantum (Exanthem Subitum; Sixth Disease)

Nature
Roseola is an acute febrile disease of infants in which the rash appears when the temperature subsides. It is rarely found in children over the age of 2 years. The incubation period is probably between 10 and 15 days.

Clinical Features
The child is feverish and irritable for 3 to 5 days. Some children have a febrile convulsion during this stage. The temperature falls rapidly and as it does so a discrete maculo-papular rash appears, first on the trunk and subsequently on the face and limbs.

Differential Diagnosis
There should be no difficulty in differentiating roseola from measles, rubella, or scarlet fever, in all of which the child is pyrexial while he has a rash. Certain entero-viral infections, especially ECHO virus, are sometimes associated with a rash, but here again the child is usually pyrexial while he is spotty.

The most frequent mis-diagnosis is a drug rash. When the child is feverish he may be given an antibiotic. The rash appears when the child looks better, and it is wrongly assumed that the antibiotic cured the infection (whatever it was) and that the rash is due to drug allergy.

Management
No specific treatment is needed. By the time the rash appears the child has recovered.

Prophylaxis

None is needed as there are no complications, other than the possibility of a febrile convulsion.

Rubella (German Measles)

Nature

There is no connection between ordinary measles and German measles, except that both are virus infections producing a skin rash. The average incubation period is 17 days with a range of 14 to 21 days.

As a childhood infection it is almost free of complications. Thrombocytopenia has been reported, manifesting itself as a purpura. Polyarthritis as a sequel to an attack of rubella is rare in adults and very rare in children; so, too, is a post-infectious encephalitis.

The only important complication is the hazard to the fetus if the mother gets an attack during the first trimester in pregnancy. The earlier in pregnancy the mother is infected, the more severe are the effects likely to be. Congenital rubella is associated with a multiplicity of defects, prominent among which are deafness, cataracts, microphthalmus and heart defects (especially patent ductus and ventricular septal defect). A low birth weight is a common finding.

Incidence

It is difficult to assess the precise incidence because of the considerable clinical variation, but about 90 per cent of adults in Britain have acquired rubella antibodies at some period in their life.

Infectivity

One attack almost always produces life-long immunity. Transmission is probably by droplets in the early stage of the illness. It is not as contagious as some of the other exanthemata and attempts to artificially induce attacks in young girls before they were old enough to become pregnant were often unsuccessful.

Clinical Features

In children there are usually no prodromata. The rash is usually the first symptom; pink macules appear on the face and spread rapidly over the body. The macules often coalesce to give the characteristic appearance but there is considerable variation in the pattern which makes the clinical diagnosis difficult in some cases. Usually there is some cervical lymphadenopathy, especially the posterior nodes. Enlargement of the sub-occipital gland is a helpful diagnostic feature. The rash may last only a few hours or even be absent, but it usually persists 2 to 5 days. The glands may remain enlarged a little longer. The temperature rarely rises above 38°C. and may even be normal in children. Very occasionally part of the rash may be purpuric.

Differential Diagnosis

It is not usually difficult to recognise measles if one sees the case early enough to identify Koplik's spots, and in measles the child looks more ill. Roseola infantum only affects infants; rubella is rare at that age (except for the congenital variety, which is devoid of a rash). Also in roseola the rash appears as the temperature subsides. Perhaps the most difficult differential diagnosis to make clinically is glandular fever.

Because of the risks to an expectant mother, if there is any doubt she has the disease or has been in contact with it, the diagnosis can be confirmed by estimating the rubella antibody titre at the onset of the disease and again 2 to 3 weeks later. A fourfold or greater increase in antibody titre confirms the diagnosis of rubella. Glandular fever can be identified from a white blood count and Paul Bunnell reaction. However, there may be a delay in the Paul Bunnell reaction converting to positive and it may remain positive long after the attack.

Other virus infections, for example the ECHO virus, can sometimes also be associated with a rash not unlike that of rubella. Few family practitioners in Britain have yet got access to virus laboratories where cultures can identify the aetiological agent.

Management

No treatment is needed, nor is any available. The only precaution is to protect any pregnant or potentially pregnant woman from coming in contact with an affected child, which is much easier said than done.

Prevention

The availability of a vaccine should eliminate most of the risks to a fetus in the future. Every girl should be vaccinated at the age of 11 or 12, though even this may be too late to avoid all pregnancies. Women not vaccinated at puberty should have their rubella antibodies estimated. If the titre is low they should be offered rubella vaccine immediately after delivery of their first pregnancy, or at any time they can be sure not to fall pregnant within three months of the injection.

Those exposed to special risk, for example nurses, should be tested for antibodies and, if necessary, offered the vaccine subject to a similar warning.

Scarlet Fever

Nature

Scarlet fever is a streptococcal pharyngitis accompanied by a rash.

Pathology

The rash is due to an erythrogenic toxin produced by Lancefield Group A β-haemolytic streptococci. One attack of scarlet fever produces a life-time immunity to the rash but not to further streptococcal infections. There used to be an increased risk of post-streptococcal rheumatic fever and nephritis but this has declined, together with the severity of the illness.

Clinical Features

In the past, when streptococcal infections were more virulent, the child was often extremely ill. Nowadays he may not even be in bed. The temperature and pulse are both raised. The pharyngitis usually precedes the rash by 48 to 72 hours. The rash — bright red pinpoint papules — starts in the groin and axillae and is most prominent there. It spreads to cover the whole of the body, except for a pale area around the mouth (circumoral pallor).

The tongue is at first heavily coated with bright red papillae showing through (white strawberry tongue). As the coating disappears the red papillae are more prominent (red strawberry tongue). The appearance of the tongue is said to be diagnostic, but similar, though less marked changes, can be seen in some other non-streptococcal upper respiratory infections.

If the disease is untreated, the rash will fade over the next 3 to 4 days and as it does so the skin will desquamate, often in large plaques.

Otitis media often accompanies the infected throat and the lower respiratory tract may also sometimes be involved.

Differential Diagnosis

There is usually no difficulty in differentiating measles and rubella though, not unnaturally, the parents may frequently make this mistake. It goes without saying that every child with a rash should be fully examined, preferably in daylight. The rash which sometimes accompanies glandular fever can be misleading but the story is usually different. A blood film will identify the mononucleosis and a Paul Bunnell test will confirm the diagnosis. The rash of meningococcal meningitis is usually purpuric but the rash which accompanies some ECHO and other virus infections may be misleading. In roseola infantum, the rash appears after the fever subsides.

The diagnosis of scarlet fever can be confirmed if, in a suspected case, a throat swab is taken before starting an antibiotic.

Management

β-haemolytic streptococci are almost always sensitive to penicillin. Unless the child is hypersensitive to this antibiotic, a course may be started immediately after a throat swab has been taken to confirm the diagnosis. Alternatively, erythromycin may be given, but not tetracyclines, to which many streptococci are resistant. (Tetracyclines should not, in any case, be given to children under the age of 10 years.)

It is a wise precaution to check the urine for protein 3 weeks after an attack of scarlet fever, though post-streptococcal nephritis is nowadays rare and probably occurs no more frequently after scarlet fever than after an ordinary streptococcal tonsillitis.

HEART DISEASE IN CHILDREN

The almost complete absence of rheumatic fever in Britain has led to the disappearance of new cases of rheumatic heart disease. Whereas in past generations this was a major cause of chronic morbidity in children, few family practitioners will now see a child whose mitral or aortic valves have been damaged in this way. Today it is the congenital heart diseases (CHD) which have assumed major importance, especially as many are now amenable to surgery.

From a practical point of view, CHD can be classified into those with symptoms and those without. The main symptoms are a failure to thrive and shortness of breath, which may vary from tachypnoea at rest to a mild degree of dyspnoea only noticeable after exertion. Very occasionally the parents may also consult their doctor because they have detected a discolouration of the lips or extremities, but usually cyanosis is first detected by a doctor or nurse examining the child. Only a small proportion of children with CHD have any symptoms at all and about 90 per cent of these present during the first year of life. Most cases are asymptomatic and remain unrecognised until the child is examined.

Estimation of the blood pressure is not often performed routinely in children. The commonest cause of a raised blood pressure in this age group is a coarctation of the aorta which is more likely to be suspected from the discovery of absent femoral arterial pulses, the sound of a heart murmur over the back of the chest or the presence of rib notching on a chest X-ray, than it is from the discovery of hypertension.

Cardiac enlargement, when present, is usually easier to detect in children than in adults because the chest wall is thinner. Other physical signs of congenital heart disease include an excessively rapid or slow heart rate and anomalies of rhythm. However, the most frequently encountered disorder of rhythm is sinus arrhythmia, which is physiological and entirely benign. The heart rate in many children and a number of adolescents increases with each inspiration and slows down on expiration.

The most common symptom is a heart murmur but only a small proportion of children with a murmur have significant heart disease; most of the murmurs heard are associated with an excellent prognosis and may, therefore, be described as innocent. Some of these murmurs are due to delayed closure of a ventricular septal defect and others are associated with a minor degree of pulmonary stenosis.

Obviously every child with a heart murmur must be carefully assessed. As a general rule it may be said that the softer the sound the more likely the murmur is to be innocent; so too are those murmurs which are localised.

If necessary the opinion of a cardiologist should be sought, preferably one with paediatric experience. The decision to investigate must be weighed carefully, not so much because of the hazards — cardiac catheterisation is today a relatively safe procedure — but because of the psychological affect upon the child and the family. It is rarely possible to explain away as 'routine' such a major investigation. Many parents, unfortunately, take the view that there is no smoke without fire and assume the worst, irrespective of what is said after the tests have been carried out. As a result they may overprotect the child with possibly harmful effects upon his future emotional stability.

For this reason the family practitioner must carefully assess the benefits of investigation against the risks of creating a cardiac neurotic. Unfortunately it is not always possible to hide the existence of a heart murmur from the parents. If the family practitioner does not tell them, a school doctor may later do so, at which stage the family practitioner will find it virtually impossible to explain away his concealment of the facts.

Herein lies the need for all the family doctor's skill and tact in explaining the significance of his problem to the family. The words first used to describe the significance of a murmur, especially one that is innocent, are the words most likely to be remembered by the family.

24

Care of the Aged

M. K. Thompson

INTRODUCTION

As a result of the progressive elimination of random causes of death, advanced industrial societies show a rising increase in the proportion of elderly individuals which has imposed considerable stresses on the available medical services. To deal with the special problems of this age group it has been found necessary to erect a parallel system of medical care, called 'Geriatrics', based on the recognition that the medicine of old age is a separate specialty, a fact recognised even in the time of Galen, but now having more compelling implications.

The primary care physician, who will therefore be considerably involved with the care of elderly people, will encounter problems occupying an adjacent, but separate spectrum from that of the specialist geriatric physician. Not only will he discover that some people of advanced years remain healthy, but he will be involved less with the problems of the merely aged than with the effects of the ageing process and the diseases associated with it. Endeavour has hitherto been lacking by the failure to distinguish between biological ageing and the results of accumulated pathologies. This distinction is not always clear, and makes the management of elderly patients extremely complex, but this is a field where progress is being made through a more active endeavour based upon new concepts, and knowledge made available through advances in gerontology. Old ideas of irreversible degenerative change, with the pessimism they engender, are disappearing *parri passu* with the passing of a generation that had low requirements and poor expectations of medical care.

There are, in later life, much greater discrepancies between biological and chronological age than in childhood. Not only are these of prime clinical importance in as much as they affect the natural history of diseases, but those who rely on clinical criteria as developed on younger subjects may be misled. Diseases regarded as clear-cut entities, capable of being revealed by a battery of tests, defy recognition because they present atypically, so that text-book signs are often absent, or notoriously unreliable. Diagnosis, while remaining of the utmost importance, is more valuable in its quantitative than qualitative aspects, needing to take account of plural pathology and to be all inclusive rather than to throw a brilliant light on isolated components. Diagnosis once reached leads straight on to prognostic considerations. These must be formulated by considering not only how one disease may affect another, but also a realistic assessment of the patient's social expectations. It is obvious that the comprehensive care of the whole person that is required cannot be achieved by a series of separate interventions, by one individual, but requires the combined skills of a team able to provide nursing care, advice on health maintenance in later life, and estimates of and provision for social needs. The undoubted place of the family practitioner in this team is that of clinician.

The common complaints of the elderly are frequently described in terms of lost function, are usually of multifactorial aetiology, and may be listed as follows:

anorexia/constipation	vertigo, syncope and falling
failing vision	fatigue
failing hearing	dyspnoea
	nocturnal frequency
	sleep disturbance
	shakiness and tremor

PHYSICAL APPEARANCE IN OLD AGE

There are common physical changes with age that should be understood as indicating geriatric anatomy, rather than disease. The face of elderly people is very revealing. Deterioration is often associated with changes of contour, such as hollowing of the cheeks, or sagging of the corner of the mouth. Pallor of the cheeks, however, is commonly due to a poor capillary field rather than anaemia. Dilated venules may, even in the anaemic, give an impression of plethora. Myxoedema may be suggested by puffy wrists, sparse hair and eyebrows, and slow cerebration; while muscle shrinkage, weakness and ptosis may be misinterpreted as indicating a myopathy. Guttering between the metacarpals is common, especially in thin subjects, while the loss of subcutaneous fat and atrophic epidermal changes make the usual tests of tissue turgor useless. 'Senile' purpura may appear on the dorsal aspects of the hands and forearms due to shearing forces on the capillaries for the same reason. Small raised red Campbell de Morgan spots are often seen on the trunk, and seborrhoeic warts, which although often black in colour, are of no pathological significance. Grey hair is more common than white. Heberden's nodes, and osteoarthritis of the knees with audible crepitus affect the majority of old subjects.

Anatomical changes, such as loss of stature due to shrinkage of the intervertebral discs is common in the eighth decade, although there is retention of the span. Kyphoscoliosis is common, especially in females. This in conjunction with contraction of the thoracic cage, reduces the vital capacity, and increases the cardiothoracic ratio. The surface anatomy of the liver and heart may be altered, giving a false impression of hepatomegaly and cardiac enlargement. Inspection of the neck veins on the left side may be rendered valueless in the assessment of cardiac failure due to an unfolded and rigid aorta producing fullness of the left external jugular vein. On the other hand, especially in hypertensive subjects, aortic distortion may produce a pulsating swelling behind the clavicular part of the right sternomastoid muscle as the innominate artery is brought up into the neck. This should not be misinterpreted as an aneurysm.

The body temperature, as traditionally measured in the mouth by a thermometer, varies considerably in people over the age of sixty. Old people with feeble lips, tremulous and edentulous mouths cannot hold the instrument in place for long. In general, levels tend to be normally lower than the traditional $37°C$.

In the nervous system there are many apparent abnormalities which are quite compatible with health and activity, but which in younger subjects would be regarded as 'abnormal', such as the absence of vibration sense in the lower limbs, or the progressive loss of some tendon reflexes with age, those in the upper limb being easier to obtain than those in the lower. There is furthermore, a progressive failure of the pupil of the eye to react to light, so that an absent response is not infrequently found in nonagenarians. The accommodation reflex is even more affected than the light reflex.

The three decades which come under the general heading of old age are those in which fit and active old men and women may present physical signs on careful examination which are anomalous, and which may appear abnormal but may be compatible with health and activity. The connotation of the term 'normal' must therefore be correctly understood when dealing with this age group, and constantly borne in mind by the examining physician.

EXAMINATION OF THE ELDERLY PATIENT

In assessing the elderly, diagnosis is often of critical importance, and the axiom that the old invariably harbour plural pathologies requires examination to be complete enough to evaluate the contribution made by each in the total clinical picture. Diagnosis in this age group is not only important as the basis for treatment, but often has its greatest significance in the formulation of the prognosis. The practitioner will encounter difficulty with patients with impaired cognition and memory, who are often deformed anatomically, wearing voluminous clothing and with restricted mobility. Yet, the home situation provides him with many opportunities to understand patients that are denied to secondary assessors in the more auspicious surroundings of a hospital, and indeed, removal there from the familiar entrenchment can be expected to cause some degree of disorientation. It is important to aspire to a systematic approach, bearing in mind always that in old people common conditions presenting atypically are the rule, and may pose more diagnostic difficulty than rare diseases. I have found the following methods to have been helpful, and I offer them in the hope that others may avoid those pitfalls into which I have not infrequently stumbled.

The History

There is little doubt that history-taking is most fruitful in the patient's familiar surroundings. He should be addressed always by his proper name, and not by affectionate impersonal terms, such as 'old fellow'. This is not just good manners, but will reinforce the sense of personal identity which may, through loneliness or depression, have been eroded. Full allowance must be made for failing mental powers, hostility or loquacity, and indeed, the discerning physician will find in irrelevant talk much of value concerning spontaneous thought, mood and preoccupations, and should not at first be discouraged. The slow tempo of the old must be patiently accepted, for attempts to hurry the patient are self-defeating, and lead only into frustration which may be detected by the appearance of inappropriate motor responses, such as clearing the throat, scratching the head, or losing temper. Because of uneven performance in the elderly, a second consultation may be required, when a better result can be obtained.

Old people are inclined to attribute the onset of illness to particular events, such as a fall or a bereavement, but it is unwise to follow the patient in his speculations, since the onset of disease in old age tends to be insidious rather than precipitate. Symptoms are described in terms of lost function, so that complaints are made of being unable to climb the stairs, or of inability to drink without spilling.

It is important to establish a time scale on which to place events leading up to the present, if possible by defining the age at which illnesses and operations happened, rather than as subtractions from the present. The home will often provide talking points, and even photographs by which the patient's present state may be compared with what he was like in his hey-day. Depressed and inert patients will often respond to questions about their family, the army days or sporting achievements. The presence of a third party is welcome in confirming the statements made, but should not be allowed to take over the interview.

The Examination

It is rarely possible to follow the sequence of examination taught in medical school, or to match its perfection. Intelligent modifications must be made with due regard to the patient's ability to co-operate.

It is reasonable to begin by testing the special senses of sight and hearing, since little progress will be made without integrity of the patient's perceptual apparatus. Complicated methods of testing are not required, and much can be learned at the bedside with nothing more than a newspaper, which can be found lying to hand in almost any home, printed in letters of various sizes. By asking the patient, without gesture, to pick up the paper and read a passage aloud, a process is set in train with opportunity to make clinical observations concerning hearing, language function, praxis, co-ordinated movement, the presence of senile or intention tremor, visual acuity, articulation and vocal quality. A short discussion on the material read will give some indication of comprehension and ability to recall information.

The Eyes
Conjugate eye movements may reveal nystagmus, but it is not uncommon to find in extreme deviation irregular eye movements of no pathological significance: or, that the full range of upward movement is restricted as a sign of general weakness or, in the absence of raised intracranial pressure, some compromise of the cerebral bloodflow. The reactions of the pupils to light and accommodation are often absent in advanced age, or they may show abnormalities due to ocular hypertension, cataract, or other intraocular disease. Cataract may be diagnosed by ophthalmoscopic examination (using the +12 lens) and not assumed to be present if a grey reflex is seen on direct inspection, for this is commonly due to altered refraction of light due to the increased optical density that arises in late age.

Examination of the fundus is difficult because of opacity of the media, wandering attention, and the dangers of using mydriatic drops to dilate a small pupil. More may be gained from observing normal healthy vessels than a persistent search for the varying degrees of narrowing and tortuosity. Pathological changes should lead to a request for specialist examination.

The Ears
Having made sure that the auditory canals are free from wax, simple tests of hearing are sufficient, and carried out by asking the patient to repeat words at varying distances, at first with the normal, and then with the whispered voice. If a hearing aid is worn, it should be inspected as part of the body. In a high proportion of cases, the aids are found to be defective, or incorrectly used.

The Limbs
Attention is directed next to the upper limbs, for signs of wasting, spasticity, rigidity of the Parkinsonian type, flaccidity, or tremor, but with care to recognise and exclude that paratonic type of rigidity occasionally met with in old people as a defensive reaction that appears immediately the limb is grasped,

and resists all efforts at persuasion to relax. The radial pulse is felt, and visible brachial pulsation looked for lateral to the medial epicondyle, after which the hand is carefully inspected.

In the lower limbs, adductor spasm is noted if, when one limb is adducted, the other follows it across the bed. The skin temperature is felt with the dorsal aspect of the fingers which give quite accurate thermographic impressions, for comparative purposes. The feet are inspected for colour changes, oedema, digital health, the state of the nails, callosities, and the speed of capillary flow back into the white zone produced by pressure on the pad of the great toe. Reflexes are tested in the usual way, but it is as well to bear in mind the anomalies that may be produced by local disease, such as hallux rigidus which may mechanically reduce, or even abolish, the plantar response. As age increases the tendon reflexes are more difficult to elicit distally, while superficial reflexes, such as the abdominals, are rarely present in the lower quadrants over the age of 75 years. Sensory testing is seldom successfully carried out, not only because it depends upon patient response, but patchy losses of sensation are often present without necessarily signifying ill health. Vibration sense is commonly absent below the mid-dorsal spine, and in the lower limbs, due to degeneration of the posterior columns.

The Spine

If possible the patient can now be asked to stand out of bed so that the spine may be examined for curvatures, or pelvic tilt. An opportunity occurs also for testing the strength of the quadriceps, while they resist gravity, and note can be made of the presence of contractures such as flexion deformity of the knee joint. One of the most important physical signs in old people, the gait, can be observed by taking the patient for a walk around the bed, and although this is difficult in small rooms, circumduction of the leg at the hip, scissor gait, or *marche à petits pas* may be looked for.

The Chest

For examination of the chest the patient is asked to sit on the edge of the bed. On inspection it is usual to see some degree of thoracic cage deformity, the importance of which may be to cause real or apparent displacement of organs in relation to it, so that erroneous conclusions may be arrived at, such as cardiomegaly, and hepatomegaly. Inspection from above is advisable in addition to lateral and frontal views. In the female, the breasts are palpated as she sits, and following this she may be asked to stand in order to carry out inspection from the front, when a transverse sulcus may be seen across the upper abdomen, indicating osteoporotic change with lower dorsal vertebral collapse. One can then proceed to examine the heart and lungs in the usual way.

Arrhythmias are of common occurrence, and the dominant arrythmia found in late life is atrial fibrillation, commonly associated with acute infections, cardiac ischaemia, pulmonary embolism, surgical operations, thyrotoxicosis, and heart failure, especially when due to rheumatic heart disease. The presence of altered rhythm will direct the examiner to look for peripheral oedema, which, in bedridden patients, may be localised to the sacral region. Although the incidence of ischaemic heart diseases rises with age, the diagnosis may be rendered difficult due to the lesser severity of cardiac pain which may be present only as a sensation of chest tightness. Special note must be made of any sudden development of heart failure, left atrial or ventricular gallop rhythm, or elevation of the venous pressure.

Aortic ejection murmurs are common as the result of aortic valvular sclerosis, or from true stenosis with definite obstruction to outflow. Though often asymptomatic, aortic stenosis may cause dyspnoea, angina or syncopal attacks, and obstruction to flow reveal itself by an anacrotic pulse, reversed splitting of the second sound and left ventricular hypertrophy. It is important to attempt to distinguish this condition from valvular sclerosis, where the ejection murmur is less loud and harsh. The possibility of bacterial endocarditis must be borne in mind, for old patients may present with mental symptoms, or progressive renal failure, instead of the classical manifestations. Pulmonary embolism is increasingly to be found in the later decades in association with heart failure, obesity, fractured femur, and chronic disease of the leg veins.

The Neck
The patient should then be returned to bed for inspection in a good light of the neck veins. The thyroid gland may also be examined, but in elderly kyphotic women it may have come to occupy a retrosternal position. The patient may be asked to demonstrate the degree of movement retained in the cervical joints. Because of their importance to the cerebral circulation, particular attention should be paid to the quality of pulsation in each carotid artery, and auscultated for bruit.

The Alimentary System
Careful examination of the mouth, with inspection of the tongue and teeth is important. Many old mouths are neglected and edentulous, and if false teeth are worn, they should be examined in situ for an evaluation of their usefulness. This often reveals them to be ill fitting due to alteration in the mandibular contour and angle with natural ageing.

Before turning down the bedclothes to examine the abdomen it helps to engage the patient in conversation in order to encourage relaxation. Sitting at the bedside the practitioner can inspect the abdominal contours, and take visual note of lax skin, scars, herniae, or the presence of visible masses or peristalsis. The possibility of malabsorption will be suggested by any scar that might indicate partial gastrectomy, and the presence of small scars will bring to mind the possible presence of a transistorised pacemaker.

The pulsation of the abdominal aorta, so prominent in thin people, should be a reminder that occasionally aneurysmal dilatation may be found at this point. Firm masses felt in the left iliac fossa are often puzzling until their identity is revealed by ability to indent them with the examining finger per rectum, pressing laterally into the sigmoid. The presence of an impacted faecal mass in the rectum, with distension of the lax sphincter, is a not uncommon cause of spurious diarrhoea, especially where the patient has been dehydrated over a long period by the unwisely protracted use of diuretic drugs. The prostate gland is often enlarged in elderly men, and in many instances biochemical tests are required before its benign character can be assured. It is wise to look at the abdomen at this point to see if there is distension of the bladder. If possible, the patient should be asked to pass urine, for one may be fortunate enough to be able to observe the act of micturition for signs of hesitancy, interruption, and *vis a tergo*. After emptying the bladder, it is advisable to perform a bimanual examination for two reasons: in the first place, middle lobe enlargement can only be felt in this way and, secondly, a rough idea of the amount of residual urine present may be gained by feeling distension of the retroprostatic pouch.

In the elderly female, vaginal examination should precede the rectal examination, after inspection of the vulval area and the vaginal walls for prolapse.

By arranging for the patient to be ready for the examination, valuable time can be saved in practice, since much time can be wasted trying to get old people in and out of their clothes.

ANAEMIA IN THE ELDERLY

Normal Haematological Values

Although anaemia is common in the aged, there is no characteristic anaemia, so that the old require the same aetiological evaluation as in younger people. When effective treatment exists, the elderly individual will respond with gratifying results. Failure to do so indicates the presence of a complicating factor, such as a nutritional disorder, chronic infection or malignant disease. Haematopoeisis is hardly affected by age, so that values for Hb, W.B.C. and platelets remain unchanged. For practical purposes the practitioner may define anaemia as a Hb of less than 12.0 g per cent.

There are conflicting reports in the literature concerning the interpretation of the E.S.R. in the elderly, for in apparently healthy old people 40 mm/hr. may be recorded. In practice, adherence to normal values is advised. Those patients showing raised values should be kept under review.

Iron Deficiency Anaemia

This is the most common anaemia, as at other ages. The major diagnostic considerations are chronic overt, or occult blood loss, particularly from the gastro-intestinal tract. Unfortunately the clinical features are often accepted as the expected result of advancing age, and are borne without complaint. Since the course is insidious, presenting symptoms are commonly related to impaired cardiac or cerebral function. Women often reach old age with chronically diminished iron stores due to menopausal loss and childbearing. Low income, impaired mobility, and simple ignorance of food values may create conditions leading to primary dietary disease, of which iron deficiency is but a part, along with deficiencies in protein, vitamins, and mineral salts. The practitioner may recognise the presence of anaemia in the family practice setting when patients experience increased circulatory demand, as in intercurrent illness, or change in the daily routine. Breathlessness, ankle swelling, myocardial failure, dizziness and non-specific mental changes, all result from impaired tissue nutrition. This may also be seen in epithelial changes, such as dry inelastic skin, thin and brittle hair and nails, and a smooth pale tongue. The cheeks become avascular in late life, and mere facial pallor may then mislead, but dilated venules can, on the other hand, create a mistaken picture of plethora in the presence of anaemia. The nail beds and conjunctivae, though more reliable, are uncertain indicators. Associated signs such as enlarged lymph nodes, spleen, liver, abdominal mass, bone tenderness and peripheral neuropathy should be sought.

Investigation

There is therefore no substitute for Hb estimation, but this in itself is meaningless without examination of the blood film. This is a simple procedure, and requires only the use of Leishman's stain, buffered distilled water and a microscope. The blood smear shows contracted red cells deficient in Hb, but not uniformly so, and showing anisocytosis. Additional information may be obtained from the mean corpuscular haemoglobin concentration (MCHC), serum iron, and total iron binding capacity (TIBC). The cause of the iron deficiency should be sought, with particular reference to lesions of the gastro-intestinal tract, such as hiatus hernia and haemorrhoids. Barium studies may therefore be needed, and a chest x-ray, urine microscopy, tests of serum B12 and folate, and the Schilling test in the assiduous search for the cause.

Treatment

While achlorhydria may prevent absorption of iron from dietary sources, it does not prevent absorption of medicinal iron. This may be given once daily, an hour before a meal, in the greatest amount available in the ferrous state of a slow release preparation, and continued for three months after the Hb has become normal in order to replenish iron stores, or for longer should chronic blood loss continue. Parenteral iron is rarely needed, and is indicated only where oral iron is not tolerated, or where rapid replenishment is important.

Pernicious Anaemia

This disease is almost exclusive to old age, with half the cases developing over the age of 60. It is relatively uncommon, and seems to occur in blue-eyed individuals with white, rather than grey hair. It should be regarded as a general systemic illness, in which autoimmune mechanisms cause disturbances in cellular integrity, producing in addition to the anaemia, atrophy of the tongue and other epithelial surfaces. A lemon yellow colour is imparted to the skin both from the anaemia, and its mildly haemolytic component. The classical neurological lesion, with which it may present, is patchy demyelination of the posterior and lateral columns. Being due to vitamin B12 deficiency, it may rightly be regarded as a true nutritional anaemia.

Clinical Features

The anaemia is often severe when the patient presents, due to the insidious development of the disease. Clinical signs may be observed in the cardiovascular system, with glossitis, and hepatomegaly. The presence of a laparotomy scar, especially for partial gastrectomy, should arouse suspicion. Mental symptoms may predominate, or the patient may present with the features often ascribed to 'senility', such as unsteadiness, dragging of the feet, peripheral neuropathy and sensory ataxia. It is important to realise that subacute combined degeneration of the cord is not a feature of severe cases of pernicious anaemia.

Diagnosis

The blood picture shows a pancytopenia. The Hb may be at normal levels, or reach surprisingly low levels. The red cells are macrocytic and normochromic. The macrocytes are oval, with some aniso- and poikilocytosis. The presence of neutrophils with multiple lobes (shift to the right) is almost diagnostic. Mean red cell volume (MCV) levels are increased, while MCHC is normal, unless iron deficiency is also present. Confirmation may be gained by finding low serum B12 levels, and the demonstration of pentagastrin-fast achlorhydria. Demonstration of the impaired B12 absorption by the Schilling urinary excretion test is not to be relied upon in elderly patients in whom renal function may be impaired. It must always be borne in mind that megalocytic anaemia may occur in patients with myxoedema, or gastric carcinoma, which many authors have reported as more likely to develop in the stomach affected by atrophic gastritis.

Treatment

Treatment must be continued for life, commencing with 1000 micrograms of vitamin B12 (hydroxycobalanin) on alternate days for one week, followed by 250—1000 micrograms every second month, or more frequently if signs of subacute degeneration are present. Delay in treatment may result in impaired response of neurological signs, but haematological response may be quickly detected by a marked reticulocytosis at the end of the first week of treatment. Oral iron therapy is advisable for the first month of treatment.

Folic Acid Deficiency

This is an uncommon nutritional anaemia, which develops in patients on a deficient diet, particularly alcoholics. There are no body stores, as in Vitamin B12, and deficiency strikes at DNA synthesis, so that requirements increase in conditions of increased cell turn-over as well as malabsorption. Serum folate levels below 2 ng indicate deficiency, and treatment consists of a return to an adequate diet of fruit and vegetables, the major sources, with folic acid tablet supplementation for a month.

Symptomatic Anaemias

The response of elderly patients to adequate treatment based on accurate diagnosis is the same as with younger subjects. Cases will be encountered, however, of refractory anaemia. Consideration must then be given to the presence of chronic disease processes, such as carcinoma, myelo- or lymphoproliferative processes, renal failure, chronic infection, or rheumatoid arthritis, in which the degree of anaemia is proportional to the activity of the disease.

Conclusion

The practitioner may go far in the diagnosis and treatment of anaemia in the elderly with simple apparatus. A haemoglobinometer, a box of slides, microscope and bottles of Leishman's stain and buffered distilled water, finger cots and Occultest tablets, are sufficient to make satisfactory penetration of many clinical conditions in elderly patients. The ability to estimate the ESR is also very useful, and in practice the micro method has several advantages, not the least of which is the ease with which it can be set up in the home and recorded by the patient himself.

CARDIORESPIRATORY DISORDERS

Although one is obliged, for the purposes of description, to describe functions separately, the reader should never lose sight of the reciprocity of action and interaction between the heart and lungs. Thoracic and intrathoracic dynamics must be regarded, in patients of advanced years, as a single function.

There is probably no area in geriatric medicine where accurate diagnosis plays a more important part than in heart disease. Under ordinary conditions, the normal aged heart can provide adequate output, due to reduced requirements, lower metabolic rate, and body atrophy. Heart/body ratio is an important prognostic factor, and the loss of weight, often reported in late years, may be regarded in a favourable light once wasting diseases have been excluded. Although heart failure is often attributed to myocardial senility, age-related changes result from vascular insufficiency rather than ageing of the heart muscle. The atherosclerotic process appears first, often under the age of 20, in the brachiocephalic trunk and the left common carotid, and progresses in a stepwise fashion, with considerable increases in the third and fifth decades. The same risk factors, heavy smoking, hyperlipidaemia, hypokinesis, apply to arterial occlusion of the limbs as to coronary disease, but obliterative peripheral atherosclerosis is not correlated with hypertension.

Ischaemic Heart Disease

Since coronary disease is almost universal after the age of 70, the clinical distinction between the anginal syndrome, acute coronary insufficiency and myocardial infarction, may not be made so precisely as with younger groups. Other causes of chest pain multiply with rising age, such as hiatal hernia, pulmonary embolism, cervical and gall bladder disease, while atypical presentations of myocardial infarction predominate, such as dyspnoea from left ventricular failure, symptoms of reduced cerebral blood flow, abdominal distress from visceral congestion, and less commonly syncope due to heart block.

Prognosis
Although absolute survival of the elderly is shorter, a comparison with younger groups similarly affected may show that life expectancy is less adversely affected in the aged. The hormonal protection afforded to females before the menopause, once lost, brings equality of incidence after a few years, but a worse prognosis in

elderly females, who show increased incidence of sudden death due to cardiac rupture. Unfavourable factors are advanced age, associated chest or renal disease, cardiogenic shock, cyanosis, arrhythmias, and acute mental failure.

Management
While treatment of myocardial infarction is in general similar to younger patients, heavy sedation must be carefully avoided, especially if mental changes are present. Old patients are better nursed in a bedside chair, rather than in bed. Early ambulation is to be looked for, but must be measured against other factors that may be found to demand undue exertion such as obesity, stiff joints, general weakness, or inadequate assistance for lifting. Specialist advice should be sought where there is severe heart failure, shock, or embolic phenomena. Anticoagulants are best not used, because of increased susceptibility of elderly patients to vascular haemorrhage, even with normal prothrombin times. The aim should always be to treat at home.

Hypertension

Because of his longitudinal association with the patient the family practitioner is in a specially favourable position to manage problems of blood pressure. The new entrant to practice will note with surprise the frequency of systolic hypertension among fit and active old men, with figures of 200/100 mm Hg being common. He may attribute this to the well-known tendency for the blood pressure, especially the systolic, to rise with age. Over the age of 70, however, this upward trend is arrested, and blood pressure levels become more stable, especially the diastolic. There is some reassurance to be gained from the absence of malignant hypertension in this age group, and the ability to tolerate high levels of blood pressure for many years with little discomfort by many old people, especially females.

It is important, however, to remember that each elderly patient poses an individual problem in respect of blood pressure level. It is a mistake to assume that old normotensives are immune to heart disease or, because one has become accustomed to disregard the height of the systolic pressure in the young, to imagine that the same insouciance can be maintained with elderly subjects; when the systolic pressure remains above 190 mm Hg the risk of cerebral haemorrhage is greatly increased.

Clearly then, frequent measurements are desirable to know what is happening in the individual case. Over a period of years it will then be noticed that sudden spells of hot weather may cause the systolic pressure to drop by as much as 40 mm Hg which may account for the fact that many elderly patients complain at these times, while some even display mental confusion, or syncope. A fall in the systolic pressure will also occur in acute infections, such as enteritis, or pneumonia, or will herald a failing heart, or metastasising carcinoma. Less commonly, a rising blood pressure may indicate renal impairment or polyarteritis.

Assessment

Before treatment is commenced, an assessment should be made of any patient whose blood pressure lies outside the normal range, say 180/100 mm Hg for men, and 190/110 mm Hg for women. The blood pressure should be taken with the patient lying down, and then after one minute's standing, when about a quarter of elderly patients will show a drop of 20 mm Hg or more in the systolic pressure, and this is most marked over the age of 75. Orthostatic hypotension is usually related to varicose veins, or a combination of factors such as organic brain disease, low serum sodium, anaemia, valvular or ischaemic heart disease or potentially hypotensive drugs.

Much can be learned from the past history, and of the family history, particularly that of siblings. Enquiries should be made concerning stroke illness, heart failure, and ocular or renal disease, and the ages at which these events occurred. A urine test, and estimation of the blood urea, or creatinine clearance, is essential. The serum electrolytes should also be measured, especially if diuretic drugs are to be used. An attempt should be made to view the fundus oculi, for the appearance of normal vessels is not unusual, even in long-standing hypertension, and may reinforce a resolve to withhold treatment. Pathological changes, when present, are often mixed, and difficult to interpret without considerable experience, in the aged.

Management

It cannot be too greatly stressed that reduction of blood pressure in old people is a considerable hazard, and should only be undertaken occasionally, and for definite indications. The presence of angina pectoris, renal or cerebral failure, are contraindications, while dizziness and headaches are rarely if ever symptoms to be relieved by the prescription of hypotensive drugs. The presence of orthostatic hypotension is a further warning before considering drug therapy.

The dangers of drug induced hypotension are considerable. When levels are rapidly reduced in patients with sclerotic vessels, there is a real danger of producing cerebral insufficiency, coronary infarction without thrombosis, or senile gangrene. In addition, the thiazide diuretics, frequently used in the treatment of hypertension may precipitate the diabetic state, or less commonly hyperuricaemia, or pre-renal uraemia.

The chief indication for treating hypertension in the elderly is hypertensive left ventricular failure. Less commonly, it is necessary to treat those patients where hypertension is producing retinal vascular damage. The object of treatment in the elderly is to lower the diastolic pressure gradually to levels of about 100 mm Hg. Much can be accomplished if reduction of weight and salt intake can be achieved.

The drugs which are of greatest service are those which are the least likely to produce side effects. In the anxious, hyperkinetic patient, rauwiloid, two tablets at night may be all that is required. The beta-adrenergic blocking drugs are of much value in selected patients. Other drugs, such as methyldopa, clonidine and thiazide diuretics may be used in various combinations. The benefits of treatment must be closely balanced against the production of side effects, and potassium supplementation or the use of amiloride becomes increasingly important in the late decades.

Pulmonary Heart Disease (Cor Pulmonale)

The reduction of pulmonary function with age, resulting from distortion of the thoracic cage, interstitial fibrosis, emphysema, infection and emboli, all place an added burden on the right ventricle. Few patients are found in practice to have reached the age of 75 with chronic *cor pulmonale*, but the typical patient is usually one reaching retirement age, from industrial employment, addicted to cigarette smoking, and having a persistent cough, with wheezing and dyspnoea. During winter these patients are pushed into congestive cardiac failure, by acute pulmonary infection, to which they are increasingly susceptible. The heart failure is of secondary importance to the pulmonary insufficiency which requires close monitoring of the blood gases, best achieved in hospital. Recovered patients should be urged to stop smoking, and are helped by postural drainage if fit enough. Breathing exercises are of little help, but much benefit may result from assisted expiration by manual compression of the thoracic cage. These patients have a much reduced pulmonary blood flow, so that drug therapy is disappointing. But, since even marginal improvement is to be looked for, a bronchodilator, such as salbutamol, and the occasional use of a diuretic, may relieve respiratory distress. The use of Bisolvon for a period of not less than a month may be helpful for patients unable to cough away tenacious mucus from the bronchi.

Murmurs

It has to be remembered at the present time that, while rheumatic heart disease has become a rarity in the young, established cases of rheumatic carditis are now to be found relatively more commonly in the older age groups. In elderly persons undergoing surgery bacterial endocarditis remains a threat, and antibiotic cover should be offered for minor procedures, such as dental extraction, or instrumentation for genito-urinary conditions, as well as major procedures. The presentation is often atypical, but blood culture should always be carried out in patients who present with weight loss, pyrexia, mental confusion, and a raised ESR, especially where a mitral murmur is present. The diagnosis is often missed simply because the symptoms suggest the popular picture of 'senility'.

Murmurs at the aortic area may be due to dilatation of the aorta, or due to increased emotion or hyperthyroidism. Most commonly over the age of 75 one encounters the patient with fibrous thickening of the aortic cusps, which become increasingly calcified with age. When these cusps remain separate, and mobile, they cause no functional change, but inflammatory changes may cause fusion, and stenosis, with dizziness, syncope, angina, and left ventricular failure.

The mitral valve may be affected at a later age by similar changes, and murmurs may result from this cause, as well as from cardiac dilatation, or the involvement of papillary muscle by infarction, with consequent dysfunction. The variety of cardiac murmurs, and their causes, make this an aspect of cardiology in which specialist advice is often extremely important. Similarly, the variety of cardiac arrythmias and conduction disturbances encountered, some of which are asymptomatic and only encountered on electrocardiograms, require more than usual expertise in interpretation and management. The more aggressive approach to cardiology in the elderly means that many are now treated with pace-makers for heart block and sick sinus syndrome with the possibility of recovery from cerebral failure.

Cardiac Failure

Cardiac failure, particularly of the congestive type, is quite commonly found present in the ambulatory aged. It is important in this age group to be aware that a single cause is rarely responsible, though ischaemic and hypertensive heart disease predominate. In the management it is important to consider the role of extra-cardiac causes which may be present, such as anaemia, anoxia, thyrotoxicosis, and less commonly, Parkinsonism, Paget's disease and thiamine deficiency.

Diagnosis

Diagnosis is not always easy in the elderly patient, when difficulty may be experienced in hearing the heart sounds, and in whom oedema is present not uncommonly from non-cardiac causes. Whereas breathlessness may be confused with dyspnoea, and arise from obesity, emphysema and the generally reduced ventilatory capacity that develops in advanced age, orthopnea should be enquired about, and provides a better indicator of failure.

Management

Whole Body Rest   This is perhaps the most important basis of treatment. The well-known dangers of bed-rest apply to cardiac patients no less than to others, and a suitable chair with arms in which the patient can sleep with comfort, and from which he can rise with ease, has considerable advantages. Prolonged rest is unwise, and the patient should be mobilised after one week. A failure in response during the first week is a grave sign, and attention should be directed to elimination of extra cardiac causes, such as anaemia, anoxia and thyrotoxicosis. The recovered patient should be advised to climb stairs only once a day, and to stop frequently if distress arises. Many old patients are enabled to remain reasonably active if they plan to remain in bed for one day each week, or if they arrange to sleep downstairs.

Digoxin   The other main treatment is the use of digoxin. Digitalization may be begun with 0.25 mg twice daily for three days, and then reduced by half. Usually 0.25 mg daily will be adequate for maintenance dosage, but a careful watch must be kept for toxic effects of this drug in the elderly, usually shown as arrythmias and conduction defects, which are most likely to arise in conditions of potassium depletion. Many elderly patients will not require long continued use of digoxin, and the practitioner should seek to discontinue its use whenever it seems practical to do so.

Diuretics   The use of diuretic drugs is much abused. These drugs can be likened to the practice of blood-letting in the eighteenth century. They are life saving when used intravenously in cases of acute pulmonary oedema, and play an important rôle in the treatment of hypertensive heart disease. In the elderly, however, vulnerability to electrolyte depletion, dehydration, pre-renal uraemia and constipation are serious clinical side effects. Many physicians fail to realise the social restrictions these drugs may cause, or indeed, that facilities for passing urine must be quickly accessible. It is quite obviously not the intention to have the patient toiling up the stairs a dozen times each morning to micturate. Where diuretics are used, potassium supplementation is standard in the elderly, where lean body mass, and total body potassium are proportionately reduced.

Oxygen and Fluid Intake   Bed rest, salt restriction, and digoxin are the main lines of treatment. The wise use of diuretics, and the use of oxygen where hypoxia is present are also very important. It must be remembered that since iron deficiency anaemia is not uncommon in the elderly, cyanosis may not occur. Patients may have reduced their fluid intake voluntarily in an attempt to mitigate the bother caused by nocturia, while old people lose the sense of thirst. The practitioner should therefore encourage patients to continue to take sufficient fluid for physiological requirements.

Potassium   Where potassium supplements are poorly tolerated, or where there is difficulty in avoiding potassium depletion, use may be made of amiloride which augments sodium loss, while sparing loss of potassium, when given with a thiazide.

Cardiac Pacing   Complete heart block is often due to isolated disease of the conduction tissues. Provided there is normal myocardium and healthy coronary arteries, old age should not be considered a contra-indication to artificial pacing. Such control of ventricular rate may well result in several more years of active life. The commonest indication is for Stokes-Adams attacks, but congestive cardiac failure or heart failure refractory to medical treatment are other reasons for offering treatment which may be undertaken under local anaesthesia. Reversal of chronic brain failure has been reported in patients where the cause was a combination of low cardiac output with slow heart rate. Artificial pacing must be considered an advantage over drug therapy, in suitable cases.

VASCULAR DISEASE

The pathology of old age is becoming increasingly dominated by that of vascular degeneration and diseases, which are so common that they occupy a place in the dim borderline separating biological from pathological ageing. Yet arteriosclerosis is not an inevitable accompaniment of ageing. Furthermore, all or only a part of the vascular tree may be affected by it, a fact revealed by recent advances in arterial radiography. Environmental factors outweigh ethnic and other factors in importance in its production. Males appear to be affected earlier in life than females, especially those in the lower social classes, or those who have undergone prolonged mental and physical stress, such as former prisoners of war. Arteriosclerosis is usually a combination of Monckeburg's sclerosis and atherosclerosis, and is clearly multifactorial in origin, being hastened in its evolution by tobacco, alcohol, diabetes, gout, and renal disease. Atherogenic factors are generally held to be operative in earlier life, so that preventive advice by the practitioner may be directed at young patients whose life style involves a combination of risk factors.

Current diagnostic methods, and advances in reconstructive surgery, have greatly improved the outlook of elderly patients in whom the disease has become established.

Aortic Changes

Elongation and thickening of the thoracic aorta are frequently reported to the practitioner in chest radiographs. Although this is usually symptomless, it is important to note it, since in some patients it may cause dysphagia due to pressure on, or displacement of the oesophagus. This can be verified by the compression visible in the lateral view of a barium swallow. It is important also to be aware that buckling of the innominate artery may produce a pulsatile swelling in the right sternoclavicular angle, which might be thought to be a tumour or aneurysm (p. 583). Widening of the arch will also be liable to cause pressure on the left innominate vein, preventing the external jugular vein on that side from emptying freely, which, if observed by itself, may cause a mistaken diagnosis of congestive cardiac failure to be made.

Acute Occlusive Arterial Disease

Arterial embolism involving visceral, mesenteric, cerebral or renal territory is not uncommon in old age, following the development of atrial fibrillation, or a myocardial infarction, which may have been silent, but creating a site where mural thrombus can form. Diagnosis is usually simple, but it must be remembered that the onset is not always sudden, or painful; but coldness and numbness are always present in a limb. The lower limb is affected four times as commonly as the upper limb. Emergency treatment before admission to hospital is important. The patient should be supported in a sitting position, and the affected limb kept at rest, and free from pressure. Elevation and the application of heat must be strictly avoided. Intravenous heparin (10 000 units) may be given as soon as possible.

Chronic Obliterative Arteriosclerosis

The average age of onset of intermittent claudication is 50, and the high mortality associated with it reduces the number of elderly patients seen with this disease. Nevertheless, the practitioner will usually have one or two patients at any one time, with threatening gangrene of the foot. Severe ischaemia and gangrene are more likely to follow involvement of the femoral artery, or arteries distal to it, than where aortoiliac disease alone is present. Examination should include auscultation for bruit below Poupart's ligament. Ischaemic rest pain suggests advanced disease and a poor prognosis, but in elderly diabetics this may be masked by neuropathy. The presence of diabetes, which should always be looked for, increases the gravity of the vascular process, because lesions tend to be widely disseminated.

Management
Strict control of diabetes, particularly by dietary restriction of carbohydrate, is of cardinal importance.
Amputation Because of his closer supervision of such patients, the practitioner rather than the vascular surgeon, will find himself called upon to advise on the matter of amputation. The following advice may be found helpful in these agonizing decisions. Age, alone, is not a contraindication to fitting a patient with a prosthesis after amputation of the lower extremity, if the patient

has been able to walk up to the time of the amputation, especially if this is a below-knee, or even a through-knee procedure. Contraindications are:

> mental deterioration, which will preclude retraining;
> advanced neurological disease, with loss of function;
> cardio-pulmonary disease, limiting exercise tolerance;
> impending gangrene, ulcers, or infection of the other limb;
> contractures fixing hip or knee in flexion.

Nevertheless, many patients, through poor follow up at home, appear to wear their prostheses only for visits to the clinic, especially where the amputation is of the above-knee type. Motivation, based upon continued social expectation, dominates the follow-up period. Failure to consider all aspects of the patient's situation, and to present these realistically to the surgeon, is a main cause of poor results. It is also essential for a patient to receive daily follow-up visits at home, preferably from a rehabilitation nurse who can supervise stump exercises, and give encouragement. The advantage of attending a physiotherapy unit, apart from the material facilities and professional expertise of the staff, is the element of competition provided by other patients.

Limb Salvage   The early referral of patients with ischaemic limbs to the vascular surgeon offers the best opportunity for saving the limb by reconstructive surgical procedures. Where short segmental occlusions are found on angiography in the common iliac or common femoral arteries, thromboembarterectomy may be successful, and removal of the occluding block restore arterial flow to the entire lower extremity.

Arterial flow may be achieved by means of synthetic or autogenous vein grafts to by-pass the aortoiliac, or femoropoliteal segments. These procedures may be combined with lumbar sympathectomy which is designed to promote the development of collateral circulation.

Vasodilator Drugs   The use of vasodilator drugs has fallen into disrepute. Mackenzie long ago pointed out that no vasodilator action is superior to that produced by ischaemic tissue. A rigid vessel wall will not dilate, but since arteriosclerosis is patchy in distribution, blood is diverted away from the ischaemic limb and into tissues capable of response to adrenolytic drugs. Side effects may be produced, chief among which is postural hypotension. Valuable time may be spent in their administration during which the disease process advances beyond surgical relief. Benefit reported from their action should be an indication to revise the diagnosis. The use of alcohol is often urged by surgeons when they can do no more. The practitioner should be in no doubt that what benefit the patient derives from it is central, rather than peripheral. Increasing faith in the 'water of life' prompted by a moment of brief authority may have unwanted effects, unless the dose is accurately prescribed as for any other drug.

Medical Management   This is best confined to care of the general health, and good results may derive from correction of anaemia, cessation of smoking, and attention to diet and obesity. Meticulous local attention to the ischaemic foot, drainage of necrotic lesions, debridement, and wet dressings of Eusol, outweigh the benefit of systemic antibiotics which cannot reach effective tissue concentrations. Control of pain, particularly at night, is essential, for pain is felt less in the dependent position while sitting, and where the mind is diverted.

Vascular Aneurysms

Aneurysms of the abdominal aorta are found usually in males in the 7th and 8th decades. The presence of pain indicates rapid expansion, and requires immediate referral. More commonly, a pulsatile and expansile tumour is felt in the umbilical region. Prognosis is poor, for most will die of rupture within 1 or 2 years. Where there is x-ray evidence of calcification of the aneurysm wall, the prognosis may be more favourable. Abdominal aneurysmectomy can be successfully performed at any age for patients in reasonable health.

Aneurysms may also be found along the course of the femoral and popliteal arteries, and the hazard in these more peripheral lesions is thrombosis and resultant loss of limb.

Venous Thrombosis

Venous thrombosis and pulmonary embolism occur frequently in geriatric patients, probably due largely to progressive enlargement of the calf veins with increasing years. The signs of deep vein thrombosis are often minimal, or entirely absent. Presumptive diagnosis may be made more readily in post-operative patients, those confined to bed, the obese, the anaemic, and those with heart disease or carcinoma. Symptoms are more likely to be noted in the active ambulant patient. Good support of varicose veins is important.

While diagnosis may be easily missed in the calf veins, the manifestations of ileofemoral, or inferior vena cava thrombosis are obvious, with swelling, and aching pain in the whole lower extremity, cyanosis, and tenderness to pressure in the midline of the upper thigh.

It is not surprising that the source of emboli proves elusive in about half the cases of pulmonary embolism. Focal segmental or lobar involvement in a lung, gradual deterioration, acute hypotension, rapid onset of congestive cardiac failure, or sudden collapse may all therefore arise mysteriously in an elderly patient. One of the most difficult clinical problems in pulmonary embolic disease is to decide upon the minimal diagnostic criteria for the institution of therapy. It is advisable always to seek hospital admission for patients with deep venous thrombosis, or where pulmonary embolism is a possible diagnosis. Old patients reluctant to enter hospital, or where there are other cogent reasons against it, may be nursed at home. The position to be adopted should be with the trunk flat, and the head supported on one pillow. Both legs may then be elevated. Venous return is maximal in this position. Crepe bandages may be applied to the legs, and heparin 12 500 units given twice daily intramuscularly for 72 hours, and coumarin 20 mg given concurrently in twice daily doses for six weeks. A weekly prothrombin time should be estimated, and bed exercise encouraged. It is safe to allow patients to sit out after a week, and to do a little walking at the end of two weeks.

CEREBRO-VASCULAR DISEASE

The pathogenesis of cerebro-vascular disease is discussed in Chapter 14, p. 265.

Strokes

A family practitioner will encounter on average a new case of stroke every two months, but, because the winter incidence is twice that in summer, in the northern hemisphere most will occur during the months of January and February. In addition to the five or six new cases arising each year, the practitioner will also have a similar number of patients with varying degrees of long-term impairment resulting from a previous stroke. Three quarters of all strokes will be in those who are over the age of 65, a significant number of whom have developed a major stroke during the difficult period of readjustment to retirement, so that the degree of strain on the married partner, or close companion, is severe, and may be devastating. Stroke is a common and seriously disruptive illness, and one about which there has been a distressing lack of interest, and a feeling that little can be done, though this seems quite irrational, when one considers the prestige of the organ involved.

It is probably true to say that all stroke patients should be admitted to hospital other than those who are going to die. This is a severe illness, and even the mild stroke will require investigation, which may prevent a second or more severe one. This decision will depend on the proximity of a Stroke Unit, or a general medical ward with facilities for monitoring, intravenous feeding and radiological and neurological diagnosis. Inevitably, for some years to come, many stroke cases will have to be treated at home.

Beyond the general epidemiological datum that women tend to cerebral thrombosis, and men, through the androgenic drive, to haemorrhage, the family practitioner is able to offer real help from his past knowledge of the patient.

Diagnosis

The call to the doctor often mentions suspicion of a stroke. It is a diagnosis clear to the layman. The practitioner will first ask himself: who is this patient; has he been seen before; what is known of his medical history; is he hypertensive; has he a history of rheumatic heart disease, or coronary thrombosis; has auricular fibrillation occurred; what kind of man is he, and how does he deal with trouble?

On arrival, it is important to establish that this is a stroke, for one patient in 20 will have an alternative diagnosis of chronic subdural haematoma, or cerebral tumour, with the possibility of a good prognosis (see Chapter 14). The question of head injury, personality change, and minor symptoms preceding the illness must not be forgotten.

The practitioner should assess the posture, the pupil reaction, and the presence of lateral deviation. He should attempt to develop a degree of sophistication in neurological examination that allows localization of the lesion, even in the unconscious patient, since this knowledge confers an ability to make some prognosis for functional recovery. This is particularly important where an old person, living alone, has been found unconscious in a house, so that there is no eye witness of the mode of onset.

Investigation
Wherever possible the following investigations should be carried out: urinalysis, haemoglobin, ESR, chest x-ray, skull x-ray for possible shift of calcified pineal and to exclude head injury.

Management
This will depend on many factors. In severe strokes, the first action is to maintain the essential functions, with attention to the airway. Skilled nursing is required to prevent pressure sores and chest infection. Hypertension well above recently recorded levels may indicate cerebral oedema, causing cerebral compression. Raising the head, and injections of intravenous frusemide (40 mg) and dexamethasone (10 mg) may prevent the development of a pressure cone. The steroid should be repeated 6 hourly; 4 mg dexamethasone by mouth if and when consciousness returns.

Adverse factors are advanced age, severity of stroke, the presence of homonymous hemianopia, the presence of associated disease and notably a prior history of declining health.

The patient who is conscious, but unable to communicate, due to dysphonia or dysarthria, presents a special problem. He will be helped in the early stages if the practitioner carries the Word and Picture Chart, supplied for a minimal charge by the Chest and Heart Association, London, England.

Rehabilitation   This can be achieved in the home. Before deciding on this, the suitability of the home, the quality of help proffered by relatives, and the motivation of a patient relatively free from locomotor, cardiac or other disorder must be assessed. It is essential that the practitioner should recognise the mental barriers to recovery that arise from focal lesions. The patient who displays anosognosia, or denial of half of space, cannot be expected to co-operate in a programme of rehabilitation. Unco-operative patients should be reassessed by an interested specialist. In general, it can be said that a patient can compensate for loss of power in a limb more easily than for proprioceptive loss of inco-ordination.

The rehabilitation of a stroke patient is a skilled matter, and patients should be referred wherever possible to those with special experience. All too often patients are lifted up the bed by untrained nurses, using the axilla on the plegic side as a fulcrum, causing permanent damage to the brachial plexus. The increase in the number of Geriatric Day Centres brings almost every patient within the ambit of an enthusiastic multidisciplinary team, where physiotherapy, occupational therapy, psychometric evaluation, and speech therapy are available.

During this time, the practitioner may ask the health visitor or social worker to assess the home for modifications such as hand rails, and bath seats. Because of transport difficulties and dependency on day centres, many patients are unable to continue a rehabilitation programme for long enough. Since improvement may continue for five years, it is important that the practitioner should continue to encourage, and supervise these patients. Cerebrovascular accident is the third greatest cause of death and the greatest cause of disturbed consciousness. As a clinical problem, it offers more interest than coronary occlusion, showing little distinction between the sexes, social classes and races, except in the Japanese.

Minor Strokes

The difference between a transient and completed stroke may be marginal, but two thirds of transient ischaemic attacks lead on to completed stroke at a later date.

Diagnosis

Little strokes are rich in symptoms, but poor in signs. They often come to the family doctor's notice through the report of a wife or colleague. The story is of sudden loss in function or anti-social behaviour. Common manifestations are confusion, loss of good judgment, inability to work, failure of memory, increased irritability, pseudo-Meniere's syndrome, sudden ageing and fatigue, poor grooming, swallowing difficulties, falling, clumsiness, speech difficulties and vile tastes or smells. A case of my own was the lady of 73 who fell going upstairs to bed, bruising her forehead, about which she was concerned. Her sister, who accompanied her, reported the significant fact that getting her up again was like lifting a dead weight. It was then that I became aware of the slight droop at the corner of the mouth.

It is important to remember that systemic disorders will cause reduction of cerebral blood flow, such as cardiac arrhythmias and Stokes-Adams attacks. What one has to decide is whether there is a state of cerebro-vascular insufficiency, and, if so, what is the trigger mechanism of the ischaemic attacks. Investigation at this stage may reveal a treatable cause, such as giant cell arteritis, or a careful history may direct attention to brain stem dysfunction, or show patterns of recurrent symptoms, such as is found in syndromes of internal carotid insufficiency. Anticoagulant therapy has now been established as a valid treatment of transient ischaemic attacks provided always that there is no severe hypertension.

Sudden decrements in elderly people in whom gradual functional decline is to be expected, should always alert the practitioner to consider the diagnosis of little stroke. A high index of suspicion of this common but often missed condition is needed, for it presents to the family doctor for recognition, rather than to the specialist.

Rehabilitation in the Home
Many patients will continue to be treated at home. Although recovery from stroke is spontaneous, the role of the practitioner is important, in several ways.

Motivation
Little progress can be expected unless the patient is encouraged to maximal effort. This does not mean deploying the kind of blind enthusiastic drive in which the patient is considered either as a co-operator, or something less. The clinical features of the stroke, the character of the patient and his social expectations, and the facilities of the home, all impose limiting conditions which demand recognition, and which create a framework within which to work. The practitioner must also recognise the role played by other conditions which may be present, such as ischaemic heart disease, or locomotor difficulties.

Nursing Care and Rehabilitation
Nurses with special experience in home rehabilitation are greatly needed. There is much to be learned by watching them at work. The patient should be set a target of attainment to be reached at the next visit. Urgently needed are aids for toilet, walking and bathing purposes. Grab rails, ramps, and alterations to the home should be requisitioned for early. The conscious patient should be properly dressed in daytime wear, and sit in a chair of the 'carver' type, with a high seat, and arms for support when standing. Bed-end exercises depend on the style of bed and the presence of a rail, but a pulpit walking frame may easily be stabilised for this purpose. The nurse may teach relatives how to put the limb through a range of passive movements. Simple pulleys may be erected in doorways so that the patient may elevate the paralysed arm himself, or bicycle

pedals modified for exercising the lower limbs, which recover earlier as a rule. Apparatus, as well as new ideas, can often be loaned by visiting the local Geriatric Day Hospital.

Social Assessment

There is always a need for the practitioner to set in motion this type of assessment, for urgent financial needs must be met, and entitlement to statutory allowances brought to the attention of the patient's family. These matters require the special skills of the Social Worker. Families who feel initially unable to cope with the stroke patient are often helped by the knowledge that care may be shared with the hospital, in certain areas, and a consultation with the local consultant physician may achieve flexibility in these arrangements.

Continuing Support

If stroke illness is under-diagnosed, it is also often undertreated. There is probably no other illness in which follow-up by the family doctor is more important. Failure to do so implies abandonment to hopelessness. Follow-up visits should not, however, be of the 'tea and sympathy' type, nor merely for the patient to demonstrate his progress. There are many points to be noted, such as nutritional status, the correction of anaemia, treatment of urinary tract infection, and attention to cardiac function, which lie within the province of the family physician, and which, if neglected, may retard or nullify the recovery of function. Again it is helpful to expect much of the patient, and never to be quite satisfied: but then, it is a good attitude to adopt concerning one's self also when dealing with this type of patient.

CRANIAL ARTERITIS

The term 'temporal arteritis' to describe one local manifestation of this condition may divert attention from the involvement of the visual system. This is a true arteritis with a predilection for the aged, and presents with persistent and severe headache, which is often unilateral (see page 268). The temporal arteries are tender, and are often felt as pulseless cords, whose thickness is easily felt under the hot overlying skin. This is an emergency condition, since vision may fail at any time. Bilateral fundal abnormalities may be detected, such as optic atrophy, retinal haemorrhages, or retinal artery thrombosis. The ESR is markedly raised, usually above 50 mm in one hour, and treatment with prednisolone should be started promptly, with large initial doses of 40 mg daily, with slow reduction to maintenance levels of 5–10 mg daily.

A significant proportion of cases demonstrate this disease to be a general one. The occurrence of cranial arteritis in association with polymyalgia rheumatica is well-known. It is important to be aware of the manifestations of polymyalgia rheumatica (described on page 203) which characteristically occur in the early morning and may have passed off completely by the afternoon. The response to moderate doses of steroid is dramatic, and 5 mg prednisolone given three times daily may banish symptoms in one day. Slow reduction of dosage over a period of 12—18 months is to be aimed at. Patients treated with analgesics and physiotherapy only always carry the risk of developing sudden eye complications.

NEUROLOGICAL DISORDERS

The nervous system is of special importance in relation to the ageing process. Neurones, if they degenerate and die before the death of the organism are not replaced, and undergo progressive attrition with time. The changes thus produced in a governing and communicating system will inevitably affect many organs and other systems, and lead to the disruption of functions that are delicately balanced. Abnormalities may be found in old people who are in apparently good health. With advancing age both the tendon reflexes and vibration sense disappear in the lower limbs, and superficial reflexes, such as the abdominals, are frequently lost. There is reduced acuity in the special senses, with a corresponding reduction in awareness. There is little alteration with age in the velocity of peripheral nerve impulses, but there is a definite retardation of response in the central nervous system. Loss of muscle bulk is common, and guttering of the small muscles on the back of the hand are frequently noted, although grip strength is well maintained. Sensory testing becomes impossible when the distinction between neurological deficit and imperfect comprehension can no longer be made.

Assessment

Despite these impedimenta, the assessment of neurological disorders must proceed, as in the young, on a good history and examination. A sudden onset will usually suggest a disorder of vascular origin, while slowly progressive evolution is more indicative of neoplastic, degenerative, neuropathic, or endocrine pathology. Where cerebral symptoms such as faintness, dizziness, or giddiness, are mentioned, more specific information must be sought concerning the circumstances in which the symptoms were provoked, their duration, and whether a sense of rotation was noted. In cases where a true loss of consciousness has been established, it is important to ask if recovery was rapid, or slow. A careful examination of the nervous system is required in order to avoid missed diagnosis of treatable illness which might otherwise pass as an incurable degenerative condition. Where tendon reflexes are difficult to elicit reinforcement techniques are essential.

Senile Tremor

The hands are most commonly affected, but rarely with equal severity. Later the head and tongue may become tremulous. The condition is usually familial, and akin to intention tremor, being aggravated by stress, social occasions and voluntary movement. The effect of the adrenergic component may be inhibited by oxprenolol, but patients often find for themselves the beneficial effect of alcohol. In case the use of alcohol cannot be disciplined, it is unwise to suggest its use, except for the important social occasion. Patients need to be reassured that this type of tremor is different from that of Parkinson's disease, which is a more progressive disorder.

Parkinsonism

Although Parkinson's syndrome frequently begins in the early fifties, the clinical features are little different when it develops in elderly patients. Since surgery has little part to play in patients over the age of 65, medical treatment is advised. The treatment of choice is the combined use of levodopa and carbidopa, the latter substance working as a peripheral decarboxylase inhibitor that permits a reduction in levodopa dosage and the side-effects. Less frequent dosage is needed than with Levodopa alone, and an earlier therapeutic plateau is achieved. All signs and symptoms of Parkinsonism respond to this treatment, the bradykinesia being the first symptom to be modified. A low dose is given initially, and gradually increased. It is important to bear in mind that the patient, who was formerly inactive, may now encounter the difficulties of increased mobility, such as the development of angina. In some instances, what appears to the practitioner as a therapeutic triumph may precipitate a family crisis! The few patients who develop extra-pyramidal tremor on an arteriosclerotic basis show a poor response to medical treatment. Difficulties which may not be mentioned to the practitioner, but which need sympathetic attention, are constipation, speech and swallowing difficulties and the strange symptom of 'freezing'. The deterioration in handwriting may be compensated for by the use of a felt tip pen, lifting it between each letter, and adopting the italic script which uses this technique. It is important in management to realise that every case is different, and that much benefit will derive from attention to the universal emotional aspects of the illness. Patients become dehydrated from loss of saliva through dribbling, and in severe cases, from inability to hold a drinking vessel. Physiotherapy once or twice a week is of no value, but exercises that stretch the rigid muscles around a joint can be carried out by a member of the family with improvement in function. The most valuable asset a patient with this disease can have is an understanding spouse. Instruction in the nature of the disease is important if this is to be achieved, and the patient's slowness and feeding and walking difficulties correctly understood, and not interpreted as unwillingness.

Herpes Zoster

Probably because of lowered immunity to varicella in the elderly, herpes zoster is found predominantly in this age group. Cases of ophthalmic and geniculate herpes are more frequently encountered, and post-herpetic pain is almost always to be expected. The diagnosis and management of herpes zoster is described in Chapter 18, page 427.

Temperature Regulation and Hypothermia

It is often difficult to take the oral temperature of an old person with tremulous mouth, feeble lips and no teeth. Denied the accuracy of this method, and the fact that the mean of axillary temperature lies only 1°C above the lowest calibrated mark of the clinical thermometer, there is much advantage in using an electrical thermometer. It is obvious that the traditional 37°C is not the true normal mouth level in patients over the age of 65. The temperature of the extremities show wide variations due to changes in the peripheral circulation, either from arterial obstruction, or from individual efficiency in autonomic control over vasoconstriction. The elderly person can be expected to have impaired thermoregulatory reflexes and to react as a poikilothermic individual of inconstant internal temperature. The finding of warm hands when an old person is in a cold ambient temperature will alert the visitor to the presence of defective vasoconstriction, and impaired thermoregulation.

Accidental Hypothermia
This insidious and widespread hazard may affect patients even in reasonably warm surroundings, and the most likely time for its occurrence is in the early morning hours when physical activity, metabolic rate, and ambient temperatures are lowest. As is typical of disorders of late life, hypothermia is produced by many factors: advanced age; prolonged exposure; intercurrent illness; subnutrition; impaired thermoregulatory reflexes; immobility; hypothyroidism; the effect of drugs.

Diagnosis may need to be made independently of a history due to inability to feel or communicate. The most striking feature is skin cold to the touch in regions such as the abdomen and axilla, which usually remain warm. Once body temperature has passed below 32°C (90°F) tissue metabolism is progressively depressed, with reduction of the level of consciousness, increased muscle tone, falling blood pressure due to sinus bradycardia, which may progress to heart block and dangerous arrhythmias. The colour is greyish pallor, with puffy features. Speech, if present, is slow and husky.

Confirmation, if needed, is based on the finding of a rectal temperature below 90°F, using a low-reading thermometer left in situ for 10 minutes.

Treatment is best carried out in hospital and the patient transported in a warm ambulance with oxygen administration. In rural districts, where removal to hospital is prevented by severe winter conditions, slow rewarming may be carried out at home. External heat should be applied with great care as in excess it may relax the vasoconstriction, and thereby lead on to cardiovascular collapse. As emergency treatment the patient may be sustained by intravenous dextrose and hydrocortisone (100 mg), oxygen, and broad spectrum antibiotic therapy repeated 12 hourly. The conscious patient may be given hot sweetened drinks, and nursed between blankets in a room kept at 70°F. The head should always be covered.

Miscellaneous Neurological Disorders

Alcoholic Neuropathy
While authorities vary in describing the incidence of alcoholic addiction, and even suggest that it is not conducive to longevity, it must be considered where access to alcohol is free. Alcoholic neuropathy is uncommon, but cases of Korsakoff's psychosis are occasionally met with, usually in elderly women.

Diabetes
Diabetes occasionally presents with neuropathy of the lower limb, and even trophic ulceration. It may be confused with peripheral vascular disease, but the feet remain warm, and pain is relieved by exercise instead of increasing with it.

Degenerative Neurological Disorders
Degenerative neurological disorders of uncertain aetiology, such as senile tremor, trigeminal neuralgia, facial hemispasm, and motor neurone disease, are more common in the elderly. With the exception of trigeminal neuralgia, treatment of these conditions is unsatisfactory. It must be remembered that progressive muscular weakness can be the first sign of hypothyroidism. Neurological changes may occur in association with other common conditions of the elderly, such as vitamin B1 and B12 deficiencies, Paget's disease (page 620), and cervical spondylosis, while in cases of obscure aetiology, carcinomatous neuropathy must always be considered.

THE VISION OF ELDERLY PEOPLE

Although, in exceptional persons, normal visual acuity may be retained in the ninth decade, losses of visual acuity and colour vision are to be expected in old persons. Good vision is threatened by many factors, and specialist referrals for ophthalmic problems are more common than to other specialties. Yet, four out of five elderly people retain useful vision commensurate with their limited activities, and tests of each eye separately not infrequently demonstrate that useful vision is confined to one eye only.

The preservation of good vision, so vital to independence, may owe much to the vigilance of the family practitioner. Regular examination of the eyes is essential, and lesions may be prevented by knowledge of the patient's behaviour. In elderly females, corneal damage can occur from uncut nails, or the claws of domestic cats. The amateur gardener must take care when spraying fruit trees. Corneal damage from lid atrophy, giving rise to entropion or ectropion, is preventable by early tarsorrhaphy. The widespread use of eyebaths should be discouraged, but dry eyes should be treated with instillation of 0.5 per cent methyl cellulose drops.

The Lens

The practitioner is concerned in the diagnosis of cataract and the referral of patients as soon as misted vision is noted. Ignorance of the meaning of cataract is widespread among the public, who either fear it overmuch, or are too sanguine in respect of operative cure. Patients need guidance in the early post-operative phase when vision in the corrected aphakic eye is enlarged, and very brilliant, and leads them to suppress the smaller of unequal images. Later, when the second cataract is removed, adjustment must be made to contraction of the visual field.

Glaucoma

In the absence of criteria to define glaucoma, early diagnosis by the practitioner, so essential in preventing further irreversible blindness, is difficult. Patients should be questioned about pain around the eyes, and blurring of vision after reading, or seeing haloes around streetlights. Symptoms are more likely to be noticed in low light intensity. All patients with a family history of glaucoma should be screened by an ophthalmic specialist. It should be remembered that the pupil is small in old age, and a shallow anterior chamber, predisposing to angle closure, is common, so that atropine preparations, anticholinergic drugs, and even levodopa, must be given with caution, especially in hypermetropic subjects. Special experience is required to screen for glaucoma with the opthalmoscope, over which the tonometer has little advantage.

The Retina

Those who suffer from degeneration of the macular area do not become totally disabled, because peripheral vision is retained. The physician may suspect the condition in any elderly patient who looks at him obliquely. Treatment is unsatisfactory, but may be directed against associated conditions such as diabetes or hypertension.

Vascular occlusions causing sudden loss of vision should be seen by a specialist within two hours if treatment is likely to be effective. Heavy pipe smokers occasionally develop poor vision in both eyes due to tobacco amblyopia, a condition that is improved by injection of 1000 micrograms of hydroxy-cobalanin on alternate days for a week, so that differentiation of this condition is worthwhile.

Visual Aids

Though these are well-known and in Britain are supplied to people placed on the Blind Register, the most valuable action is to advise on light distribution within the home. Most old people are ignorant of the inverse square law. It is helpful to spend a little time to explain how a 60 Watt bulb close to one's work or reading is more effective than a 200 Watt bulb up near the ceiling, and that while electric lighting may be expensive, illuminating dark regions of the house is an important factor in home safety.

HEARING LOSS IN THE ELDERLY

The rehabilitation of the elderly deaf patient is an important function of the family practitioner, for loss of human communication constitutes a potent threat to social health and mental stability. As in all organ deficiencies in the older subject it is important to distinguish between impairment due to ageing, and the accumulation of pathologies that may be treatable, such as chronic infection, trauma, ototoxic drugs, and wax occlusion.

It is generally recognised that from middle age on there is a general decline in sensitivity and in the range of sounds heard, in particular of the higher frequencies (Presbyacusis page 137, paralleling the sensineural loss occurring in the other specialised input-sensory systems, like taste and smell.

Hearing loss in the elderly however involves not only decreased receptive capacity, but also reduction in the ability to discriminate between sounds.

Because the consonants, which supply so much speech information, are of short duration, and in the higher frequency range, speech sounds distorted rather than attenuated to the elderly. Furthermore, against the background noise of a social gathering, speech may be distorted beyond understanding through an inability to select the encoded information provided by consonants, so that reliance is placed increasingly on lip reading. The third element which makes heard speech difficult to understand is a general slowing of speech analysis in the brain. Thus rapid speech, or complex constructions, are not understood by many elderly people even in optimal circumstances. The comprehension of speech is thus related very indirectly to the results of pure tone audiograms, and sound amplitude.

The practitioner has a duty to estimate the inherent hearing difficulties of elderly patients (see Chapter 10). Where the hearing loss is predominantly in the middle ear, minor surgical procedures are often effective. Lesions of the inner ear may be helped by hearing aids where all sounds have become attenuated. Insertion of a speaking tube in the affected ear will identify the type of patient who will benefit. Unfortunately, aids are frequently supplied to patients who in fact rely upon lip-reading for understanding, and in whom the amplification of distorted sound merely adds to their communication difficulties. The practitioner has a responsibility to explain the use and limitations of hearing aids, to help patients adjust to their use, and to encourage care in their maintenance, for too many aids are found on routine inspection to be discarded or derelict.

Provided he has reasonable visual acuity, simple rules will help the patient whose hearing is seriously impaired to be reintegrated within the family. The speaker should sit, facing the patient, in a position that places him on the same level, with his face well illuminated. Once the deaf person has adopted an alert, listening posture, he should speak slowly, with exaggerated consonants, the free use of facial expression aided by meaningful gestures. It is often helpful to teach this technique when it is observed that the deaf person has become a source of irritation to a spouse or other relative.

ENDOCRINE DISORDERS

Diabetes

Diabetes is a condition the clinical effects of which resemble accelerated ageing. Ageing also predisposes to its development, and the glucose tolerance test, as developed on younger people, will reveal abnormalities in 25 per cent of people over the age of 70. Very often these dysglycaemic patients are thrown into frank diabetes by an intercurrent infection. There is a preponderance of obese female cases, though the incidence of new cases declines rapidly over the age of 75, suggesting that the very old are genetically an élite.

The term 'maturity onset diabetes' suggests a disease of insidious onset, likely to be discovered incidentally, by investigation of ungual infection, dry mouth, or the perspicacious observation of crystallised glucose on the shoes or floor. Occasionally, however, keto-acidotic disease occurs dramatically in the course of pulmonary or renal infection, with the need for insulin and fluid replacement. On the other hand, many are diagnosed when they exhibit one of the long term complications. It has been suggested that screening would prevent such morbidity but this assertion is open to much doubt.

Confirmation of diagnosis is best made by finding a fasting blood sugar raised above 130 mg/100 mL. Diminished renal blood flow and high renal threshold in elderly people makes negative urine testing unreliable. Once diabetes has been diagnosed examination for complications, particularly in the lens, retina, and peripheral circulation, should be made.

The aim of treatment should be control of the diabetes by carbohydrate restriction alone. There is a real danger that concomitant treatment by dietary restriction with oral hypoglycaemic agents may produce hypoglycaemic coma, difficult to reverse, and refractory even to intravenous 50 per cent glucose. Since brain damage may be caused, tolbutamide, with a shorter half life, is safer than other sulphonylurea drugs. Experienced practitioners will find much satisfaction in the management of elderly diabetic patients. The management of diabetes is fully discussed in Chapter 20.

Thyroid Function

Disorders of thyroid function are common in the elderly, frequently offering few clinical grounds for suspicion, so that some have advocated that tests of thyroid function should become routine. Hypofunction of insidious onset may be suspected less easily by the family doctor than by an unfamiliar physician. Furthermore, endocrinopathy may be confused with age changes such as loss of body hair, dry skin, and slow cerebration. Hypofunction may arise as an autoimmune phenomenon, or secondary to treatment for thyrotoxicosis or hypopituitarism. The well-known reduced speed of the ankle jerk in hypothyroidism, short of myxoedema, is difficult to observe in a class of patient in whom these tendon reflexes are frequently absent from other causes. The gland itself is difficult to palpate, and clinical impressions of nodularity in it misleading. In shrunken kyphotic females, it may come to occupy a retrosternal position.

Hypothyroidism

Hypofunction shows a female preponderance of at least four to one, and the increased vulnerability to hypothermia, liability to ischaemic heart disease, and occasional florid psychiatric manifestations are well known (see page 471).

Tests of thyroid function have become complicated in recent years, but the Free Thyroxine Index is probably the most useful test in old people, since it is unaffected by changes in plasma protein level, and exogenous sources of iodine are known to raise the protein bound iodine.

Replacement therapy should be introduced cautiously, beginning with 0.05 mg L-thyroxine daily, and increased by 0.05 mg every two weeks to a maximum of 0.2 mg daily.

Hyperthyroidism

Hyperthyroidism nearly always presents atypically in elderly patients, and while its clinical features may be mono-systemic, they are more likely to resemble the syndrome of 'failure to thrive' (if this useful paediatric term may be borrowed). Indeed, a picture is sometimes presented which suggests apathy and hypo-function, while weight loss, muscular wasting around the limb girdles, tachy-arrythmias, diarrhoea, confusional psychosis and accelerated osteoporosis may suggest 'senile deterioration'.

This is one of those conditions in which a high index of suspicion is needed, for it is more common among the elderly, and one of the most satisfactory of the treatable conditions in this age range (see page 472). Treatment is preferably with carbimazole, when an effect is noted in 3—4 weeks. During this time a beta-adrenergic blocking drug, such as practolol propranolol 40 mg t.d.s., is a useful adjuvant in the control of somatic symptoms, particularly of tremor and palpitation.

THE SKIN IN OLD AGE

While the elderly patient is subject to all the skin diseases found in the young, skin problems are modified by changes resulting from the cumulative effects of exposure and insult. Thinning, drying, wrinkling, and hair redistribution are well recognised changes that sometimes cause distress in certain individuals. Dermatoses in the elderly are more likely to occur on exposed skin surfaces, while the covered skin often differs little from that seen in youth.

In considering the complex dermatological problems in late life, the practitioner must note other pathologies, and their frequently plural therapies, the patient's emotional adjustment, previous dermatological problems, and occupational history. The ability to carry out a prescribed self-treatment may be limited by joint stiffness, poor vision, and mental change, while the ability to heal after trauma and infection may be reduced by circulatory and immunological deficiency.

Many skin disorders are preventable by the avoidance of physical agents, such as heat, cold drying wind, excessive use of soap and water, all of which may produce fine mosaic fissuring. The addition of suitable bath oils, or their inunction after bathing retains moisture in the skin. Regular washing and powdering beneath pendulous breasts will help to prevent fungal infection.

Generalised Pruritus

Generalised pruritus is one of the commonest and most baffling problems met with in this age group, when no rash, or signs of infestation are present. All that may be observed is a fine branny scaling. The widespread involvement suggests a systematic cause, such as neoplasia, reticulosis, blood dyscrasia, biliary disease, or chronic renal failure. Diabetes more usually presents as a local vulval or anal irritation, associated with fungal infection. Neurodermatitis, usually in the nuchal region, may recur during periods of stress. The principles of management are restriction of bathing, emollient bath additives, clothing which is light and non-frictional, avoidance of temperature changes, especially in winter, and the encouragement of mental occupation.

Pigmentary changes are often noted in older patients. The creamy hue in myxoedema, and the lemon tint in pernicious anaemia, may be diagnostic, although depigmentation is sometimes seen in the latter condition.

The aged skin is more likely to be the seat of malignant change. Precancerous lesions such as leukoplakia, and actinic keratoses (see page 451) should be referred immediately for biopsy. The good results of early treatment place on the family doctor the responsibility of detecting malignant lesions at an early stage. Any indurated lesion, showing rolled edges, and telangectasia that persists for three weeks or longer must be suspected. The commonest lesion is basal cell epithelioma. Cases in practice are found in sailors, farmers, winter sportsmen, and more recently in retired people returning home from villas on the 'Costa Geriatrica' in the Mediterranean sunbelt. Any lesion that grows, bleeds or shows darkening pigment, demands histologic diagnosis. The prognosis depends on the duration of the lesion, and its site, and is generally favourable, except for lesions situated on the pinna.

Pressure Sores

The patient confined to bed or chair for long periods is always in danger of developing pressure sores. Responsibility for their prevention cannot be delegated to nurses. The time honoured practice of buttock rubbing, or the traditional fear of wet beds, are quite unimportant considerations. A man may lie for weeks on his back and not develop a pressure sore until he is allowed to sit up. The most important preventive measure is reduction of pressure so that it does not remain maximal over a few bony points, and this is best achieved by nursing the bed-fast patient on a ripple mattress. Yet it must be admitted that some patients will develop pressures sores despite every precaution.

GENITO-URINARY FUNCTION

Interest becomes concentrated on genito-urinary function in elderly patients. Shame and fear accompany urinary disorders, personal dignity is eroded, and continued ability to live at home is constantly threatened by their emergence. Understandably, old people are slow to report such disorders, or accept them as part of the folklore of normal ageing. The smell of stale urine on the clothing should begin a direct line of enquiry, whatever else is invoked as a reason for consultation.

Bladder Function in the Elderly

The history should not omit simple matters such as the volume and type of drink taken, and the hour of its consumption. The diuretic action of beer and tea, often taken in the evening, should not be forgotten, nor the long-lasting action of the diuretic Chlorthalidone. Other drugs, particularly those with an anti-cholinergic effect, may cause retention. Incontinence may be due to faecal impaction, and a wet bed may indicate no more than slowness in moving from bed to toilet, or an inability to handle a urinal in bed. The volume of urine passed on each occasion is significant, for the frequent voiding of small amounts indicates lower tract irritation, while large volumes suggest the presence of uncontrolled diabetes, or chronic renal failure. In elderly patients with several pathologies bladder function is highly complex, being vulnerable to local anatomical changes and remote neuropathic influence.

Examination

It is important to palpate the bladder, and whenever possible to watch the act of micturition in the male patient. The enlarged bladder may be tense and easy to feel, imparting a fluid thrill and increasing the urge to micturate when pressed upon. When the wall has become atonic, as the result of chronic obstruction, its detection may depend entirely on alteration of the percussion note in the midline.

Careful examination of the external genitalia in the male may reveal hydrocele, phimosis, or testicular swellings in the male and signs of prolapse, urethral caruncle, and senile vaginitis in the female.

In both sexes, bimanual examination of the bladder and its adenae is helpful. Apart from identifying pelvic tumours in the female, it is possible in thin male subjects examined in the dorsal position to gain far more information regarding prostatic size and form, and occasionally an idea of residual urine in the retroprostatic pouch.

The Role of Infection

While chronic pyelonephritis may progress asymptomatically to uraemia, without detection of bacteria in the urine, a dilemma is created by the recognition that chronic bacteriuria in the elderly is usually a benign condition, related in many instances to residual urine. Treatment with antibiotics produces temporary results only, and prolonged use frequently causes skin eruptions and other side effects. Nocturnal and diurnal frequency must not be attributed to infection unless dysuria or precipitancy are also present. The significance of infection can be assessed by serial estimations of urine deposit, the blood pressure and blood urea, or serum creatinine. Straight radiography of the abdomen will generally reveal renal or bladder stone shadows.

The Management of Incontinence

While incontinence is common in geriatric hospital patients, it is rare in family practice. Such cases as do occur are usually of short duration, and referable to a cerebro-vascular accident or intercurrent infection. Relatives usually consider a wet bed an indication for hospital admission, so that an explanation of the temporary nature of the disorder by the family doctor is essential. These patients often recover well at home, while removal to hospital at this juncture may aggravate a confusional state.

Much of the dysuria and incontinence in very old people results from inability to inhibit spontaneous contractions of the bladder. Loss of control is presumed to result from frontal lobe, or spinal cord lesions, or simply from reduction of functional neurones associated with ageing. Patients may attempt to influence this condition by limiting their fluid intake to dangerously low levels.

No age barrier should be set for patients needing pelvic floor repair or prostatectomy. Although elderly men require encouragement during the post-operative weeks until control is regained, oestrogen treatment of senile vaginitis and prostatic carcinoma produces excellent results.

Before resort is made to protective clothing, incontinence pads, bags, catheters and drugs can be tried. It is always important to correct minor degrees of cardiac failure by giving a medium-acting diuretic, such as bendrofluazide 5 mg each morning. Emepromium bromide 100 mg two hours before retiring may be given for a few nights, or anticholinergic drugs, such as propantheline 15 or 30 mg combined with orphenadrine. Drugs should be withdrawn if real benefit has not resulted in a week.

Cases of acute retention, due to faecal impaction, or prostatic hyper-trophy, may be seen less often if regular geriatric health checks are carried out.

Chronic Renal Failure

Chronic renal failure is usually associated with vascular changes, and may occur in diabetes, despite good control. General deterioration, drowsiness and loss of weight occur, insidiously at first. The diagnosis is difficult in family practice, but a rising blood pressure, increasing blood nitrogen levels, and an inability to produce a concentrated early morning urine are confirmatory clinical findings. The first principle in treatment is to reduce or stop all drugs the patient may be taking. Protein intake should be reduced to about 50 g daily. Anabolic steroid by injection may be given, and sodium bicarbonate solution to prevent renal acidosis. Frusemide may be given in heroic doses where urine output is falling. Antibiotics, especially tetracycline, should be avoided in the management of chronic renal failure. Only when dysuria, foul smells, and significant bacteriuria are present, may it be permissible to give short courses of cephalexin at night.

MUSCULO-SKELETAL DISORDERS

Osteoporosis

This means usually an osteopoenia or loss of bone substance. The atrophy occurs as a result of advancing age, more in caucasians than negroes, more in the short than the tall, and particularly in females past the menopause. It is largely a symptomless condition, the significance of which lies in an increased liability to fracture. The aetiology of the condition is multiple, but factors which hasten it are the prolonged use of corticosteroids, prolonged immobility, hyper-thyroidism, malabsorption, especially after gastrectomy, presumably due to negative calcium balance.

The condition advances to produce loss in body height, kyphosis, and the appearance of a transverse skinfold across the upper abdomen. The role of the practitioner is to delay the appearance of this end picture by encouraging mobility, ensuring an adequate intake of calcium and vitamin D in the diet, by considering oestrogen replacement in the postmenopausal woman, and non-virilizing anabolic steroids in older age.

Osteomalacia

Although rare, this condition is more common among the elderly, particularly in the heavily clothed female recluse who never sees the light of day. Apart from simple intake deficiency, malabsorption may result from jejunal diverticulae, post-gastrectomy syndrome, gluten enteropathy, and the abuse of alcohol or liquid paraffin.

Diagnosis
Unlike osteoporosis, symptomatology is marked, the patient complaining of increasing limb weakness, and pains all over, especially around the rib cage,

usually with severe exacerbations. Deformities of the trunk eventually occur if treatment is not instituted.

Diagnosis is made by finding low serum calcium and phosphorus levels with a product below 27 mg per cent, and a raised serum alkaline phosphatase. Radiographic demonstration of pseudo-fractures in ribs, pubis, or humerus (Looser's zones), is pathognomonic. Diagnosis may be missed because many patients suffer from cerebral failure, and isolate themselves; or, being unable to localise their aches and pains, present to their doctors an unappealing picture of neurotic disgruntlement.

Treatment

This deficiency disease is eminently treatable by replacement therapy. Calciferol 0.1 mg is given daily for 2—3 months, together with calcium supplements.

Paget's Disease of Bone

The practitioner with an average-sized mixed practice can expect to have one diagnosed and two undiagnosed cases of Paget's disease. It is unlikely he will have made a direct diagnosis, but will have had it reported to him when X-raying a person for another condition.

Diagnosis

Paget's disease of bone develops from the 5th decade, and is more common in males. Since the usual presenting symptom is pain patients are frequently diagnosed as having osteoarthritis, and treated with simple analgesics. It is possible that the finding of local warmth and a raised alkaline phosphatase would raise the suspicion of a disease whose advance may be arrested by calcitonin. Paget's disease of bone develops asymmetrically, and never involves the entire skeleton. It may remain confined to one bone, and in its early stages decalcification and destruction of trabecular bone takes place in circumscribed areas, which may be thought to be a metastatic bone lesion. More widespread involvement, producing a picture of thickened cortical bone, which is soft despite its appearance, gives rise to the picture of classical deformity, at which stage one third of cases become diagnosed. Widespread involvement may produce complications. The outward growth of cortical bone in the skull not only produces the cotton wool appearance on X-ray, but may produce deafness and other CNS involvement through cranial nerve compression. The highly vascular bone may act as an arteriovenous shunt causing high output cardiac failure. Secondary osteoarthritic changes arise from malalignment of weight bearing joint surfaces. The development of an effective therapy makes early diagnosis important, but initial treatment and dose stabilization should be conducted in hospital.

Persistent bone pain, particularly in the lower spine must always be investigated, because of the high incidence of metastasizing carcinoma in older subjects, and the occasional finding of multiple myeloma.

RHEUMATIC DISORDERS

The elderly seem to be more sensitive receptors of arthritic pain than other age groups, and more inclined to accept it as their lot in life. Yet, so great is the threat to social capacity posed by this group of disorders, that the practitioner must assist the patient to retain mobility by every means.

It is important to think of joints and muscles as a functional entity. Divided attention may adversely affect the other component of integrated movement, as for instance where prolonged bed rest of an inflamed knee joint results in muscle shortening and flexion deformity. Consideration of the patient's life style is valuable, as is increasing his understanding of his disease, about which many misconceptions abound. Patients may be advised against:

1. Persisting in heavy occupation;
2. Stoically working on through pain;
3. Attributing fluctuating symptoms to the weather, or 'acid';
4. Preferring patent to orthodox medical treatment;
5. Raising the whole body weight on the flexed finger joints rather than the palm;
6. Resting in beds and chairs that offer no skeletal support.

Assessment

The fact that osteoarthritis or 'osteoarthrosis' has a large female preponderance, and is diagnosed by clinical observation without any laboratory tests to confirm it, may lead to an approach to rheumatic problems which is too superficial. The practitioner must often assess disability which is the result of several pathologies. Erosion may be present within a joint, as well as extra-articular deposits of calcium salts. All elderly patients can be assumed to have some degenerative joint change, though not all complain of pain. Elderly obese females with apparent osteoarthrosis of the knees are not infrequently discovered to have a raised ESR, and to become mobile on small doses of corticosteroid. Both gout and rheumatoid disease are encountered more frequently with advancing age. The ESR is raised in most patients with rheumatoid disease, alpha-globulins are increased, and C-reactive protein is positive almost as frequently. Anaemia is present in proportion to the activity of the disease.

Management

Treatment of elderly arthritics often requires antidepressant drugs. Physiotherapy, to be effective in this age-group, should be daily and intensive, and therefore admission to the wards or daily day hospital attendance is justifiable.

The effectiveness of surgical intervention has produced a more optimistic outlook in the management of arthritis. Synovectomy, reconstructive surgery to the hands, tibial plateau prosthesis, and low friction arthroplasty, or total hip replacement, are highly effective operations on patients with sufficiently good general health and social expectation to be successfully rehabilitated. It is the practitioner who must select patients in this category for surgical consultation.

Polymyalgia Rheumatica

Brief, but special, mention must be made of this syndrome, which occurs almost exclusively over the age of 60. Patients complain of pain and stiffness, which radiates symmetrically in the neck and shoulder girdles, and, less frequently, around the pelvic girdle, and sometimes into the limbs. Symptoms are most pronounced in the early hours of the morning, when they may be severe enough to prevent turning in the bed. By mid-day, the patient is often symptom free, so that a case has been reported of a doctor revisiting a patient at that time because he obtained no reply on an earlier visit, and discharging her from his list in the belief that she was abusing his services.

It is usual to find some general systemic disturbance and weight loss, and the ESR is usually markedly raised. Since in a proportion of cases, associated giant cell arteritis involves the temporal artery, treatment should begin at once with cortico-steroids, to which response is immediate and dramatic. A reasonable dose is prednisolone 5 mg three times a day, which should be reduced after a week to 10 mg daily. After a month a maintenance dose of 7−8 mg is usually achieved. Treatment should be continued for some 2 years, with 6 monthly reduction of dosage which may be effectively lowered to 2.5 mg at night.

Muscle Disorders

Old people who have continued in good health and active occupation, usually retain much of their muscular strength. Where significant muscular weakness occurs, disuse, reduced hormone levels, and loss of anterior horn cells may be responsible. Conditions leading to hypoxia, or potassium deficiency, may be responsible, while other common factors are endocrine disorders, nutritional deficiencies, neoplasia, or prolonged steroid therapy.

Nocturnal cramps are a common cause of sleep disturbance. The most satisfactory treatments are quinine sulphate 300 mg nightly, Paroven 2 tablets twice daily, or tablets of effervescent calcium taken before retiring.

CLINICAL PSYCHIATRY IN THE ELDERLY

Intellectual Decline

It is a strange fact that, if asked to write down the number of elderly demented patients in his practice, the average family doctor will call to mind very few. The consultant psychiatrist, on the other hand, will complain that the number of old people with structural brain changes is stretching the capacity of his staff to the utmost.

Nothing is more likely to engender pessimism than the mechanistic theories of neuronal 'fall out' to explain defective mental function in old age. Fortunately, experimental studies of the effects of sensory deprivation have shown that certain aspects of senile mental functioning can be quite easily induced in the young also. Behavioural characteristics commonly perceived as signs of old age are indicators of social maladjustment, and not specific to the late years of life. Unusual nervousness, irritability, depression, unaccountable anger, personality change, apathy or withdrawal are considered clear indications for psychotherapy in the young. In the elderly person they are frequently considered to be part of the course of old age.

Tests of intellectual function must take the patient's situation into account. The pressures on the young to learn are persistent, and highly organised. When tested, therefore, children love to shine: the old may feel only a fear that they may fail.

Memory disorder is usually a disorder of learning, and registering information. A distinction between faulty learning due to adverse factors at the time, and the type of memory loss in which the slate is, as it were, wiped clean by organic disease, must be distinguished.

Assessment

Mental assessment is a highly skilled technique, and the tester should be fully acquainted with the patient's past educational status, his present state of health, motivation, and habitual social environment. This is vouchsafed to few besides the family practitioner who must yet not invade the field of the clinical psychologist.

Mental Status Questionnaire   This is a simple and quick assessment, which is acceptable to the patient. If care is taken to allow for degrees of deafness, it will at one point in time disclose and roughly measure intellectual impairment, but the application of such questionnaires and reliance on their scores are not simple matters. It is an advantage that the patient is led into the test situation by items which arise naturally as collection and identification data. The questions are:

1. What town is this?
2. In which month were you born?

3. What is this place?
4. What is your age?
5. What month is it now?
6. In what year were you born?
7. What is the name of the present Prime Minister?
8. What year is it?
9. What is to-day's date?
10. Who was the previous Prime Minister?

The Set Test This is another simple test where the patient is asked to recall items in four different common categories. He should be led into the test as a challenge, with an invitation such as 'Let us see how good your memory is' and then asked to name as many colours, towns, fruits, birds, flowers, or articles as he can that can be purchased in a certain shop. Although occasional retrieval may be encouraged by the subject's educational and cultural background, this provides a useful short test, in which speed of retrieval, as well as the number of items recalled, is significant. The test can be regarded as complete when the subject has offered ten different items, or has stopped short of this number, making a maximal score of 40.

These tests are useful in detecting cerebral failure in patients who fail to reveal it by the retention of verbal fluency, which can mislead. The clinician must not in turn be misled into coming to firm conclusions regarding the patient's performance, which, when faulty is an indication for further investigation.

Memory Disorder

Dysmnesia, almost universal over the age of 60, progresses slowly in senescence, often in a setting of relatively good preservation of the other higher cerebral functions. Its presence should be regarded as the presenting symptom which should lead to assessment of other higher cerebral functions, such as language function, praxis and gnosia, and abstract thought. Psychological testing shows a different pattern between normal ageing, and dementing disease, which carries a poor prognosis.

Confronted with a patient with memory disorder, the practitioner should first exclude aphasia, agnosia, and apraxia. Then he should seek to discover whether the memory loss is old or new, partial or total. Finally, he should seek neurological signs which may indicate Korsakoff's psychosis, general paresis of the insane (GPI), subdural haematoma, ventricular dilatation, or frontal tumour.

Cerebral Failure

Geriatric medical practice is dominated by mental breakdown, and to a lesser extent, urinary disorders. While old people with poor vision, locomotor disorders, and chronic heart failure can often manage their domestic life, mental status is the dominant consideration in the decision whether an old person may continue to live at home.

The family doctor will know that what was formerly put down to 'senility' is more often the result of some specific disease that may occur also in earlier life, and the occurrence of mental symptoms in an elderly person need not appear therapeutically unpromising.

Chronic cerebral failure is very common in elderly people living at home as revealed by psychometric testing. These people constitute a huge reservoir of potential problems, but none arise so long as they are supported in their cultural environment, or environmental demands are reduced to manageable proportions. In these individuals cerebral failure is compensated.

Decompensated cases present as social problems. Those living at home alone cease to be responsible for fuel and power devices, while those living in a family setting may cause distress by their deviant behaviour.

Chronic cerebral failure may be further complicated by extra-cerebral disease, such as thyroid disorder, electrolyte imbalance, nutritional pseudo-dementia (e.g., Korsakoff's syndrome and pernicious anaemia), subdural haematoma, or insulin hypoglycaemia.

The reintegration of many elderly patients with symptoms of mental failure is therefore well within the competence of the family physician. Vulnerable old people may be identified by the following indices:

1. Advanced age.
2. Poor physical health.
3. Impaired special senses.
4. Reduced mobility and capacity for self-care.
5. Pre-morbid personality — moody, anxious, hypochondriacal.
6. History of mental illness in patient or relative.
7. Low sociability and limited range of interests in the past.
8. Few or decreasing social contacts.

Social Variables and Loneliness

It must be recognised that in a rapidly changing society isolation is not always harmful, nor indeed a sign of personality deviation. There always exist lifelong isolates for whom living alone represents a way of life, and a necessary condition making for stability. One must be able to discern, however, in the complaints of loneliness the symptoms of lifelong personality traits that have led to maladjustment in old age. Here the need is not the provision of more social contacts, but to be concerned with the feelings of neglect and their underlying causes. It is unwise to see these situations as simple moral issues, for old people are rarely neglected by their children if their role was that of a true parent.

Experiments in sensory deprivation have shown the need for continual confrontation with reality, and in particular for conversation which enables differentiation to be made between intrinsic and extrinsic stimuli when verbalizing the sensory input. Like lone sailors, widows hallucinate, because of the projection of inner feelings into a fantasy reality, a not uncommon or unpleasant late aspect of bereavement. More commonly, depression and hypochondriacal delusions are the reactions to the painful perception of inner disorganization as morbid feeling is introjected. Less commonly, but often associated with the sensory deprivation from hearing loss, senile paranoia, with emotion externalised and thrust at the environment, results in feelings of imagined persecution by others.

Sleep-Awake Rhythms

Bad sleep and unrest during the night are early signs of age disturbance, and the ability to influence the sleep pattern is of great importance in management. While sedatives may stimulate, it is paradoxical that small doses of amphetamine or methylphenidate can have a calming effect in the aged patient with reversed sleep rhythm.

Regressive Behaviour

Extreme reactions to a feeling of inadequacy in the face of abnormal stress may cause regressive behaviour, especially in old people. Hoarding compulsions as security-seeking strategies, incoherence as an expression of doubt about self-assertive ability, and senile autism, with food refusal, and intolerance of any form of intervention from outside, are common patterns of behaviour regression. They are often quickly reversed when social support is provided.

Psycho-somatic Illness

In old age so many somatic and social equilibria are broken that it is difficult to identify a dominant cause of the growing feeling of uncertainty, insecurity and failing homeostasis. The complaint of dizziness is probably one of the most unwelcomed by physicians, and one is inclined at first to think in terms of vestibular pathology. But it is important to understand that old people develop a fear of their unsupported vertical stance once proprioceptive mechanisms begin to fail, and many of the vague complaints of 'dizziness' need more than advice against sudden postural changes, and the provision of walking aids. The vogue for prescribing vasodilators is of dubious value. The action of such agents is likely to be exerted on tissues remote from physiological need, and is markedly inferior to substances produced naturally in response to regional ischaemia. These patients do in fact require total assessment, leading to an enhanced sense of security based on improved function, or environmental support.

Emotional Disturbance

Emotional disturbance, both as prime cause, and as a complicating factor in many conditions, occupies a dominant place in medicine, regardless of age. In the elderly in particular emotional changes possess the ability to influence the intensity with which a belief about the environment is held. Depression, which may be obvious in some, is more protean and difficult to recognise in late life, when diminution of spontaneity, increased caution and resistance to change are normal patterns of adaptation. Nevertheless, among the mental disorders of the elderly, depressive illness is of importance second only to the dementias, from which it may be dissociated only with extreme difficulty. A significant percentage of admissions to geriatric units for ostensibly physical conditions also testify to depression as the great mimic, since the sources of emotional energy are undirected. Nevertheless, for a favourable outcome, early diagnosis is vital, before physical deterioration and social breakdown ensue. Symptoms, such as diminishing energy and enjoyment, loss of interests and ability, and poor concentration, are useful diagnostic pointers, as well as impairment of sleep and appetite. But the practitioner must not fail to recognize the frequently expressed hypochondriacal fears, and morbid preoccupations with bodily functions, especially of the bowel, as manifestations of introjected emotion. Clearly it is often wiser in many instances to postpone the panoply of investigations until after a therapeutic trial with an antidepressant drug.

Personality Disorders

While a high proportion of aggressive patients become better adjusted with age, inadequate personalities fail to do so, and drift downwards in the social scale as advancing age imposes its challenges. Alcoholism in elderly patients is usually the result of a life-long drinking problem, but occasionally in the circumstances of bereavement, or chronic ill health, the abuse of alcohol as a sedative or analgesic may lead to dependency, with consequent damage to the central nervous system and subnutrition.

Sexual deviations, however, while uncommon, occur in ageing males who were usually previously well adjusted in marriage, and result more from the effect of increasing impotence, than as the result of organic brain changes. Whereas depression is most responsive to treatment, the elderly neurotic has a long history of intractable illness refractory to drugs. Reassurance that the doctor realises the patient is ill, investigation of physical complaints sufficient to reassure medical opinion, and the prescription of a placebo to bring the interview to its expected conclusion are all that is usually required. The appearance of psychoneurosis *de novo* in the elderly patient must arouse a suspicion of organic disease as the cause.

Confusional States

Mental confusion, usually encountered in family practice as a toxic confusional state of sudden onset, is one of the most challenging problems of geriatric medicine. The patient has a disordered awareness of the surroundings fluctuating with his level of consciousness and the complexity of his environment. Delusions or erroneous percepts, which appear as reality to the patient, may be an accompaniment of a confusional state more readily where dementia is present, but may also be manifestations of depressive or paranoid states. Common conditions to look for are acute infections, cardio-respiratory disease, falling haemoglobin, dehydration, and urinary or faecal retention. Drug therapy should be reviewed, and intoxication by digitialis, barbiturates, sulphonamides, hyoscine and steroids ruled out.

There is a skill in handling both the patient and the anxious relatives (see Chapter 22, page 513). It is important not to deny to the patient the reality of his percepts, but to gain his confidence by recognizing the menace they may pose to him. Thus the old lady hanging out of the window calling in naughty children at two in the morning may be comforted by the one person who ceases telling her 'not to be silly', but who says rather 'This is most distressing for you. Please allow me to go down, and bring them in. Meanwhile, you sit down and rest.'

The toxic agent must be eliminated. If drugs have to be used, 20 mg diazepam may be given intravenously in an emergency, or a phenothiazine given early in the evening to avoid drowsiness next day.

The Role of the Psychiatrist

It is impossible to overrate the importance of domiciliary assessment of problems before admission to hospital. The current trend of thinking is towards removing the care of the elderly from the ambit of psychiatric hospitals except for the short-term treatment of affective disorders. Home visiting by psychiatric social workers, boarding out schemes, hostels for the mentally frail, and psychiatric day hospitals are alternatives provided in some areas, but at present involve small numbers.

The Maintenance of Mental Health

The family practice team can do much to prevent mental breakdown in the elderly by:—

1. encouraging the maintenance of a high state of physical health;
2. encouraging the prevention of mental stagnation by attendance at clubs, outings, holidays and workrooms;
3. providing pre-retirement courses and acclimatization advice;
4. helping those with inadequate incomes to claim allowances.

MANAGEMENT

Selecting the Environment

It is generally agreed policy to strive to keep elderly people independent, and in their own homes. In fact in the UK such 'independence' consists of highly complex social buttressing, with mobile meals, and the provision of various services. It is, furthermore, very rare for the milieu of the home to be suitable for an old person's needs, other than on a basis of sentimental attachment. Much reluctance to move from cold, damp, insanitary rooms is in fact due either to inertia, or the fear of something worse, not infrequently encouraged by unsympathetic handling. Old people should not be persuaded to move from their homes without an opportunity to visit the alternative accommodation first.

Very often the suitability of the home is assessed by a social worker or an experienced health visitor. The assessment should include not only the siting of the house in relation to shops and other amenities, but also the internal comfort and safety, the facilities available, and the family and neighbours as a medical resource. It is useful to have a check-list (Table 24.1) of the various points to be noted in such an assessment.

The profile of the patient presented, following the completion of such a report, will in almost every case expose deficiencies in health status, or of the social needs of the individual assessed. In the majority of cases, medical examination by the practitioner will reveal opportunities for effective therapy, or for discarding treatments that have outlived their effectiveness. At the same time, simple modifications to the home may be recommended, such as hand rails and bath seats, which can enable the patient to regain self-reliance.

Of the supportive services in the UK, the Home Help service is the most important. Yet, because of the need to recruit to it people of high quality, it is always stretched tight, and in many areas is deficient. Unfortunately, as a result of deficient help from within the neighbourhood, many old people are sent to hospital on purely social grounds. To prevent this, the concept of shared care has

Table 24.1　Check list of points to be noted in assessment of the suitability of the home.

Identification Data
　　　Name, date of birth, marital status.
　　　Address, date of interview.
　　　Family Doctor, Health Visitor.
　　　Spouse: alive/dead, next of kin, principal helper.
　　　Living alone/household composition.
　　　Occupation: present/previous.
Social Dimension
　　　Family/neighbours/friends.
　　　Church, clubs, day centre, workshop.
　　　Financial: pension state/other, supplementary, other income.
Housing
　　　Site, type, number of rooms.
　　　Heating: living room/bedroom, cooking facilities.
　　　Bath, WC inside.
　　　Reasons for rehousing: medical/faulty/dangerous.
Self Care and Domestic Care
　　　Feeding, washing, dressing, use of WC, shaving, hair care.
　　　Cooking, housework, laundry, shopping.
　　　Able to pick object from the floor.
　　　Fully mobile/dependent/disabled.
Known Diagnoses
Drugs Taken
　　　Recognition, ability to repeat dosage.
　　　Ability to read prescribed instruction.
Services Provided
　　　Social Worker, Health Visitor, District Nurse.
　　　Home Help, Meals-on-Wheels, voluntary help.
Physical Condition
　　　Feet, eyesight, hearing, teeth, nutrition.
　　　Appearance: pallor/obesity/emaciated/pulse rate, rhythm/breathlessness oedema/
　　　　　anxiety/depression/walking/balance.

been developed in some areas of the UK. The Day Hospital has been one of the most successful ventures, providing many nursing needs and opportunities for rehabilitation. The day hospital for the elderly is the logical evolution of the geriatric hospital to provide a bridge with the community. Those patients likely to benefit are those who have suffered cerebro-vascular accidents, arthritis, recent fractures, and amputees. There is also a case for offering rehabilitation to certain patients recovering from depressive illness, in whom physical deterioration has resulted from inertia and subnutrition. It is important in referring patients that the practitioner should be able to set out clearly and fully the patient's medical status, and also to indicate the specific reason for the referral. Medical investigations, such as ECG, haematology and diagnostic cardiology can be carried out on one instead of several visits, and functional assessment for physiotherapy can be made in the best surroundings. One of the chief gains felt in the community is of course the relief and support afforded to relatives who can look forward to one or two days in the week when they are freed from their responsibilities. This is frequently all that is needed to enable the relatives to maintain the patient at home. There are other schemes that allow of this, such as the half-way homes, and 5-day ward schemes. It is important that the hospital day centre should not be looked to for the relief of loneliness, since this is not the main concern of trained personnel.

The practitioner will encounter a small group of patients who require full medical assessment rather urgently on account of physical deterioration, disturbances of function, diffuse or localised pains, or disordered cerebration, where full diagnostic facilities are urgently required. It is this class of patient, where several contributory pathologies are present, that admission to the Geriatric Assessment Unit of a hospital should be sought. With so many alternatives, blind referral to a consultant colleague with a request to take over does not flatter with its implication of faith, nor is it very satisfactory for the family doctor to labour in his vineyard too long, and at a certain point cast his patient into a sort of limbo. The timing and direction of the referral procedure, particularly in respect of elderly patients, is a skill of cardinal importance among the arts of family practice. It can only be exercised if the practitioner has familiarised himself with the facilities available, and how these may be matched to the patient's needs.

ABDOMINAL SURGERY IN THE AGED

The ability to distinguish between chronological and anatomical age acquires particular importance in the field of surgery, and the art may be practised by the examples that may be observed at all college reunions. In the past the barriers commonly thought to be imposed by old age prevented the elderly from the benefit capable of being conferred by operative techniques. Surgically correctible lesions were allowed to progress to an irreversible stage. Recent years have witnessed improvement in all aspects of pre-operative and post-operative care, surgical skills, anaesthetic agents, and rehabilitation units. Although surgery carried out beyond the eighth decade is still often hazardous, of greater importance is the general health of the patient. So far as risk is concerned, emergency procedures carry more than twice the risk of elective procedures. There is therefore every reason to avoid delaying referral of patients for surgery, and there is now an increasing proportion of elderly and unfit patients among the general surgeon's case work. Since the surgeon rarely sees a patient without reference from the family practitioner the quality of family practice will have a decisive bearing on the consultant's work. Delay will, in most cases, only enhance the surgical risks of spreading infection, and obstruction to various systems. However, procrastination may be understandable due to the difficulty of differential diagnosis, and where difficulty in describing symptoms, lowered pain threshold, and diminished muscle spasm distort the clinical picture.

Strangulated Hernia

The most common abdominal emergency in family practice is a strangulated hernia. This dangerous emergency would be greatly reduced if earlier referral were the rule, especially when inguinal and femoral herniae are accompanied by persistent pain or discomfort, recurrent incarceration, and the truss habit. Surgeons will show little hesitancy to proceed with surgical repair, which can be carried out under local anaesthesia, the use of non-absorbable sutures, and followed by early ambulation. When the patient can be persuaded to accept orchidectomy, hernorrhaphy with a rectus sheath graft does not lead to recurrence.

Gallstones

The largest percentage of gallstones occurs in the 6th and 7th decades, and the well-known female preponderance is reversed in late life, and they are then more common in men. Stones *per se* are not a danger, and the occurrence of acute cholecystitis may be regarded as an urgency, rather than an emergency. Cholecystectomy is only carried out if the surgeon can demonstrate the biliary structures in a good risk patient, so that the operation most usually performed is cholecystotomy. If the obstructing agent can be removed with removal of the fundus, recurrence is unlikely. A large barrel-shaped cholesterol stone may lie for many years in the gall-bladder, and erode through into the duodenum, performing an auto-cholecysto-duodenal fistula. Since the small bowel narrows distally, the stone passes along it, and impacts or obstructs in the region of the terminal ileum. The patient is usually a female, between the ages of 65 and 75, showing signs of small bowel obstruction, with vomiting, but no abdominal scar to suggest the more common cause of post-operative adhesions.

Obstruction of the Large Bowel

Obstruction of the large bowel, on the other hand, rarely causes vomiting, except perhaps as a terminal phenomenon. Tumours of the right side rarely obstruct, and grow to a large size, due to the large lumen, and fluid contents of the ascending colon. Such patients present with profound anaemia and weight loss. On the other hand, obstruction occurs earlier when the left colon is the site of a tumour.

Abdominal Pain

Pain in the left iliac fossa is usually attributable to diverticular disease, yet occasionally, a redundant sigmoid can permit an inflamed diverticulum to reach over to the right, and confuse the clinical picture of acute appendicitis. Appendicitis, however, is not rare in the aged, but carries with it a higher rate of perforation.

Pancreatitis must be considered in the differential diagnosis of abdominal pain. There are two broad aetiologies, the gall bladder type, which carries a benign prognosis, and is easily treated by gall bladder removal. Those with an alcoholic aetiology (pancreatic cirrhosis), carry a less favourable outlook. The diagnosis of acute pancreatitis may be suspected if there is a raised serum bilirubin combined with hypocalcaemia. Clinical jaundice may not be present, especially when the hyperbilirubinaemia is moderate.

Volvulus

The practitioner must bear in mind the increasing likelihood of thrombotic and embolic phenomena affecting branches of the coeliac axis, the superior and inferior mesenteric arteries. Elderly men are prone to develop volvulus, and present with extreme abdominal distension, hiccup and flatulence. The distension is mainly left-sided, but vomiting is not present until a late stage is reached. They should be admitted early before circulatory changes develop in the affected viscus.

The entire field of acute abdominal diagnosis is rendered difficult in the elderly by the frequent role played by constipation, and the increasing use of prostheses for aneurysm of the abdominal aorta which may eventually erode, adding a fresh cause to the differential diagnosis of upper gastro-intestinal bleeding.

25

Care of the Chronic Sick and Vulnerable

E. Wilkes

THE ECCENTRIC PATIENT

In family practice one is perpetually meeting diseases and syndromes never described in the standard textbooks. Some of these patients may be suffering from highly individual personality disorders, they may be eccentrics or recluses, sometimes – but by no means always – of low intelligence, and they can be a major socio-medical problem much more popular, for example, with the local rats than with the neighbours. These people are more than ever unacceptable in our hurried and crowded communities and despite the pressures on his time the general medical practitioner must somehow maintain a relationship, no matter how intermittently, with these difficult or deviant social isolates.

These patients may have had reasonably normal patterns of behaviour until middle life. As one ages one tends to become more the person one always was, so the careful become miserly and the unfriendly become frankly hostile. Similarly these eccentrics become more so and alienate their neighbours, their relatives, the local ministers and the local doctors. Often enough the more they need the doctor, the more they will manipulate him into rejecting them. If they ever leave their homes they do not keep their appointments; if they do not leave their homes they will not necessarily let the doctor in, even if they have been reported unwell.

Other patients use the doctor to provide the only meaningful personal relationship they have left. One patient gave herself several hundred abscesses over the years to ensure repeated visiting by a local practitioner, but when he left the practice the abscesses ceased.

They may also produce unusual attitudes to their own disability. An elderly man told to rest up for a week or two after a mild coronary episode was bed-fast for months with anxiety. When he had a similar episode a year or two later he was told to stay out of bed but not to fetch the coal in. On this occasion he was mobilised more appropriately after only three or four weeks. A more flagrant example of this exaggerated response was that of a lady who was advised late in her pregnancy to rest up in bed because of her mild pre-eclamptic toxaemia. Many years later she was still refusing to leave her bed save for minimal toilet purposes. The doctor who had given her the original advice tried hard to mobilise her again. Her spurious invalidism continued for years, acting as a protective mechanism against her family duties and her husband's sexual demands. Many visitors made a pilgrimage to her bedside and praised her for the courage and fortitude with which she bore her long-standing disability. When a new practitioner took over her case he asked both husband and wife if they wished her to have in-patient treatment in an attempt to mobilise and rehabilitate her. Both had adjusted well and they firmly, and indeed indignantly, rejected any suggested change. For these sort of people the family practitioner must keep his channels open and must, albeit realistically and without any illusions, have some respect for the adjustment attained by these patients, however psychopathic or sociopathic this may be at times.

THE NERVOUS PATIENT

A far commoner category of patients who need a special and durable relationship with their doctor are those who are emotionally vulnerable although hardly ever frankly disturbed. These people are usually women, often with a family history of nervous disability, and who may be either under excessive stress with young children or the even greater stress of no longer having a vital role to play in their early middle age. Their children have grown up, and the husband's working and social life permits him almost unconsciously to neglect the supportive role of earlier years. It is typically these patients who come repeatedly to their doctor with headache and with backache, with muzziness and anorexia, with a feeling of weakness and a lack of zest for life which may be an early depressive psychosis but is far more frequently a lack of respect for their own life-style. They no longer need to be imprisoned in the routine of housework but they have no other existing responsibilities to take its place. Their children may be independent, unattractive, rebellious, or demanding. The garden is too big, their husbands are inattentive, the old world has atrophied and nothing has replaced it. Over the years they have tried to cope with these routine burdens and have succeeded in doing so but at a greater than average effort. These are the patients who especially need the re-assurance of their doctor and counselling towards a new pattern of behaviour.

These are also typically the patients for whom tranquillisers on a massive scale are being prescribed. It is the role of the doctor to aid in any way he can their tolerant awareness of their own limitations. The tranquillisers and the anti-depressives may help with the more acute phases but the only possible cure lies in the emotional adjustment of the patient to her real situation; in this adjustment repetitively and unspectacularly the family practitioner has a vital role to play.

A knowledge of the family history, and of the tantrums of preceding generations can be a tremendous help here, as can the recall of adolescent stresses. This area of practice is perhaps more menaced and threatened than any other by the depersonalisation of primary medical care consequent on a high through-put appointments-system approach.

The sheer size of this problem in family practice is indicated by the results of many surveys. Taylor and Chave[1] found that in every 1000 patients 1.9 were psychiatric in-patients, 4.4 were psychiatric out-patients, 81 needed treatment from the family practitioner and a further 330 had symptoms with a major neurotic component. Certainly most practices would include a figure of between 15 and 35 per cent of all their consultations as containing some component of psychiatric need. It is chastening to see that in one survey[2] it was thought that the family practitioner missed a psychiatric diagnosis in 20 per cent of men and 25 per cent of women. The majority of these psychiatric cases however are not the traditional material for referral. They are people who need help in a more simple, basic, and friendly way. It may be possible for the family practitioner to find some local facility, a voluntary group, a health visitor, or a social worker, to undertake this supportive role for him. Local lay counselling services seem to be increasing and although variable in their quality may be a most helpful adjunct to the traditional resources.

Sometimes such patients are not necessarily very demanding and yet still are doctor-dependent and will resist any attempt to replace him.

THE CHRONICALLY DISEASED OR DISABLED PATIENT

A third category of chronic and vulnerable patients are those suffering from major life-dominating but chronic disease processes. In the young the commonest reasons for this predicament are accidents and multiple sclerosis. Among older age groups severe chronic bronchitis, rheumatoid arthritis, or strokes tend to hold the field. Ischaemic heart disease, despite its prime importance as a cause of death, is not necessarily associated with very many dreary years of disability, although it can last over many decades. One patient died in congestive cardiac failure after a history of angina that had apparently been authenticated over the preceding 40 years.

Certainly chronic diseases and their social implications are now a major factor in the inability of the health-care system to cope with the demands being imposed on it. We must pay greater attention to the many years of disability which we can palliate but not cure.

Multiple Sclerosis

The detailed management of multiple sclerosis is dealt with elsewhere but it needs perhaps to be said yet again that the loneliness and deprivation of the case of multiple sclerosis and the economic as well as intellectual deterioration which usually accompanies the progressive physical handicap are among the most disturbing and burdensome of community-based problems. Admission of such cases to hospital may, for some acute episode, be strongly indicated, but normally the transfer of such cases to hospitals is a prelude to further deterioration. The quality of nursing care in an acute unit is not always geared to the vulnerable pressure areas of the paraplegic. The intense mobilisation of such patients necessary after an acute abdominal emergency may be beyond the routine capacity of hard-pressed staff operating well below their full establishment. The chronic sick wards may be far from home and make visiting a tedious and laborious chore. Isolation from the family as the unit of care will accelerate and enhance deprivation and loneliness. The medical profession has tended to be more interested in the detailed investigations of these patients and these are of course important: we must however also look at the general quality of life of these patients and see how we can help improve that.

Day centres for the chronic sick, social gatherings bringing together varied kinds of disability, holidays for handicapped patients, occupational therapy, or sheltered employment for those more able to control their limbs, these are rarely suggested to those who regularly but infrequently attend neurological out-patient departments. They must therefore be part of the spectrum of care of the family practitioner. He must be interested in the social life of these patients, encouraging them, and also the spouse, to have stimulus, change, meaningful occupation. For this they may need various aids or gadgets, alterations to the house in the way of downstairs lavatories, hand-rails, or ramps. The Housing Department will do what they can, and the Social Services Department also. But all the members of the primary health care team must know about these patients in the practice and be involved in their various ways in improving the quality of life, both for the patient and for the family. We have learned from the handicapped children that they so often are part of a handicapped family. The situation is just the same for the multiple sclerosis patient, and the family needs help as well as the patient.

Rheumatoid Patients

The restricted life of the rheumatoid patient is another common problem and one is repeatedly impressed — and depressed — by the severity of the contractures obtained only after decades of kind and good-natured neglect. These patients, too, need high quality supervision and need to be considered for the more novel aspects of treatments now available for them. We do not claim that every family practitioner should be qualified to produce splints for these patients or to consider their suitability for penicillamine or immuno-suppressive regimes. What we must do in family practice however is to assess the degree of pain and disability and if this is gradually eroding the morale of the patient and the family, a short-term admission to a rheumatology unit may well prove of tremendous benefit to everyone concerned, even though more dramatic intervention is not found necessary. A rest and a change, or alterations in the analgesic regime can be just as helpful in many patients as synovectomy or potent drugs.

Awareness of Deterioration

In a stable practice population, the doctor is tempted to adjust and accept the disability of his chronic patients without realising that gradually and subtly over the years they have deteriorated to a state where intervention is now necessary. We may be proud of our unique capacity to maintain continuity of patient care. In fact this very continuity of patient-care has its own traps and pitfalls. One can live with patients whose myxoedema or thyrotoxicosis is apparent at a glance to the most callow and inexperienced registrar and yet, because they have 'always been like that' one can in family practice fail to recognise the syndrome because they are so much a long-term and accepted part of ones patient.

This is even more likely to happen in patients where the diagnosis is quite apparent and has been obvious for many years. It may even be worth asking such chronic rheumatic patients to fill in each six or twelve months a short questionnaire about their capacity to cope with the activities of daily living: how do they manage the stairs, dressing, toilet, cooking, or shopping; how do they sleep; how depressed do they get; how many friends do they see; how often have they got out for some social purpose?

It is common for such patients to smoke too much and to eat too much and obesity can further complicate and exacerbate any and every chronic disability. Prevention is easier than cure, but a major part of prevention will be to give them some company and some pastime still within their physical and mental capacity. The family practitioner must have as much interest in all such local clubs and organisations as in the pre-school play-groups so important for the mental health of the young mothers and the stimulation of their young children.

Strokes

Strokes have perhaps been neglected by the medical profession. We have relied too much on our reasonably justifiable hope that such patients will either die or get better, and indeed this is generally true. There is a tremendous wastage in the two or three months following a major cerebro-vascular accident and most of those who are totally dependent will be dead in a month or two. Many, especially among the more minor attacks, will be able to fight their way back, if not to total, at any rate to a reasonable, state of independence. We are left, therefore, with a small minority who neither die nor get better and who are a tremendous burden either on the geriatric services or on the families attempting to support them. We in family practice must guard against leaving attempts to rehabilitate our strokes too late. If in fact the patient proves unrehabilitatable, here too is an area of activity appropriate to primary medical care. Such stimulus as can be relevant to the patient – physiotherapy, occupational therapy, or a visit to the local day centre, should be organised. Local nursing services must be called in and the morale of the caring relative must be maintained and safe-guarded by the organisation of holidays, preferably for a fortnight at a time and two or three times a year, through temporary admission of the patient to geriatric or community hospital facilities or by temporary transfer to another suitable relative if such exist.

PROVIDERS OF CARE IN THE COMMUNITY

The isolation of families with a chronically ill member is one of the problems that needs to come under the scrutiny of the family practitioner. In Britain there are three main headquarters from which help can be obtained: the Health Service, the Social Services Department and various voluntary organisations.

The Health Service

The Health Service provides district nurses, day hospitals, physiotherapists and occupational therapists, and consultant colleagues with their special areas of expertise.

The Social Services Department

The Social Services provide a home help service, old people's accommodation, special housing and has the ability to instal into the patient's home the ramps, handrails or other aids helpful in the maintenance of a reasonable quality of independent life. The ability of the social worker to deliver a case-work type of help and support is, of course, possible only on rare occasions, because resources are so scarce that they tend still to be deployed on a crisis-intervention service. On occasion, however, even the most hard-pressed social services department will try and help in preventive care rather than in merely patching up the ruins. The doctor too may find his own involvement and his own contribution in the forming of local clubs for old people, in using different activities in the help of the handicapped through youth clubs and other organisations; all this should be part of his interest.

Voluntary Organisations

The voluntary organisations are available in amazingly varied situations. Citizens Advice Bureaux and local Councils for Social Service will be able to advise practitioners about what is going on in their particular area. Such knowledge should be an inseparable part of the on-going vocational training of the practitioner. There are also many specialised organisations concerned, for example, with the spastic, the old, multiple sclerosis, migraine, spinal injuries, limbless ex-servicemen – the list is long. The Rheumatism and Arthritis Council, for example, produce helpful pamphlets on everything from sex to gardening. The addresses of these different organisations can be obtained from local Social Services Departments and many are listed in 'Coping with Disablement' published by the Consumers Association in 1974.

Institutional Care

It is of course a major preoccupation of the family practitioner to keep his patients going at any reasonable level of achievement or enjoyment in the community for as long as possible. There comes, inevitably, a time when institutional care is essential. It may not be perfect, it may even at times be unsatisfactory in its standards, but even at this stage the family doctor should try and visit, should try and see fair play, and seek to act as a link between the past and the future of his institutionalised patient. If he permits isolation to seal off his handicapped patient, and very many times he must resign himself to just this, he must accept, in spite of the pressures on his day, some feeling of responsibility for the patient and the relatives, even if he can no longer be directly responsible for adequate standards of care himself. One of the tragedies of an ageing society dealing with increasing numbers of dependent people is that there should be such a poor interchange of resources and places, between hospital and hostel, and between the patient's home and the home of relatives. We can only even hope to improve the integration of these different resources if the family doctor tries to see the problem as a whole and tries to milk suitable resources for his patient all along the line, so that the willing horses are not routinely over-burdened and the rejection of the elderly is not seen as the prudent norm.

SCREENING THE OLD

There is increasing agreement that so far as the older people are concerned — say those over seventy five years of age — that it is no longer good enough to await contact from the patient. The request for a visit or for an appointment often does not come easily from those in greatest need. Contact needs to be initiated by the primary care team.

Screening procedures, profitable but of unproven value despite their large-scale use in the USA, seem to be gaining increasing trust and respect from the general public. Most doctors still regard them as an expensive placebo, wasting scarce medical time and skill, unless fined down very specifically to areas susceptible to this approach. Screening of the old people may well prove to be one of these especially suitable areas: whether done by health visitor or doctor or even well-trained lay personnel seems to matter little. Much may be done by the chiropodist or rehabilitation professionals to maintain safe but mobile independence. Chiropody is the greatest need, but help in neutralising stiffness, weakness, ataxia or the bad lay-out of domestic facilities can prove vital. The treatment of urinary infections or anaemia, the correction of ill-fitting or antique dentures, of deafness or visual defect may be more effectively performed in this way than by the hurried, valued but rarer social call paid by the doctor. These visits are a help, but rarely delve below the corsets. On the other hand, screening procedures require an age-sex register readily enough available yet possessed by less than a fifth of practitioners.

DEFORMITIES AND MUTILATIONS

There is yet another category of patient who must form part of the family doctor's interest: these are the deformed or mutilated. Ours is a profession soaked in an ancient and honourable tradition of care for these people, but we need to alter our ideas since these are still perhaps geared too much to the picturesque mutilations of the beggar in the oriental bazaar and not enough to the more stoical self-rejection of western suburbia.

The woman who desperately wants plastic surgery for a nose or a bust that is somewhat unfashionable in silhouette may need help with her insecurity or her depression: this help must include at least consideration of the answer on which she has fixed her hopes.

More often however in family practice the mutilation is real enough but we ourselves have become less sensitive through familiarity. The woman with a recent mastectomy will not be helped by any excessive sympathy from her practitioner. She will be tremendously helped by his brisk and practical help with her prosthesis, by his suggestion that bikinis are not quite as reliable as bathing suits, and perhaps most of all by his detailed discussion, best done while she is still in hospital, with her husband. Here is a major role that must be done by the family doctor or it may not be done at all. Unless the briefing is adequate, the discreet and patient lack of sexual demands on a convalescent woman inevitably unsure and fearful can be interpreted wrongly as rejection. If the husband can be advised to see the mastectomy scar as soon as possible after the return home, to admire the engineering ingenuity and tidiness of the procedure, to joke about it and demonstrate his undiminished affection, the battle is half-won and precious months may be saved that would otherwise be spent in shyness or an unhelpful and premature resignation.

The patient after a hysterectomy is in a similar though less obvious situation and a similar approach is needed for the colostomy or the rarer ileostomy patient. Many hospital teams use in a most helpful way other patients as teachers of the routines usually attained successfully by stoma cases. The practitioner must try and keep up to date with the stoma appliances in use locally, he must be willing to learn from his patients, and he must be ready to organise self-helping contacts in his practice if he should have two or three suitable patients who can share experiences and expertise. Unless supervised and supported, active and stable patients may withdraw from the outside world and give up valuable activities purely through a lack of confidence. On the other hand, with support and after-care many limited or aged patients succeed in getting back to a fully normal range of activities.

CONCLUDING REMARKS

These then are the chronic and the vulnerable — the aged and the eccentric, the nervous, those suffering from major chronic diseases and those who see themselves as abnormal as a result of some mutilating procedure. Even these are not a total catalogue. The incontinent and the head injury, the disturbed adolescent and the chronic schizophrenic, the bad burn case, or the mentally retarded, all may require his care and support spread over years or even decades, but they are rather rarer.

In a society so obviously admiring skills more than motivation, these patients need more, and are threatened with less, personal care from their doctor than ever before. In any self-evaluating judgements that may be inaugurated and accepted in the years ahead, the attention and regard paid to these patients should, perhaps unfashionably, be a central criterion in assessing the value not only of the individual practitioner but also of the whole area of primary medical care.

References

1. Taylor, Lord and Chave, S. P. W. (1964). *Mental Health and Environment*, (London: Longman).
2. Eastwood, M. R. (1971). *Psychol. Med.* 1, 197.

26

The Care of the Dying

E. Wilkes

INTRODUCTION

Ours is a death-denying society. The whole of medical training tends to assume that dying occasionally happens but is not part of the universal prognosis. Relatives have to be led gently towards acceptance of death. The funeral baked meats are no longer a joyous occasion commemorating the life and health of the newly dead. The anonymous and furtive routine at the crematorium symbolises our inadequacies with a world of canned music and a highly abbreviated service geared to synchronise with the next funeral. There is little here for comfort and consolation.

Changes in medical care have accentuated and sharpened these problems. Save for the occasional catastrophe and for accident, death occurs mainly at the extremes of life and most people have little contact with it. They are frightened and inexperienced in its management. They try to shield their relatives from the knowledge of their own illness. Every doctor will similarly have heard pleas from a husband or wife not to tell the dying spouse the real situation because 'they could not stand it'. Children, even in their teens, are grossly over-protected. The dying child, who is as upsetting to the doctors and nurses as to the parents, must feel that dying is something very terrible since it is never mentioned.

There are, however, slowly, signs of change. In a recent survey of family practitioners 13 per cent of terminally ill patients had had their situation frankly explained and discussed with their family doctor. Furthermore the family practitioner thought that up to 50 per cent of his patients who were dying had a good idea of their real situation. Predictably enough, the doctors found it easier to communicate with patients who approximated to their own socio-economic status.

This is not invariable however and the younger patient seems to be wanting to know more of the truth about his own case, although often he tolerates that truth badly.

The family needs a good deal of training and support to do their best to look after the dying relative at home. We have ceased to have unrealistic expectations of high-quality care in all our hospitals and realise now that they are short of staff and of money and harassed by their acute responsibilities. The tradition of dying at home 'in one's own bed' still is given great respect by both relatives and family doctors. However, most deaths occur these days from heart disease, cancer or stroke, and these tend to be, with some exceptions of course, long and tedious illnesses. They are occurring in a more mobile society which is also an ageing society. Housing is compact and expensive, the part-time job is very much the way of life for married women, and what is possible for the forty year old daughter is not possible for the seventy five year old daughter or wife.

As a consquence of these purely social changes, dying at home is becoming a little rarer each year and now only about one third of deaths occur at home, and two thirds in acute hospital units which are not designed for this purpose. Specialised terminal care units can be most helpful centres of excellence but will not in the foreseeable future be a major resource on any scale that can deal with this problem. We seem, therefore, to have attained a pattern in which most of the illness is spent at home until the family can cope no longer and then admission to an acute hospital is sought for the last week or so. Even among patients dying in hospital, however, most of their last month − two thirds on average − is spent at home, and in a terminal care unit operating in a provincial city no less than 40 per cent of the admissions were indicated to give respite to tired relatives. Ten per cent of admissions were because the patients were true social isolates, often literally people who had outlived all their close friends and relatives, and another 10 per cent were isolates who may have had children in other areas or cities who for good reasons could not possibly be involved in their care.

MAJOR SYMPTOMS OF THE DYING PATIENT

The ten major symptoms in a series of 296 terminal cases recently analysed are shown in Table 26.1 and it is perhaps worth discussing briefly each of these in turn.

Pain

Pain was a major symptom in 58 per cent of cases. Patients dying at home from cancer have only a 50 per cent incidence of pain, but this is likely to be a little

Table 26.1   The 10 major symptoms in 296 terminal cases after admission to hospital.

Symptom	Per cent	Symptom	Per cent
Pain	58	Bedsores	15
Incontinence	38	Vomiting	13
Confusion	21	Open wounds	13
Dyspnoea	17	Cough	5
Nausea	16	Dysphagia	3

Note: Symptoms such as insomnia, anorexia, depression and anxiety are excluded since, although often diagnosed, they were rarely complained of even when present, nor did they often impress the observer as a major symptom.

higher among those going into hospital and indeed pain was a major indication for admission among those patients who also needed transfer to give their relatives a break. In many of these cases psychological and social factors are greatly potentiating the pain. Pain will be much more acutely felt if the patient is living as a full-time invalid undistracted and alone in a small room without company and without support. It is therefore a prime duty of the doctor in attendance to train and to mobilise the family resources so that they operate on some kind of shift system if necessary, that they know very roughly what to expect in the way of problems and so in consequence can either treat or accept them. This is extremely important in the arrangement of effective pain control since this problem is mishandled very frequently in both family and hospital practice.

Analgesics
It is often felt by the doctor that the opiates and mixtures of the 'Brompton cocktail'* type should be delayed and deferred until the very end of the illness, since the patient may have more distress and will need gradually increasing doses. This, in fact, happens only rarely. The majority of pain felt by terminal cancer patients is largely consequent on an undue reliance on the less effective synthetic morphine analogues which mostly do not compare in their clinical effectiveness with the traditional opiate mixtures. To exhibit morphine or heroin (diamorphine) when a terminally ill patient is uncomfortable can greatly enhance the quality of the patient's life and only rarely does the patient need a gradually increasing dose. Many patients can have their pain stabilised and controlled for months on the same dose. Indeed there is on occasion so much improvement in morale and in attitude that after a few weeks of genuine freedom from pain the analgesic dosage can be reduced.

* A mixture popularised by the Brompton Hospital, London, England and containing opium, cocaine and a sedative in an alcohol base.

Such a reduction obviously implies a pain controlling regime geared to the individual needs of the patient with the right drug in the right dose given at the right frequency for that particular patient. In 90 per cent of patients a mixture of 10 mg of cocaine and 10 mg of diamorphine on a 3 hourly or 4 hourly dosage schedule will control the pain until the last few hours of life. Longer acting preparations may be helpful in domiciliary management and a 60 mg morphine suppository may give genuine control of pain for a full 8 hours.

The patient and the family need careful instructions so that the blasphemy of everyone waiting for the clock before the pain can be relieved is never allowed to happen. Patients and relatives must be clearly told that if the patient is sleepy the dose can be delayed but if the patient is in pain it can be brought forward or extra doses inserted, so long as the pain merits the extra dosage. The regular schedule of potent analgesics to prevent pain, with extra occasional dosage, will combine to maintain a high quality of control. It is an unfair burden on patient, relative, or nurse, to rely entirely on 'as required' dosages or regular and inflexible dosages to give fully effective control of pain. Both these types of schedule are usually indicated.

Sites which quite often give rise to intractable pain are primary neoplasms of cervix and rectum infiltrating the lumbo-sacral plexus, the Pancoast tumour of the lung infiltrating the brachial plexus, any tumour invading bone, and occasional exceptionally painful tumours arising from the head of the pancreas. These tumours may well merit a routine of 30—60, or even 100 mg of diamorphine for full control and it must be remembered that the duration of effective action of diamorphine is shorter than that of morphine. A 3 hourly schedule will therefore often be indicated, but is a more effective treatment than the even shorter or less effective help afforded by pethidine or dextromoride or lesser analgesics.

Neurosurgery

Neurosurgical procedures to relieve intractable pain take up a disproportionate amount of the literature and are needed by only a small proportion of patients. Probably the commonest of the special measures for pain control is nerve block by phenol, and this can have a valuable place in the management of the exceptional problem. Specialised clinics in pain control are now organised in many teaching centres in big cities, but the quality of these clinics, and the expertise and the enthusiasm of the consultants involved, must of course vary and the difficult case for the family practitioner is very often a difficult case for the pain clinics also.

Psychological Support

At all times the family doctor must remember that pain mirrors the spiritual situation of the patient. Diminished need for diamorphine has been shown in patients who are enthusiastically involved in occupational therapy or who are having a hair-set or are involved in visitors or the television. Deprivation is a far more potent potentiator of pain than ever chlorpromazine is of analgesics. This is why so often the loneliness of home is where the pain is, and transfer to a stimulating friendly community in a ward can prove of great value, even without major changes of treatment.

One of the commonest problems of great pain is with the patient who knows the real situation but has not yet shared it or come to terms with it. Patients who have been quite out of control on 50 mg of heroin (diamorphine) every 2 hours can, when they are ready to accept their predicament, be relaxed and supported quite free of pain on a lower analgesic dosage. Clearly this demands a deep personal relationship which can be attained very quickly by an experienced family doctor, but it also implies a need for continued involvement and support which is not always easy to organise in the present circumstances.

This involvement and support is extremely important too in the management of the depression which often accompanies this difficult situation. It will be remembered furthermore that a considerable incidence of severe and intractable pain is a correctable feature of depression and this severe pain closely resembles, clinically, the demoralising tension pain described above. The tricyclic anti-depressives have only a limited role to play in most cases needing terminal care but occasionally can produce a magical improvement after a few weeks if given in appropriate dosage. This is always worth trying therefore when there is doubt as to the precise diagnosis.

Incontinence

Incontinence, occurring in 38 per cent of patients, can become a major indication for transfer to an institution in a household where the caring is being done by elderly relatives with limited laundry facilities. A British survey from a North Midlands city demonstrated that 14 per cent of cancer patients dying at home were being cared for by relatives themselves over 70 years of age and incontinence understandably can be the last straw for domiciliary management. Sterile disposable catheters for control of urinary incontinence are inserted by family practitioners or district nurses with surprising and disappointing rarity. Certainly such catheters can be a nuisance, for they will need changing every few weeks and may become blocked because of the presence of infection or blood clot or tumour. A high fluid intake, routine chemo-therapy or antibiotics and the use of epsikaproic acid will help or prevent or diminish these problems and a bladder wash-out is, after all, not impossible even in the home.

Faecal incontinence is an even bigger problem. Quite frequently this is a complication of faecal impaction in inactive patients who are eating little, who are elderly, and who are routinely on opiates. Energetic clearing of the lower bowel with enemata or laxatives may well transform this situation. Furthermore the mobilisation of cases who have been made pain-free yet are not over-sedated can allow the re-establishment of good sphincter control in a proportion of elderly patients. Indeed in a terminal care unit's analysis of evacuations it was found that 2 per cent were voided out of bed and out of control, 12 per cent occurred in the bed, 14 per cent in a bed pan but the remaining 72 per cent of evacuations, even in a series of dying patients, occurred in either bedside commode or W.C.

Incontinence consequent on the presence of malignant fistulae is usually an indication for admission and the nursing burden can be very heavy for these patients because of the perpetual seepage of urine and faeces per vaginam, per rectum, or per urethram. Even at a late stage in the disease, a palliative colostomy can be of inestimable value to the quality of life in the patient's remaining days and more rarely, if the patient is stronger, an ileal bladder operation can also be performed.

Although in family practice terminal cases receive antibiotics in only some 10 per cent of cases, the control of smell with phthalyl sulphthiazole and the control of urinary infection with a suitable preparation can be generally helpful. Toxic and expensive antibiotics for the control of infections due to proteus or pseudomonas will not often be required, although on occasion the patient's clinical state may lead one to use them.

Confusion

Although incontinence can be a major worry to the caring relatives, and although it is nearly twice as common as confusion, it is confusion of the patient that can even more speedily demoralise the family.

An acute paranoid disturbance in terminal patients has been noted in some 1 per cent of patients. These patients formerly had a close relationship with their nurses but suddenly became frightened and convinced that doctors and nurses were going to kill them. They respond well to the cessation of all drug therapy and to their transfer home into the care of trusted relatives. If this is not possible, but relatives do exist, the most trusted spouse or daughter or other relative should be admitted to the unit to stay with the patient day and night until the paranoid episode is over. Phenothiazines can be helpful but are less helpful than a relative. In an exactly similar way district nurses and health visitors and doctors sometimes hear, after many decades of happy marriage, the dying patient accuse in a whisper the spouse of trying to poison him. If phenothiazine or haloperidol fail to control this confusion, paradoxically such patients are best helped by admission to a unit which can have the time to look after their emotional as well as physical needs. Frequently one hears bewilderment expressed by harassed wives as to how happy and normal their husbands have become simply by transfer to changed surroundings. As always in medicine, however, there are many exceptions and transfer to the care of strangers and to a wholly unfamiliar environment can create far more confusion in debilitated and elderly patients than any other set of circumstances. If necessary this price will have to be paid but one is perpetually in the situation of having to weigh the physical needs of the patients against the emotional and physical resources of the family, and no matter how sensitive and experienced the clinican may be, he must be resigned perpetually to making errors of judgement.

Mental confusion due to primary or secondary cerebral tumours is often controllable by steroids — dexamethasone injections of 8 mg two or three times daily have a good reputation in this respect — until the patient is comatose and diminished cerebral oedema is no longer associated with any worthwhile improvement.

Dyspnoea

Dyspnoea is most frequently met with in the terminal stages of lung cancer. Chronic bronchitis is so common in our society, especially in the more industrialised areas, that the shortness of breath on exertion and the broncho-spasm frequently precede by many years any malignant change. These symptoms are thus wholly acceptable to the patient because, although slightly worse, they are by no means a novel or frightening experience for him, and he may be resigned to taking spasmolytic preparations or steroids for some help. In spite of this, breathlessness is associated with severe anxiety even more frequently than is pain. It is, for example, the breathless patient who needs company. A young nurse to sit by the bedside holding his hand is more often necessary with those fighting for breath than for those in great pain. Company and support can be of more value here than most drugs. Piped oxygen, so helpful in many other acute states of dyspnoea in routine practice, is mostly a placebo in terminal care. The aspiration of large pleural effusions is, of course, extremely helpful if the patient's state permits this. But tapping small effusions does not make much difference when both lungs are heavily infiltrated with malignant disease. The most valued drugs in this situation are diamorphine and diazepam. Diamorphine is used for the control of breathlessness in rather smaller and more carefully controlled doses than when it is being used as a pure analgesic. Five or 10 mg every two or three hours will in many cases give a minor and wholly acceptable degree of drug-induced respiratory depression while greatly relieving the patient's distress. Frequently rather smaller doses of diamorphine can be used in conjunction with 2 to 10 mg of diazepam and this combination rarely fails. In cases exhibiting breathlessness of fairly rapid onset and known to have large bilateral pulmonary metastases, it is important to warn the relatives that the patient may suddenly perish much sooner than seemed likely a short time before. This seems especially the case with cases of disseminated mammary carcinoma and it is important that the relatives should at least be aware of this possibility or the shock can be extremely damaging for them.

Nausea and Vomiting

There have been no dramatic advances in the control of nausea and vomiting and most doctors probably still use well-established drugs such as prochlorperazine. This is useful since it can be given in both tablet, syrup, suppository, or injection forms. Cyclizine is again a valued anti-emetic of long standing and valuable in both oral and intramuscular use. Lesions of the upper gastro-enterinal tract can often be helped by metoclopramide, and this drug is often used in conjunction with the other preparations. One of the most widely used anti-emetics is chlorpromazine and this drug is also most helpful in the control of hiccoughs. It is important, however, not to over-use this drug. It can make the patient very drowsy and as a consequence liable to premature pressure sores. Therefore it is advisable to use it, valuable though it is, rather as a second line and to use prochlorperazine or cyclizine routinely as the first line of treatment. Chlorpromazine can be used in heavily jaundiced patients when the jaundice is, as it usually is, due to malignant obstruction.

Bedsores

It is a trite saying that bedsores are better prevented than treated. It is also widely accepted that it does not matter what you put on the bedsore as long as it is not the patient. Patients with spinal metastases are especially liable to this complication and the disseminated breast cancers are the frequent candidates. If the patient is young and the tissues are in fair condition, high quality nursing care and 2-hourly turning can, even in a dying patient, be associated with a most rapid and satisfactory rate of healing. If the patient is grossly wasted or old, or the tissues are oedematous, then the nurses will have an even more difficult job to control the sores. Patients having high doses of steroids are liable to have difficulty in the healing of their pressure sores and this again affects a proportion of breast cancer cases.

Wounds, Sinuses and Fistulae

The open wounds of disseminated malignant disease can present a most distressing and intractable burden for the patient. Painful sinuses in the neck, discharging fistulea in the perineum or on the abdominal wall, fungating wounds around the eye or jaw or face generally can be treated with nothing more than reassurance and high dosage diamorphine. Perhaps the commonest of these open wounds, however, even today, is in the elderly lady, often living alone or belonging to a generation that does not like doctors or hospitals, and who has an enormous ulcerated area on the chest wall arising from breat cancer. Radiotherapy or cytotoxic drugs, as well as hormonal management, have a great deal to offer these patients even if they are clearly never ever going to be fit enough for surgery. It must be remembered that many of these patients will conceal their symptoms from their doctors for years and that even when they have shared their problem they may refuse treatment, or default from it. Proudly and independently they will often not communicate to their doctor their pain or their humiliation. Another, and one of the commonest symptoms which may be dominating the household, but which will be concealed from the doctor and about which complaints are only rarely made to him, is the smell from some of these unhappy cases. The doctor himself must see what can be done to improve ventilation. Broad spectrum antibiotics may help and one of the most effective smell-controlling measures for the fungating breast lesion is an application twice daily of plain live yoghurt directly on to the ulcerated area. This may possibly work by replacing the smell-producing bacteria on the wound by the more innocuous lactobacilli. Certainly patients who could be smelt many yards away can become socially acceptable after a few days on this simple regime.

Cough

The control of cough is a special need in only a small proportion of cases if diamorphine is used routinely for their pain control. Clearly if some other analgesic agent is used and this agent has a less potent anti-tussive effect, cough suppressant treatment will be needed by far more patients. Diamorphine or methadone linctus are extremely potent anti-tussives and are indicated in cases not controlled by routine codeine linctus.

Sleeplessness

Although not necessarily a major symptom, sleeplessness has been reported as the most frequent of all symptoms in the terminally ill and this surely is unnecessary. If the patient has been long dependent on barbiturate hypnotics then these should, for so long as is necessary, be continued during the terminal illness. If the symptom is of early waking due to pain or associated with depression, then clearly extra analgesics or anti-depressives are indicated. If the mind is active and the body not naturally tired by any normal activities, then a chloral derivative for the elderly or nitrazepam should be used.

There is a tendency to give nitrazepam in 10 mg dosage. This can be excessive for light or aged patients, but there is no real excuse for allowing terminally ill patients to spend pointless hours alone in the early hours of the morning when they need all the rest they can manage to carry the burdens of the day. A patient who has had a decent night's sleep can tolerate far more discomfort far more cheerfully. If the night is bad the battle of the day may already be lost, and when the days are few, they are precious.

SOCIAL MANAGEMENT

One of the most subtle factors in the successful management of the terminal illness is that of timing. It is clearly improper to isolate an intelligent and involved executive prematurely when he still has much to offer. He may demoralise the whole household while he sits around waiting for the end. It is equally improper to over-burden a patient with a mountain of everyday responsibilities with which they are no longer able to deal. This is most acutely seen in the mother of young children, with a home to look after. Despite the grief involved in leaving the home and children, if reasonable arrangements can be made for the care of the family such mothers are best transferred to institutional care, since they tend to worry much less about the inadequacies that they can no longer see with their own eyes. One is perpetually impressed by mothers, previously judged to be rather emotionally immature and unsophisticated, but who respond so bravely to the true situation and put the children first. The most unlikely parents can cooperate in planning, with guidance and support, the future management of their childrens' lives, and become much less self-centred if they are allowed to share the real problems consequent on the fatal illness. This cannot be lightly done and the general principle that no patient should be given a burden which they are unable or unwilling to carry must also be respected. In the majority of cases, when there has been a difficult relationship between the caring doctor and the family this is because too few people were told too late rather than because too many people were told too early. The older doctor is the more cautious, for he will have noted in his past experience how information once given cannot be taken back.

BEREAVEMENT

We are accustomed now to treating bereavement as a social problem but it does have a medical area also. The rather difficult marriage does not prevent the widow from canonising retrospectively her rather tedious spouse. Friends loyally support her until, after a few months, they get bored and leave. Children assiduously visit for two or three months, and as the need for their continued support grows, their assiduity of visiting is eroded by the increasing demands of their own lives. Sleeplessness among the bereaved is a major cause of psychological dependency on hypnotics. Many women can benefit from simple help in social adjustment or by a new commitment. Church groups and voluntary organisations and widows' groups and societies all have a part to play, but for the majority of people who are bereaved the family will remain the unit of care and it is the practitioner's role to explain the problems of bereavement, with its natural elements of aggression, resentment, loneliness and fear. The tendency to think of the long-dead husband as still upstairs, the children's thoughtlessness, the dangers of rigid self-pity should all be calmly discussed; much preventable morbidity can at least be modified by full and frank discussion with surviving members of the family circle. The health visitor may well have a more important role to play here in the years that lie ahead, but now it must be the responsibility of the family doctor to involve all the relevant organisations, be they private charities, voluntary organisations, or statutory services, in the care of his patients and their families.

Despite the unnecessary pain and the hurried and inevitably inadequate support, the family practitioner has not too much to be ashamed of in this area. Again and again one is hearing patients say that they do not know how they would have got through it all without the help of their family doctor. Despite the increasing hospitalisation of terminal care, this responsibility for the dying and the bereaved will remain one of the most difficult, demanding, and worthwhile elements of family practice.

References

1. Wilkes, E. (1974). *Proc. roy. Soc. Med.* **67**, 1001.

Index

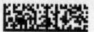